Percutaneous Interventions for Congenital Heart Disease

Percutaneous Interventions for Congenital Heart Disease

Edited by

Horst Sievert MD
Professor of Internal Medicine, Cardiology, Vascular Medicine
CardioVascular Center Frankfurt
Sankt Katharinen
Frankfurt
Germany

Shakeel A Qureshi FRCP
Department of Congenital Heart Disease
Evelina Children's Hospital
Guy's and St Thomas's Hospital Foundation Trust
London
UK

Neil Wilson FRCP
Consultant Paediatric Cardiologist
Department of Paediatric Cardiology
John Radcliffe Hospital
Oxford
UK

Ziyad M Hijazi MD MPH FACC FSCAI
George M Eisenberg Professor of Pediatrics and Medicine
Staff Cardiologist, Section of Pediatric Cardiology
University of Chicago, Pritzker School of Medicine
Chicago, IL
USA

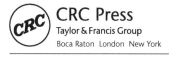

CRC Press
Taylor & Francis Group
Boca Raton London New York

CRC Press is an imprint of the
Taylor & Francis Group, an **informa** business

CRC Press
Taylor & Francis Group
6000 Broken Sound Parkway NW, Suite 300
Boca Raton, FL 33487-2742

First issued in paperback 2019

© 2010 by Taylor & Francis Group, LLC
CRC Press is an imprint of Taylor & Francis Group, an Informa business

No claim to original U.S. Government works

ISBN-13: 978-1-84184-556-2 (hbk)
ISBN-13: 978-0-367-38936-9 (pbk)

**Visit the Taylor & Francis Web site at
http://www.taylorandfrancis.com**

**and the CRC Press Web site at
http://www.crcpress.com**

Contents

Contributors

Mazeni Alwi MRCP
Department of Paediatric Cardiology
National Heart Institute
Kuala Lumpur
Malaysia

Zahid Amin, MD
Professor and Medical Director
Children's Hospital of Omaha
Omaha, NE
USA

Ramesh Arora MD DM FICC FACC(USA)
Chief Cardiologist-Metro Hospitals &
    Heart Institute
Formerly Director Professor
    & Head of Cardiology
GB PANT Hospital
New Delhi
India

Vasilis Babaliaros MD
Assistant Professor of Medicine
Emory University Hospital
Atlanta, GA
USA

Yves Laurent Bayard MD
Cardiovascular Center
Sankt Katharinen
Frankfurt
Germany

Reinhardt M Becht MD
Cardiovascular Center Frankfurt
Sankt Katharinen
Frankfurt
Germany

Lee Benson MD FRCPC FACC FSCAI
Professor of Pediatrics (Cardiology)
Director, Cardiac Diagnostic and Interventional
    Unit (CDIU)
Department of Pediatrics, Division of Cardiology
The Hospital for Sick Children
University of Toronto School of Medicine
Toronto, ON
Canada

Peter C Block MD
Principal Investigator
School of Medicine
Emory University Hospital
Atlanta, GA
USA

Philipp Bonhoeffer MD
Chief of Cardiology and Director, Cardiac
    Catheterisation Laboratory
Great Ormond Street Hospital
London
UK

Mark M Boucek MD
Joe Dimaggio Children's Hospital
Hollywood, FL
and
University of Colorado
Denver, CO
USA

Grazyna Brzezinska-Rajszys MD
The Heart Catheterization Laboratory
The Children Memorial Health Institute
Warsaw
Poland

Franziska Buescheck
Medical Student
Cardiovascular Center Frankfurt
Sankt Katharinen
Frankfurt
Germany

Haran Burri MD
Division of Cardiology
University Hospital
Geneva
Switzerland

Gianfranco Butera
Paediatric Cardiology Center
Istituto Policlinico San Donato
San Donato
Milanese
Milan
Italy

Patricia Campbell
Mater Misericordiae Hospital
Dublin
Ireland

Qi-Ling Cao MD
Senior Research Scientist
Section of Pediatric Cardiology
University of Chicago,
    Pritzker School of Medicine
Chicago, IL
USA

Mario Carminati MD
Pediatric Cardiology Center
Policlinico San Donato
Milan
Italy

Francesco Casilli MD
Division of Cardiology
Humanitas Gavazzeni Clinic
Bergamo
Italy

John P Cheatham MD
Director, Cardiac Catheterization and
    Interventional Therapy
The Heart Center, Columbus Children's Hospital
and
Professor, Pediatrics and Internal Medicine,
    Cardiology Division
The Ohio State University
Columbus, OH
USA

Jonathan M Chen MD
Director, Pediatric Cardiac Surgery
Weill Cornell Campus
New-York Presbyterian Hospital
New York, NY
USA

Massimo Chessa
Pediatric Cardiology Center
Policlinico San Donato
Milan
Italy

Alain Cribier MD
Professor of Medicine (Cardiology)
Chief, Department of Cardiology
Charles Nicolle University Hospital
Rouen
France

Ryan R Davies MD
Pediatric Cardiac Surgery
The Morgan Stanley Children's Hospital of
    New York – Presbyterian
Columbia University College of Physicians
    and Surgeons
New York, NY
USA

Joseph V De Giovanni MD FRCP FRCPCH
Heart Unit
Birmingham Children's Hospital
Birmingham
UK

Makram R Ebeid MD
Department of Pediatrics (Cardiology)
University of Mississippi Medical Center
Jackson, MI
USA

Helene Eltchaninoff MD
Professor of Medicine (Cardiology)
Director, Cardiac Catheterization
    Laboratory
Department of Cardiology
Charles Nicolle University Hospital
Rouen
France

Yun-Ching Fu MD PhD
Section of Pediatric Cardiology
Taichung Veterans General Hospital
Taichung City
Taiwan

Mark Galantowicz MD
Co-Director, Columbus Children's
    Heart Center
Columbus Children's Hospital
Columbus, OH
USA

Marc Gewillig MD
Professor, Pediatric Cardiology
University Hospital Gasthuisberg
Leuven
Belgium

Motoya Hayase MD
Skirball Center for Cardiovascular
    Research
Cardiovascular Research Foundation
Orangeburg, NY
USA

William Hellenbrand MD
Professor of Pediatrics
Director Pediatric Catheterization Laboratory
Columbia University College of Physicians
    and Surgeons
Children's Hospital of New York Presbyterian
New York, NY
USA

Ziyad M Hijazi MD MPH FACC FSCAI
George M Eisenberg Professor of Pediatrics
    and Medicine
Staff Cardiologist, Section of Pediatric Cardiology
University of Chicago, Pritzker School of Medicine
Chicago, IL
USA

Hüseyin Ince MD
Division of Cardiology
University Hospital Rostock
Rostock School of Medicine
Rostock
Germany

Frank F Ing MD
Associate Professor of Pediatrics
Baylor College of Medicine
Director, Cardiac Catheterization Laboratories
Texas Children's Hospital
Houston, TX
USA

Vladimir Jelnin
Department of Medicine
Section of Cardiology
University of Illinois at Chicago
Chicago, IL
USA

Sachin Khambadkone MD DCH DNB MRCP
Consultant Pediatric Cardiologist and Honorary
    Senior Lecturer
Great Ormond Street Hospital
London
UK

Stephan Kische MD
Division of Cardiology
University Hospital Rostock
Rostock School of Medicine
Rostock
Germany

Charles S Kleinman MD
Professor of Clinical Pediatrics in Obstetrics and
    Gynecology
Columbia University College of Physicians and Surgeons
Weill Medical College of Cornell University
New York, NY
and
Chief, Pediatric Cardiac Imaging
Morgan Stanley Children's Hospital of
    New York- Presbyterian
New York, NY
USA

Peter R Koenig MD
Associate Professor of Pediatrics
Section of Pediatric Cardiology
Director, Echocardiography Laboratory
Comer Children's Hospital
University of Chicago, Pritzker School of Medicine
Chicago, IL
USA

Paul Kramer MD
Interventional Cardiologist
Shawnee Mission Medical Center
Shawnee Mission, KS
USA

R Krishna Kumar MD DM FACC FSCAI
Chief Pediatric Cardiologist
Amrita Institute of Medical Sciences and
    Research Centre
Kerala
India

Michael Landzberg MD
Director, Boston Adult Congenital Heart
    (BACH) Group
Children's Hospital, Brigham and
    Women's Hospital
and
BIDMC
Harvard Medical School
Boston, MA
USA

Larry Latson MD
Department of Pediatric Cardiology
Cleveland Clinic Foundation
Cleveland, OH
USA

Trong Phi Lê MD
Department of Pediatric Cardiology
University of Hamburg
Hamburg
Germany

Martin B Leon MD
Professor of Medicine and Associate Director
Center for Interventional Vascular Therapy
Columbia University Medical Center
and
Chairman, Cardiovasular Research Foundation
New York, NY
USA

Gerald R Marx MD
Children's Hospital Boston Department
    of Cardiology
Boston, MA
USA

Audrey Marshall
Associate in Cardiology
Department of Cardiology
Children's Hospital Boston
Boston, MA
USA

Sibyl C Medie
Research Asistant
Peditric Cardiology
University of Illinois at Chicago
Chicago, IL
USA

Bernhard Meier MD
Professor and Chairman of Cardiology
Swiss Cardiovascular Center Bern
University Hospital
Bern
Switzerland

Haverj Mikailian MRT(R)
Department of Medical Imaging
Department of Pediatrics, Division of Cardiology
The Hospital for Sick Children
University of Toronto School of Medicine
Toronto, ON
Canada

Diana Negura
Paediatric Cardiology Department and GUCH Unit
Istituto Policlinico San Donato
San Donato Milanese
Milan
Italy

JP Morales MD
Department of Interventional Radiology
Guy's and St Thomas' Hospital
London
UK

Christoph A Nienaber MD FACC
Division of Cardiology
University Hospital Rostock
Rostock School of Medicine
Rostock
Germany

Eustaquio Onorato MD FSCAI
UO Cardiologia 1
Humanitas Gavazzeni
Bergamo
Italy

Stephan H Ostermayer
Cardiovascular Center Frankfurt
Sankt Katharinen
Frankfurt
Germany

Igor F Palacios MD
Director, Cardiac Catheterization Laboratories
Director, Interventional Cardiology
Massachusetts General Hospital
Boston, MA
USA

Manuel Pan MD PhD
Assistant Professor
Department of Cardiology
University Hospital Reina Sofia
Córdoba
Spain

Djordie Pavlovic MD PhD
Assistant Professor
Department of Cardiology
University Hospital Reina Sofia
Córdoba
Spain

Michael Petzsch MD
Division of Cardiology
University Hospital Rostock
Rostock School of Medicine
Rostock
Germany

Luciane Piazza
Department of Pediatric Cardiology and Cardiac Surgery
Instituto Policlinico San Donato
San Donato Milanese
Milan
Italy

Jean-François Piéchaud MD
Institut Hospitalier Jacques Cartier
Massy
France

Shakeel A Qureshi FRCP
Department of Congenital Heart Disease
Evelina Children's Hospital
Guy's and St Thomas's Hospital Foundation Trust
London
UK

P Syamasundar Rao
Professor and Director, Division of Pediatric Cardiology
The University of Texas/Houston Medical School
Houston, TX
USA

Oleg Reich MD PhD
Kardiocentrum
University Hospital Motol
Prague
Czech Republic

John F Reidy MD
Department of Radiology
Guy's and St Thomas' Hospital
London
UK

Tim C Rehders MD
Division of Cardiology
University Hospital Rostock
Rostock School of Medicine
Rostock
Germany

Miguel Romero MD PhD
Assistant Professor
Department of Cardiology
University Hospital Reina Sofia
Córdoba
Spain

Carlos E Ruiz MD PhD
Professor of Medicine and Pediatrics
Chief, Division of Cardiology Department of Pediatrics
University of Illinois
Chicago, IL
USA

Martin BE Schneider MD
Chief, Department of Congenital Heart Disease
German Paediatric Heart Centre
Sankt Augustin
Germany

José Segura MD PhD
Assistant Professor
Department of Cardiology
University Hospital Reina Sofia
Córdoba
Spain

Peter Sick MD
University of Leipzig, Heart Center
Leipzig
Germany

Horst Sievert MD
Professor of Internal Medicine, Cardiology, Vascular Medicine
CardioVascular Center Frankfurt
Sankt Katharinen
Frankfurt
Germany

Ulrich Sigwart MD FRCP FACC FESC
Professor and Head of Cardiology
University Hospital
Geneva
Switzerland

Vladimir Jelnin
Department of Medicine
Section of Cardiology
University of Ilinois at Chicago
Chicago, IL
USA

José Suárez de Lezo MD PhD
Professor of Cardiology
Department of Cardiology
University Hospital Reina Sofia
Córdoba
Spain

Alejandro J Torres MD
Assistant Professor
Division of Pediatric Cardiology
Columbia University College of Physicians and Surgeons
Children's Hospital of New York Presbyterian
New York, NY
USA

Wayne Tworetzky MD
Associate in Cardiology
Department of Cardiology
Children's Hospital Boston
Boston, MA
USA

Michael Tynan MD FRCP
Emeritus Professor of Paediatric Cardiology
Kings College
London
UK

Kevin P Walsh MD
Consultant Paediatric Cardiologist
Mater Misericordiae Hospital
Dublin
Ireland

Neil Wilson FRCP
Consultant Paediatric Cardiologist
Department of Paediatric Cardiology
John Radcliffe Hospital
Oxford
UK

Evan M Zahn MD
Department of Cardiology
Miami Children's Hospital
Miami, FL
USA

Mario Zanchetta MD FSCAI
Director, Department of Cardiovascular Sciences
Cittadella General Hospital
Cittadella
Padua
Italy

Foreword

This book is the offspring of the annual Frankfurt course of interventional cardiology which has focused strongly on congenital heart disease. This course has, year by year, gained in reputation. It is essentially a practical course. The live case demonstrations are the heart of such meetings. This book reflects the course and is a practical book; a 'how to' book. A quick scan of the 60 or so chapters reveals the galaxy of talent operating and lecturing during the courses and who are now giving their accounts in writing.

As one who was in at the beginning of catheter interventions in congenital heart disease I am filled with wonderment at what is now on offer to the patients. As a young trainee in the late 1960s, Bill Rashkind's introduction of balloon atrial septostomy marked a milestone in the treatment of transposition. Not only did it transform the outlook for babies with this malformation but it marked the start of the quest for practical minimally invasive types of treatment of structural cardiac anomalies. It was admittedly a slow start, with few innovations until the 1980s, but since then the treatment of cardiovascular diseases has been transformed. The advances that have been made have been due, in great part, to the partnership of physicians and industry and it would be hard to overstate the importance of the contribution of our colleagues in industry.

With the rapid incorporation of advanced technologies into this field we have seen procedures and devices come and go. We can expect this dynamic to continue; so this book is a statement of where we stand in 2006 and I am sure that by 2016 a similar book will have many new techniques to offer.

Michael Tynan MD FRCP
Emeritus Professor of Paediatric Cardiology
Kings College
London
UK

Foreword

Most knowledgeable interventional historians would argue that the era of lesser-invasive non-surgical cardiovascular therapy began almost 30 years ago when Andreas Gruentzig performed the first successful coronary angioplasty, fulfilling his dream to accomplish catheter-based percutaneous treatment of vascular disease in alert, awake patients. Undoubtedly, Andreas would have delighted in the astounding developments of the ensuing decades, as disciples of his 'simple' procedure applied creativity, technical acumen, and scientific rigor to sculpt the burgeoning interdisciplinary subspecialty of interventional cardiovascular medicine. Importantly, over the years, a typical development pattern has emerged – early stage well characterized procedures involving a restricted lesion subset and patient cohort became generalized to the mainstream patient population after equipment innovations and refinement of physician operator skills. Thus, coronary intervention, beginning with 'plain old balloon angioplasty', begat bare metal stents, atherectomy devices, and drug-eluting stents, finally resulting in a procedure with safe, predictable, and definitive clinical outcomes which could be generalized to most patients with obstructive coronary disease. Soon thereafter, peripheral vascular and neurovascular intervention underwent a similar renaissance, 'borrowing' ideas, technology templates, and operator skills from coronary platforms to extend catheter-based treatments to other regions of the extracardiac vascular system.

The third chapter of this interventional odyssey applies to the current textbook, entitled *Percutaneous Interventions for Congenital Heart Disease*. This newest and most diverse branch of the inteventional tree embraces a potpourri of congenital and acquired cardiovascular disorders, previously left untreated or relegated to surgical therapy alternatives. We have employed the term 'structural heart disease' to encompass a wide variety of non-atherosclerotic and generally non-vascular disease entities, ranging from intracardiac septal defects to valvular lesions. This newcomer on the interventional horizon is unique for several reasons. First, the diversity and complexity of interventional skills required to safely and successfully treat both neonates and octogenarians with advanced cardiac lesions are unprecedented. Second, the intersecting physician groups are far-reaching, spanning pediatric and adult interventional cardiology, imaging specialists (not just angiography, but also echocardiography, MR imaging, and CT angiography), and hybrid surgical therapists. Finally, since many of the cardiac anomalies targeted for catheter-based treatment occur rarely, the focused interventionalists working in this rarified zone have clustered into a small, well bonded fraternity. The purpose of this textbook is to highlight the practical teaching experiences of this congenital and structural interventional fraternity.

For almost a decade, an international live case demonstration workshop has convened in Frankfurt, Germany for the purpose of observing and discussing interventional procedures in this eclectic subspecialty. Directed by Dr Horst Sievert (and more recently with Drs Neil Wilson and Shakeel Qureshi as co-directors), this clinical symposium has become the definitive 'how to' educational event for practicing congenital and structural interventionalists. The current textbook serves as a comprehensive syllabus including a virtual 'who's who' author list, representing the thought leaders from all allied fields under the umbrella of congenital and structural heart disease. The organizational structure is both authoritative and intuitive with easy to navigate sections beginning with the catheterization laboratory environment, new imaging modalities for diagnosis and procedural guidance, and fetal and infant interventions, and marching through an orderly progression of every conceivable congenital and structural lesion category which has been managed using existing or proposed interventional therapies. As with the clinical symposium, this textbook has a familiar stylistic consistency emphasizing clinical treatment indications and practical operator technique issues with helpful procedural 'tips and tricks' and careful descriptions of potential complications. The breadth of this textbook is impressive, extending from commonly recognized conditions to less well established domains, such as exciting new transcatheter valve therapies and intraoperative hybrid VSD closure and stent implantation.

Lest one think that this textbook is merely a compendium of obscure interventional oddities, the subspecialty exploding from the predicate symposium and this textbook represents the greatest potential growth area in all of interventional cardiovascular medicine. Just imagine the consequences if adult transcatheter valve therapy becomes commonplace in patients with aortic stenosis and mitral regurgitation, or if patent foramen ovale closure becomes a treatment option in patients with refractory migraines, or if left atrial appendage closure becomes an important alternative for patients with atrial fibrillation. In 5–10 years it is entirely conceivable that this small fraternity of interventionalists focused on congenital and structural therapies will multiply into an army of catheter-based therapists with specialized operator skills, an advanced appreciation of cardiac imaging modalities, and a thorough clinical understanding of multi-varied cardiac disease states. This first edition of *Percutaneous Interventions for Congenital Heart Disease* fills a medical literature void and should be heartily embraced by all cardiovascular healthcare professionals, from the curious to the diehard interventional practitioner. I expect as this

field continues to transform in the future that subsequent editions of this textbook will help to define the unpredictable progress of this unique subspecialty.

Martin B Leon MD
Professor of Medicine and Associate Director
Center for Interventional Vascular Therapy
Columbia University Medical Center
and
Chairman, Cardiovascular Research Foundation
New York, NY
USA

Preface

This book is intended as a practical guide to the interventional treatment of congenital and structural heart disease for invasive cardiologists in the pediatric and adult fields. Where possible we have tried to emphasize practical aspects of the procedures including the important issues of indications and patient selection, potential pitfalls, and complications. Greater understanding, technical know-how, and wider availability of catheters, balloons, delivery systems, and devices have spread intervention into the realm of acquired valve disease, degenerative disease of the aorta, paravalve leakage, post-infarction ventricular septal defects, and closure of the left atrial appendage. Some of the procedures covered in the book are emerging techniques representing the forefront of interventional treatment today, and will not be practiced in every catheter laboratory.

We have collated contributions from a team of expert interventionists throughout the world in an effort to draw together, via the common link of catheter technology, an approach to congenital and structural heart disease which results in a new emerging specialist, the cardiovascular interventionist.

This book, by complementing practical experience, will be valuable as a practical procedural reference guide to catheter lab staff of all levels and disciplines.

HS, SAQ, NW, ZMH

Color plates

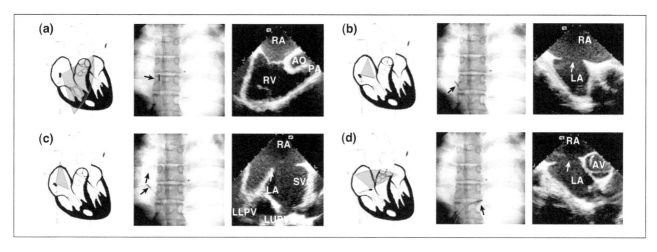

Figure 4.2

(a) Images in the home view. Left, sketch representing the heart with the position of the intracardiac catheter inside the heart with the ultrasonic array box in the neutral 'home view' position. The shaded area represents structures seen in this view. Middle, a cine fluoroscopy image showing the position of the ICE catheter (arrow) in the mid-right atrium with the transducer facing the tricuspid valve and parallel to the spine. Right, an actual intracardiac echocardiographic image with the ultrasonic box in the neutral home view position. The tricuspid valve, right ventricle out, and inflow are well seen in this position. The aortic valve and pulmonic valve can also be seen. AO, aortic valve; RA, right atrium; PA, pulmonary artery; RV, right ventricle. (b) Images in the septal view. Left, sketch representing the heart with the position of the intracardiac catheter inside the heart with the ultrasonic array box in the posterior flexed position looking at the atrial septum 'septal view'. The shaded area represents structures seen in this view. Middle, a cine fluoroscopy image showing the position of the ICE catheter (arrow) in the right atrium with the transducer flexed posterior looking at the septum. Right, an actual intracardiac echocardiographic image with the ultrasonic box in the septal view. The atrial septal defect is well seen (arrow), as are the left and right atria. (c) Images in the long-axis 'caval view'. Left, sketch representing the heart with the position of the intracardiac catheter inside the heart with the ultrasonic array box in the posterior flexed position with a cephalad advancement looking at the atrial septum and the superior vena 'cava caval view'. The shaded area represents structures seen in this view. Middle, a cine fluoroscopy image showing the position of the ICE catheter (black arrow) in the right atrium with the transducer flexed posterior looking at the superior vena cava (white arrow). Right, an actual intracardiac echocardiographic image with the ultrasonic box in the caval view. The atrial septal defect (arrow), the left and right atria, the left pulmonary veins, and the superior vena cava are all well seen. SVC, superior vena cava; LLPV, left lower pulmonary vein; LUPV, left upper pulmonary vein. (d) Images in the 'short-axis view'. Left, sketch representing the heart with the position of the intracardiac catheter inside the heart with the ultrasonic array box in the flexed position and the entire handle rotated clockwise until the imaging transducer is above the tricuspid valve looking at the aorta from below. In this position, fine rotation of the knobs can demonstrate different parts of the atrial septum. The shaded area represents structures seen in this view. Middle, a cine fluoroscopy image showing the position of the ICE catheter (black arrow) in the right atrium with the transducer above the tricuspid valve. Right, an actual intracardiac echocardiographic image with the ultrasonic box in the short-axis view. The atrial septal defect (arrow), the left and right atria, and the aortic valve are all well seen. This view is similar to a TEE short-axis view with the left atrium in the far field (opposite to the TEE).

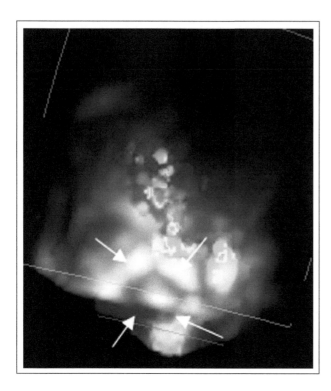

Figure 6.4
Three-dimensional color flow echocardiogram in a 41-year-old woman with a paravalvar leak. The arrows depict the annulus of the prosthetic mitral valve. The specific position of two paravalvar leaks is seen outside the prosthetic mitral valve annulus.

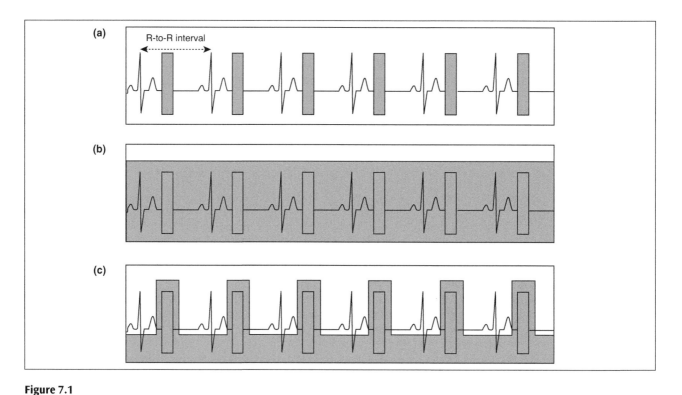

Figure 7.1
(Pink shading represents radiation exposure during cardiac cycle) (a) Prospective ECG triggering utilized by EBCT. The patient is exposed to X-rays only during pre-selected times (100 ms) of the cardiac cycle, routinely at 40% of the R–R interval, at the moment of minimum heart velocity. (b) Retrospective ECG triggering utilized by MDCT. X-rays produced continuously and data acquired during all phases of the cardiac cycle together with ECG recording. Same phase images are reconstructed using retrospective ECG gating. The reconstruction window can be positioned at any phase of the cardiac cycle. (c) Prospective triggering of X-ray tube output modulation by MDCT. The output of X-ray tube is at nominal exposure only at the phase which is used for image reconstruction and is decreased during the cardiac phase, which is not used for image reconstruction. ('pulse' X-ray tube modulation).

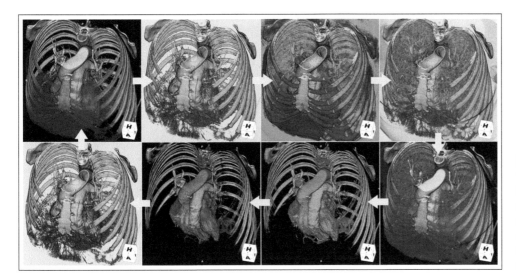

Figure 7.8
The volume rendering technique allows extensive color and opacity manipulation, which can be effectively used by the operator to view specific anatomic structures.

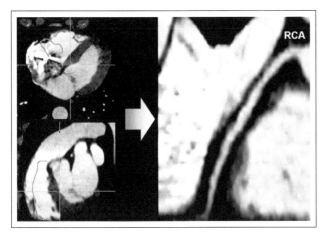

Figure 7.9
The blue line drawn follows the path of the right coronary artery (RCA) on the axial cross-sectional images (top, left) or sagittal images (bottom, left), creating the curved plane. The image on the right is a flattened view of this plane, showing the right coronary artery (RCA).

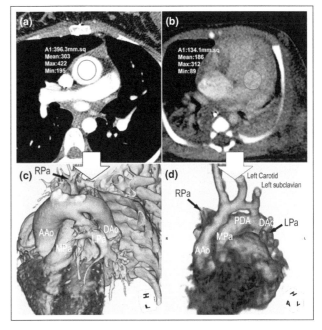

Figure 7.14
(a) A 23-year-old female with pulmonary artery anomaly – LPa originates from the aortic arch. Mean CT density in Pa: 303 HU. (b) A 4-day-old male with complex congenital heart disease (CHD) VSD, tricuspid atresia, transposition of great vessels. … Mean CT density in the aorta: 189 HU. (c), (d) Three-dimensional computer reconstructed images from the source data, demonstrating quality differences depending on the level of contrast enhancement. AAo, ascending aorta; MPa, main pulmonary artery; LPa, left pulmonary artery; DAo, descending; aorta; PDA, patent ductus arteriosus; RPa, right pulmonary artery; HU, Hounsfield units.

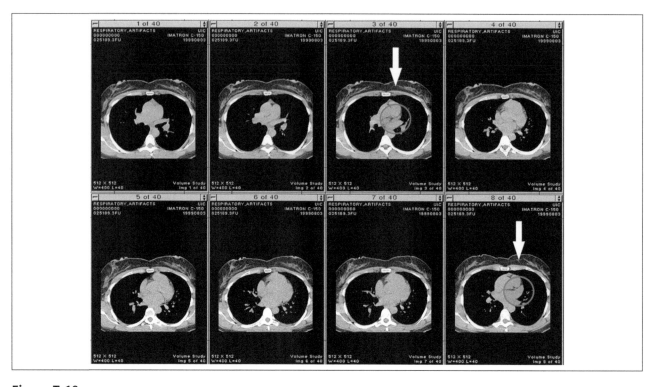

Figure 7.10
The picture shows eight contiguous slices of transaxial tomograms of the heart. Slice thickness is
3 mm, with 3 mm table increments between image acquisition by EBCT. Arrows pointing at image 3 and 8 display similar anatomic levels, however due to breathing motion, the image of slice 8 moved to the level of image 3, resulting in a motion amplitude of 15 mm between inspiration and expiration.

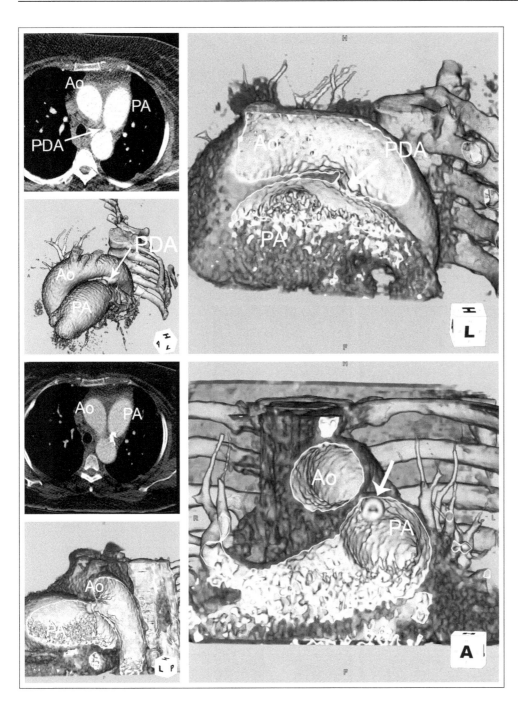

Figure 7.19

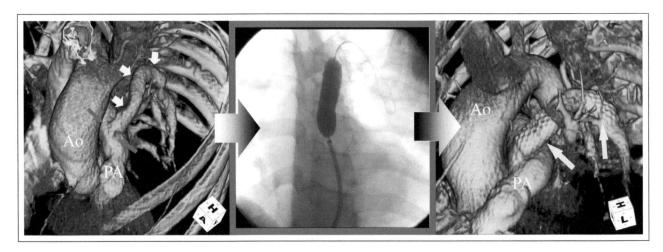

Figure 7.20

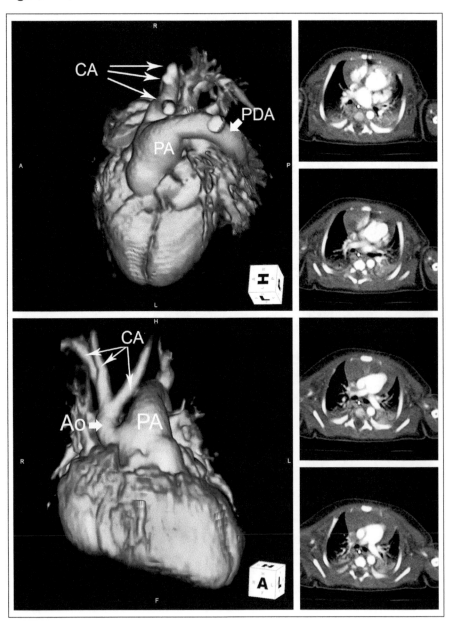

Figure 7.21

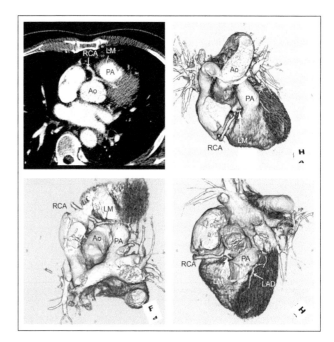

Figure 7.22

Figure 7.23

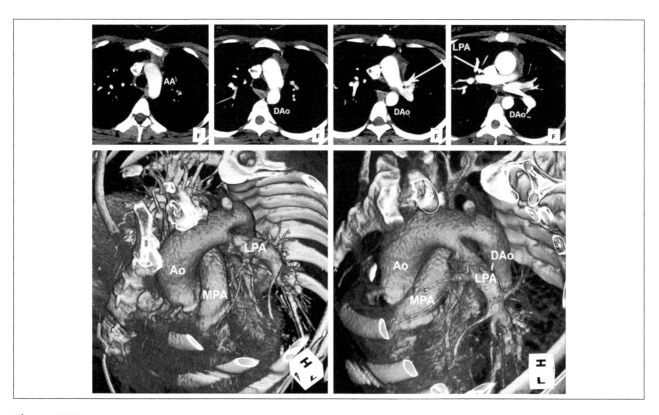

Figure 7.24

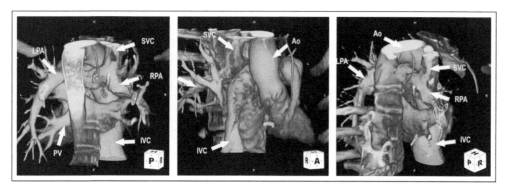

Figure 7.25

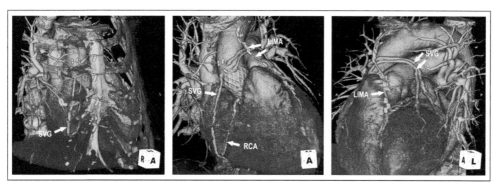

Figure 7.26

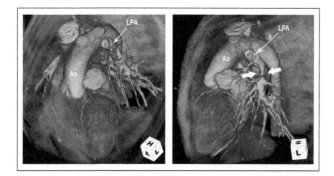

Figure 7.27

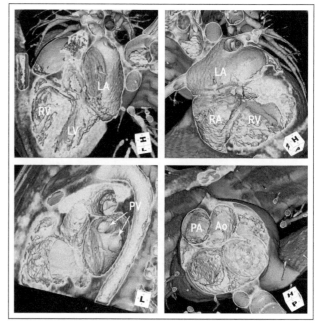

Figure 7.28

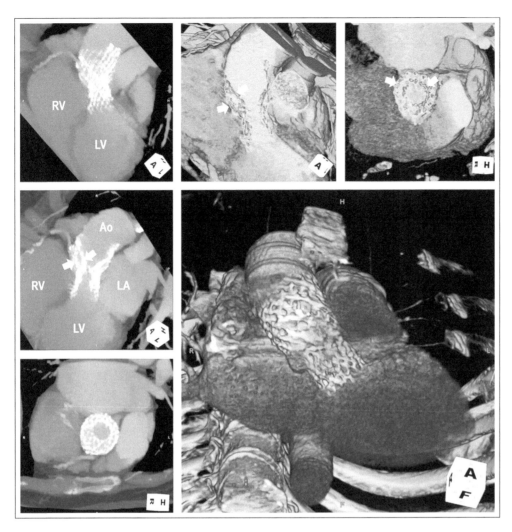

Figure 7.29

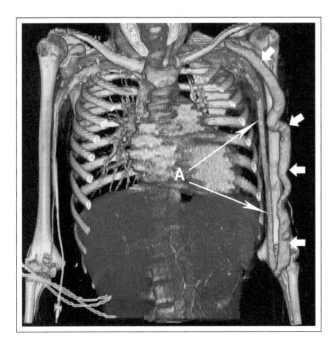

Figure 7.30

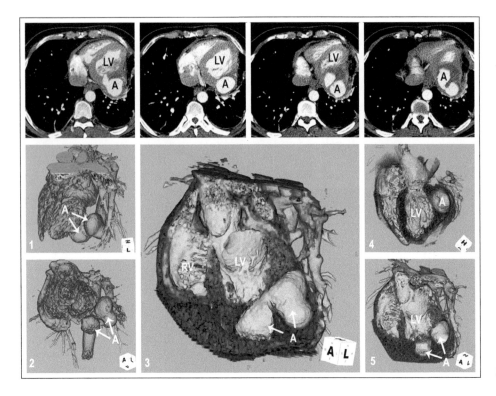

Figure 7.31

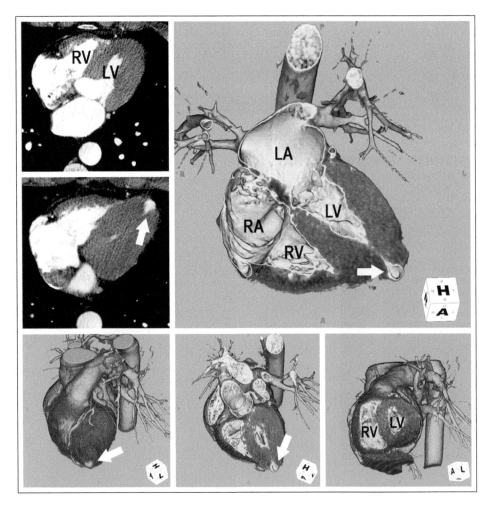

Figure 7.32

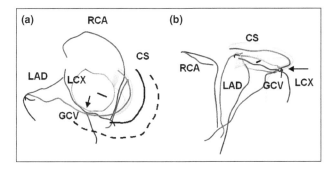

Figure 25.2
Multi-slice CT 3D model data. Overlay of anatomy from multi-slice CT data from 10 human subjects with ischemic mitral regurgitation with chronic heart failure.Panel (a) is a short axis view and panel (b) shows the long axis. Red lines show the coronary arteries; the blue line is the coronary vein, and the yellow line indicates the mitral annulus. The long arc (broken line) is the length between the ostium of the CS and distal GCV. The short arc (solid line) is the distance between the CS ostium and the cross-over between the GCV and LCX. The short line in the mitral annulus is a 1 cm calibratio. An arrow indicates the crossover between the GCV and LCX. LAD, left anterior descending coronary artery; LCX, left circumflex coronary artery; RCA, right coronary artery; Coronary sinus; GCV, great cardiac vein; (Reproduced courtesy of Viacor Inc., Wilmington MA)

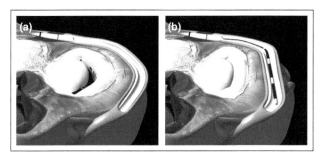

Figure 25.6
Straight shape percutaneous mitral annuloplasty device. (a) Catheter placed in the CS. (b) Reshaping of the mitral annulus via the coronary sinus utilizing a 'rigid bar'. The device pushes forward the posterior annulus, thereby increasing leaflet co-aptation. (Reproduced courtesy of Viacor Inc., Wilmington, MA, USA.)

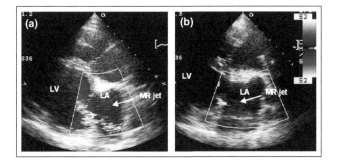

Figure 25.10
The PTMA device significantly reduced the MR jet area (b), compared to baseline (a) in chronic IMR. LV, left ventricle; LA, left atrium.[30] (Reproduced courtesy of Viacor Inc., Wilmington, MA, USA.)

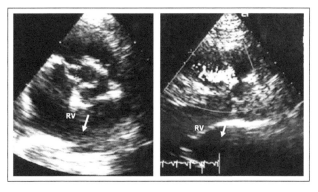

Figure 27.1
Two-dimensional echo and color flow mapping showing PSOV from right coronary sinus into right ventricle. RV, right ventricle.

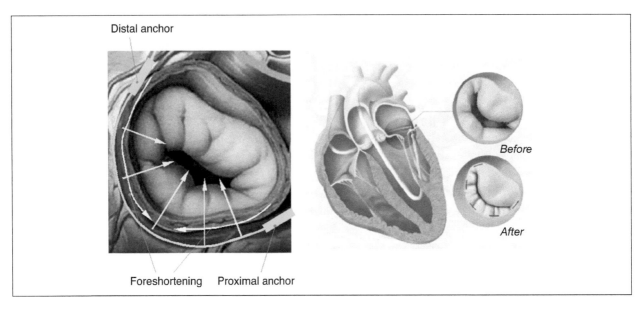

Distal anchor

Before

After

Foreshortening   Proximal anchor

Figure 25.12

New Techniques for percutaneous mitral transvenous annuloplasty. This method proposed a C-shaped percutaneous mitral annuloplasty device that was fixed at the CS ostium and reduced the arc of the mitral annulus. (a) Schematic drawing of the prototype annuloplasty system (C-Cure, ev3, Plymouth, MN). (b) This system is a wire-based percutaneous mitral annuloplasty device. Distal and proximal anchors are collapsed before insertion and the device is delivered to the CS via a guide catheter. A distal anchor is deployed in the distal CS or GCV and locked in place. Tension is then applied via the delivery system until satisfactory acute efficacy with stable coronary perfusion is documented. The proximal anchor is then deployed and locked in the proximal CS and then the delivery system is uncoupled and removed. This device is proceeding towards initial human implants. (Reproduced courtesy of Cardiac Dimensions, Kirkland, WA, USA.) (c) This device is a stent-based percutaneous mitral annuloplasty device. The device consists of three elements: two anchor stents to be deployed into the CS and GCV respectively, and a middle stent or constricting device for shortening to make the posterior leaflet attach to the anterior leaflet. Among the embodiments proposed is a delayed constriction device disposed between the two anchoring stents. By this method, the stents would endothelialize for several weeks before treatment effect would be induced via the constricting device. (Edwards Lifescience, Irvine, CA). (Reproduced courtesy of Edwards LifeScience, Irvine, CA, USA.) (d) Transventricular suture-based annuloplasty. This procedure entails, first, positioning one magnet-tipped guidance catheter in the CS adjacent to the posterior side of the mitral valve and an opposite pole magnet-tipped catheter retrograde into the left ventricle. Magnetic attraction guides the catheter in the left ventricle into position under the mitral valve annulus. There, catheters deliver a series of implants into the annulus. The implants are tensioned together to cinch down the annulus then they are locked into place, reducing the circumference of the dilated valve and eliminating mitral regurgitation. The catheter in the CS, since used for guidance only, is removed, leaving nothing behind in that critical vessel. CS, coronary sinus; GCV, great cardiac vein. (Reproduced courtesy of Mitralign, Salem, NH, USA.)

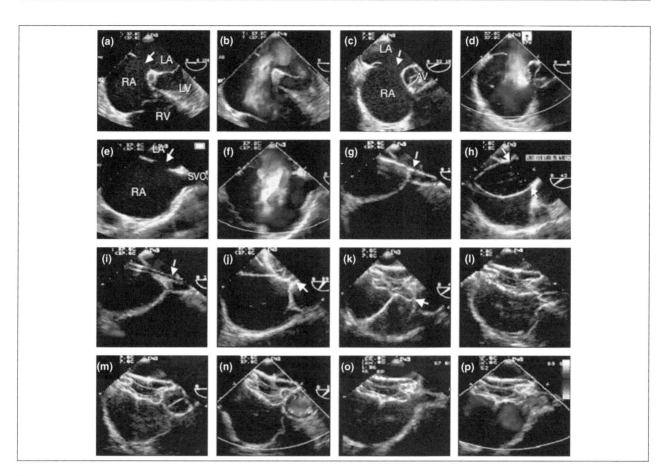

Figure 28.3

Transesophageal echocardiographic images in a 53-year-old patient with a secundum atrial septal defect measuring 30 mm demonstrating the various steps of closure. (a) and (b) Four-chamber view (0° omniplane) showing the defect (arrow), the inferior/anterior rim is deficient, the inferior/posterior rim is adequate, and the left-to-right shunt. (c) and (d) Short axis view at about 15° demonstrating the defect (arrow), the anterior rim, the posterior rim, and the left-to-right shunt. (e) and (f) Bicaval view at about 120° demonstrating the superior rim, the inferior rim, and the defect (arrow). (g) and (h) Wire passage and balloon sizing indicating the stretched diameter (arrows). (i) Passage of the delivery sheath (arrow) through the defect. (j) Deployment of the left disk (arrow) of a 38 mm Amplatzer device in the left atrium. (k) Deployment of the right disk (arrow) in the right atrium in short axis view. (l) Bicaval view after the device has been released. (m) and (n) Short axis views without and with color Doppler after the device has been released indicating good device position and no residual shunt. (o) and (p) Bicaval views without and with color Doppler after the device has been released indicating good device position and no residual shunt. LA, left atrium; RA, right atrium; LV, left ventricle; RV, right ventricle; SVC, superior vena cava.

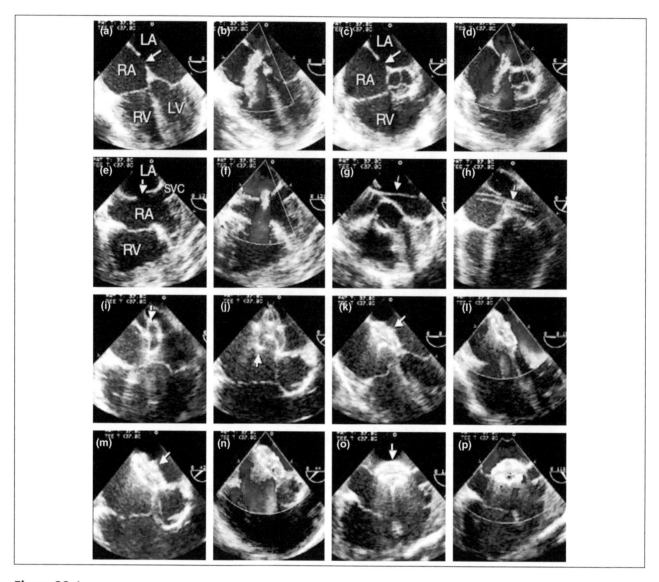

Figure 28.4

Transesophageal echocardiographic images in a 1.2-year-old patient with a secundum atrial septal defect measuring 7 mm demonstrating the various steps of closure. (a) and (b) Four-chamber view (0° omniplane) showing the defect (arrow), both inferior-anterior and inferior-posterior rims are adequate, and the left-to-right shunt. (c) and (d) Short axis view at about 15° demonstrating the defect (arrow), the anterior rim (deficient), the posterior rim (adequate), and the left-to-right shunt. (e) and (f) Bicaval view at about 120° demonstrating the superior rim (adequate), the inferior rim (adequate), and the defect (arrow). (g) and (h) Wire and delivery sheath passage (arrows). (i) Four-chamber view demonstrating deployment of the left disk (arrow) of a 8 mm Amplatzer device in the left atrium. (j) Short axis view demonstrating deployment of the right disk (arrow) in the right atrium. (k) and (l) Four-chamber view without and with color Doppler after the device has been released demonstrating good device position (arrow) and no residual shunt. No mitral or tricuspid valve regurgitations. (m) and (n) Short axis view without and with color Doppler demonstrating good device position and no residual shunt. (o) and (p) Bicaval view without and with color Doppler demonstrating good device position and no residual shunt. LA, left atrium; RA, right atrium; LV, left ventricle; RV, right ventricle; SVC, superior vena cava.

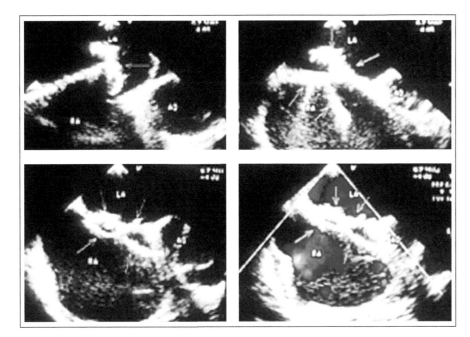

Figure 29.2
Transesophageal monitoring of device implantation. Top right: the distal umbrella is deployed in the left atrium. Top left: both umbrellas are deployed, with the device still attached to the delivery cable. Bottom right: the device was released; note the flat appearance of both umbrellas, as a 'sandwich' on the atrial septum. Bottom left: no evidence of residual shunt at color flow interrogation.

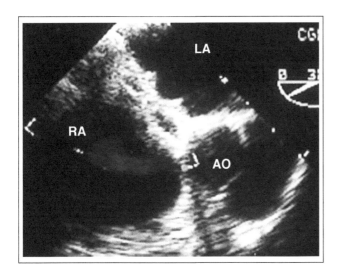

Figure 29.3
TEE short axis view of a well positioned device, with no residual shunt.

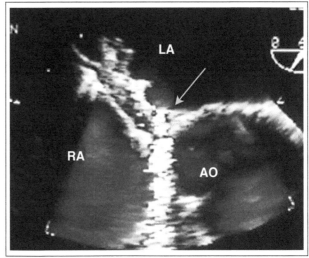

Figure 29.4
TEE short axis view in another case with deficient anterior rim and small residual shunt as assessed by the color flow jet.

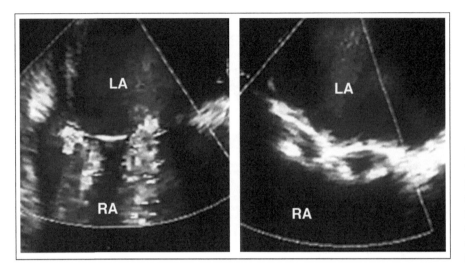

Figure 29.7
TEE image of a case of multi-fenestrated atrial septum (right part of the figure), as clearly demonstrated by multiple color flow jets. A single large device (left part of the figure) is covering all the fenestrations, with no residual shunt.

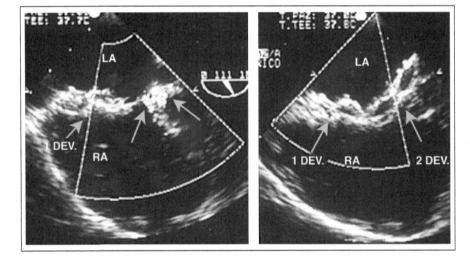

Figure 29.8
TEE of a case of double defects. One defect was closed with a device, but there was evidence of a large additional hole, as shown by the color flow (right part of the figure). A second device was successfully implanted, closing the second hole (left part of the figure).

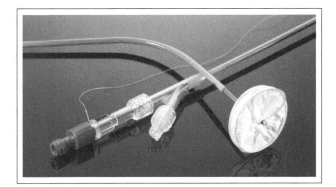

Figure 30.4
Helex device presented attached to the integral green delivery catheter. The control catheter is seen attached to the red cap. The safety suture is seen locked into position by the red safety cap. The mandrel is controlled by the short side arm, which can be locked into position using the Luer lock.

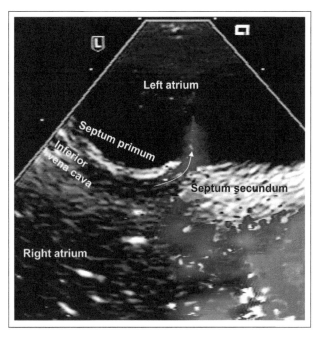

Figure 31.2
Transesophageal echocardiogram performed for suspicion of paradoxical stroke through a PFO immediately after a prolonged Valsalva maneuver. A flame of red color indicates a temporary right to left shunt through the PFO (curved arrow).

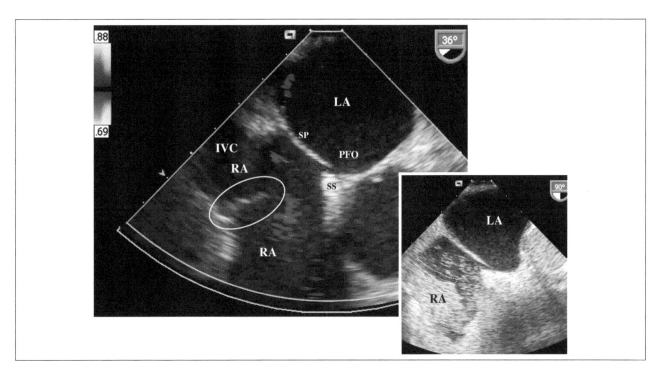

Figure 31.9
Transesophageal echocardiogram showing a Eustachian valve (circle), similar to the one in Figure 31.8, in the presence of a PFO. There is a spontaneous left to right shunt through the PFO (red Doppler flow signal). The flow from the inferior vena cava (IVC) through the right atrium (RA) following the Eustachian valve is shown by blue color Doppler flow signals. The insert in the right bottom corner shows the situation during a bubble test with the Eustachian valve (outlined by a dotted line) separating the almost bubble-free inflow from the IVC from the bubble-laden blood coming from the superior vena cava (lower part of the right atrium). Some of the bubbles still manage to cross the PFO. It is understandable that, in the presence of a Eustachian valve, a bubble studied through the arm may be falsely negative and fail to diagnose a PFO. LA, left atrium; SP, septum primum; SS, septum secundum.

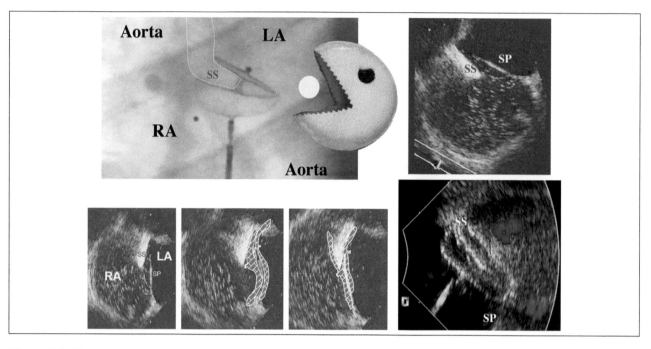

Figure 31.17
Pacman sign for correct placement of PFO occluder. The top left panel shows a 25 mm Amplatzer PFO occluder placed correctly. Even without dye injection the V-shape of the two disks can be appreciated. Separation of left side of the disks is caused by the muscular septum secundum (dotted outline), while the paper-thin septum primum to the right does not separate the two disks ostensibly. The right panels show the transesophageal echocardiographic picture in an analogous projection without (top) and with (bottom) the device. The bottom left panels show the echocardiographic situation in the projection used angiographically with an incorrectly (center) and correctly (right) placed superimposed Amplatzer PFO occluder. LA, left atrium; RA, right atrium; SP, septum primum; SS, septum secundum.

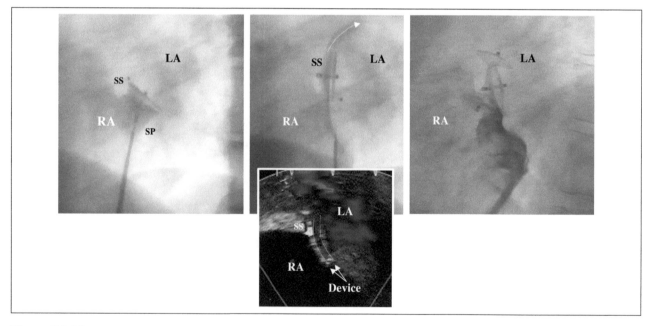

Figure 31.20
Amplatzer 18 mm PFO ocluder erroneously released without a reliable Pacman sign. Left panel: the right atrial disk of the device is barely indenting (rather than embracing) the septum secundum (SS). After release from the pusher cable, the right atrial disk slips into the PFO tunnel, resulting in a significant residual shunt (center panel, arrow). The device should have been replaced for a 25 mm PFO occluder to safely embrace the septum secundum before release. The residual shunt was still present at the 6-month follow-up transesophageal echocardiogram (bottom insert). At that time it was remedied with the implantation of a second Amplatzer PFO occluder (right panel). LA, left atrium; RA, right atrium; SP, septum primum.

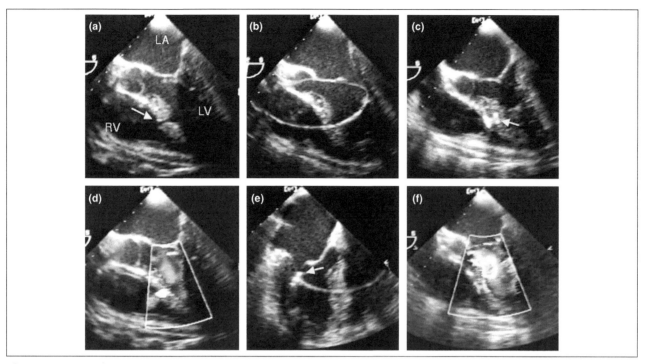

Figure 35.2

Transesophageal echocardiographic images in modified four-chamber views in a 31-year-old male patient with a 5 mm anterior muscular VSD and left-to-right shunt. (a) View demonstrates the VSD (arrow). LV, left ventricle; RV, right ventricle; LA, left atrium. (b) Similar view to (a) with color Doppler demonstrating the shunt. (c) View demonstrating the arteriovenous wire loop (from the aorta, left ventricle, VSD, right ventricle, and out the jugular vein. (d) Deployment of the LV disk of a 6 mm Amplatzer muscular VSD device in mid-LV cavity (arrow). (e) The device has been released (arrow) in the ventricular septum. Note, for an adult the connecting waist is not long enough, but it achieves closure. (f) Final image with color Doppler demonstrating good device position and no residual shunt.

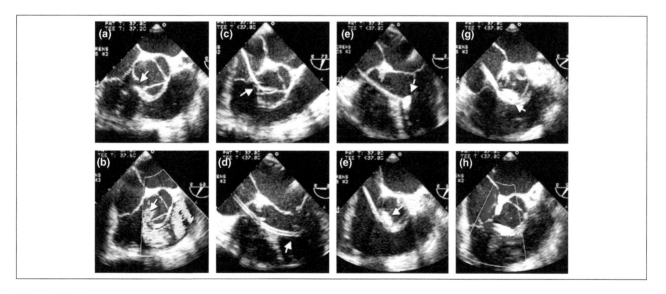

Figure 37.4

Transesophageal echocardiographic images of a 34-year-old male patient with an 8 mm perimembranous VSD. (a) and (b) Short axis view without and with color Doppler at the subaortic level demonstrating the defect (arrow) with left to right shunt (arrow). (c) Short axis view demonstrating passage of the wire forming an arteriovenous loop (wire is passing from the aorta through the VSD to the right atrium. (d) Four-chamber view showing the delivery sheath in the left ventricular apex. (e) The left ventricle disk is deployed. (f) Short axis view showing good position of the LV disk (arrow) in short axis view. (g) Short axis view showing the two disks of the device in good position (arrow). (h) Short axis view with color Doppler mapping showing no residual shunt with a trivial tricuspid regurgitation.

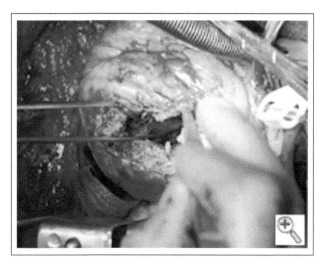

Figure 39.1
Ruptured interventricular septum. A ragged perforation (forceps holding it open) seen at the the time of surgical repair.

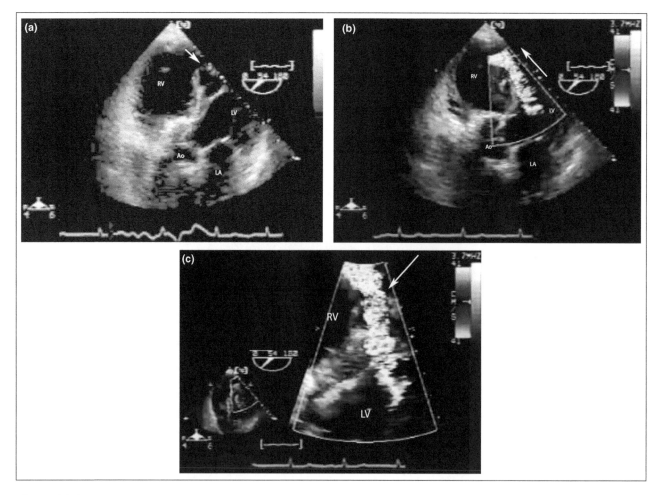

Figure 39.3
Transesophageal echocardiographic (TEE) images of an acute post-infarct ventricular septal defect (VSD). The transgastric view (a) shows the ragged margins of the ruptured (arrow) septum. Color-flow mapping (b) shows a high velocity flow exiting the tunnel-like VSD (arrows) (c). RV, right ventricle; LV, left ventricle; LA, left atrium; Ao, Aorta.

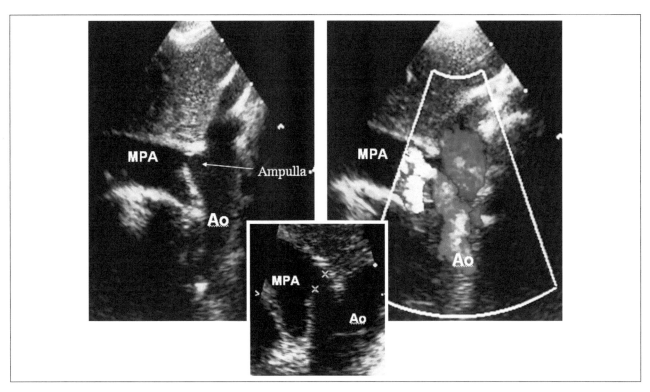

Figure 42.3

Echo definition of the patent ductus arteriosus. This is a high left parasternal view (ductal view) obtained in an infant. The duct insertion as well as the ampulla is clearly defined. Measurement of the duct insertion site is made in the magnified view (bottom insert). Note the retrograde flow of blood in the color Doppler picture (right). MPA, main pulmonary artery; Ao, aorta.

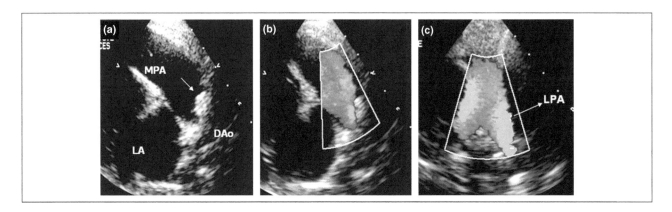

Figure 42.9

Echocardiographic assessment after free coil delivery. (a) High parasternal view of a duct after coil occlusion. (b) The color Doppler picture in the same view. (c) Short-axis view with the same transducer position. It is important to demonstrate a laminar flow in the origin of the left pulmonary artery (LPA).

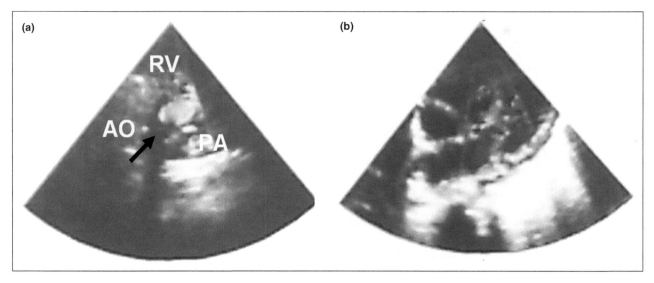

Figure 43.1
Two-dimensional Echo and Doppler color flow imaging in the high parasternal short-axis view in a 2-year-old with severe pulmonary artery hypertension. (a) Showing APW defect with low velocity colour flow; (b) after oxygen inhalation – high velocity color flow (arrow). AO, aorta; PA, pulmonary artery; RV, right ventricle.

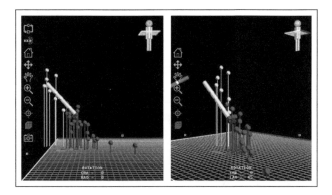

Figure 56.7
LocaLisa images with no cranial or RAO rotation in (a) but with LAO rotation of 45° in (b). The His and left bundle are shown in aquamarine and the areas where radiofrequency has been applied is shown by the red markers. The ablation catheter in aquamarine with white strips and red tip indicates the position at the time of energy application without requiring fluoroscopy.

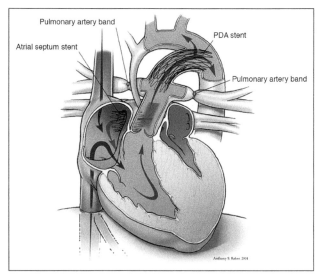

Figure 59.2
The hybrid Stage I palliation. Note pulmonary artery (PA) bands on the left and right PAs, proximal to the upper lobe branches. Stents span the length of the PDA and atrial septum (if necessary).(Reproduced from[2])

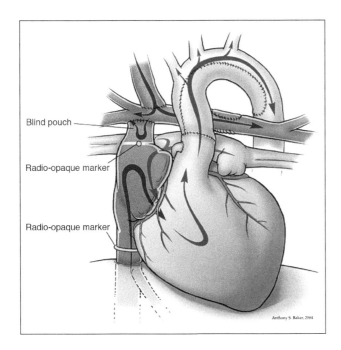

Figure 59.11
Illustration of the anatomy after the Comprehensive Stage 2 procedure.

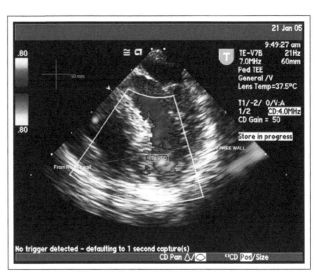

Figure 61.1
Echocardiographic still frame from a patient with a muscular VSD. It is crucial to measure the distance from the free wall of the right ventricle to the VSD, and, from the free wall of the right ventricle to the free wall of the left ventricle.

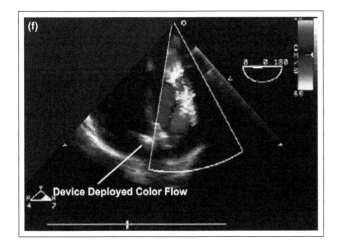

Figure 61.2 (f)
Echocardiographic still frames of muscular VSD closure. See text for detail. LV, left ventricle; RV, right ventricle; VSD, ventricular septal defect.

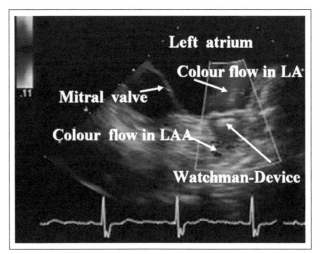

Figure 65.10
Echocardiographic control 45 days after implantation of the device. The color Doppler demonstrates very little flow behind the device in the LAA, thus coumadine therapy can be stopped.

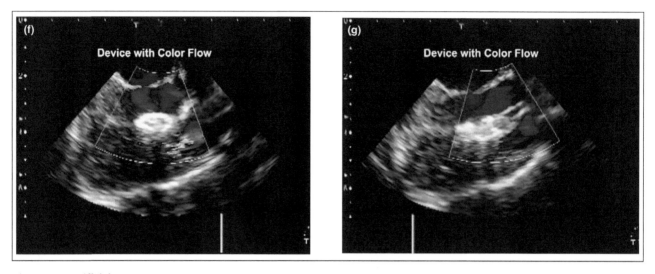

Figure 61.3 (f) (g)
Echocardiographic still frames from a patient who underwent device closure of a perimembranous VSD. (f) and (g) Color flow evaluation after device deployment. LV, left ventricle; RV, right ventricle; VSD, ventricular septal defect.

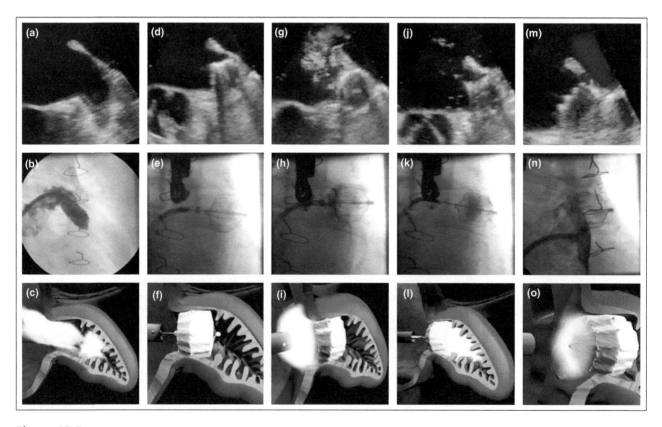

Figure 63.5
Device implantation step by step. (a)–(c) Assessment of LAA morphology. Measure the LAA orifice diameter by TEE (a) and angiography (b) to choose appropriate device size (see Table 63.1). Exclude possible thrombi in the LAA. (d)–(f) Positioning and expansion of the device. Make sure that at least two rows of anchors are engaged in the LAA tissue. Perform proximal (g–i) and distal (j–l) dye injections to assess the seal quality of the occluder (see Table 63.3). After a successful device stability test, the PLAATO™ occluder is released from its delivery catheter. To assess the final leak status, color Doppler (m) is used and a final dye injection (n, o) is performed. LAA, left atrial appendage; TEE, transesophageal echocardiogram.

Section I

1

The ideal cardiac catheterization laboratory: not just for cardiologists anymore – it is hybrid time!

John P Cheatham

Introduction

What would Werner Forsmann say about what has happened since that fateful day, so long ago, when he performed the first cardiac catheterization on himself? Of course, he never actually reached his heart with the catheter the first time *and* he was banished from his promising career as a young surgeon. However, his spirit exemplifies what has now become the modern day interventional cardiologist. Since there is a distinction between the cardiologist trained to treat adults with predominant coronary artery and acquired cardiac disease and those cardiologists specially trained to manage congenital heart disease, the same can be said for the cardiac catheterization laboratories in which these patients are treated. For the purpose of this chapter, the design, equipment required, necessary inventory, and personnel requirements for the modern day lab dedicated to advanced transcatheter therapy for the smallest newborn to the largest adult with complex congenital heart disease will be discussed. The author readily acknowledges the biases instilled in him by his mentor and idol, Charles E (Chuck) Mullins, MD, who has taught many of the congenital heart interventionalists across the globe (Figure 1.1a and b).

A new era

Historically, cardiothoracic surgeons and interventional cardiologists have had a somewhat competitive relationship. This is especially true with physicians treating coronary and acquired cardiac disease in adults. However, a 'team concept' has always been important when establishing a center of excellence for the treatment of complex congenital heart disease. The collaborative spirit between the cardiac surgeon and the entire cardiology team has advanced therapies offered to patients. More recently, the unique relationship

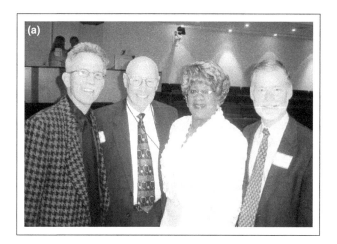

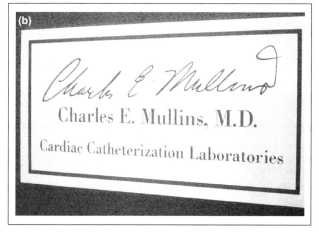

Figure 1.1
Charles E. (Chuck) Mullins MD has taught and inspired many interventionalists specializing in congenital heart disease all over the world. (a) During the dedication ceremony at Texas Children's Hospital, Dr Mullins gathers with some of his 'aging' pupils and his long time cath lab assistant. (b) The new cath labs were named in Chuck's honor – an honor well deserved.

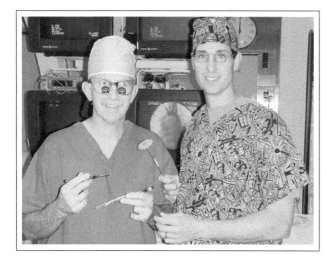

Figure 1.2
The unique and collegial relationship between the interventional cardiologist and cardiothoracic surgeon has fostered new hybrid treatment strategies for complex congenital heart disease. However, sometimes the members of the team get confused and want each other's job!

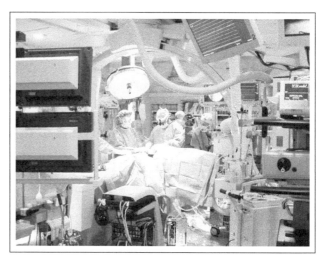

Figure 1.3
During a hybrid cardiac procedure involving the surgical and interventional teams, as well as the perfusionist for cardiopulmonary bypass, the hybrid suite gets crowded very quickly. Space and proper ergonomics in design will overcome many obstacles in a traditional cath lab or operative suite.

between the interventionalist and surgeon has fostered combined transcatheter and surgical therapeutic options – so called 'hybrid' treatment (Figure 1.2).[1–3] This innovative spirit mandates a fresh and open mind to create the 'ideal' venue, or hybrid suite, to expand the capabilities of the traditional cath lab and operating room.[4]

Hybrid suite design

In planning an ideal hybrid suite, there are five major considerations: (1) personnel that will be participating in the procedure, (2) adequate space for the equipment and personnel, (3) equipment that is necessary, (4) informational management and video display, and (5) necessary inventory and consideration of costs.

Personnel

Traditionally, the team responsible to perform both diagnostic and interventional cardiac catheterizations in children and adults with congenital heart disease consists of the interventional cardiologist, an assisting fellow or cath lab nurse, and technicians and nurses who are responsible to monitor the physiologic recorder, the X-ray imaging equipment, and to 'circulate' in the room to assist with the procedure. These team members are former ICU nurses, radiologic technicians, respiratory therapists, and paramedics who receive 'on-the-job training'. Specially trained registered cardiovascular invasive specialists (RCISs) are quite valuable in today's lab, as they are trained in all aspects of cath lab procedures

and frequently have adult interventional experience. They are particularly helpful in treating adults with CHD and in the use of coronary stents, vascular closure devices, and small diameter guidewires. All staff are 'cross trained' to be able to run the imaging and hemodynamic equipment and rotate into any job necessary during the procedure. However, as the complexity of transcatheter procedures has evolved, many changes have been necessary to ensure safety and success.[5] A highly trained and competent assistant to the primary operator is imperative. A general pediatric cardiology fellow is usually inadequate to serve in this role today with the higher risk and complicated interventional procedures now performed. Therefore, it is becoming more common to have an advanced level interventional cardiology fellow in the lab. However, many institutions do not have a general or advanced level cardiology fellowship program, therefore, the role of a specially trained interventional nurse practitioner has evolved and offers many advantages.

In addition to the team members mentioned above, dedicated cardiac anesthesia and cardiac ultrasound imaging is mandatory. This requires a staff anesthesiologist with assisting trainee or nurse anesthetist. A staff echocardiographer is also in attendance along with a fellow or technician. One gets the sense that the room is rapidly becoming crowded. By the way, dedicated anesthesia and echo equipment must find a home as well. With the new hybrid procedures, the cardiothoracic surgeon and team will be present which may include an assisting surgeon or resident, a scrub nurse, as well as the perfusionists and accompanying cardiopulmonary bypass machine (Figure 1.3). Now the suite really is shrinking! The electrophysiologist and equipment when electrical therapy or a pacemaker is required can add

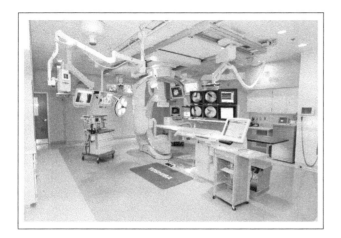

Figure 1.4
The appropriate space, design, and equipment are shown here in one of the hybrid suites at Columbus Children's Hospital. Note the flat screen monitors, ceiling mounted equipment, and video and equipment booms to allow easy access to the patient and informational imaging for all personnel.

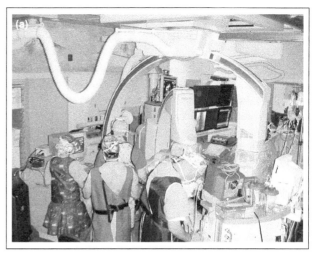

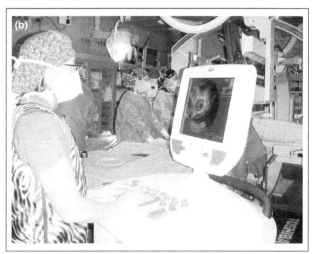

up to 18 people, all with their specialized equipment, during a single hybrid cardiac catheterization intervention for CHD! So, we have to design the suite to accommodate all of the personnel and the equipment.

Design: space and ergonomics

The space required for a modern day hybrid cardiac catheterization suite is significantly more than a single plane, adult coronary cath lab, or for that matter, the traditional biplane CHD cath lab built 10–20 years ago.[6–9] The suite design must account for the actual working space or procedure room, the control room, a computer 'cold' room, an adjacent inventory supply room, and a new space very important to the modern suite – the induction room, where all of the 'team' can assess the patient and discuss the procedure, as well as administer sedative/anesthetic agents. With dedicated personnel now being assigned to the suites, it is desirable to also plan for administrative office space, personnel offices and workspace, a conference and editing room, a 'break' area, and dressing rooms with bathroom and shower facilities. For the purpose of this chapter, we will confine our remarks to the essential space dedicated to the actual procedure being performed.

Ideally, the hybrid suite should be a minimum of 800 square feet, and preferably 900 square feet (Figure 1.4). A square room, rather than the conventional rectangular suite, allows equal space around the catheterization table for complete patient accessibility – 30′ × 30′ would be 'ideal'. This is especially important when interventional procedures may be performed from either femoral, jugular, or subclavian sites, and let's also not forget about transhepatic access. In the majority of hybrid procedures, access is

Figure 1.5
It is important to design appropriate space for the echo and anesthesia teams to be involved in transcatheter or hybrid therapy for congenital heart disease. (a) The echo and anesthesia teams have a completely free space at the head of table during TEE guidance of device closure. (b) In addition, during IVUS or ICE examination, the space at the foot of the table must also allow the team to do their job.

required through a median sternotomy and personnel will be on both sides of the table. There must be room for the anesthesiology team and anesthesia equipment at the head of the patient and to either side, while space must also be available for the echocardiography personnel and echo machine at the head of the patient during transesophageal echo (TEE), and at the end of the table for intracardiac echo (ICE) or intravascular ultrasound (IVUS) (Figure 1.5a,b). The perfusionist and cardiopulmonary bypass machine will usually be positioned on the side opposite the surgeon and/or interventionalist, making the width of the room extremely important and different from a traditional cath lab – hence, a square room.

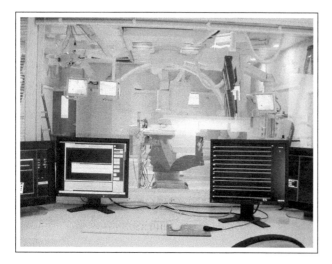

Figure 1.6
The control room should be designed to allow personnel to view the catheterization procedure without obstruction. Note the clear line of view down the table during the final phase of hybrid suite construction.

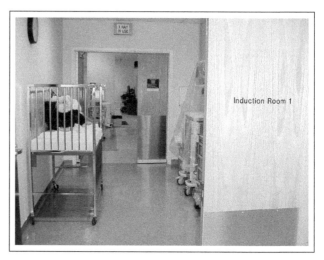

Figure 1.7
A relatively new concept is the use of an 'induction room', which allows access to the patient and family by all team members in a quiet environment. Wall mounted anesthesia equipment conserves space and allows sedation or induction of anesthesia as needed. The room should be directly connected to the hybrid suite, as shown here.

The control room should be as wide as the hybrid suite (25–30 feet) and approximately 10 feet in depth. This will allow all of the personnel, along with the physiologic and digital X-ray imaging equipment and monitors, to be strategically placed. In addition, the digital review station and archiving system should be located in this room. In the combined interventional/electrophysiology suite, appropriate electrophysiology (EP) recording, pacing, radiofrequency ablation, and three-dimensional (3D) mapping equipment must also be placed in the control room. This room should be designed in order for the personnel to view the procedure directly by looking down the table from the foot to the head of the patient (Figure 1.6). This ensures an unobstructed view of the procedure, regardless of the position of the biplane equipment or the team. Therefore, the patient table should be parallel to the viewing angle of the control room. The adjacent computer or 'cold room' size will be dependent on the manufacturer's specifications, but should allow easy access for maintenance or repair work to be performed. When building multiple suites, this room can be shared to conserve space.

The suite should also have an adjacent and ample supply room to store the extra inventory and consumable equipment that is not located in the cabinet storage within the procedure room. A blanket warmer is placed here, as well as other non-consumable equipment. If possible, the adjacent supply room should be approximately 100–120 square feet and should be directly accessible from the procedure room for maximum efficiency. If there are multiple suites, then a larger central supply room could be used that is accessible to both suites.

A relatively new concept in both surgery and interventional cardiology is the use of an 'induction room' adjacent to the hybrid suite (Figure 1.7). This room becomes very important since it allows the interventional, anesthesia, and surgical teams direct access to the patient and family, while maintaining a quiet and comforting environment to explain the procedures, perform history and physical examination, and to administer sedation. By installing small, space efficient, anesthesia machines that can be mounted on the wall, induction can be performed here as needed. In addition, this room may serve as a separate TEE room while an interventional catheterization is being performed, allowing maximum efficiency of the anesthesiology team. Ideally, this room should be approximately 12 feet by 17 feet, which will allow the appropriate family members and personnel to interact in a comfortable environment.

Not mentioned is the mandatory soil or 'dirty' room, where reusable equipment is washed, and which must be separate from the 'clean' scrub room, as per occupational safety and health administration (OSHA) standards. Also, when building two hybrid suites, it becomes apparent that a centrally located scrub area with two separate sinks be located immediately outside the procedure rooms with open access from both control rooms, but with appropriate barriers for infection control. This allows maximum efficiency and entry into both suites, while maintaining safety and a sterile environment.

Equipment

What used to be a pretty simple list of equipment needs 10 years ago has mushroomed into a huge cloud of needs, wants, and money! Biplane X-ray imaging equipment and a physiologic monitoring system with recording and reporting capabilities occupied most of the capital expense requirements of the traditional lab 10 years ago. However, the new hybrid suite's capital equipment list has grown proportionally, incorporating many services within a Heart Center.

Beginning with X-ray equipment, we certainly live in a new age of imaging. While some might argue the merits of biplane versus single plane fluoroscopic and angiographic units, no one would dispute the clear advantages of displaying complex spatial anatomy using biplane cameras. This is especially true when performing transcatheter procedures in the tiniest preterm neonate to the 200 kg adult with complex CHD. So in a perfect world and without consideration of costs or space requirements, a modern biplane, digital cath lab is mandatory to achieve optimal imaging for the complicated interventional procedures of today.

Today, no one would argue the merits of digital (film free) radiographic systems. However, for some interventionalists over the past 10 years, it was a slow process to 'give up' cine film, X-ray processing rooms, and splicing lessons for fellows. The obvious advantages of digital technology are real time access and viewing, no deterioration of angios, ease of storing, managing, and retrieving image data, and labor savings for the procedure. The digital images are easily accessible both inside and outside the hospital using a web server, as well as by remote satellite transmission. Yet, just as the 'digital age' in cardiac catheterization began over a decade ago, we now live in the world of PC-based digital platforms and flat panel detectors (FPDs). This began with General Electric Medical's introduction of a single plane FPD approximately 5 years ago, then the PC-based digital platform for hemodynamic monitoring systems arrived in 2004, and culminated with the introduction of biplane FPD technology in 2005 by Siemens Medical and Toshiba Medical Systems Corporation. The targeted specialties for this new equipment are centers specializing in CHD cardiac catheterizations, advanced electrophysiology laboratories, and neuroradiology treatment centers.

We must ask, what are the advantages of FPD technology?[10,11] The definition of FPD is a compressed or flat detector which uses semiconductors or thin-film transistors (TFTs), converts X-ray energy into electrical signals, and creates X-ray images. Currently, indirect conversion FPD technology is used for biplane systems. Eventually, direct conversion technology may be used, once the 'blanking' and frame rate limitations are overcome in the biplane configuration. Direct conversion will improve resolution as the image is never converted to light. The FPD will likely replace all existing X-ray detectors, such as image intensifier (II)-TV cameras and spot film cameras, as well as film screen systems. For cardiovascular work, the small profile of the detector size will allow a more compact design and facilitate improved patient access. In addition, high image quality with improved blood vessel detectability by high modulation transfer

function (MTF) and no distortion will be an advantage. Finally, 3D digital tomography and interventions may be possible. If there has been a downside to this technology, it has been the lack of appropriate Windows™ software programs being provided by all manufacturers during this introductory phase. This should improve with time, as more software programming specialists are incorporated into the research and development teams of manufacturers.

In the dedicated CHD hybrid suite, patient accessibility is equally important to high quality imaging. Therefore, since the 3D gantry positioner was introduced by General Electric Medical over a decade ago, other companies have now realized the importance of patient access in a biplane lab. Since a 3D gantry allows rotation of the C-arm in the x, y, and z axes, this allows additional space at the head of the table to accommodate the anesthesia and interventional teams. However, with the original design by General Electric and later Siemens Medical, the space was still crowded. The most recent and innovative design has come from Toshiba Medical Systems Corporation with a 5 axis C-arm positioner with biplane FPD (Infinix CF-i/BP), which allows movement in five axes around the patient, with rotation of the C-arm base to −135° or +135°, which actually places the C-arm on the 'foot' side of the lateral camera (Figure 1.8). This allows a completely 'head free zone' of 180° while in a biplane configuration, allowing easy access to the patient by the anesthesia, echo, and interventional teams (Figure 1.9). It is also highly beneficial to the electrophysiology service during complex studies with transvenous pacemaker implantation.

All teams must have not only free access to the patient, but also a clear line of site to the image display monitors. Speaking of monitors, the days of the CRT monitors are coming to an end. Flat screen monitors are achieving comparable black-white and line resolution, and are ergonomically more versatile in a biplane laboratory. They take up less space, are lighter, and can be mounted on a 6 monitor gantry that can be strategically placed around the procedure table to allow optimal viewing by all personnel participating in the procedure, regardless of location (Figure 1.10). This gantry should be able to be placed on either side of the table, as well as over the table at the head or foot of the patient. In the hybrid suite, it is also important to install a surgical light mounted strategically on the ceiling. We also prefer to mount all other accessory equipment from the ceiling, i.e., contrast injector with wall mounted controls, local spotlight, and radiation shield.

The other components of X-ray imaging equipment found in the hybrid suite are fairly standard by today's standards. TV cameras using the charged coupled device (CCD) technology, developed by Toshiba Medical Systems Corporation, to improve brightness and resolution; X-ray tubes using spiral-grooved and liquid metal bearing technology, introduced by Phillips Medical, Inc to eliminate noise and reduce the delay in fluoro/digital acquisition; and

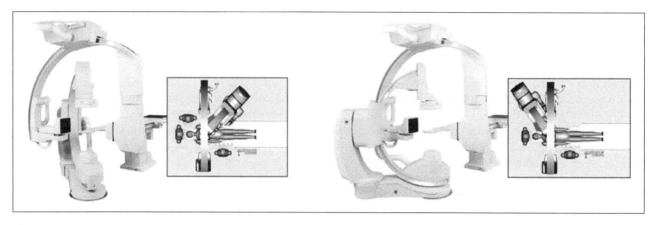

Figure 1.8
The new design of the Toshiba Infinix CF-i/BP positioners allows rotation of the C-arm base from −135° to +135°. This schematic drawing demonstrates the 180° of 'head free zone' afforded by this new design.

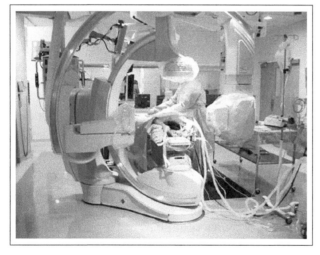

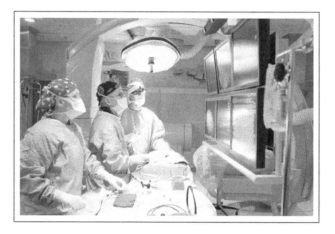

Figure 1.10
Flat screen monitors have now approximated CRT monitors in terms of resolution. The lighter, more compact configuration of the flat screen monitors allows a gantry holding six monitors to be easily positioned at any location for the hybrid team to view the images, as depicted here during a stage I hybrid palliation for hypoplastic left heart syndrome (HLHS).

Figure 1.9
During a cardiac catheterization procedure, the open space at the head of the table is nicely demonstrated here. There is plenty of room for the interventional, echo, and anesthesia teams to perform their jobs.

high frequency generators are now uniformly offered by all manufacturers. Furthermore, while using different technology, radiation dose management is a priority with all manufacturers to protect the patient and all of those participating in the longer interventional catheterization procedures being performed today.[12]

An important, but forgotten, component of the new hybrid suite is the procedure table. Traditional cath lab tables have certain features that are well suited for X-ray imaging, patient positioning, and quick and easy 'free float' movement, and that are electronically integrated into the manufacturer's X-ray imaging equipment. In addition, some tables have the ability to be placed in the Trendelenburg position. In comparison, the traditional operating room

table is narrower, shorter, less 'fluoro friendly', and does not provide 'free float' capabilities. Additionally, the table has the very important feature of 20–30° lateral tilt which provides the cardiothoracic surgeon with exposure to the desired operative field ergonomically, while the Trendelenburg position is also possible. So, currently, either the surgeon or the interventionalist must make sacrifices while performing hybrid procedures in the traditional operative or catheterization suite. A new hybrid table is essential to facilitate new hybrid management strategies for complex CHD. The table must be manufactured by the X-ray equipment companies in order to provide 'connectivity' to the imaging equipment and possess tableside controls. This table must possess all of the above mentioned specifications, so will require input

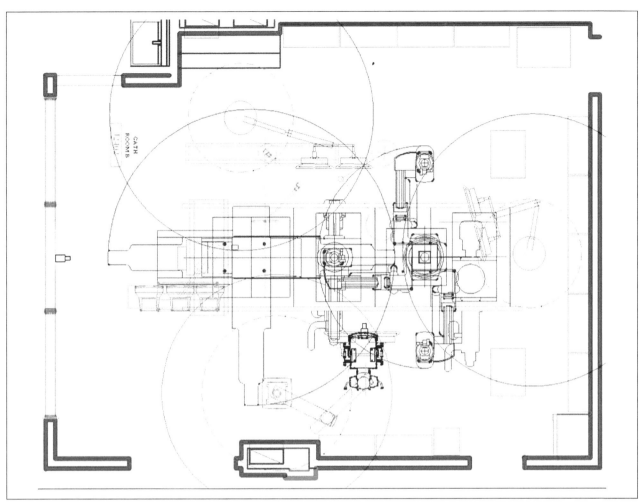

Figure 1.11
The schematic drawing of our hybrid suite demonstrates the importance of careful planning, input from multiple members of the Heart Center, and collaboration with several industry representatives. Note the video monitor and equipment boom design to ensure all personnel can view the appropriate images during the procedure, regardless of their location in the suite.

from both cardiothoracic surgeons and interventional cardiologists as they are being designed. Such a hybrid table is being planned by both Toshiba Medical Systems Corporation and Siemens Medical. Stay tuned!

Informational management, video display, and transport

Staggering amounts of information are generated in today's healthcare environment and these data need to be readily available during the procedures. In our Heart Center, we attempted to provide access for angiography, echocardiography (including TTE, TEE, ICE, and IVUS), and the PACS system (CT, MRI, and chest X-ray) from any computer inside or outside the hospital with a dedicated web server and VPN access. This same information must be readily available in the new hybrid suites where complex procedures and decision-making are being performed by

the multidisciplinary team. The information needs to be accessible to all participants in the suite and must be specific to their assigned tasks. If the staff moves around the room, so must the displayed images. Furthermore, all of this information should be able to be transmitted to other sites within the hospital, i.e. operative room, teleconference center, or research lab, as well as to sites anywhere in the world, i.e. educational conferences, outside referring physicians for patient care, and teaching workshops. A dedicated and expansive archiving system is imperative for the digital technology of today. The data must be sent 'seamless' from the archived source to the active procedure and/or educational site.

In an ideal world, money, space, and hospital administrative support would be unlimited. So, let's begin with the video display within the hybrid suite. Flat screen monitors are strategically placed around the room, mounted to ceiling booms with a rotational axis that provides viewing from any location (Figure 1.11). We chose to enlist the expertise of

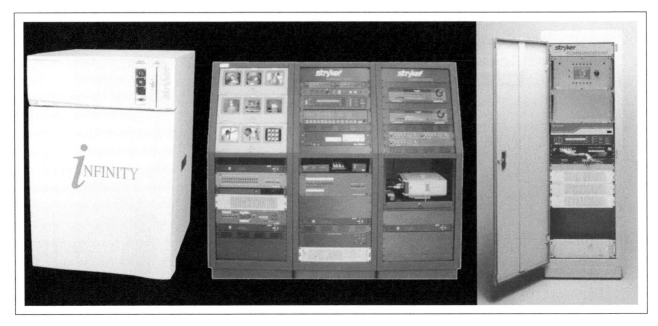

Figure 1.12
A large video router and informational management unit is located in our teleconference center and provides interconnectivity to the hybrid suites through the smaller video router and cameras within each suite. In turn, the operative suite and research laboratory can also be connected through the teleconference center, providing a 'video network topology' for worldwide education and patient care.

Stryker Communications to fulfill these needs. Two monitors are mounted on three video booms, while one of the booms also serves as an equipment boom. Mounted on the equipment boom is a defibrillator, fiber optic surgeon's headlight, electrocautery, and a pan/tilt/zoom video camera. A second camera is mounted on the wall above the control room, providing expansive views of the suite and the procedures being performed. A video router is located within each suite and allows any image to be displayed on any video monitor, giving each staff member optimal viewing of the information pertinent to their job. In turn, the video router in the hybrid suite is connected to a larger management and routing unit within the teleconference center, serving as the 'mother ship' (Figure 1.12). All information can be transmitted anywhere in the world from this location. We believe this 'video network topology' to be the framework of the future.

Inventory

Every cardiac catheterization procedure in patients with CHD requires a large inventory of 'routine' consumable items. In addition, each interventional procedure requires an additional inventory of special and very expensive consumable materials. Words from my mentor, Dr Mullins, are etched in my mind. 'In a congenital heart laboratory, all consumable items must be available in a very wide range of sizes in order to accommodate every patient's size, from the tiniest premature neonate to the largest adult patient. A cardiac catheterization procedure *never* should be compromised or

terminated because of the lack of a necessary piece of consumable equipment.' However, these special consumables will vary with the individual operator's experience and credentials, as well as with the availability of a particular device or material in any particular part of the world. Equally important in determining the inventory is the individual hospital administrator's 'budget' control. We are very fortunate with tremendous hospital support, which seemingly allows unlimited access to all available consumables, i.e. balloon catheters, devices, delivery systems, stents, guidewires, RF perforating systems, all imaging equipment (TTE, TEE, ICE, IVUS), etc. – which are justified and 'reasonable'. Accordingly, our inventory consumable costs are over $1 million, so it is incumbent upon the cath lab manager and medical director to maintain strict inventory control and management. New 'bar coders' can be used to scan all consumables used during the procedure to maintain an accurate accounting for billing purposes, as well as maintaining a computerized inventory and order management system. Most new hemodynamic systems have an inventory management program that can be used for this purpose. Unfortunately, economics, rather than necessity, will continue to dictate the practice of medicine.

Summary

In conclusion, collaboration between the interventional cardiologist and cardiothoracic surgeon continues to increase as the hybrid strategies for complex CHD evolve. Making informational resources available when and where they are needed can have a dramatic impact on patient care. The implementation of a hybrid cardiac catheterization suite is a result of careful planning involving multiple disciplines, including Heart Center medical staff, equipment manufacturers, architects, contractors, and information technology specialists. Specially designed equipment and trained personnel are paramount to success. A huge inventory of consumables is required and must be judiciously managed. However, there is no substitute for a collegial and professional relationship and understanding among the Heart Center staff of the ultimate goals of success. Finally, it must be recognized that a progressive and forward thinking hospital administrative staff is a prerequisite for the planning, building, and financial support necessary for the ideal hybrid cardiac catheterization suite to become a reality.

REFERENCES

1. Diab KA, Hijazi ZM, Cao QL, Bacha EA. A truly hybrid approach to perventricular closure of multiple muscular ventricular septal defects. J Thorac Cardiovasc Surg 2005; 130(3): 892–3.
2. Galantowicz M, Cheatham JP. Lessons learned from the development of a new hybrid strategy for the management of hypoplastic left heart syndrome. Pediatr Cardiol 2005; 26(2): 190–9.
3. Holzer R, Hijazi ZM. Interventional approach to congenital heart disease. Curr Opin Cardiol 2004; 19(2): 84–90.
4. Melvin DA, Chisolm JL, Lents JD et al. A first generation hybrid catheterization laboratory: ready for 'prime time'. Catheter Cardiovasc Interven 2004; 63(1): 123.
5. Mullins CE. History of pediatric interventional catheterization: pediatric therapeutic cardiac catheterizations. Pediatr Cardiol 1998; 19(1): 3–7.
6. Mathewson JW. Building a pediatric cardiac catheterization laboratory and conference room: design considerations and filmless imaging. Pediatr Cardiol 1996; 17(5): 279–94.
7. Verna E. Evolution of the catheterization laboratory: new instruments and imaging techniques. Ital Heart J 2001; 2(2): 116–17.
8. Bashore TM, Bates ER, Berger PB et al. Section on Cardiology and Cardiac Surgery: American Academy of Pediatrics. Guidelines for pediatric cardiovascular centers. Pediatrics 2002; 109(3): 544–9.
9. Moore JWM, Beekman RH, Case CL et al. American College of Cardiology/Society for Cardiac Angiography and Interventions Clinical Expert Consensus Document on cardiac catheterization laboratory standards. A report of the American College of Cardiology Task Force on Clinical Expert Consensus Documents. J Am Coll Cardiol 2001; 37(8): 2170–214.
10. Holmes DR Jr, Laskey WK, Wondrow MA, Cusma JT. Flat-panel detectors in the cardiac catheterization laboratory: revolution or evolution – what are the issues? Catheter Cardiovasc Interven 2004; 63(3): 324–30.
11. Chotas HG, Dobbins JT, Ravin CE. Principles of digital radiography with large-area, electronically readable detectors: a review of the basics. Radiology 1999; 210: 595–9.
12. Ross RD, Joshi V, Carravallah DJ, Morrow WR. Reduced radiation during cardiac catheterization of infants using acquisition zoom technology. Am J Cardiol 1997; 79(5): 691–3.

Section II

Imaging modalities in the cath lab

2

Angiography

Lee Benson and Haverj Mikailian

Introduction

Accurate anatomic and physiologic diagnosis is the foundation of a successful catheter based therapeutic procedure. As such, a number of complementary imaging modalities have been developed to define, in real time, specific aspects of the heart and circulation for interventional applications. In the evolution of our understanding of the cardiovascular system, angiography with fluoroscopy was the first to be developed, and the angiography suite remains the cornerstone around which the interventional suite is built.

This chapter will include a discussion of standard angiographic approaches and how to achieve them. Emphasis will be placed on the application of these projections as applied to interventional procedures. A detailed description of the physical principles of image formation is beyond the scope of this chapter and the interested reader is referred to other sources for more detailed information.[1]

Angiographic projections

In the therapeutic management of the child with a congenital heart lesion, the spatial orientation and detailed morphology of the heart and great vessels are of critical importance. As the operator enters the laboratory, an overall understanding of the anatomy should have been synthesized, based upon information from other imaging modalities such as chest roentgenography, echocardiography, and computed tomographic and magnetic resonance imaging. As such, the angiographic projections used in the procedure will be 'tailored' to outline the lesion to allow appropriate measurements and guide the intervention.[2]

In most children, the heart is oriented obliquely, with the left ventricular apex being leftward, anterior and inferior, then the heart base (Figure 2.1). The interventricular septum is a complex geometric three-dimensional structure that takes an 'S' curve from apex to base (Figure 2.2), the so-called sigmoid septum. From caudal to cranial the interventricular septum curves through an arc of 100° to 120°. The right ventricle appears as an appliqué to the left.

To address this unique topology, today's angiographic equipment allows a wide range of projections, incorporating caudocranial or craniocaudal angulations to outline or profile specific structures. The up-to-date laboratory of today consists of independent biplane imaging chains which, with the proper selection of views, minimizes overlapping and foreshortening of structures.

Terminology

Angiographic projections are designated either according to the position of the recording detector (image intensifier or flat panel detector) or the direction of the X-ray beam toward the recording device. Generally speaking, in cardiology, the convention is the former, and all terminology discussed henceforth will be using that convention. For example, when the detector is directly above a supine patient, the X-ray beam travels from posterior to anterior and the *angiographic projection* is designated postero-anterior (PA), but based upon detector *position* it is called frontal, and the position of the detector is by convention at 0°. Similarly, when the detector is moved through 90°, to a position besides and to the left of the patient, a lateral (LAT) projection results. Between 0° and 90° there are a multitude of projections termed left anterior oblique (LAO), and when the detector is moved to the right of the patient, a right anterior oblique projection (RAO) is achieved. As in the LAO projection, there are numerous RAO projections depending on the final angle from the midline. When the detector is posterior to the patient (the X-ray tube is anterior), then a right (RPO) or left (LPO) posterior oblique projection occurs (Figure 2.3).

Standard detectors mounted on a C-arm or parallelogram not only allow the above positions, but the detectors can be rotated around the transverse axis, toward the feet or head, caudal or cranial (Figure 2.4).

In summary, the conventional terms RAO, LAO, PA, and left-LAT designate the position of the recording detector. The LAT position usually will have the detector to the left of the patient by convention, and will be so implied throughout this chapter. Finally, for clarification, while the

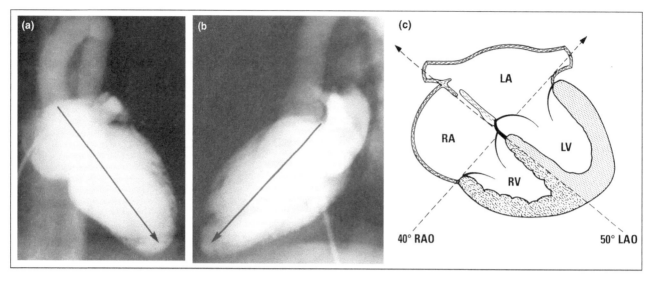

Figure 2.1

The typical lie of the heart in the chest. (a) Frontal and (b) lateral projections of a left ventriculogram demonstrate the axis of the heart. The apex points anteriorly, inferiorly, and leftward. Panel (c) is a diagram of how a standard mid-RAO and a standard mid-LAO profile images of the axes of the heart. The RAO profiles the atrioventricular groove, and presents the ventricular septum *en face*. The mid-LAO view profiles the intraventricular septum, and separates the left and right ventricular and atrial chambers. (Modified from Culham[1] with permission.)

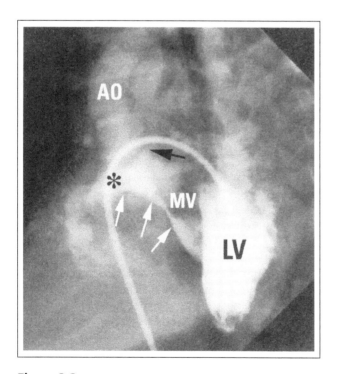

Figure 2.2

The sigmoid septum. A venous catheter is in the apex of the left ventricle through the mitral valve, in the long axis oblique projection. The sigmoid configuration of the septum is well seen (white arrows). Aortic–mitral continuity is noted (black arrow). Contrast is seen mixing across a ventricular defect (asterisk). (Modified from Culham[1] with permission.)

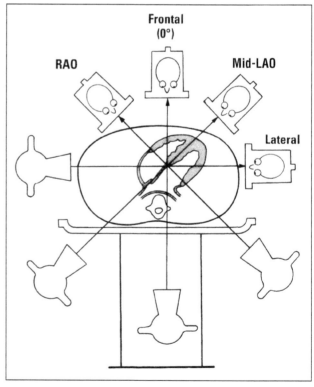

Figure 2.3

Naming the standard projections with the X-ray tube under the table. This diagram illustrates the various positions of the detector/X-ray tube. The patient is supine, and the view is from the patient's feet, looking toward the head. (Modified from Culham[1] with permission.)

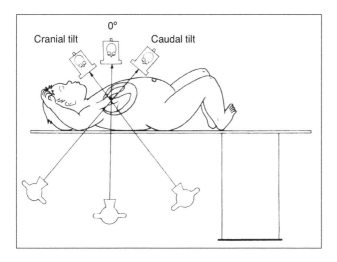

Figure 2.4
Naming the standard projections with the X-ray tube under the table. Cardiologic convention is such that cranial and caudal tilt refers to the detector position. (Modified from Culham[1] with permission.)

term projection refers to the path of the X-ray beam, to be consistent with cardiologic practice, projection or view will refer to the position of the detector.

Biplane angiography

As outlined in an earlier chapter discussing the ideal catheterization suite, dedicated interventional catheterization laboratories addressing congenital heart defects require biplane facilities.[3,4] Biplane angiography has the advantage of limiting contrast exposure and of facilitating the assessment of cardiac structures in real time in two projections simultaneously. However, this is at a cost, as these facilities are expensive, and with existing image intensifiers and newer flat panel detectors, extreme simultaneous angulations can be compromised. The choice of a set of projections will depend upon the information required, equipment capabilities, and the physical constraints to patient access. Standard biplane configurations include RAO/LAO, and frontal or lateral projections, with additional cranial or caudal tilt. The possible combinations are endless (Table 2.1 and Figure 2.5).

Cranial-LAO projections

A clear working understanding of these projections is of critical importance in developing a flexible approach to congenital heart defect angiography, and intervention. The practice of using 'cookbook' projections for each case *may*

Table 2.1 *Summary of projections*		
Projection	Angles	
Single plane projections		
Conventional RAO	40° RAO	
Frontal	0°	
Shallow LAO	1° to 30°	
Straight LAO	31° to 60°	
Steep LAO	61° to 89°	
Left lateral	90° left	
Cranially tilted RAO	30° RAO + 30° cranial	
Cranially tilted frontal (Sitting up view)	30° or 45° cranial	
Cranially tilted shallow LAO	25° LAO + 30° cranial	
Cranially tilted mid-LAO (Long axis oblique)	60° LAO + 20° to 30° cranial	
Cranially tilted steep LAO (Hepatoclavicular view)	45° to 70° LAO + 30° cranial	
Caudally tilted frontal	45° caudal	
Biplane combinations	*A plane*	*B plane*
AP and LAT	0°	Left lateral
LXO	30° RAO	*60° LAO + 20° to 30° cranial*
Hepatoclavicular view	*45° LAO + 30° cranial*	*120° LAO + 15° cranial*
Specific lesions		
RVOT-MPA (sitting up)	*10° LAO + 40° cranial*	Left lateral
Long axial for LPA (biplane)	30° RAO	60° LAO + 30° cranial
LPA long axis (single plane)		60° LAO + 20° cranial
ASD	*30° LAO + 30° cranial*	
PA bifurcation and branches	*30° caudal + 10° RAO*	*20° caudal*

Primary projections are in italics. RAO, right anterior oblique; LAO, left anterior oblique; AP, antero-posterior; LAT, lateral; RVOT, right ventricular outflow tract; MPA, main pulmonary artery; LXO, long axis oblique; LPA, left pulmonary artery; ASD, atria septal defect; PA, pulmonary artery.

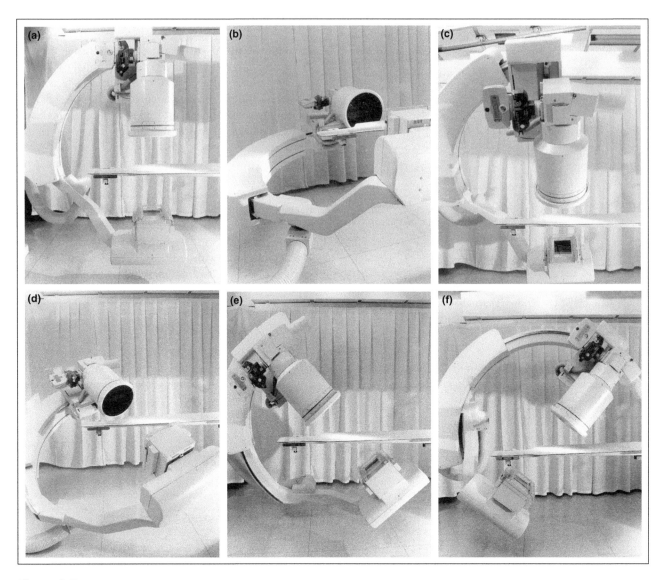

Figure 2.5
Standard projections. (a) Frontal (PA), (b) Lateral (LAT), (c) RAO, and (d) mid-LAO with cranial tilt. (e) Cranially tilted frontal (sitting up);
(f) caudally tilted frontal. (Modified from Culham[1] with permission.)

allow acceptable diagnostic studies, but will fall short of the detail required to accomplish an interventional procedure. However, a comprehensive understanding of normal cardiac anatomy, especially the interventricular septum, allows the operator to adjust the projection to optimize profiling the region of interest.

There are a number of 'rules of thumb' that allow the operator to judge the steepness or shallowness of an LAO projection. Of importance is the relationship of the cardiac silhouette to the spine, the ventricular catheter, and the ventricular apex.

To optimize the profile of the mid-point of the *membranous ventricular septum* (and thus the majority

of perimembranous defects), two-thirds of the cardiac silhouette should be to the right of the vertebral bodies (Figures 2.6 and 2.7). This will result in a cranially tilted left ventriculogram showing the left ventricular septal wall, the apex (denoted by the ventricular catheter) pointing toward the bottom of the image. A shallower projection will have more of the cardiac silhouette over towards the left of the spine and profile more the infero-basal component of the septum, ideal for *inlet type ventricular defects*. This projection allows for evaluation of atrioventricular valve relationships, inlet extension of perimembranous defects, and posterior muscular defects. A steeper LAO projection can be used to profile the *outlet extension of a perimembranous*

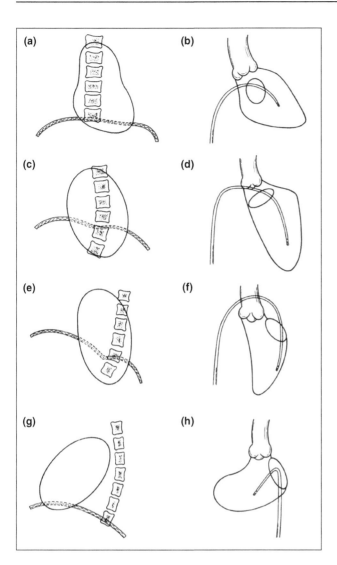

Figure 2.6
Setting up a standard LAO projection. To achieve the LAO projection, attempt to adjust the detector angle such that two-thirds of the cardiac silhouette is to the left of the spine, as in (e). If a catheter is through the mitral valve in the left ventricular apex, it will point to the floor, as in (f). In this view, the intraventricular septal margin points toward the floor. The so-called 4-chamber or hepatoclavicular view is achieved by having half the cardiac silhouette over the spine, as in (c). A catheter across the mitral valve will appear as in (d). A steep LAO projection will have the cardiac silhouette shown in (g), and a transmitral catheter in the left ventricle will appear as in (h). (a) and (b) show the frontal projection. (Modified from Culham[1] with permission.)

defect, and anterior muscular and apical defects. As noted in Figure 2.6, the ventricular catheter in the cardiac apex can be used to help guide the projection, but only if it enters the chamber through the mitral valve. If catheter entry is

through the ventricular defect or retrograde, it tends to be more basal and left lateral.

Modification of the cranial LAO projection will have to be made if there is a discrepancy in chamber sizes, and the septum rotated, such that a steeper or shallower projection may be required. Also, it is assumed that the patient is laying flat on the examining table, but if the head is turned to the right, or a pad is under the buttocks, it will rotate the thorax such that the LAO projection is steeper and the detector caudal. This has to be compensated for during the set up for the angiogram. The clue in the former case is that more of the heart silhouette is over the spine.

The first step in setting up a cranial-LAO projection is to achieve the correct degree of steepness or shallowness. After that, the degree of cranial tilt has to be confirmed, so that the basal–apical septum is elongated. This can be estimated by seeing how much of the hemidiaphragm is superimposed over the cardiac silhouette – the more superimposition, the greater the cranial tilt. Additionally, the degree of cranial tilt can be determined by looking at the course of the ventricular catheter, it appearing to be foreshortened or coming directly at the viewer as the degree of cranial angulation is decreased (Figure 2.8).

Specific lesions
Ventricular septal defect (Figure 2.9)

The imaging of specific ventricular defects is beyond the scope of this review, but is commented upon in detail by various authors.[5] The injections to outline the septum and the lost margins which circumscribe the defect(s) are best performed in the left ventricle using a power injector. Two orthogonal (right angle) projections will give the best chance of profiling the lesion. However, pre-catheterization, the location of the defect should be well characterized by other imaging modalities, such that the projections chosen would give the optimal profile, with little modification. Table 2.1 lists single and biplane angulations for the various projections. For the perimembranous defect the mid-cranial LAO projection, at about 50° to 60° LAO, and as much cranial tilt as the equipment and patient position will allow (Figure 2.10) should be attempted. Additional projections can include a shallow-LAO with cranial tilt (so-called four-chamber or hepatoclavicular view) to outline the basal septum or inlet extension of a perimembranous defect. The RAO view will outline the high anterior and infundibular (outlet) defects.[6]

Coarctation of the aorta (Figure 2.11)

Biplane angiography should be used to outline the arch lesion. Projections that can be used include LAO/RAO,

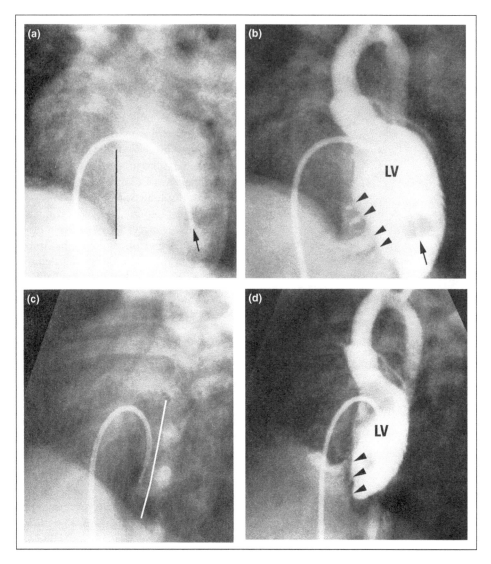

Figure 2.7
Achieving an LAO projection. (a) For a hepatoclavicular view, half of the cardiac silhouette is over or just left of the spine, with the catheter pointing toward the left of the image. (b) During the injection, the apex and catheter (arrow) will point toward the bottom and left of the image. In this example, the basal (inlet) portion of the septum is intact. Multiple mid-muscular septal defects are not well profiled (arrowheads). In (c) the LAO projection is achieved with the catheter pointing toward the bottom of the frame, and the cardiac silhouette well over the spine. During the contrast injection (d), the mid-muscular defects are now better profiled. (Modified from Culham[1] with permission.)

PA and LAT, or a shallow- or steep-LAO. Our preference is a 30° LAO and left-LAT, with 10° to 15° caudal tilt to minimize any overlapping structures, such as a ductal bump or diverticulum. Modifications to accommodate a right arch are generally mirror image projections (i.e., 30° RAO and left-LAT). The operator must be cautious to examine the transverse arch for associated hypoplasia, and this may be foreshortened in the straight left-LAT projection. In such an instance, for a left arch, a left posterior oblique projection may elongate the arch. This is particularly important if

an endovascular stent is to be implanted near the head and neck vessels.

Aortic valve angiography (Figure 2.12)

Assessment of the diameter of the aortic valve in the setting of normally related great arteries with ventricular arterial concordance for balloon dilation is best performed using biplane in the long axis and RAO projections (Table 2.1).

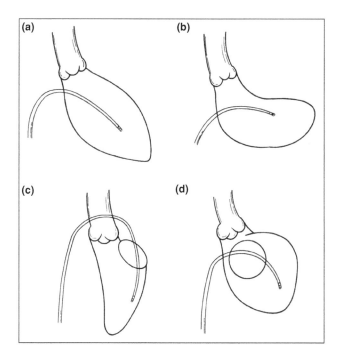

Figure 2.8
Obtaining the cranial tilt. In the standard RAO view, (a), the left ventricular apex points caudally and to the left. The LAO view will open the outflow from apex to base, as in diagram (c). If there is an upturned apex, as in Fallot's tetralogy, the RAO view will appear as in (b). Adding cranial tilt to a mid-LAO projection will not effectively open the apex to base projection, and the appearance will be as looking down the barrel of the ventricles, as in (d). (Modified from Culham[1] with permission.)

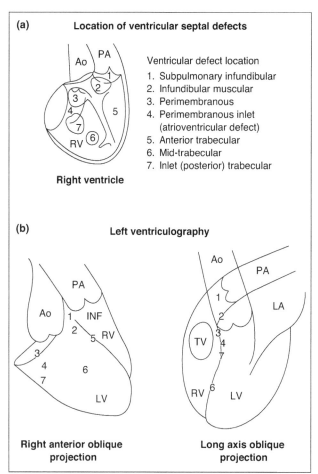

Figure 2.9
The locations of various ventricular defects are shown in panel (a) viewed from the right ventricle. In panel (b), the locations of these defects are noted as seen in an RAO or LAO projection.

Our preference is to obtain the diameter of the aortic valve from a ventriculogram, which profiles the hinge points of the leaflets. Caution must be observed when using an ascending aortogram, as one of the leaflets of the valve may obscure the margins of attachment.

The Mustard baffle (Figure 2.13)

Children who have had a Mustard operation may, over time, develop obstruction to one or both limbs of the venous baffle. As atrial arrhythmias are not uncommon in this population, particularly as adults, pacing systems are frequently required for management. In this regard, enlargement of a stenotic, although at times asymptomatic, superior baffle is frequently required. The optimum projection to outline superior baffle obstruction, for potential stent implantation, is a cranial angulated LAO projection (30° LAO and 30° cranial). This view will elongate the baffle pathway allowing accurate measurement prior to stenting. For inferior baffle lesions, a frontal projection will allow adequate localization of the lesion. Leaks along the baffle are more problematic, and require modification of the

projection. The initial approach should be a PA projection, with modifications in angulation made thereafter to best profile the lesion for device implantation, not too dissimilar to that of Fontan fenestration closure.

The secundum atrial septal defect and the fenestrated Fontan (Figures 2.14 and 2.15)

Secundum atrial septal defects are best profiled in the 30° LAO with 30° cranial tilt. With the injection made in the right upper pulmonary vein, the sinus venous portion of the septum can be visualized, and anomalous pulmonary venous return ruled out. Additionally, any associated septal aneurysm can be outlined. With the application of transesophageal or intracardiac echocardiography, there is less fluoroscopic reliance on device positioning. When

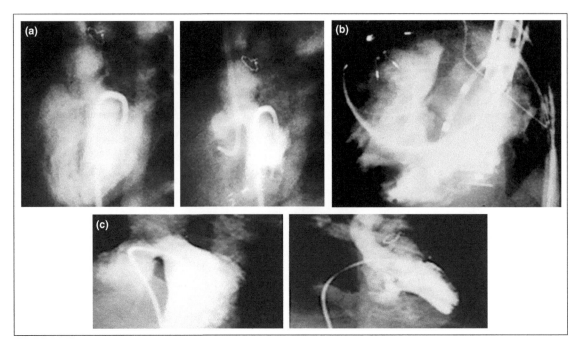

Figure 2.10
Panel (a) shows a left ventriculogram taken in the cranial-LAO projection. Note the apical, mid-muscular, and perimembranous septal defects. In panel (b), a modified hepatoclavicular view profiles a mid-muscular defect. Panel (c), left pane, is a left ventriculogram taken in the cranial-LAO view, with the catheter entering the ventricle through a perimembranous defect. Right pane, taken in the hepatoclavicular view with the catheter through the mitral valve, defines an inlet muscular defect, in a child with a pulmonary artery band.

balloon sizing is performed, this projection will elongate the axis of the balloon, for proper measurements.

The interventional management of the child with a fenestrated Fontan, whether a lateral tunnel or extracardiac connection, generally requires selective studies of the superior and inferior caval vein and pulmonary circulations, to determine the presence or absence of obstructive or hypoplastic pathways, and whether venous collaterals have developed. As such, they must be addressed by angioplasty, stenting, or embolization techniques before consideration of fenestration closure. Venous collaterals after an extracardiac Fontan will generally develop either from the innominate vein or from the right upper hepatic/phrenic vein, toward the neo-left atrium, less frequently from the right hepatic veins to the pulmonary veins. The optimum way to outline these lesions is in the AP and LAT projections, with selective power injections in the appropriate vessel. The location and dimensions of the fenestration may also be defined in these views, but for ideal profiling some degree of right or left anterior obliquity may be required.

The bidirectional cavopulmonary connection (Figure 2.16)

Second stage palliation for a number of congenital defects consists of a bidirectional cavopulmonary connection (aka,

the bidirectional Glenn anastomosis). Because the caval to pulmonary artery connection is toward the anterior surface of the right pulmonary artery (rather than on the upper surface), an AP projection will result in overlapping of the anastomotic site with the pulmonary artery. Therefore, to determine whether the anastomosis is obstructed, a 30° caudal with 10° LAO projection will generally open that region for better definition. Furthermore, this projection will outline the full extent of the right and left pulmonary arteries. The left-LAT projection with or without 10° caudal angulation will profile the anastomosis for its anterior–posterior dimension. Contrast injection must be made in the lower portion of the superior caval vein. Examination of venous collaterals can be performed from the AP and LAT projections in the innominate vein.

Pulmonary valve stenosis, Fallot's tetralogy, and pulmonary valve atresia with intact ventricular septum (Figures 2.17 and 2.18)

Percutaneous intervention on isolated pulmonary valve stenosis was the procedure which assured in the present era of catheter based therapies. While angiographic definition of the right ventricular outflow tract and valve is not

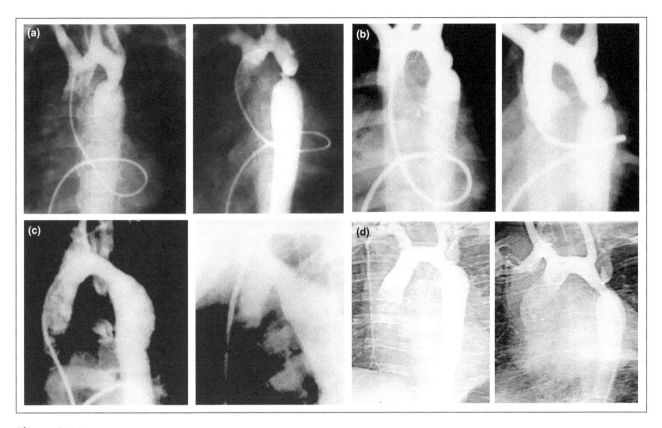

Figure 2.11

Panel (a), left pane, shows an ascending aortogram taken with a shallow-LAO projection without caudal angulation. The catheter was placed through a transeptal entry to the left heart. While the area of the coarctation can be seen, it is the caudal angulation which identifies the details of the lesion, including a small ductal ampulla, right pane. In panel (b), similar information is obtained, by employing caudal angulation to the frontal detector, right pane, while in the shallow-LAO projection in contrast to that information obtained without caudal angulation, left pane. In panel (c), left pane, hypoplasia of the transverse arch can be identified. However, in contrast, in the right pane, the degree of foreshortening is obvious. Panel (d), right pane, shows the standard LAO projection of an ascending aortogram. In this case there is overlap of the area of obstruction, transverse arch hypoplasia, and stenosis of the left subclavian artery, not defined until cranial angulation is employed, right pane.

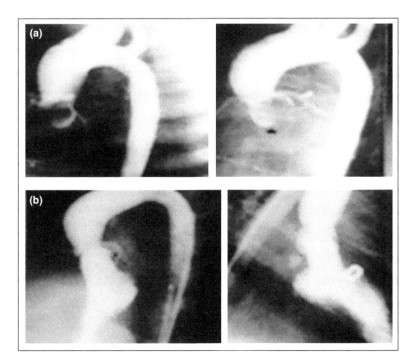

Figure 2.12

Intervention on the aortic valve requires accurate definition of the hinge points of the leaflets. In panel (a), long axis oblique views from an ascending aortogram do not define the margins of the leaflets due to overlap of the cusps (bicuspid in these examples). In panel (b), long axis oblique (left) and RAO views, the left ventriculogram allows easier identification of the leaflet hinge points, where measurements can be made.

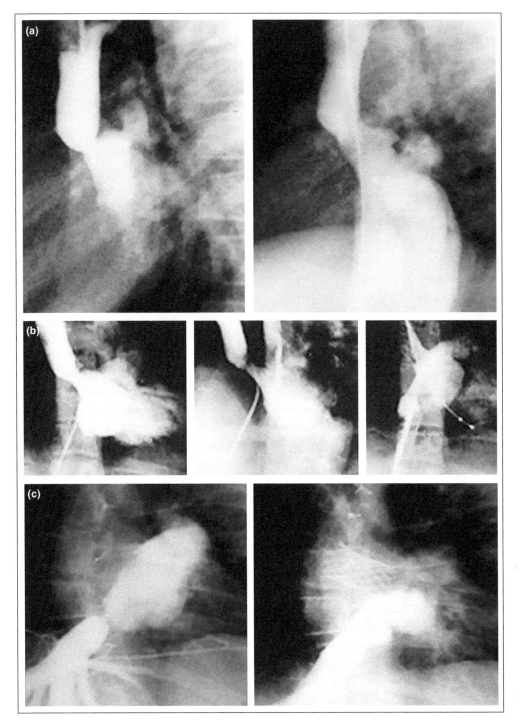

Figure 2.13
Baffle obstruction after a Mustard operation is, as the population ages, an increasingly common event. This is particularly so, with the need to manage such patients with transvenous pacing devices. In panel (a), left pane, the presence of a superior baffle obstruction can be identified from the left-LAT projection. However, only with cranial angulation (cranial-LAO view, right pane) will the full extent of the lesion be detailed. This is particularly critical, as shown in panel (b), where the frontal view, left pane, does not show the full extent of the obstruction, and only from the angulated view will the length and diameter of the lesion be outlined (middle pane). A stent is placed, followed by a transvenous pacing system, shown in the right pane from a frontal projection. For an inferior baffle lesion, the frontal (PA) projection is optimal, panel (c), before (left) and after (right) a stent is placed.

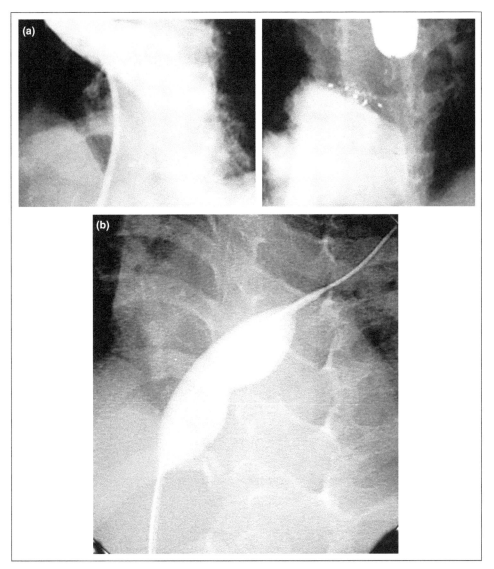

Figure 2.14

Use of angiography for septal defect definition and device placement in the setting of a secundum atrial septal defect has been supplanted by intracardiac and transesophageal techniques (panel a). However, fluoroscopy is still required for initial device localization, and in many laboratories a short cine-run records the diameter of the static balloon diameter to choose the device size. In this case, we find the 30° LAO with 30° cranial tilt best to elongate the balloon to avoid foreshortening (panel b).

complicated, several features must be kept in mind when approaching the angiography for an interventional procedure. In the case of isolated pulmonary valve stenosis, and other right ventricular outflow tract lesions, because the outflow tract can take a horizontal curve, a simple AP projection will foreshorten the structure. Therefore, a 30° cranial with 15° LAO will open up the infundibulum, and allow visualization of the valve and the main and branch pulmonary arteries. The best definition of the hinge points of the valve, to choose the correct balloon size, is from the left-LAT projection. Occasionally, 10° or 15° caudal angulation of the LAT detector can be used to separate the overlap of the branch vessels seen on a straight left-LAT projection.

However, this is not recommended, as it will also foreshorten the outflow tract and the valve will appear off plane, giving incorrect valve diameters.

Branch pulmonary artery stenosis (Figures 2.19–2.21)

Pulmonary artery interventions are most common, and represent the most difficult angiographic projections to separate out individual vessels for assessment and potential intervention. A cranially tilted frontal projection with a left-LAT or RAO/LAO projections is frequently the first

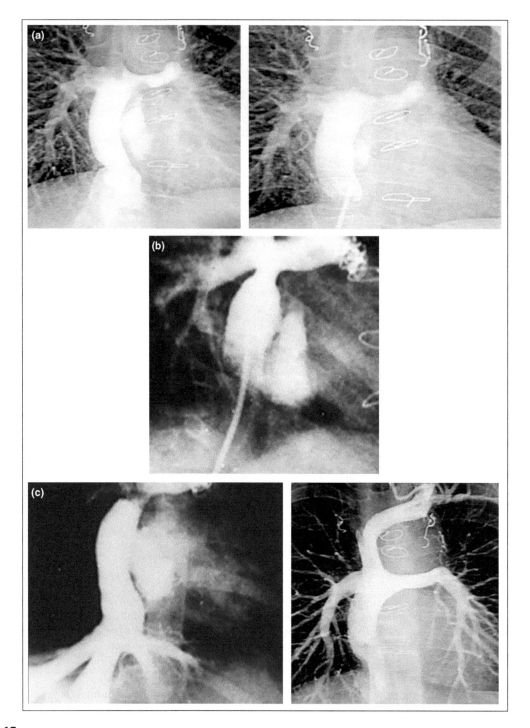

Figure 2.15

Panel (a) shows the appearance of a fenestrated extracardiac Fontan in the frontal projection, and its appearance after device closure. Generally, a frontal projection profiles the defect adequately, but at times some angulation is required, as seen in panel (b), where the defect is best profiled in a shallow-RAO view. Also note coils in the left superior caval vein which developed after the Fontan procedure and required embolization. Occasionally, collateral vessels develop from the hepatic/phrenic vein (panel c, left) or innominate vein (panel c, right), where coils have been placed. The primary view being frontal (PA) and left-LAT.

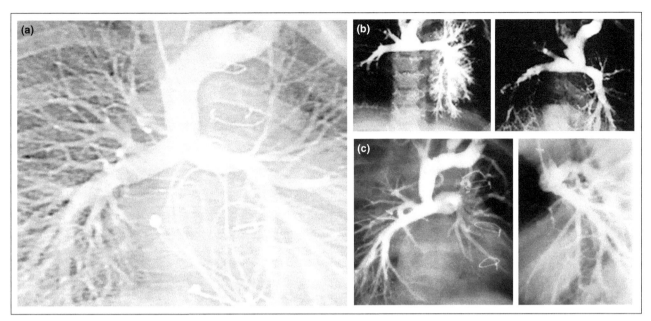

Figure 2.16

Because of an offset in the anastomosis between the superior caval vein and right pulmonary artery, the optimal view to see the anastomosis without overlap is a shallow with caudal tilt, as seen in panel (a). Panel (b), left pane, is in the frontal projection, where overlap of the anastomosis obscures a potential lesion, as seen in the angulated view, right pane. The combination of an angulated frontal detector and caudal angulation of the lateral tube will allow definition of the anastomosis (left pane) and the pulmonary artery confluence (right pane), panel (c).

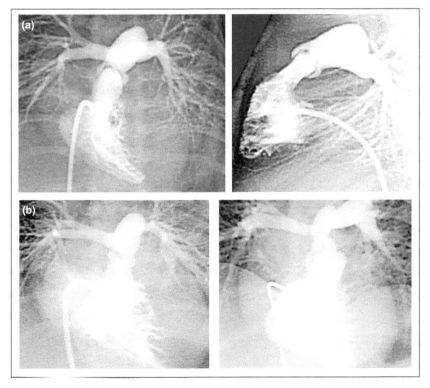

Figure 2.17

Panel (a) depicts a case of typical isolated pulmonary valve stenosis in a neonate. The outflow tract is profiled in the cranially angulated frontal projection, with a slight degree of LAO angulation (left pane). The right ventriculogram outlines the form of the ventricle, the main pulmonary artery (and ductal bump) as well as the pulmonary artery confluence, and branch dimensions. The LAT view (right pane) outlines the valve leaflets (thickened and doming) and allows accurate delineation of the valve structures for balloon diameter determination. In panel (b), two right ventriculograms in the cranially angulated slight LAO view depict the size of the annulus and main and branch pulmonary arteries (typical valve stenosis with left pulmonary hypoplasia, left pane; dysplastic valve stenosis, small non-dilated main pulmonary artery and proximal left branch pulmonary artery stenosis with post-stenotic dilation, right pane).

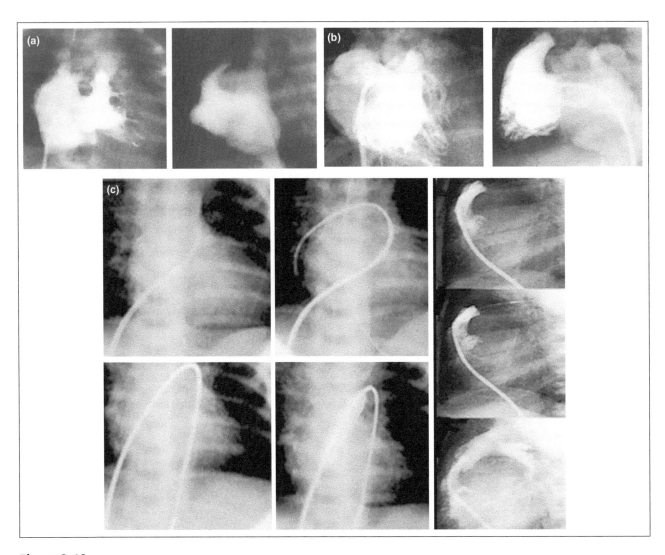

Figure 2.18

Angiographic projections for intervention in pulmonary atresia with intact septum are similar to that of isolated pulmonary valve stenosis. In panels (a) and (b), cranial angulation is critical to image the valve plate (left panes), while a left-LAT will suffice for imaging the anterior–posterior aspects of the outflow tract. In valve perforation, it is critical to have visual control in 2 orthogonal planes, to avoid inadvertent infundibular perforation. A series of images during valve perforation is seen in panel (c). The left upper pane shows the catheter position; right upper pane, perforation and wire in the right pulmonary artery; left lower pane, the wire guide across the duct for stability; and in the right lower pane, balloon dilation of the valve. In the accompanying panel, viewed from the left-LAT projection, is a series of images taken during perforation: top pane, position confirmation; middle pane, radiofrequency perforation; lower pane, angiography in the main pulmonary artery.

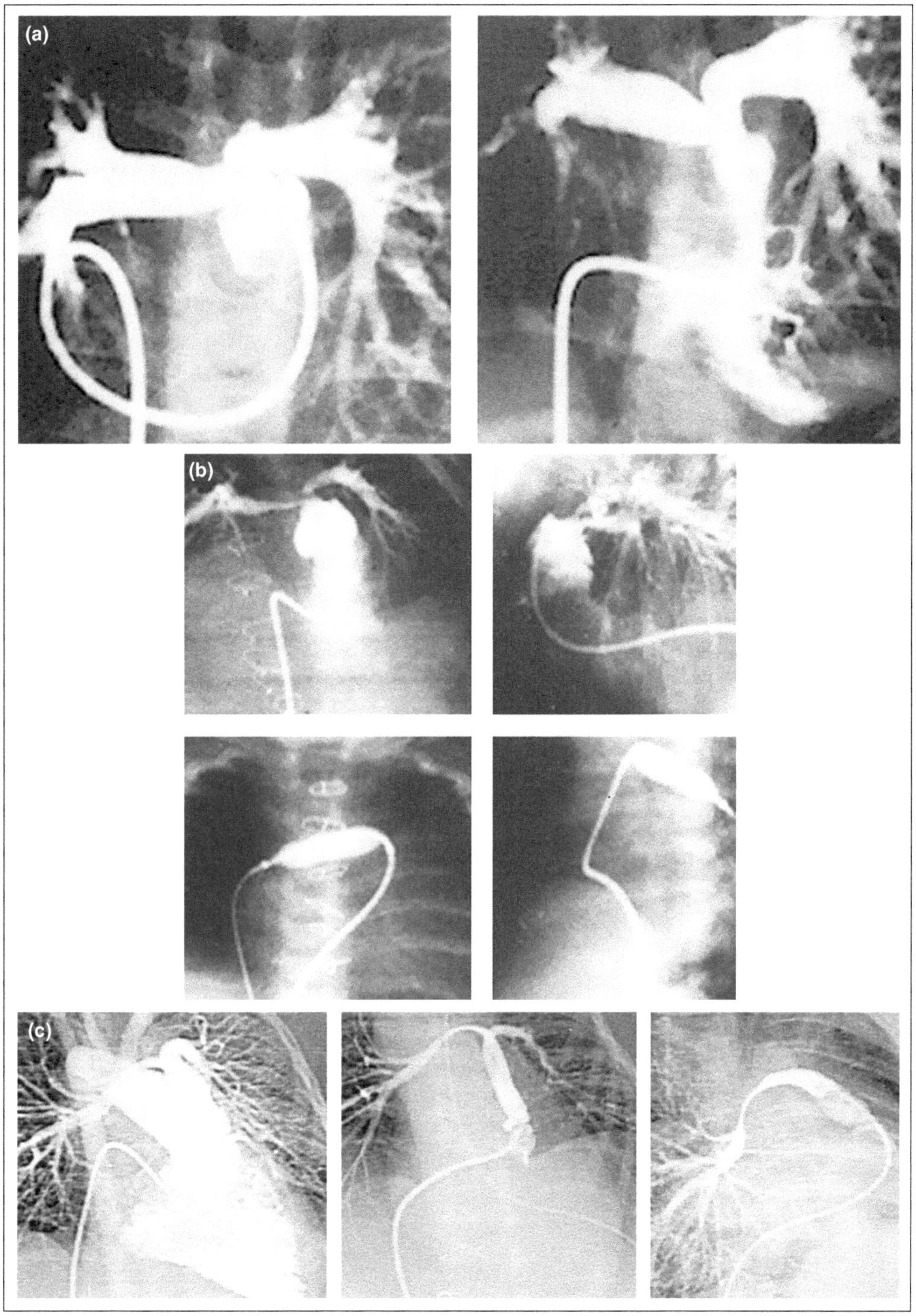

Figure 2.19
Angiography for selective intervention on the branch pulmonary arteries can be most difficult due to overlapping of structures. No single projection is totally representative and frequently multiple views are required. In panel (a), left pane, a scout film is taken in the main pulmonary artery, and in the right pane, the right ventricle. Both images are taken in the cranial-LAO projection and, in these examples, clearly outline the outflow tracts and branch confluences. In panel (b) the dilated main pulmonary artery would have obscured the branch pulmonary artery confluence, and this cranial-LAO (left upper pane) and caudal left-LAT (right upper pane) nicely details the anatomy for subsequent intervention (lower panes). In panel (c), ventriculography obscures the details of the crossed pulmonary vessels (left pane), while selective injection in the cranial (middle pane) and RAO (right pane) projections details the anatomy.

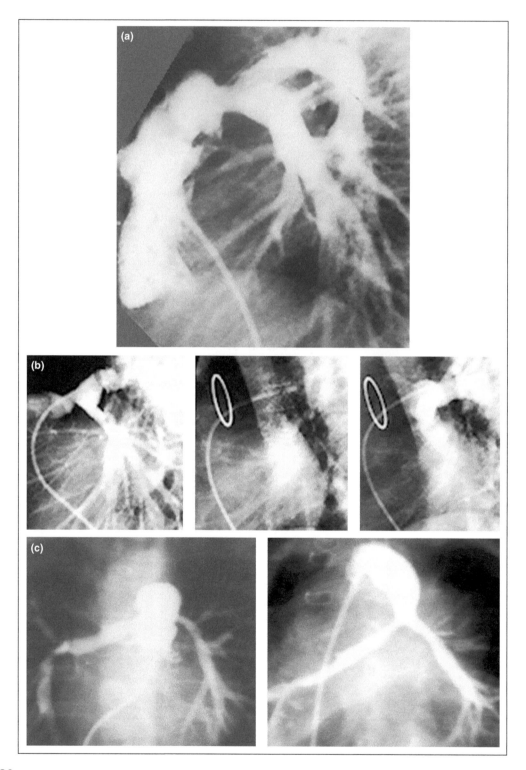

Figure 2.20
In panel (a), the image is taken from a left-LAT projection with caudal tilt. This will separate the proximal right and left pulmonary artery branches, and detail the main pulmonary artery. The outflow tract is foreshortened, and this view will mislead the operator when examining the diameter of the valve, and infundibulum. If such detail is required, a straight left-LAT should be performed. In the caudal-LAT projection, the left pulmonary branch will sweep superiorly and towards the upper right corner of the image, while the left pulmonary artery will appear more medial and in the center of the image. In panel (b) the child had severe bilateral branch stenosis (left pane), which persisted after surgical repair and valve insertion. Using the left-LAT view, stents could be placed in each branch (middle and right panes). In panel (c), severe main pulmonary artery dilation has obscured the confluence and very hypoplastic pulmonary arteries (left pane) in this child shortly after surgery. In this case, steep caudal angulation of the frontal tube with 10° or 15° LAO has detailed the lesion for the intervention (right pane).

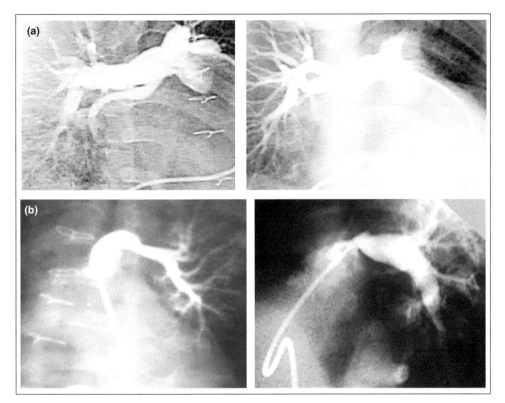

Figure 2.21
Selective injection into a branch pulmonary vessel will give the best detailed image. Overlap of the intrahilar branching vessels, however, will interfere with interpretation of the lesion as seen in panel (a), left pane, taken in the RAO projection. By adding caudal tilt, as in this example, the tortuous path of the intrahilar vessel can be seen. In panel (b) (left and right panes), cranial-LAO projections detail the length of the left pulmonary artery and proximal areas of potential stenosis.

series of views that can be performed, as scout studies to map the proximal and hilar regions of the pulmonary circulation. The injection may be performed in either the ventricle or main pulmonary artery. Since there is frequent overlap as seen in viewing the right ventricular outflow tract (see above), these standard views can be modified by increasing or decreasing the degree of RAO or LAO, and adding caudal or cranial tilt. Selective branch artery injections are best for detailed visualization, to plan the intervention. For the right pulmonary artery, a shallow-RAO projection with 10° or 15° cranial tilt will separate the upper and middle lobe branches, while a left-LAT with 15° caudal tilt will open up all the anterior vessels. Similarly, to maximize the elongated and posterior leftward directed left pulmonary artery, a 60° LAO with 20° cranial is very effective, with a caudal tilt on the lateral detector. Occasionally, in small babies after surgical reconstruction of the branch pulmonary arteries, the main pulmonary artery is aneurysmal and obscures the confluence. In this case, a steep 30° caudal projection with the frontal detector with 10° to 20° RAO will open up the bifurcation.

Summary

This short introduction to interventional angiography will allow the reader a point of departure to visualize the most

common lesions. However, many cases occur that do not fall into a standard categorization and the operator must be prepared to alter the imaging projection to optimally define the lesion. Successful outcomes require patience, perseverance, and the learned experience of others.

References

1. Culham JAG. Physical principles of image formation and projections in angiocardiography. In: Freedom RM, Mawson JB, Yoo SJ, Benson LN, eds. Congenital Heart Disease Textbook of Angiocardiography. Armonk: Futura Publishing, 1997: 39–93.
2. Freedom RM, Culham JAG, Moes CAF. Angiocardiography of Congenital Heart Disease. New York: Macmillan, 1984: 7–16.
3. Beekman RH 3rd, Hellenbrand WE, Lloyd TR et al. ACCF/AHA/AAP recommendations for training in pediatric cardiology. Task force 3: training guidelines for pediatric cardiac catheterization and interventional cardiology endorsed by the Society for Cardiovascular Angiography and Interventions. J Am Coll Cardiol 2005; 46(7): 1388–90.
4. Qureshi SA, Redington AN, Wren C et al. Recommendations of the British Paediatric Cardiac Association for therapeutic cardiac catheterisation in congenital cardiac disease. Cardiol Young 2000; 10(6): 649–67.
5. Ventricular septal defect. In: Freedom RM, Mawson JB, Yoo SJ, Benson LN, eds. Congenital Heart Disease Textbook of Angiocardiography. Armonk: Futura Publishing, 1997: 189–218.
6. Brandt PW. Axially angled angiocardiography. Cardiovasc Intervent Radiol 1984; 7(3–4):166–9.

3

Transesophageal echocardiographic guidance of transcatheter closure of atrial septal defects

Charles S Kleinman

During the past several years the cardiac catheterization laboratory has evolved from a primarily diagnostic venue into a setting in which cardiac therapy is provided to patients with a large variety of congenital cardiac malformations. To some extent, the decreased number of diagnostic procedures is related to the availability of alternate means of assessing cardiac anatomy and physiology, including echocardiography and magnetic resonance imaging. Echocardiography has also evolved as a technique for providing an imaging modality that is, at once, complementary to angiography and fluoroscopic imaging, while providing unique imaging that allows radiolucent structures such as the atrial and ventricular septum and intracardiac valves to be imaged. Such images may be critical for the assessment of the candidacy of patients who are referred for transcatheter treatment of atrial or ventricular septal defects, and may also be used to monitor the placement of devices for the closure of these defects.

In the late 1980s the introduction of the Rashkind atrial septal defect closure device offered the potential for a relatively non-invasive option for the closure of ostium secundum atrial septal defects. It was immediately recognized, however, that the effort to replace a relatively safe and well established surgical procedure with a new, and untried, transcatheter therapy would only be acceptable if the attendant risks could be minimized.

That device consisted of multiple wire 'legs' with fish-hook-like ends for anchoring on the atrial septum, at the rim of the defect. The fish-hooks made placement of the device a harrowing experience, and made dislodgement of the devices an unacceptable risk. For this reason, we argued that visualization of the size and position of the defect within the atrial septum, and assurance of appropriate placement within the atrial septum, with adequate clearance from neighboring structures such as the atrioventricular valves or pulmonary venous entry, would be advisable.[1] In the years since, transesophageal (TEE) and intracardiac echocardiography (ICE) have evolved as essential components of the interventional catheterization protocol for the guidance of transcatheter closure of atrial septal defect.[1–27]

The purpose of this chapter is to discuss the echocardiographic findings that identify patients who are candidates for transcatheter closure of an atrial septal defect. The anatomic features of an atrial septal defect that is 'closable' by device and the use of TEE for the guidance of these procedures will be described.

The potential availability of a 'less invasive' means of defect closure than open heart surgery might well tempt referring physicians to relax the criteria for referral of patients for defect closure. Nonetheless, the criteria for referral for transcatheter closure of atrial septal defect should include whether the patient would otherwise have been referred for surgical closure. This includes the detection of physical findings suggestive of right heart volume overload, including a right ventricular impulse at the lower left sternal border, and murmurs consistent with relative pulmonary and tricuspid stenosis. Symptoms are almost never a characteristic of atrial septal defect during early childhood, and almost always are reserved for patients in the 40+ age group. In infancy, atrial septal defect may complicate the management of patients with chronic pulmonary insufficiency, including bronchopulmonary dysplasia. Echocardiographic findings that characterize a 'significant' atrial septal defect include right atrial and right ventricular dilation, and secondary to left-to-right atrial shunting. In addition, the motion of the ventricular septum is often paradoxical. The latter is secondary to contraction of the ventricular muscle mass toward the center of mass. The latter may be displaced toward the left ventricular side of the septum in cases of significant right ventricular volume overload. In such cases the ventricular septum may move toward the right ventricular free wall during systolic contraction.

Two-dimensional echocardiography may be used to visualize the position of the atrial defect within the atrial septum. The characteristics of an atrial septal defect that is potentially 'closable' by device include an ostium secundum defect, in the position delineated by the fetal fossa ovalis. The 'closable' defect characteristically has an adequate rim to separate the defect from the orifice of the right upper pulmonary vein in the left atrium, the posterior wall of the atrial septum, the orifices of the superior and inferior vena cava in the right atrium, the atrioventricular valves, and the retroaortic rim, behind the aortic root.[28]

Typically, the rims of the atrial septal defect may be evaluated from subxiphoidal and transthoracic imaging windows, or through the use of multiplane transesophageal imaging. Intracardiac echocardiography may provide imaging of the atrial defect, and may allow individual rims to be examined. The ICE approach may be particularly effective for imaging of the posteroinferior rim of the ostium secundum atrial septal defect, near the insertion of the inferior vena cava to the right atrium. Transesophageal echocardiography provides a more extensive anatomic image of the atrial septum than does intracardiac echocardiography.[11,29–33]

Anatomic characteristics

The ostium secundum atrial septal defect represents a persistently patent defect at the site of the fetal fossa ovalis.[34–38] This is anatomically distinct from the superior or inferior sinus venosus defect. The latter represent defects of the venae cavae. The superior sinus venosus defect is commonly associated with partial anomalous drainage of the right upper pulmonary vein, which usually enters the superior vena cava. Defects of the coronary sinus usually involve partial unroofing of the coronary sinus, with potential right-to-left shunting at this level, with persistent drainage of the left superior vena cava to the coronary sinus. Ostium primum atrial septal defects are a form of atrioventricular septal defect, with the defect at the lower aspect of the atrial septum, immediately above the ventricular septum. These defects characteristically are associated with abnormalities of the atrioventricular valves, including a cleft of the septal leaflet of the mitral valve (Figure 3.1).[34–36]

The remainder of this chapter will focus on the characteristics of the fossa ovalis and ostium secundum atrial septal defect that render such defects candidates for transcatheter occlusion. It should be noted, for example, that the superior rim of the fossa ovalis represents an infolding of the junction between the superior vena cava and the right

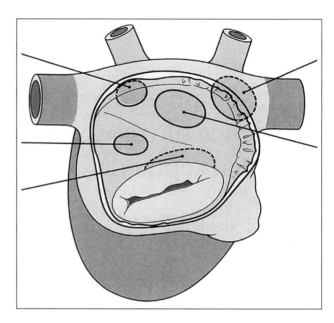

Figure 3.1
Schematic diagram of the right atrial aspect of the atrial septum, with the locations of various forms of atrial septal defect demonstrated. Ostium secundum defects, at the site of the fetal foramen ovale, are the only defects that are considered potentially 'closable' using currently available devices (SSV, superior sinus venosus; ISV, inferior sinus venosus; CS, coronary sinus; ostium 1°, ostium primum; ostium 2°, ostium secundum). Note the proximity of the inferior and superior sinus venosus defects to the respective vena caval insertions to the right atrium. The superior sinus venosus defect is virtually always associated with partially anomalous drainage of the right pulmonary vein. The coronary sinus defect is associated with the entry of the coronary sinus to the right atrium, and is almost always associated with persistent drainage of a left superior vena cava, and some degree of coronary sinus unroofing. The ostium primum defect is at the central fibrous body, with close proximity to both atrioventricular valves. (Reproduced from Anderson et al[34] with permission.)

upper pulmonary vein, rather than a true 'secondary septum' (Figure 3.2). This infolding abuts the aortic root (Figure 3.3 and Figure 3.4).

Characterizing a defect 'closable' by device

The characteristics of a defect defined as 'closable' by device have evolved with increasing experience and with alterations in device design. Using the 'Clamshell' or 'Star-Flex' devices, which consist of two sets of articulated wire arms, with Dacron patches, connected by a central wire 'post,' small to moderate defects, in a central position within the atrial septum, could be closed. Devices were chosen that

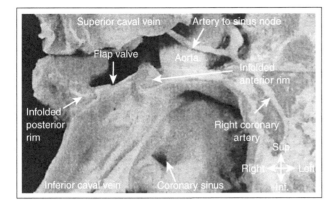

Figure 3.2
Development of the atrial septum includes an infolding of the atrial roof, at the superior aspect of the atrial septum. This area, near the aortic root, does not represent true septal formation, and results in a potential space between the superior and anterosuperior aspect of the atrium and the aorta. (Reproduced from Anderson et al[29] with permission.)

were twice the diameter of the defects to be closed. This two-to-one ratio of diameters imposed limitations on the size of the defects that could be closed. Such devices are not 'self centering,' within the atrial defects. The devices closed the defects through apposition of the two sets of wire arms to the opposing sides of the septal rims of the defects. Thus, it was initially thought that only secundum defects of less than 20 mm diameter would be closable by devices. It has subsequently been accepted that, with the use of devices that close defects through the use of a central 'stent' with apposing disks, defects approaching 40 mm in diameter and those with rim deficiencies in the retroaortic (anterosuperior rim) area could also be closed.

The latter design, introduced by AGA Medical Corporation as the Amplatzer Atrial Septal Occluder® (ASO), includes a central stent within the atrial septal defect. The disks on either side of the central occluder anchor the device in place. The 'size' of the device is defined as the central stent diameter, in mm. The disks on either side extend 6–8 mm beyond the margins of the central occluding stents.

The rims of septum surrounding the ostium secundum atrial septal defect are defined as superoposterior (superior vena caval), inferoposterior (inferior vena caval), inferior (atrioventricular valve), posterior, and anterosuperior (retroaortic).[39]

Transesophageal imaging of atrial septal defect

Utilizing the multiplane TEE probe, ostium secundum (Figure 3.5) defects may be characterized[10] Figueroa et al

(Table 3.1) have defined the angulation required to visualize the rims surrounding these defects. Multiplane imaging has been defined as important, predominantly for providing adequate imaging of the anterosuperior (retroaortic) rim of the defect, with a median TEE angle of 34°, with a range from 0° to 98°.

The anatomic characteristics of the ostium secundum atrial septal defect have been defined by Podnar and associates, who examined 190 consecutive patients who presented for consideration for transcatheter treatment (Table 3.2).[39]

Centrally placed defects, without rim deficiency, represented only 24.2% (46) of these patients, whereas 42.1% (80) had deficiency of the retroaortic (superoanterior) rim. Most centers do not consider retroaortic rim deficiency to represent an absolute contraindication to device placement. Deficient inferoposterior (inferior vena caval) (10%), inferoposterior and posterior (2.1%), inferoanterior (1%), and coronary sinus (1%) rim would be considered by many centers to be contraindications to device placement.

Transesophageal echocardiographic monitoring of atrial defect closure

Recently, reports have focused attention on the potential for late erosion of the atrial septal wall, following transcatheter closure of atrial septal defect.[41] These erosions have occurred at varying intervals, ranging from hours to 3 years, following device placement, and have been associated with varying degrees of hemodynamic embarrassment, ranging from aorto-atrial fistulas to hemopericardium with acute tamponade and death.[42] The incidence of these late complications appears to be in the range of 0.1%. After a careful review of the reported cases of late atrial erosion with the Amplatzer ASO, a review board concluded that the region most 'at risk' for late erosion is the retroaortic rim, where erosion may occur into the region representing the fold in the roof of the atrium, that is interposed between the superior vena cava and right superior pulmonary vein, and the aortic root. It was determined, however, that while anterosuperior rim insufficiency may be necessary for such erosions to occur it is not, in and of itself, sufficient to account for them. It appears that a necessary component is oversizing of the device used for defect occlusion. Such oversizing appears to have become a frequent occurrence following general availability of the Amplatzer ASO, probably relating to the desire of operators to avoid the potential for device embolization, and initial ignorance of the risk for late erosion.[41] The review board has, therefore, re-emphasized the importance of TEE monitoring of device placement. TEE is used to locate the defect and to evaluate the sufficiency of the inferoposterior, inferior, and superoposterior

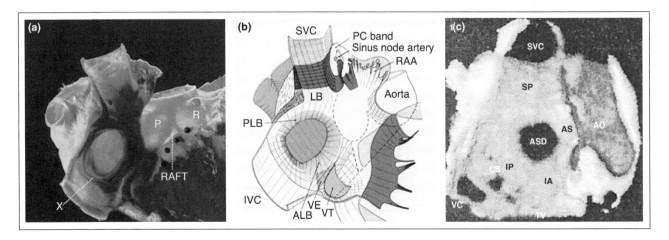

Figure 3.3

Transilluminated, waxed specimen, demonstrating right atrial aspect of the atrial septum, with three-dimensional rendering of same (a,b). Note the relationship between the region of the foramen ovale (X) and the aortic posterior sinus of Valsalva. CS, coronary sinus; IVC, inferior vena cara; LV, left ventricle; MS, membranous septum; P, posterior sinus of Valsalva; PT, pulmonary trunk; R, right sinus of Valsalva; RIPV, right inferior pulmonary vein; RPA, right pulmonary artery; RSPV, right superior pulmonary vein; RV, right ventricle; TS, transverse sinus; Valvula F ovalis, Valvula fossa ovalis. (Reproduced from McAlpine[23] with permission.) Part (c) is a reference figure for comparison with the three-dimensional echocardiographic reconstruction of the atrial septum, to the right. Note the position of the atrial septal defect (ASD), and the relationship to the superior vena cava (SVC), the inferior vena cava (IVC), the coronary sinus (CS), and the aortic root (AO). The superior vena caval rim of the ASD is also referred to as superoposterior (SP), the inferior vena cava rim of the ASD is also referred to as inferoposterior (IP). The atrioventricular valve rim of the defect, near the tricuspid valve (TV), is also referred to as the inferoanterior (IA) rim, whereas the retroaortic rim of the defect is also referred to as the posteroanterior (PA) rim of the defect.

Table 3.1 *Multiplane TEE – imaging angle and structures seen (Reproduced from[34] with kind permission of Springer Science and Business Media.)*

	TEE angle	
Rim	Median (°)	Range (°)
Superior vena cava	92	78–126
Inferior vena cava	90	51–126
Tricuspid valve	0	0–60
Mitral valve	0	0–18
Right upper pulmonary vein	0	0–69
Posteroinferior rim	90	0–120
Anterior (aortic) rim	34	0–98

Table 3.2 *Atrial septal defect morphology in 190 consecutive patients*

Morphology	Number (%) patients
Centrally placed defect	46 (24.2)
Deficient superior anterior rim	80 (42.1)
Deficient inferior posterior rim	19 (10.0)
Perforated septal aneurysm	15 (7.9)
Multiple defects	14 (7.3)
Deficient IA and SA rim	6 (3.1)
Deficient IP and posterior rim	4 (2.1)
Deficient inferior anterior rim	2 (1.0)
Deficient superior posterior rim	2 (1.0)
Deficient coronary sinus rim	2 (1.0)
Total	190 (100)

Source: Podnar et al.[39]

defect rims. Retroaortic (anterosuperior) rim insufficiency is noted, but is not considered a contraindication to device placement. Multiplane two-dimensional echocardiography is used to estimate the largest defect diameter. TEE imaging is used to monitor placement of the delivery sheath across the defect, and to evaluate the balloon sizing of the defect, using gradual inflation of a flexible sizing balloon. The echocardiogram is used to determine the point of 'stop-flow' across the atrial septal defect. The image intensifier is used to measure the balloon diameter at the point of 'stop-flow', and this is compared with the TEE measurement of the balloon diameter at this point. If the 'stop-flow' diameter exceeds the estimated largest defect diameter on

TEE a careful re-evaluation is suggested, prior to device placement.[12,17,43–45] TEE is then used to monitor the deployment of the septal occluder, documenting the placement of the left disk within the left atrium, the stent within the atrial septum, and the right sided disk on the right side of the atrial septum. TEE is used to document complete occlusion of the defect, both prior to and following release of the device from the delivery cable. TEE is used to evaluate the presence of pericardial effusion, both prior to and

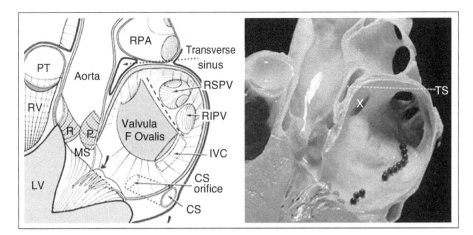

Figure 3.4
Transilluminated, waxed specimen, demonstrating left atrial aspect of the atrial septum, with three-dimensional rendering of same. Note the relationship between the foramen ovale (X) and the aortic root, the right superior pulmonary vein (RSPV), and the transverse sinus (TS).

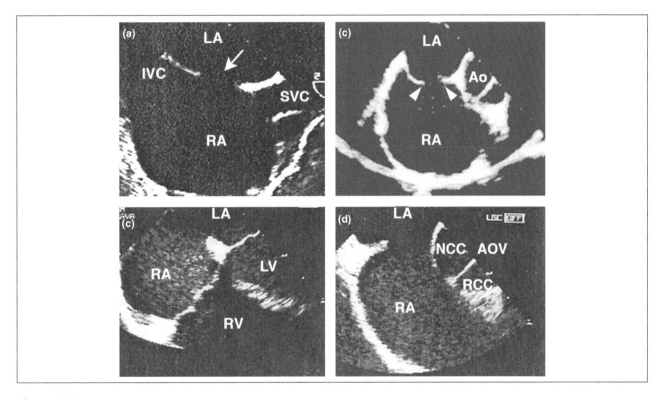

Figure 3.5
Four panels demonstrating transesophageal images of ostium secundum defects from differing vantage points. Upper left panel demonstrates centrally placed ostium secundum defect (arrow), with superior and inferior vena caval (SVC, IVC) entry points visualized. There is adequate rim at both locations. Upper right panel demonstrates atrial defect (between arrowheads). Note aortic root (Ao) in the right aspect of the figure, with adequate retroaortic rim. Lower left panel demonstrates adequate inferoanterior defect rim, near the atrioventricular valves. Lower right panel shows a large atrial defect, virtually abutting the non-coronary cusp (NCC) of the aortic valve, in a patient with a deficient (absent) retroaortic (anterosuperior) rim. (Reproduced from Du et al[17].)

following the occlusion procedure, with close follow-up recommended when a new or enlarging pericardial effusion is identified. TEE is also used to determine that the atrial septal occluder is not interfering with flow from the right superior pulmonary vein, or with the normal function of the atrioventricular valves.

Summary

In summary, transesophageal imaging provides images that are both unique and complementary to the fluoroscopic and angiographic images obtained during diagnostic and interventional catheterization procedures. By providing visualization of the soft tissue of the atrial septum, TEE affords the opportunity to assess the candidacy of specific defects for device closure. Visualization of defect rims and the relationship of the defect(s) to important surrounding structures is afforded by this technique, which adds to the safety and efficacy of device closure for atrial septal defects in the catheterization laboratory.

References

1. Hellenbrand WE et al. Transesophageal echocardiographic guidance of transcatheter closure of atrial septal defect. Am J Cardiol 1990; 66(2): 207–13.

2. Abdel-Massih T et al. Assessment of atrial septal defect size with 3D-transesophageal echocardiography: comparison with balloon method. Echocardiography 2005; 22(2): 121–7.

3. Acar P et al. Influence of atrial septal defect anatomy in patient selection and assessment of closure with the Cardioseal device; a three-dimensional transoesophageal echocardiographic reconstruction. Eur Heart J 2000; 21(7): 573–81.

4. Aeschbacher BC, Chatterjee T, Meier B. Transesophageal echocardiography to evaluate success of transcatheter closure of large secundum atrial septal defects in adults using the buttoned device. Mayo Clin Proc 2000; 75(9): 913–20.

5. Bartel T et al. Intracardiac echocardiography is superior to conventional monitoring for guiding device closure of interatrial communications. Circulation 2003; 107(6): 795–7.

6. Beitzke A et al. [Interventional occlusion of foramen ovale and atrial septal defects after paradoxical embolism incidents.] Z Kardiol 2002; 91(9): 693–700.

7. Bennhagen RG, McLaughlin P, Benson LN. Contemporary management of children with atrial septal defects: a focus on transcatheter closure. Am J Cardiovasc Drugs 2001; 1(6): 445–54.

8. Berger F et al. [Interventional occlusion of atrial septum defects larger than 20 mm in diameter.] Z Kardiol 2000; 89(12): 1119–25.

9. Bilgic A et al. Transcatheter closure of secundum atrial septal defects, a ventricular septal defect, and a patent arterial duct. Turk J Pediatr 2001; 43(1): 12–18.

10. Butera G et al. CardioSEAL/STARflex versus Amplatzer devices for percutaneous closure of small to moderate (up to 18 mm) atrial septal defects. Am Heart J 2004; 148(3): 507–10.

11. Cao QL et al. Initial clinical experience with intracardiac echocardiography in guiding transcatheter closure of perimembranous ventricular septal defects: feasibility and comparison with transesophageal echocardiography. Cathet Cardiovasc Interven 2005; 66(2): 258–67.

12. Carcagni A, Presbitero P. New echocardiographic diameter for Amplatzer sizing in adult patients with secundum atrial septal defect: preliminary results. Cathet Cardiovasc Interven 2004; 62(3): 409–14.

13. Carminati M et al. Transcatheter closure of atrial septal defects with the STARFlex device: early results and follow-up. J Interven Cardiol 2001; 14(3): 319–24.

14. Celiker A et al. Transcatheter closure of interatrial communications with Amplatzer device: results, unfulfilled attempts and special considerations in children and adolescents. Anadolu Kardiyol Derg 2005; 5(3): 159–64.

15. Deng DA et al. [Transcatheter closure of atrial septal defects in 40 pediatric patients.] Zhonghua Er Ke Za Zhi 2003; 41(7): 531–3.

16. Di Bernardo S et al. [Treatment of congential heart disease with interventional catheterization.] Rev Med Suisse 2005; 1(31): 2049–50, 2053–5.

17. Du ZD et al. Choice of device size and results of transcatheter closure of atrial septal defect using the Amplatzer septal occluder. J Interven Cardiol 2002; 15(4): 287–92.

18. Lin SM et al. Supplementing transesophageal echocardiography with transthoracic echocardiography for monitoring transcatheter closure of atrial septal defects with attenuated anterior rim: a case series. Anesth Analg 2003; 96(6): 1584–8.

19. Lock JE et al. Transcatheter closure of atrial septal defects. Experimental studies. Circulation 1989; 79(5): 1091–9.

20. Masura J et al. Transcatheter closure of secundum atrial septal defects using the new self-centering Amplatzer septal occluder: initial human experience. Cathet Cardiovasc Diagn 1997; 42(4): 388–93.

21. Durongpisitkul K et al. Intermediate term follow-up on transcatheter closure of atrial septal defects by Amplatzer septal occluder. J Med Assoc Thai 2000; 83(9): 1045–53.

22. Mazic U, Gavora P, Masura J. The role of transesophageal echocardiography in transcatheter closure of secundum atrial septal defects by the Amplatzer septal occluder. Am Heart J 2001; 142(3): 482–8.

23. McAlpine WA. Heart and Coronary Arteries. New York: Springer-Verlag, 1975: 63, 99.

24. Faella HJ et al. ASD closure with the Amplatzer device. J Interven Cardiol 2003; 16(5): 393–7.

25. Mullen MJ et al. Intracardiac echocardiography guided device closure of atrial septal defects. J Am Coll Cardiol 2003; 41(2): 285–92.

26. Pedra CA et al. Initial experience in Brazil with the Helex septal occluder for percutaneous occlusion of atrial septal defects. Arq Bras Cardiol 2003; 81(5): 435–52.

27. Pedra CA et al. Transcatheter closure of secundum atrial septal defects with complex anatomy. J Invas Cardiol 2004; 16(3): 117–22.

28. Du ZD et al. Comparison of transcatheter closure of secundum atrial septal defect using the Amplatzer septal occluder associated with deficient versus sufficient rims. Am J Cardiol 2002; 90(8): 865–9.

29. Fischer G et al. Experience with transcatheter closure of secundum atrial septal defects using the Amplatzer septal occluder: a single centre study in 236 consecutive patients. Heart 2003; 89(2): 199–204.

30. Fontes VF et al. [Initial experience in percutaneous closure of interatrial communication with the Amplatzer device.] Arq Bras Cardiol 1998; 70(3): 147–53.

31. Gao W et al. [Transcatheter closure of secundum atrial septal defect in children.] Zhonghua Er Ke Za Zhi 2004; 42(4): 287–90.

32. Kleinman CS. Echocardiographic guidance of catheter-based treatments of atrial septal defect: transesophageal echocardiography remains the gold standard. Pediatr Cardiol 2005; 26(2): 128–34.

33. Luxenberg DM et al. Use of a new 8 French intracardiac echocardiographic catheter to guide device closure of atrial septal defects and patent foramen ovale in small children and adults: initial clinical experience. J Invas Cardiol 2005; 17(10): 540–5.

34. Anderson RH, Brown NA, Webb S. Development and structure of the atrial septum. Heart 2002; 88(1): 104–10.

35. Anderson RH, Webb S, Brown NA. Clinical anatomy of the atrial septum with reference to its developmental components. Clin Anat 1999; 12(5): 362–74.

36. Ferreira SM, Ho SY, Anderson RH. Morphological study of defects of the atrial septum within the oval fossa: implications for transcatheter closure of left-to-right shunt. Br Heart J 1992; 67(4): 316–20.

37. Hausdorf G. StarFlex ASD closure: deployment, techniques, equipment. J Interven Cardiol 2001; 14(1): 69–76.

38. Gnanapragasam JP et al. Transoesophageal echocardiographic assessment of primum, secundum and sinus venosus atrial septal defects. Int J Cardiol 1991; 31(2): 167–74.

39. Podnar T et al. Morphological variations of secundum-type atrial septal defects: feasibility for percutaneous closure using Amplatzer septal occluders. Cathet Cardiovasc Interven 2001; 53(3): 386–91.

40. Figueroa MI et al. Experience with use of multiplane transesophageal echocardiography to guide closure of atrial septal defects using the Amplatzer device. Pediatr Cardiol 2002; 23: 430–6.

41. Amin Z et al. Erosion of Amplatzer septal occluder device after closure of secundum atrial septal defects: review of registry of complications and recommendations to minimize future risk. Cathet Cardiovasc Interven 2004; 63(4): 496–502.

42. Jang GY et al. Aorta to right atrial fistula following transcatheter closure of an atrial septal defect. Am J Cardiol 2005; 96(11): 1605–6.

43. Ewert P et al. Diagnostic catheterization and balloon sizing of atrial septal defects by echocardiographic guidance without fluoroscopy. Echocardiography 2000; 17(2): 159–63.

44. Ilkhanoff L et al. Transcatheter device closure of interatrial septal defects in patients with hypoxia. J Interven Cardiol 2005; 18(4): 227–32.

45. Zhu W et al. Measurement of atrial septal defect size: a comparative study between three-dimensional transesophageal echocardiography and the standard balloon sizing methods. Pediatr Cardiol 2000; 21(5): 465–9.

Additional reading

1. Kannan BR et al. Transcatheter closure of very large (> or = 25 mm) atrial septal defects using the Amplatzer septal occluder. Cathet Cardiovasc Interven 2003; 59(4): 522–7.

2. Knirsch W et al. Challenges encountered during closure of atrial septal defects. Pediatr Cardiol 2005; 26(2): 147–53.

3. Koenig P et al. Role of intracardiac echocardiographic guidance in transcatheter closure of atrial septal defects and patent foramen ovale using the Amplatzer device. J Interv Cardiol 2003; 16(1): 51–62.

4. Kong X et al. Transcatheter closure of secundum atrial septal defect with a new self-expanding nitinol double disk device (Amplatzer device): experience in Nanjing. J Interven Cardiol 2001; 14(2): 193–6.

5. Krumsdorf U et al. Catheter closure of atrial septal defects and patent foramen ovale in patients with an atrial septal aneurysm using different devices. J Interven Cardiol 2001; 14(1): 49–55.

6. Latson LA. Per-catheter ASD closure. Pediatr Cardiol 1998; 19(1): 86–93; discussion 94.

7. Ludomirsky A. The use of echocardiography in pediatric interventional cardiac catheterization procedures. J Interven Cardiol 1995; 8(5): 569–78.

8. McMahon CJ et al. Natural history of growth of secundum atrial septal defects and implications for transcatheter closure. Heart 2002; 87(3): 256–9.

9. Mehmood F et al. Usefulness of live three-dimensional transthoracic echocardiography in the characterization of atrial septal defects in adults. Echocardiography 2004; 21(8): 707–13.

10. Moore JW et al. Closure of atrial septal defects in the cardiac catheterization laboratory: early results using the Amplatzer Septal Occlusion Device. Del Med J 1998; 70(12): 513–16.

11. Omeish A, Hijazi ZM. Transcatheter closure of atrial septal defects in children & adults using the Amplatzer Septal Occluder. J Interven Cardiol 2001; 14(1): 37–44.

12. Pedra SR et al. Percutaneous closure of atrial septal defects. The role of transesophageal echocardiography. Arq Bras Cardiol 1999; 72(1): 59–69.

13. Purcell IF, Brecker SJ, Ward DE. Closure of defects of the atrial septum in adults using the Amplatzer device: 100 consecutive patients in a single center. Clin Cardiol 2004; 27(9): 509–13.

14. Rao PS, Langhough R. Relationship of echocardiographic, shunt flow, and angiographic size to the stretched diameter of the atrial septal defect. Am Heart J 1991; 122(2): 505–8.

15. Rao PS et al. Echocardiographic estimation of balloon-stretched diameter of secundum atrial septal defect for transcatheter occlusion. Am Heart J 1992; 124(1): 172–5.

16. Reddy SC et al. Echocardiographic predictors of success of catheter closure of atrial septal defect with the buttoned device. Am Heart J 1995; 129(1): 76–82.

17. Rome JJ, Kreutzer J. Pediatric interventional catheterization: reasonable expectations and outcomes. Pediatr Clin North Am 2004; 51(6): 1589–610, viii.

18. Rosenfeld HM et al. Echocardiographic predictors of candidacy for successful transcatheter atrial septal defect closure. Cathet Cardiovasc Diagn 1995; 34(1): 29–34.

19. Salaymeh KJ et al. Unique echocardiographic features associated with deployment of the Amplatzer atrial septal defect device. J Am Soc Echocardiogr 2001; 14(2): 128–37.

20. Schrader R. Catheter closure of secundum ASD using 'other' devices. J Interven Cardiol 2003; 16(5): 409–12.

21. Schulze CJ et al. Continuous transesophageal echocardiographic (TEE) monitoring during port-access cardiac surgery. Heart Surg Forum 1999; 2(1): 54–9.

22. Sievert H, Krumsdorf U. Transcatheter closure of intracardiac shunts. Z Kardiol 2002; 91(Suppl 3): 77–83.

23. Van Der Velde ME, Perry SB. Transesophageal echocardiography during interventional catheterization in congenital heart disease. Echocardiography 1997; 14(5): 513–28.

24. van der Velde ME, Perry SB, Sanders SP. Transesophageal echocardiography with color Doppler during interventional catheterization. Echocardiography 1991; 8(6): 721–30.

25. Varma C et al. Outcomes and alternative techniques for device closure of the large secundum atrial septal defect. Cathet Cardiovasc Interven 2004; 61(1): 131–9.

26. Vincent RN, Raviele AA, Diehl HJ. Single-center experience with the HELEX septal occluder for closure of atrial septal defects in children. J Interven Cardiol 2003; 16(1): 79–82.

27. Wang G et al. Transcatheter closure of secundum atrial septal defects using Amplatzer device. Chin Med J (Engl) 2000; 113(11): 967–71.

28. Wilkinson JL. Interventional pediatric cardiology: device closures. Ind J Pediatr 2000; 67(3 Suppl): S30–6.

29. Wilkinson JL. Interventional pediatric cardiology: device closures. Ind J Pediatr 2000; 67(7): 507–13.

30. Zimand S et al. [Transcatheter closure of atrial septal defects: initial clinical applications.] Harefuah 1998; 135(7–8): 276–9, 335.

31. Grayburn PA et al. Migration of an Amplatzer septal occluder device for closure of atrial septal defect into the ascending aorta with formation of an aorta-to-right atrial fistula. Am J Cardiol 2005; 96(11): 1607–9.

32. Hales WD, Sandhu SK, Kerut EK. The Amplatzer septal occluder as a standard for therapy of secundum-type atrial septal defect. J LA State Med Soc 2004; 156(2): 99–100, 102.

33. Helgason H et al. Sizing of atrial septal defects in adults. Cardiology 2005; 104(1): 1–5.

34. Hijazi Z et al. Transcatheter closure of atrial septal defects and patent foramen ovale under intracardiac echocardiographic guidance: feasibility and comparison with transesophageal echocardiography. Cathet Cardiovasc Interven 2001; 52(2): 194–9.

35. Holzer R, Hijazi ZM. Interventional approach to congenital heart disease. Curr Opin Cardiol 2004; 19(2): 84–90.

36. Hwang B et al. Transcatheter closure of atrial septal defect with a CardioSEAL device. Jpn Heart J 2000; 41(4): 471–80.

4

Imaging during cardiac catheterization: intracardiac echocardiography (ICE) using the AcuNav® catheter

Peter R Koenig, Qi-Ling Cao, and Ziyad M Hijazi

Introduction – an overview of intravascular and intracardiac imaging

Ultrasonography, with a probe placed directly in the vascular system, has been in existence for over two decades. Initial probes, mounted on intravascular catheters/sheaths, produced radial or 360° axial imaging.[1,2] In addition, relatively high frequencies were used such that images demonstrated excellent resolution of the vessels in which the ultrasound catheters were placed (e.g. coronary arteries); however, other portions of the cardiac anatomy were not well seen.[3–6] With the development of lower frequency transducers, greater depth penetration was possible allowing improved imaging of other parts of the cardiac anatomy;[7] hence the term 'intracardiac (ICE)' rather than 'intravascular (IVUS)' echocardiography to denote the location of the catheter. Axial or radial intracardiac imaging has been used to determine chamber and valve sizes, thicknesses, and function.[8–13] In addition, this type of imaging was also used for guidance of cardiac interventions such as endomyocardial biopsy,[14] trans-septal puncture,[15] and electrophysiologic studies.[16] During the latter, ICE has been used to guide the placement of electrophysiologic pacing catheters and trans-septal puncture, as well as to evaluate lesion size, anatomy, and post-procedure complications.[17–19] Since initial intracardiac imaging used an axial plane only, only portions of the two-dimensional (2D) anatomy were visualized at a time, and only a poor mental sense of the underlying 3D anatomy was possible. In addition, initial ICE catheters lacked pulse Doppler capabilities. Linear array transducers[20] and steerable catheters[20,21] were developed to enhance 2D visualization. Over the last 5 years, phased-array intracardiac transducers[22–24] have been introduced and essentially replaced other intracardiac imaging catheters. These ultrasound catheters have lower frequency as well as Doppler imaging capability. They have been used for guidance in numerous invasive cardiac procedures and interventions, including electrophysiologic studies,[25–28] balloon atrial septostomy,[29] gene insertion,[30] and closure of atrial level defects.[31–34] ICE has been shown to have imaging comparable to prior imaging modalities used during cardiac interventions,[34,35] and is perhaps a superior imaging method.[36–38] The cost of ICE had been deemed prohibitive, but investigators have shown that the costs may be equal to or less than prior imaging modalities.[39]

Description of the ICE catheter

ICE is currently performed using the AcuNav® catheter (Acuson Corporation, A Siemens company). The original catheter has a 10.5 Fr (3.2 mm) shaft that requires an 11 Fr introducer. The transducer has a frequency which varies from 5.5 to 10 MHz and contains a 64-element phased array. The sector scan of this transducer is in a longitudinal (with respect to the catheter) plane and achieves a 90° sector image with a depth penetration of up to 12 cm. Furthermore, the catheter is steerable via a four-way tip articulation allowing maneuvering in four directions. The handle is equipped with a locking knob that allows the tip of the catheter to be fixed in a desired orientation (Figure 4.1).

In adult patients, the AcuNav catheter can be introduced in the same vein used for the device delivery. However, for patients weighing less than 35 kg (i.e. children), the contralateral femoral vein is used. However, a newer catheter which is 8 Fr in diameter is now available for use. The catheter has similar imaging capability and will require only an 8 Fr introducer.

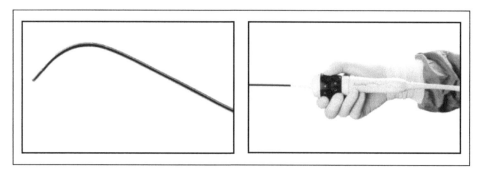

Figure 4.1
The AcuNav® catheter. Left, the tip of the catheter can be manipulated in four different directions. Right, the control handle has three knobs: one to move the tip in posterior/anterior directions, one to move the tip right/left, and the last knob is a locking one that will fix the tip in the desired orientation.

ICE imaging protocol during device placement

The use of ICE during atrial septal defect (ASD) and patent foramen ovale (PFO) closure using a phased-array transducer has been described.[31] At the start of the case, a complete evaluation of the defect(s) and surrounding anatomy is performed. The intensity of this interrogation will in part depend on the adequacy of and completeness of imaging prior to the procedure. For patients with an ASD, the size of the defect via 2D imaging (with and without being stretched by a balloon) as well as the measurement of surrounding rims is obtained. Contrast injection via agitated saline microbubbles is performed for patients with a PFO.

Step-wise protocol for ICE imaging to guide ASD or PFO closure

1. ICE imaging is initiated after advancing (under fluoroscopic guidance) the catheter to the mid-right atrium, also referred to as the 'neutral view' or 'home view'. The ICE catheter is parallel to the spine with the transducer portion facing the tricuspid valve. This is shown in Figure 4.2(a). Diagrams depicting catheter position via fluoroscopy (in the anteroposterior (AP) view) as well as the corresponding imaging planes and the image obtained by ICE are shown. In this view, the tricuspid valve, right ventricular inflow and outflow, and a long axis of the pulmonary valve are seen. The aortic valve can also be seen in a transverse (short-axis) view. The anterior part of the septum can be seen in this view.
2. The ICE catheter is flexed posteriorly using the knob so that the transducer faces the interatrial septum. Fluoroscopy showing the position of the catheter, as well as a corresponding anatomic diagram, is shown in Figure 4.2(b). The ICE image obtained shows the interatrial septum as well as the coronary sinus and pulmonary veins, depending on the exact location of the transducer. This can be referred to as the 'septal view'. One can obtain further views by locking the tip in this position and rotating the entire handle or by fine adjustments of the posterior/anterior or right/left knobs.

3. The ICE catheter itself is then advanced in a cephalad direction toward the superior vena cava (SVC). This can be referred to as the SVC or 'long-axis view'. A fluoroscopic image showing the position of the catheter as well as a corresponding anatomic diagram is shown in Figure 4.2(c). The ICE image obtained is also shown. In this plane, the transducer faces the interatrial septum and the SVC can be seen as it relates to the right atrium. The interatrial septum is shown in a superior/inferior plane and corresponds to the transesophageal echocardiography (TEE) long-axis view. Greater portions of the SVC can be seen by continued advancement of the ICE catheter in this flexed position toward the SVC. Greater portions of the inferior septum can be similarly imaged by withdrawing the ICE catheter toward the inferior vena cava in the flexed position. A defect of the interatrial septum can be well profiled, and the superior and inferior rims as well as the diameter of the defect can be measured. In this view, both the right and left pulmonary veins may also be imaged, depending on the exact angle of the imaging plane.
4. The catheter (in its locked position) is then rotated clockwise until it sits in a position with the transducer near the tricuspid valve annulus, and inferior to the aorta. A fluoroscopic image showing the catheter position and a corresponding anatomic diagram is shown in Figure 4.2(d). The ICE image obtained is also shown. In this view, the aortic valve can be seen in the short axis as well as the interatrial septum. This corresponds to the basal short-axis view obtained with TEE and is known as the 'short-axis view'. However, the right atrium is in the near field and the left atrium is in the far field, which is opposite to what is seen with TEE.

Prior to the actual device deployment procedure, the above views are obtained in order to image the ASD or PFO. Additional views can be obtained by advancing the catheter through the ASD or PFO into the left atrium (see below). From this position, an equivalent of the transthoracic four-chamber view can be obtained with views of the mitral valve, left ventricle (LV), and right ventricle

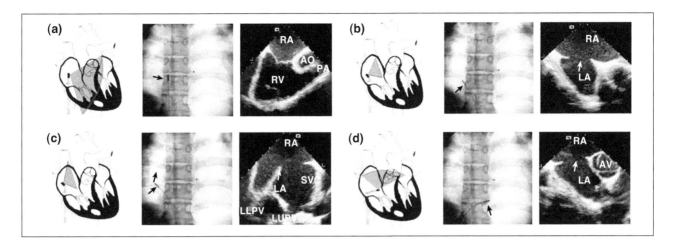

Figure 4.2
(a) Images in the home view. Left, sketch representing the heart with the position of the intracardiac catheter inside the heart with the ultrasonic array box in the neutral 'home view' position. The shaded area represents structures seen in this view. Middle, a cine fluoroscopy image showing the position of the ICE catheter (arrow) in the mid-right atrium with the transducer facing the tricuspid valve and parallel to the spine. Right, an actual intracardiac echocardiographic image with the ultrasonic box in the neutral home view position. The tricuspid valve, right ventricle out, and inflow are well seen in this position. The aortic valve and pulmonic valve can also be seen. AO, aortic valve; RA, right atrium; PA, pulmonary artery; RV, right ventricle. (b) Images in the septal view. Left, sketch representing the heart with the position of the intracardiac catheter inside the heart with the ultrasonic array box in the posterior flexed position looking at the atrial septum 'septal view'. The shaded area represents structures seen in this view. Middle, a cine fluoroscopy image showing the position of the ICE catheter (arrow) in the right atrium with the transducer flexed posterior looking at the septum. Right, an actual intracardiac echocardiographic image with the ultrasonic box in the septal view. The atrial septal defect is well seen (arrow), as are the left and right atria. (c) Images in the long-axis 'caval view'. Left, sketch representing the heart with the position of the intracardiac catheter inside the heart with the ultrasonic array box in the posterior flexed position with a cephalad advancement looking at the atrial septum and the superior vena cava 'caval view'. The shaded area represents structures seen in this view. Middle, a cine fluoroscopy image showing the position of the ICE catheter (black arrow) in the right atrium with the transducer flexed posterior looking at the superior vena cava (white arrow). Right, an actual intracardiac echocardiographic image with the ultrasonic box in the caval view. The atrial septal defect (arrow), the left and right atria, the left pulmonary veins, and the superior vena cava are all well seen. SVC, superior vena cava; LLPV, left lower pulmonary vein; LUPV, left upper pulmonary vein. (d) Images in the 'short-axis view'. Left, sketch representing the heart with the position of the intracardiac catheter inside the heart with the ultrasonic array box in the flexed position and the entire handle rotated clockwise until the imaging transducer is above the tricuspid valve looking at the aorta from below. In this position, fine rotation of the knobs can demonstrate different parts of the atrial septum. The shaded area represents structures seen in this view. Middle, a cine fluoroscopy image showing the position of the ICE catheter (black arrow) in the right atrium with the transducer above the tricuspid valve. Right, an actual intracardiac echocardiographic image with the ultrasonic box in the short-axis view. The atrial septal defect (arrow), the left and right atria, and the aortic valve are all well seen. This view is similar to a TEE short-axis view with the left atrium in the far field (opposite to the TEE).

(RV). The catheter can be further manipulated to view the left atrial appendage (LAA), which may be helpful in procedures to occlude the LAA. The catheter is then withdrawn back to the right atrium. During exchange wire and delivery sheath positioning, the long-axis view is felt to best delineate intracardiac relations. Device deployment is monitored in the long-axis view as well to demonstrate the relation of the disks to the interatrial septum. Figure 4.3(a)–(o) demonstrates the case of a patient with a large secundum ASD who underwent device closure. This figure demonstrates all the steps involved in device closure using the Amplatzer Septal Occluder. Color Doppler

imaging as well as contrast echocardiography is used to assess for the presence or absence of any residual shunts.

In summary, the routine ASD or PFO closure procedure uses ICE to demonstrate catheter, guidewire, and sheath placement across the ASD or PFO. After placement of the sheath, ICE imaging is used to show the manner in which the occluder device is advanced within the sheath. It is then used to show deployment of the device as it is advanced out of the sheath: left disk opening, positioning of the left disk toward the interatrial septum, waist deployment, and right disk deployment as these in turn are advanced out of the catheter. Finally, release of the device is imaged.

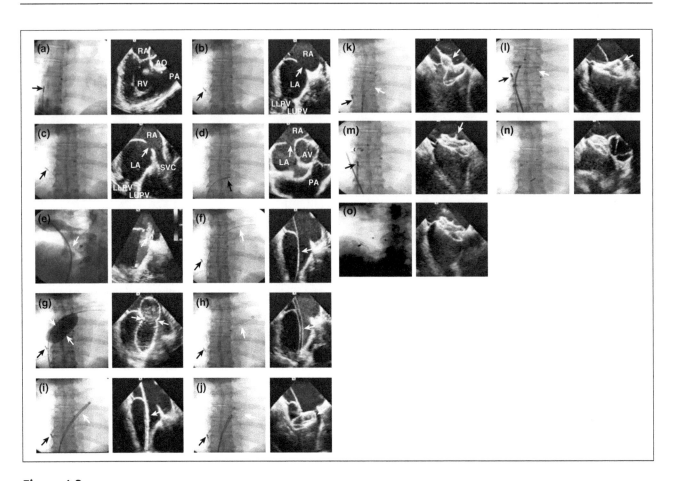

Figure 4.3

Cine fluoroscopic and ICE images in a 54-year-old female patient with a large secundum ASD who underwent closure using a 28 mm Amplatzer Septal Occluder. (a) Left, cine of the ICE catheter in the home view (arrow). Right, image obtained showing the tricuspid valve, right ventricle, aorta, and pulmonary artery. (b) Septal view images. Left, ICE transducer (arrow) facing the septum. Right, ICE image obtained demonstrating the defect (arrow), pulmonary veins and left and right atria. (c) Caval view images. Left, ICE transducer (arrow) facing the upper septum and looking at the superior vena cava. Right, ICE image obtained demonstrating the defect (arrow), SVC, pulmonary veins, and left and right atria. (d) Short-axis view images. Left, ICE transducer (arrow) above the tricuspid valve. Right, ICE image obtained demonstrating the defect (arrow), aortic valve, pulmonary artery, and left and right atria. (e) Left, angiogram in the right upper pulmonary vein demonstrating the defect (arrow). Right, ICE image with color in septal view demonstrating the defect and shunt (arrow). (f) Left, cine fluoroscopy image demonstrating the ICE catheter (black arrow) in the septal view position during passage of the exchange guidewire (white arrow) through the defect into the left upper pulmonary vein. Right, corresponding ICE image showing the guidewire (arrow) through the defect. (g) Left, cine fluoroscopy image demonstrating the ICE catheter (black arrow) in the septal view position during balloon sizing of the defect to obtain the stretched diameter (white arrows). Right, corresponding ICE image showing the indentations on the balloon (arrows). (h) Left, cine fluoroscopy image demonstrating the ICE catheter (black arrow) in the septal view position during passage of the delivery sheath (arrow) into the left atrium. Right, corresponding ICE image showing the delivery sheath (arrow) inside the left atrium. (i) Left, cine fluoroscopy image demonstrating the ICE catheter (black arrow) in the septal view position during passage of a 28-mm Amplatzer Septal Occluder within the sheath (arrow). Right, corresponding ICE image showing the device inside the sheath (arrow). (j) Left, cine fluoroscopy image demonstrating the ICE catheter (black arrow) in the septal view position during deployment of the left atrial disk (arrow) of a 28-mm Amplatzer Septal Occluder in the left atrium. Right, corresponding ICE image showing the left disk in the left atrium (arrow). (k) Left, cine fluoroscopy image demonstrating the ICE catheter (black arrow) in the septal view position during deployment of the connecting waist (arrow). Right, corresponding ICE image showing the connecting waist (arrow). (l) Left, cine fluoroscopy image demonstrating the ICE catheter (black arrow) in a modified septal short-axis view position during deployment of the right atrial disk (arrow). Right, corresponding ICE image showing the right atrial disk (arrow). (m) Left, cine fluoroscopy image demonstrating the ICE catheter (black arrow) in a modified septal short-axis view position after the device has been released from the cable (white arrow). Right, corresponding ICE image showing the device after it has been released (arrow). (n) Left, cine fluoroscopy image demonstrating the ICE catheter in a modified short-axis view position. Right, corresponding ICE image showing the aortic valve and both disks of the device. (o) Left, cine fluoroscopy image in the four-chamber view demonstrating the position of the device. Right, ICE image with color Doppler showing good device position and no residual shunt.

ICE imaging protocol for VSD closure

The use of ICE during VSD closure using a phased-array transducer has been described.[40] At the start of the case, a complete evaluation of the defect(s) and surrounding anatomy is performed. Similar to ASD or PFO closure, the intensity of this interrogation will in part depend on the adequacy of and completeness of imaging prior to the procedure.

Stepwise protocol using ICE to guide VSD

The ICE catheter is introduced in the same fashion for VSD closure as it is for transcatheter ASD or PFO closure described above. Under fluoroscopic guidance, the ICE catheter is advanced from the inferior vena cava (IVC) into the right atrium (RA). A complete ICE study then ensues.

1. ICE imaging is initiated in the RA with the 'home view' similar to ASD and PFO closure, as described above. The ICE catheter is advanced through the IVC and into the middle of the RA, with the tip of the catheter placed in a neutral position, and the orientation of the imaging plane toward the tricuspid valve, as shown in Figure 4.4(a). From this position, the RA, the right ventricle (RV) inflow, and the membranous/perimembranous portion of the interventricular septum (IVS) are seen. The defect within the IVS is noted and its relationship to the tricuspid valve is shown in Figure 4.4(a).

2. The short-axis view is obtained similar to that obtained during ASD and PFO closure. The catheter is flexed posteriorly and locked. The entire handle is rotated clockwise and advanced slightly just above the tricuspid valve until the short-axis view is achieved, with the transducer in an anterior–superior plane as shown in Figure 4.4(b). A fluoroscopic image of the catheter and the corresponding ICE image are shown. This view demonstrates the location and size of the defect, the aortic valve, and the pulmonic valve.

3. A four-chamber view is obtained by maneuvering the ICE catheter into the mid-RA with the tip positioned slightly anterior (close to the interatrial septum), and rotation such that the orientation of the imaging transducer faces the LV, as shown in Figure 4.4(c) with the accompanying fluoroscopic and ICE images. In this view, the entire left atrium and ventricle can be seen, as well as part of the right atrium and ventricle. This view is important to show disk deployment and the position of the disk in relation to the IVS.

In the patients with an associated atrial communication (ASD or PFO), the ICE catheter can be advanced across the atrial defect from the RA into the left atrium (LA) under fluoroscopic guidance. This positioning of the ICE catheter allows the following additional views:

1. The longitudinal view is obtained with the catheter in the left atrium with slight advancement of the ICE catheter in a flexed position toward the mitral valve and a 90° anterior flexion of the tip. This provides an imaging plane toward the LV long axis as depicted in the anatomic diagram in Figure 4.5(a). The corresponding fluoroscopic and ICE images are also shown. The ICE image demonstrates the LA, mitral valve, LV inflow and outflow, the long axis of the aortic valve, as well as the defect and the rim in the subaortic valve region.

2. The basal subaortic short-axis view is obtained with the ICE catheter advanced into the middle of the LA with a 45° anterior flexion of the transducer, as shown in Figure 4.5(b). This figure also shows the corresponding fluoroscopic and ICE images. The ICE image demonstrates the RA, RV inflow and outflow, and the short axis of the subaortic valve region and the defect.

3. The four- and five-chamber views are obtained by advancing the ICE catheter to the middle of the LA with a 90° anterior flexion of the tip. This provides an imaging plane facing the apex of the heart as seen in Figure 4.5(c), with the corresponding fluoroscopic and ICE images. The ICE images demonstrate a four- or five-chamber view of the cardiac structures. The latter views clearly demonstrate the subaortic rim of the defect, the relation of the defect to the aortic valve, and the relation of the device to the aortic valve.

In summary, the VSD closure procedure uses ICE to show the pertinent anatomy of the VSD including the defect and its rims, and the relation of the defect to the aortic valve. It is then used to demonstrate catheter, guidewire, and sheath placement across the VSD. After placement of the sheath, ICE imaging is used to demonstrate the manner in which the occluder device is advanced within the sheath. It is then used to show deployment of the device as it is advanced out of the sheath: left disk opening, positioning of the left disk toward the interventricular septum, waist deployment, and right disk deployment as these in turn are advanced out of the catheter. The release of the device is imaged, followed by imaging of the relation of the device to surrounding structures, especially the aortic valve and tricuspid valves.

ICE imaging for other cardiac interventional procedures

The use of ICE for other cardiac interventions precedes its use for the closure of septal defects. Its use has been well described to help guide transseptal puncture,[41] for the

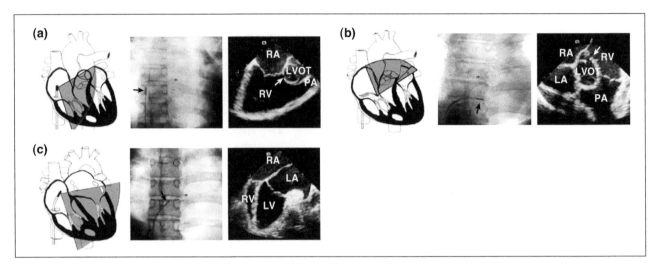

Figure 4.4

(a) Images in the home view. Left, sketch representing the heart with the position of the intracardiac catheter inside the heart with the ultrasonic array box in the neutral home view position. The shaded area represents structures seen in this view. Middle, a cine fluoroscopy image showing the position of the ICE catheter (arrow) in the mid-right atrium with the transducer facing the tricuspid valve and parallel to the spine. Right, an actual intracardiac echocardiographic image with the ultrasonic box in the neutral home view position. The tricuspid valve, right ventricle out, and inflow are well seen in this position. The aortic valve and pulmonic valve can also be seen. A perimembranous VSD can also be seen in this view (arrow). (b) Images in the short-axis view with more posterior flexion. Left, sketch representing the heart with the position of the intracardiac catheter inside the heart with the ultrasonic array box in the flexed position and the entire handle rotated clockwise until the imaging transducer is above the tricuspid valve looking at the aorta and left ventricle outflow tract from below. In this position, fine rotation of the knobs can demonstrate different parts of the membranous ventricular septum. The shaded area represents structures seen in this view. Middle, a cine fluoroscopy image showing the position of the ICE catheter (arrow) in the right atrium with the transducer above the tricuspid valve. Right, an actual intracardiac echocardiographic image with the ultrasonic box in the short-axis view. The defect (arrow), the left ventricle outflow tract, right ventricle, and relation of the defect to the aortic valve are well seen. (C) Images in the 'four-chamber view'. Left, sketch representing the heart with the position of the intracardiac catheter inside the heart with the ultrasonic array box in the anterior flexed position close to the atrial septum looking at the four chambers of the heart. In this position, fine rotation of the knobs can demonstrate different parts of the membranous ventricular septum. The shaded area represents structures seen in this view. Middle, a cine fluoroscopy image showing the position of the ICE catheter (arrow) in the right atrium with the transducer near the septum in the anterior flexed position. Right, an actual intracardiac echocardiographic image with the ultrasonic box in the four-chamber view. All four chambers are seen. LVOT, left ventricle outflow tract, RA, right atrium; PA, pulmonary artery; RV, right ventricle.

placement of electrophysiologic pacing catheters,[41] or for the hemodynamic assessment in mitral valve disease, especially with distorted atrial septal anatomy.[42] During electrophysiologic studies, ICE not only demonstrated correct catheter location for optimal ablation,[43–46] but it has also been used to demonstrate radiofrequency ablation lesion size.[47] Other potential uses have been discussed in ICE review articles.[48–50] These uses, with few reports in the literature, include its use to help guide percutaneous valvuloplasty[51] and complex biopsies within the heart.[52] For mitral valvuloplasty, the four-chamber view discussed above would be useful for guiding wires, sheaths, and valvuloplasty balloons, as would a longitudinal view of the left ventricle. The latter can be achieved by advancing the ICE catheter across the tricuspid valve and rotating the transducer until the left ventricle and mitral valve are seen with a transthoracic echocardiography (TTE) parasternal long-axis equivalent. ICE can also be potentially used for the guidance of pulmonary or aortic valvuloplasty by advancing the ICE catheter into the right ventricle and across the pulmonary valve.[53]

Summary

ICE provides imaging for the guidance of atrial and ventricular septal defect closure. The latter is a relatively new utilization of this imaging tool and shows the same promise as with ASD and PFO closure, namely, VSD closure in the cardiac catheterization laboratory without the need for general anesthesia. This would greatly advance the care of individuals requiring VSD closure. It is anticipated that experimental forays into the utilization of 3D intracardiac echocardiography[54,55] will culminate with the total elimination of fluoroscopy and any other imaging modality other than ICE for the guidance of defect closure.

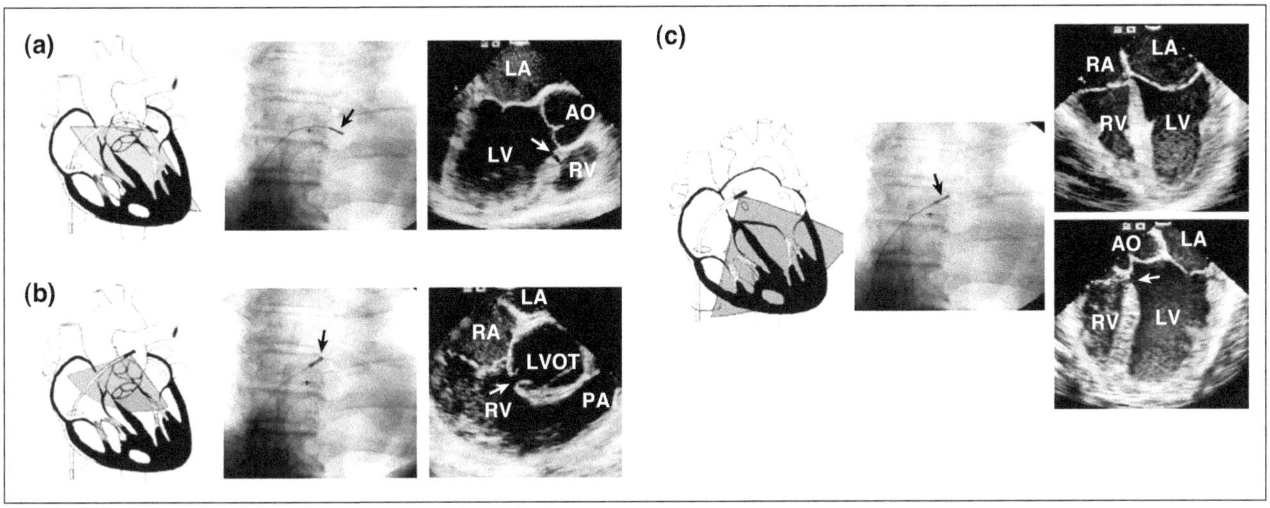

Figure 4.5

Images obtained with the transducer positioned in the left atrium. (a) Left, sketch representing the heart with the position of the intracardiac catheter and ultrasonic array box in the left atrium with a 90° anterior flexion of the tip. This provides an imaging plane toward the LV long axis and the subaortic area. Middle, the corresponding fluoroscopic image with the ICE catheter (arrow) above the mitral valve. Right, ICE image demonstrating the LA, mitral valve, LV inflow and outflow, the long axis of the aortic valve, as well as the defect and the rim of the subaortic valve region. (b) Left, the basal subaortic short-axis view obtained with the ICE catheter advanced into the middle of the LA with a 45° anterior flexion of the transducer. The imaging plane shows the right atrium and ventricle and the left ventricle outflow area with the defect. Middle, the corresponding fluoroscopic image of the catheter (arrow) in the left atrium. Right, the corresponding ICE image demonstrating the RA, RV inflow and outflow, and the short axis of the subaortic valve region and the defect. (c) Left, the four- and five-chamber views obtained by advancing the ICE catheter to the middle of the LA and a 90° anterior flexion of the tip, providing an imaging plane facing the apex of the heart. Middle, the corresponding fluoroscopic image of the transducer (arrow). Right, ICE images demonstrating a four- (top) or five- (bottom) chamber view of the cardiac structures. The latter views clearly demonstrate the subaortic rim of the defect and the relation of the defect to the aortic valve.

References

1. Glassman E, Kronzon I. Transvernous intracardiac echocardiography. Am J Cardiol 1981; 47(6): 1255–9.
2. Pandian NG, Weintraub A, Schwartz SL et al. Intravascular and intracardiac ultrasound imaging: current research and future directions. Echocardiography 1990; 7(4): 377–87.
3. Pandian NG, Schwartz SL, Weintraub AR et al. Intracardiac echocardiography: current developments. Int J Cardiol Imag 1991; 6(3–4): 207–19.
4. Pandian NG, Schwartz SL, Hsu TL et al. Intracardiac echocardiography. Experimental observations on intracavitary imaging of cardiac structures with 20-MHz ultrasound catheters. Echocardiography 1991; 8(1): 127–34.
5. Weintraub AR, Schwartz SL, Smith J et al. Intracardiac two-dimensional echocardiography in patients with pericardial effusion and cardiac tamponade. J Am Soc Echocardiogr 1991; 4(6): 571–6.
6. Pandian NG, Hsu TL. Intravascular and intracardiac echocardiography: concepts for the future. Am J Cardiol 1992; 69(20): 6H–17H.
7. Schwartz SL, Gillam LD, Weintraub AR et al. Intracardiac echocardiography in humans using a small-sized (6F), low frequency (12.5 MHz) ultrasound catheter. Methods, imaging planes and clinical experience. J Am Coll Cardiol 1993; 21(1): 189–98.
8. Fisher JP, Wolfberg CA, Mikan JS et al. Intracardiac ultrasound determination of left ventricular volumes: in vitro and in vivo validation. J Am Coll Cardiol 1994; 24(1): 247–53.
9. Chen C, Guerrero JL, Vazquez de Prada JA et al. Intracardiac ultrasound measurement of volumes and ejection fraction in normal, infarcted, and aneurysmal left ventricles using a 10-MHz ultrasound catheter. Circulation 1994; 90(3): 1481–91.
10. Vazquez de Prada JA, Chen MH, Guerrero JL et al. Intracardiac echocardiography: in vitro and in vivo validation for right ventricular volume and function. Am Heart J 1996; 131(2): 320–8.
11. Foster GP, Weissman NJ, Picard MH et al. Determination of aortic valve area in valvular aortic stenosis by direct measurement using intracardiac echocardiography: a comparison with the Gorlin and continuity equations. J Am Coll Cardiol 1996; 27(2): 392–8.
12. Spencer KT, Kerber R, McKay C. Automated tracking of left ventricular wall thickening with intracardiac echocardiography. J Am Soc Echocardiography 1998; 11(11): 1020–6.
13. Sonka M, Liang W, Kanani P et al. Intracardiac echocardiography: computerized detection of left ventricular borders. Int J Cardiol Imag 1998; 14(6): 397–411.
14. Segar DS, Bourdillon PD, Elsner G et al. Intracardiac echocardiography-guided biopsy of intracardiac masses. J Am Soc Echocardiogr 1995; 8(6): 927–9.
15. Mitchel JF, Gillam LD, Sanzobrono BW et al. Intracardiac ultrasound imaging during transeptal catheterization. Chest 1995; 108(1): 104–8.
16. Tardif JC, Vannan MA, Miller DS et al. Potential applications of intracardiac echocardiography in interventional electrophysiology. Am Heart J 1994; 127(4 Pt 2): 1090–4.
17. Ren JF, Schwartzman D, Callans D et al. Imaging technique and clinical utility for electrophysiologic procedures of lower frequency (9 MHz) intracardiac echocardiography. Am J Cardiol 1998; 82(12): 1557–60.

18. Daoud EG, Kalbfleisch SJ, Hummel JD. Intracardiac echocardiography to guide transeptal left heart catheterization for radiofrequency catheter ablation. J Cardiovasc Electrophysiol 1999; 10(3): 358–63.

19. Tardiff JC, Groenveld PW, Wang PJ et al. Intracardiac echocardiographic guidance during microwave catheter ablation. J Am Soc Echocardiogr 1999; 12(1): 41–7.

20. Tardif JC, Cao QL, Schwartz SL, Pandian NG. Intracardiac echocardiography with a steerable low-frequency linear-array probe for left sided heart imaging from the right side: experimental studies. J Am Soc Echocardiogr 1995; 8(2): 132–8.

21. Epstein LM, Smith TW. Initial experience with a steerable intracardiac echocardiographic catheter. J Invasive Cardiol 1999; 11(5): 322–6.

22. Bruce CJ, Nishimura RA, Rihal CS et al. Intracardiac echocardiography in the interventional catheterization laboratory: preliminary experience with a novel, phased-array transducer. Am J Cardiol 2002; 89(5): 635–40.

23. Bruce CJ, Friedman PA. Intracardiac echocardiography. Eur J Echocardiogr 2001; 2(4): 234–44.

24. Li P, Dairywala IT, Liu Z et al. Anatomic and hemodynamic imaging using a new vector phased-array intracardiac catheter. J Am Soc Echocardiogr 2002; 15(4): 349–55.

25. Morton JB, Sanders P, Byrne MJ et al. Phased-array intracardiac echocardiography to guide radiofequency ablation in the left atrium and at the pulmonary vein ostium. J Cardiovasc Electrophysiol 2001; 12(3): 343–8.

26. Johnson SB, Seward JB, Packer DL. Phased-array intracardiac echocardiography for guiding transseptal catheter placement: utility and learning curve. Pacing Clin Electrophysiol 2002; 25(4 Pt 1): 402–7.

27. Calo L, Lamberti F, Loricchio ML et al. Intracardiac echocardiography: from electroanatomic correlation to clinical application in interventional electrophysiology. Ital Heart J 2002; 3(7): 387–98.

28. Martin RE, Ellenbogen KA, Lau YR et al. Phased-array intracardiac echocardiography during pulmonary vein isolation and linear ablation for atrial fibrillation. J Cardiovasc Electrophysiol 2002; 13(9): 873–9.

29. Moscucci M, Dairywala IT, Chetcuti S et al. Balloon atrial septostomy in end-stage pulmonary hypertension guided by a novel intracardiac echocardiographic transducer. Cathet Cardiovasc Interven 2001; 52(4): 530–4.

30. Park SW, Gwon HC, Jeong JO et al. Intracardiac echocardiographic guidance and monitoring during percutaneous endomyocardial gene injection in porcine heart. Hum Gen Ther 2001; 12(8): 893–903.

31. Hijazi ZM, Wang Z, Cao Q et al. Transcatheter closure of atrial septal defects and patent foramen ovale under intracardiac echocardiographic guidance: feasibility and comparison with transesophageal echocardiography. Cathet Cardiovasc Interven 2001; 52(2): 194–9.

32. Hijazi ZM, Cao QL, Heitschmidt M, Lang MR. Residual inferior atrial septal defect after surgical repair: closure under intracardiac echocardiographic guidance. J Invas Cardiol 2001; 13(12): 810–13.

33. Du Z, Koenig P, Cao Q et al. Comparison of transcatheter closure of secundum atrial septal defect using the Amplatzer septal occluder associated with deficient versus sufficient rims. Am J Cardiol 2002; 90(8): 865.

34. Jan SL, Hwang B, Lee PC et al. Intracardiac ultrasound assessment of atrial septal defect: comparison with transthoracic echocardiographic, angiographic, and balloon-sizing measurements. Cardiovasc Interven Radiol 2001; 24(2): 84–9.

35. Bartel T, Muller S, Caspari G, Erbel R. Intracardiac and intraluminal echocardiography: indications and standard approaches. Ultrasound Med Biol 2002; 28(80): 997.

36. Liu Z, McCormick D, Dairywala I et al. Catheter-based intracardiac echocardiography in the interventional cardiac laboratory. Cathet Cardiovasc Interven 2004; 63(1): 63–71.

37. Bartel T, Konorza T, Neudorf U et al. Intracardiac echocardiography: an ideal guiding tool for device closure of interatrial communications. Eur J Echocardiogr 2005; 6(2): 92–6.

38. Koenig P, Cao QL. Echocardiographic guidance of transcatheter closure of atrial septal defects – is intracardiac echocardiography better than transesophageal echocardiography? Pediatr Cardiol 2005; 26(2): 135–9.

39. Alboliras ET, Hijazi ZM. Comparison of costs of intracardiac echocardiography and transesophageal echocardiography in monitoring percutaneous device closure of atrial septal defect in children and adults. Am J Cardiol 2004; 94(5): 690–2.

40. Cao QL, Zabal C, Koenig P et al. Initial clinical experience with intracardiac echocardiography in guiding transcatheter closure of perimembranous ventricular septal defects: feasibility and comparison with transesophageal echocardiography. Cathet Cardiovasc Interven 2005; 66: 258–67.

41. Epstein LM, Smith T, TenHoff H. Nonfluoroscopic transseptal catheterization: safety and efficacy of intracardiac echocardiographic guidance. J Cardiovasc Electrophysiol 1998; 9(6): 625–30.

42. Cafri C, de la Guardia B, Barasch E et al. Transseptal puncture guided by intracardiac echocardiography during percutaneous transvenous mitral commissurotomy in patients with distorted anatomy of the fossa ovalis. Cathet Cardiovasc Interven 2000; 50(4): 463–7.

43. Mangrum JM, Mounsey JP, Kok LC et al. Intracardiac echocardiography-guided, anatomically based radiofrequency ablation of focal atrial fibrillation originating from pulmonary veins. J Am Coll Cardiol 2002; 39(12): 1964–72.

44. Verma A, Marrouche NF, Natale A. Pulmonary vein antrum isolation: intracardiac echocardiography-guided technique. J Cardiovasc Electrophysiol 2004; 15(11): 1335–40.

45. Cohen TJ, Ibrahim B, Lazar J et al. Utility of intracardiac echocardiography (ICE) in electrophysiology: ICEing the CAKE (catheter ablation knowledge enhancement). J Invas Cardiol 1999; 11(6): 364–8.

46. Citro R, Ducceschi V, Salustri A et al. Intracardiac echocardiography to guide transseptal catheterization for radiofrequency catheter ablation of left-sided accessory pathways: two case reports. Cardiovasc Ultrasound 2004; 2(1): 20.

47. Ren JF, Callans DJ, Schwartzman D et al. Changes in local wall thickness correlate with pathologic lesion size following radiofrequency catheter ablation: an intracardiac echocardiographic imaging study. Echocardiography 2001; 18(6): 503–7.

48. Bruce CJ, Friedman PA. Intracardiac echocardiography. Eur J Echocardiogr 2001; 2(4): 234–44.

49. Feldman T. Intraprocedure guidance for percutaneous mitral valve interventions: TTE, TEE, ICE, or X-ray? Cathet Cardiovasc Interven 2004; 63(3): 395–6.

50. Liu Z, McCormick D, Dairywala I et al. Catheter-based intracardiac echocardiography in the interventional cardiac laboratory. Cathet Cardiovasc Interven 2004; 63(1): 63–71.

51. Salem MI, Makaryus AN, Kort S et al. Intracardiac echocardiography using the AcuNav ultrasound catheter during percutaneous balloon mitral valvuloplasty. J Am Soc Echocardiogr 2002; 15(12): 1533–7.

52. Oishi Y, Okamoto M, Sueda T et al. Cardiac tumor biopsy under the guidance of intracardiac echocardiography. Jpn Circ J 2000; 64(8): 638–40.

53. Teragaki M, Takeuchi K, Toda I et al. Potential applications of intracardiac echocardiography in the assessment of the aortic valve from the right ventricular outflow tract. J Am Soc Echocardiogr 1999; 12(4): 225–30.

54. Lee W, Idriss SF, Wolf PD, Smith SW. A miniaturized catheter 2-D array for real-time, 3-D intracardiac echocardiography. IEEE Trans Ultrason Ferroelectr Freq Control 2004; 51(10): 1334–46.

55. Ding C, Rao L, Nagueh SF, Khoury DS. Dynamic three-dimensional visualization of the left ventricle by intracardiac echocardiography. Ultrasound Med Biol 2005; 31(1): 15–21.

5

Intracardiac echocardiography by Ultra ICE

Eustaquio Onorato, Francesco Casilli, and Mario Zanchetta

Introduction

The initial work in intracardiac echocardiography (ICE) imaging appeared in the early 1960s and it was considered as the acquisition of anatomic information of structures lying beyond the confines of an intracardiac space within which the imaging device resided. However, practical implementation of clinical usefulness in humans has been limited by technological constraints, specifically the design of smaller, lower frequency transducers incorporated into small caliber catheters. Only in the last decade have miniaturized ultrasound transducers become available and this has made ICE more practical, leading to the emergence of modern ICE, which uses a catheter-based two-dimensional (2D) intracardiac ultrasound imaging modality. With the rapid development of percutaneous interventional procedures for disorders that were once approached surgically, there has been a concomitant increased interest in ICE in the clinical setting, specifically to assist transseptal left heart catheterization[1,2] or transseptal catheter placement,[3–5] radiofrequency catheter ablation of cardiac arrhythmias,[6–8] and transcatheter closure of atrial septal defect[9–11] or patent foramen ovale.[9,12] Because an extremely high level of diagnostic certainty is required before embarking on such highly innovative treatments, concurrent complementary imaging of right atrial structures is desirable in order to prevent or make an early diagnosis of complications such as aortic root perforation, pericardial effusion, and misplacement of closure devices.

At present, there are two different transducer technologies for 2D real-time intracardiac ultrasonic imaging, each of which has its own advantages and disadvantages (Table 5.1).

1. the *mechanical single-element system* (Ultra ICE[TM] intracardiac echo catheter, EP Technologies, Boston Scientific Corporation, San Jose, California)
2. the *electronic multi-element system* (AcuNav[TM] diagnostic ultrasound catheter, Acuson Corporation; A Siemens Company, Mountain View, California).

The aim of this manuscript is to provide both the clinical and interventional pediatric and adult cardiologists with a complete overview on the use of ICE by the mechanical single-element system.

Table 5.1 *Main characteristics of the two ultrasound intracardiac probes*

Ultra ICE[TM] (Boston Scientific Corporation)	AcuNav[TM] (Acuson Corporation)
• FDA approval: 20 June, 1997	• FDA approval: 15 December, 1999
• Mechanical scanning system	• Electronic scanning system
• Unique siliceous piezoelectric crystal	• Crystal matrix (64 ceramic elements)
• 8.5 Fr 'over-the-wire' catheter	• 10.5 Fr non-over-the-wire catheter
• 9 MHz frequency	• 5.0–10 MHz frequency agile
• Radial scanning at 360°	• Sector scanning at 90°
• Images on a plane perpendicular to the long axis of the catheter	• Images on a plane parallel to the long axis of the catheter
• Imaging field: 10 cm	• Imaging field: 14 cm
• Platform: ClearView Ultra, Galaxy (EP Technologies, Boston Scientific Corporation)	• Platform: Sequoia, Aspen, Cypress (Acuson Corporation)
• Single operator use	• Single operator use
• Three-dimensional reconstruction	• Doppler technique

FDA, Food and Drug Administration.

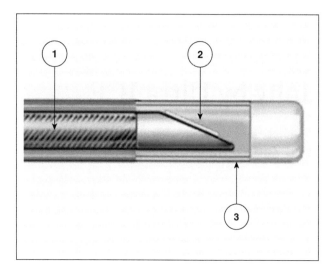

Figure 5.1
The distal end of the Ultra ICE catheter; (1) flexible wire with high torsion and rotation capacity; (2) unique siliceous piezoelectric crystal with a frequency of 9 MHz; (3) sonolucent window.

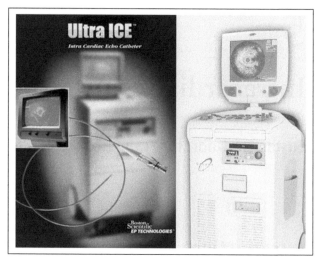

Figure 5.2
Dedicated review stations (on the left, ClearView Ultra™, version 4.22, and on the right, Galaxy™, EP Technologies, Boston Scientific Corporation).

The Ultra ICE catheter, model 9900, consists of a central inner core and of a catheter body (8.5 Fr) equipped, at its distal end, with a sonolucent window which incorporates a unique siliceous piezoelectric crystal with a frequency of 9 MHz (Figure 5.1). At its proximal end, it is equipped with a connector for the motor drive unit that allows rotation of the transducer and the transmission and reception of ultrasound waves. The central inner core consists of a flexible wire with a high torsion and rotation capacity that transfers to the transducer a circular movement with a speed ranging from 1600 to 1800 rpm. The resulting wave is propagated on a transversal plane, perpendicular to the long axis of the catheter, to create a two-dimensional imaging presented as a video tomographic session (radial at 360°) in real time on a dedicated review station, also used when performing intra-coronary ultrasound (ClearView Ultra™, version 4.22 or higher, or Galaxy™ EP Technologies, Boston Scientific Corporation) (Figure 5.2). This represents the user interface and allows modification of the image magnification, gray scale, luminosity, and contrast as well as the storage of the images in a super-VHS videotape.

Moreover, the catheter may be automatically withdrawn up to a maximum distance of 15 cm by a pullback device at a constant speed of 0.2/0.5/1.0/2.0 mm/s. The data so obtained may be stored in a personal computer (TomTec Imaging System, Unterschleinheim, Germany) (Figure 5.3) that, in turn, provides accurate measurements and a 3D reconstruction of the examined structures. In addition, it is possible to obtain a high reproducibility in spatial terms with less operator dependency, finding the same plane at successive studies with an error of just a few millimeters or even less.

With the Ultra ICE catheter, the penetration depth is about 5.0 cm, but because the scanning is radial, the useful

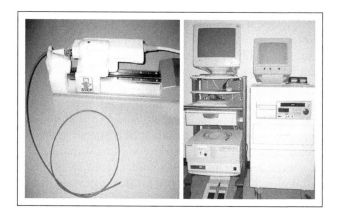

Figure 5.3
The Ultra ICE catheter may be connected to a pullback device (on the left) for an automatic withdrawal at a constant speed; the data so obtained, visualized by an ultrasound Boston Scientific console, may be stored in a personal computer (TomTec Imaging System, Unterschleinheim, Germany) for 3D reconstruction of the examined structures (on the right).

imaging field is actually about 10 cm, with axial and lateral resolutions of 0.27 and 0.26 mm, respectively.

The Ultra ICE catheter, a single-use disposable device, is introduced through the femoral vein and advanced toward the right heart with an 'over the wire' Convoy™ 8.5 Fr introducer (EP Technologies, Boston Scientific Corporation), available in several lengths and curves (distal curvature angle ranging from 0 to 140°) (Figure 5.4). This allows the operator to navigate the catheter in the right heart chambers and to manipulate the distal portion of the catheter containing the transducer in various directions. Before

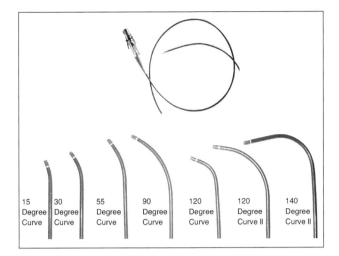

Figure 5.4
The Ultra ICE catheter is introduced through the femoral vein and advanced toward the right heart with an 'over the wire' Convoy™ 8.5 Fr introducer (EP Technologies, Boston Scientific Corporation) that is available in several lengths and curves (distal curvature angle ranging from 0 to 140°).

insertion, the Ultra ICE catheter requires an exhaustive preparation including sterile apyrogenic water rinsing of the sonolucent camera to eliminate any air which otherwise could lead to a decreased imaging quality.

Image presentation and examination technique

Although innumerable series of planes can be displayed by Ultra ICE, four views on the axial plane and only one view on the longitudinal long-axis plane have been commonly utilized for an exhaustive evaluation of the structures from the inner confines of the right atrium and great veins (Table 5.2). Because the majority of these planes bear little similarity to routine angiographic images or commonly utilized transthoracic and transesophageal echocardiography sections, the Ultra ICE images so obtained are not readily comprehended by physicians, thus there is a need to describe in detail these new unique views.

Consequently, for the identification of structures and their comprehension we employed the magnetic resonance (MR) imaging modalities, because they are superb tools for intracardiac and vascular morphology and anatomy. While cardiac MR imaging uses five tomographic views (the axial, coronal, sagittal, long-axis, and short axis ones) to study cardiac anatomy, the Ultra ICE uses only two tomographic views, that is the axial and the parasagittal long-axis planes, which are appropriate for comparative study of the morphology and relationships of the cardiac structures.

Table 5.2 *Standard scan planes during mechanical interrogation by Ultra ICE*

Scan	Transducer position
Axial	
Great vessels	T 5–6°
SVC–RA junction	T 6°
Aortic valve	T 6–7°
Cavo-tricuspid isthmus	T 8°
Para-sagittal	
Four chamber	Central on FO

T, thoracic intervertebral disk; RA, right atrium; SVC, superior vena cava; FO, fossa ovalis.

Keeping in mind that the radiologic standard format of imaging presentation gives a view on the scan plane from below, looking at the heart from the inferior vena cava upward to the cardiac base, physicians no longer need to reorient the images mentally in order to figure out the relative position of structures displayed by Ultra ICE. The imaging orientation of Ultra ICE is displayed with similar right–left and anterior–posterior MR orientation, consistent with familiar recommendations of any standard radiologic format.

Intracardiac echocardiographic axial views

The exam starts by navigating the Ultra ICE catheter and neutrally placing the transducer into the superior vena cava, and subsequently withdrawing them as a unit through the body of the right atrium toward the inferior vena cava. The axial transducer orientation will be in the horizontal plane of the body and in the short axis of the right atrium. In order to appropriately display the image in an MR imaging orientation, two specific anatomic landmarks have to be used. The first one is the crista terminalis, which appears as a bright and thick structure located at the junction between the posterior smooth wall and the anterolateral trabeculated portion of the right atrium. The second one is the right atrial auricle, which is defined as a large 'Snoopy's nose-like' structure.

During the intracardiac ultrasound interrogation, the scan section has to be rotated electronically in order to display the right atrial auricle at 12 o'clock and crista terminalis at 10 o'clock on the screen (Table 5.3). This is an essential step when interrogating the cardiac structure by ICE: so, the left-sided structures will be displayed to the viewer's right and right-sided structures to the viewer's left, whereas the anterior-sided structures to the top of the screen and the posterior-sided structures to the bottom of the screen. This orientation of the image is similar to the MR view of the

Table 5.3 *Anatomic landmarks and their spatial orientation*

Structures	Scan plan	Orientation (hour)
Aortic root	Great vessels	2:00
SVC	Great vessels	9:00
Right PA	Great vessels	6:00
Crista terminalis	SVC–RA junction	10:00
Right auricle	SVC–RA junction	12:00

SVC, superior vena cava; RA, right atrium; PA, pulmonary artery.

Table 5.4 *Great vessels axial plane: interrogated structures*

Right superior pulmonary vein
Superior vena cava
Ascending aorta
Right pulmonary artery branch
Pulmonary trunk
Transverse pericardial sinus

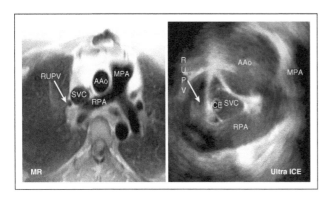

Figure 5.5
Great vessels axial plane: the Ultra ICE catheter is neutrally placed in the center of the superior vena cava and parallel to its long axis, with the transducer positioned between the 5–6° intervertebral disks of the thoracic spine, in order to achieve an ideal perpendicular angle of incidence of the ultrasound beam to the vessel wall. SVC, superior vena cava; RUPV, right upper pulmonary vein; RPA, right pulmonary artery; AAo, ascending aorta; MPA, mean pulmonary artery; ICE, intracardiac echocardiography probe.

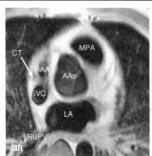
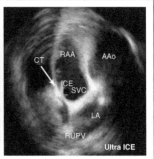

Figure 5.6
Superior vena cava–right atrium junction axial plane: the Ultra ICE catheter is neutrally positioned at the body of the 6° intervertebral disk of the thoracic spine. SVC, superior vena cava; RAA, right atrial auricle; CT, crista terminalis; RUPV, right upper pulmonary vein; AAo, ascending aorta; MPA, mean pulmonary artery; ICE: intracardiac echocardiography probe.

cardiac morphology and has never been used in the history of echocardiography until now.

Great vessels axial plane

The axial view of the great vessels is recorded with the catheter neutrally placed in the center of the superior vena cava and parallel to its long axis, with the transducer positioned between the 5–6° intervertebral disks of the thoracic spine, in order to achieve an ideal perpendicular angle of incidence of the ultrasound beam to the vessel wall (Figure 5.5). Note that, even though technique and image magnification of near and far fields differ, MR and Ultra ICE images are shown with same orientation: left-sided structures at the operator's right, anterior-sided structures at the top of the image, and so on.

The Ultra ICE axial view on the great vessels plane allows visualization of the superior vena cava, ascending aorta, and right upper pulmonary vein in their short axis, whereas the right pulmonary artery is cut on its long axis. The right ventricular outflow tract, pulmonary trunk, and left pulmonary artery are not clearly imaged due to poor lateral resolution in the far field, and they pass anterior and leftward to the aorta (Table 5.4).

On the great vessels view it is possible to evaluate the spatial orientation of the great arteries as well as to visualize the ascending aortic (enlargement, dissection) and the proximal right pulmonary branch (clot) pathologies. Moreover, the high connection pattern of partial anomalous pulmonary venous drainage may be easily identified by Ultra ICE.

Superior vena cava–right atrium junction axial plane

The axial view of the superior vena cava–right atrium junction plane is recorded by minimal withdrawal of the catheter, with the transducer neutrally positioned at the body of the 6° intervertebral disk of the thoracic spine (Figure 5.6). On the superior vena cava–right atrium junction plane, the Ultra ICE allows visualization of the right atrial auricle, crista terminalis, left atrium with right upper pulmonary veins inlet, and ascending aorta (Table 5.5).

Table 5.5	*Superior vena cava–right atrium junction axial plane: interrogated structures*

Right auricle
Superior vena cava
Crista terminalis
Ascending aorta
Left atrium
Pulmonary trunk
Right superior pulmonary vein drainage in left atrium

Table 5.6	*Aortic valve axial plane: interrogated structures*

Right atrium
Aortic valve
Left atrium
Interatrial septum:
   fossa ovalis
   superior–anterior rim
   inferior–posterior rim

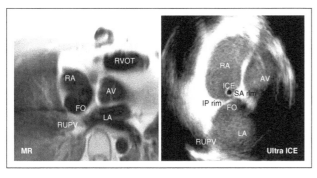

Figure 5.7
Aortic valve axial plane: the Ultra ICE catheter is positioned between the 6–7° intervertebral disks of the thoracic spine. The aortic valve is viewed in its short axis astride the right and left atria, whereas the atrial septum is transversally scanned in its entirety and the fossa ovalis with its superior–anterior and inferior–posterior rims may be well appreciated. RA, right atrium; AV, aortic valve; LA, left atrium; RUPV, right upper pulmonary vein; FO, fossa ovalis; SA rim, superior–anterior rim; IP rim, inferior–posterior rim; ICE, intracardiac echocardiography probe.

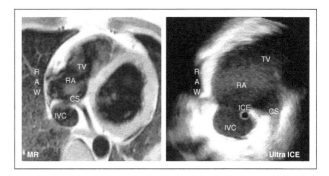

Figure 5.8
Cavo-tricuspid isthmus axial plane: the Ultra ICE catheter is positioned at the level of the body of the 8° intervertebral disk of the thoracic spine. On this plane it is possible to visualize the right lateral wall, inferior vena cava, Eustachian valve, ostium of the coronary sinus, tricuspid annulus, and tricuspid valve. RA, right atrium; TV, tricuspid valve; RAW, right atrial wall; CS, coronary sinus; IVC, inferior vena cava; ICE, intracardiac echocardiography probe.

The usefulness of the superior vena cava–right atrium junction axial plane is in evaluating the motion characteristics of the right atrial auricle, in determining the presence of intra-atrial masses and in identifying the crista terminalis. Moreover, the low connection pattern of partial anomalous pulmonary venous drainage is easy to identify on this plane.

Aortic valve axial plane

A further caudal pullback of the catheter into the right atrium with the transducer positioned between the 6–7° intervertebral disk of the thoracic spine facilitates the axial view of the aortic valve plane (Figure 5.7). The aortic valve is viewed in its short axis astride the right and left atria; the atrial septum is transversally scanned in its entirety and the fossa ovalis with its superior–anterior and inferior–posterior rims may be well appreciated (Table 5.6).

The aortic valve view is crucial in determining aortic valve abnormalities, in evaluating the origin of the right and left coronary ostium, and in providing qualitative and quantitative assessments of the atrial septum and its abnormalities (secundum atrial septal defect, patent foramen ovale, atrial septal aneurysm). In the area of the atrial septum, the fossa ovalis is qualitatively identifiable as a distinct component of the atrial septum characterized by a thin membranous region within a thicker muscular septum. Moreover, some useful parameters may be quantitatively measured, such as the systolic and diastolic transverse atrial septal diameters, the dimensions of the atrial septal defect and fossa ovalis, and the fossa ovalis distances to the inlet of the inferior vena cava (inferior–posterior rim) or to the outer aortic wall (superior–anterior rim).

Cavo-tricuspid isthmus axial plane

The inferior vena cava–right atrium junction plane is reached by further caudal withdrawal of the catheter with the transducer positioned at the level of the body of the 8° intervertebral disk of the thoracic spine (Figure 5.8). On this plane it is possible to visualize the right lateral wall, inferior vena cava, Eustachian valve, ostium of the coronary sinus with Thebesian valve, tricuspid annulus, and tricuspid valve (Table 5.7).

Table 5.7	*Cavo-tricuspid isthmus axial plane: interrogated structures*
Right atrium	
Antero-lateral right atrium parietal wall	
Inferior vena cava	
Eustachian valve	
Cavo-tricuspid isthmus	
Coronary sinus	
Tricuspid annulus	
Kock's triangle	

The cavo-tricuspid isthmus plane is frequently used during radiofrequency ablation procedures in order to perform catheterization of the coronary sinus and to identify the location and the boundaries of the Koch's right triangle with its apex pointing up. Moreover, the Ultra ICE is able to clearly elucidate the morphologic developmental deficiency that underlies the inferior vena cava types of sinus venosus defect.

Intracardiac echocardiographic parasagittal view

Long-axis four-chamber plane

The long-axis view is obtained with a 55° precurved introducer sheath advanced up to the end of the catheter and turned posterior and leftward, to longitudinally scan the atrial septum (Figure 5.9). The transducer orientation will be in the long axis of the body and oblique to the long axis of the heart. The resultant image replicates a truncated apex-up four-chamber view, without the need of image reorientation. Thus, the examiner can potentially make a transition from a transverse to a longitudinal plane without realizing the need to change the imaging orientation. Two precautions will help to avoid this problem: firstly, pay strict attention not to modify the position of the motor drive unit that interfaces between the imaging console and the Ultra ICE catheter; secondly, use the precurved long sheath to rotate the Ultra ICE catheter in order to maintain an optimal performance between the transducer and the drive shaft.

On this plane, it is possible to visualize the right and left atria, right and left atrial auricles, tricuspid and mitral valves, and the descending aorta. Moreover, the atrial septum is longitudinally scanned and the fossa ovalis with its inferior–anterior and superior–posterior rims can be well appreciated (Table 5.8). Ostium primum and ostium secundum atrial septal defects may be predictably appreciated with an optimized long-axis four-chamber view. The systolic and diastolic longitudinal atrial septal diameters, the dimensions of the atrial septal defect and fossa ovalis, and

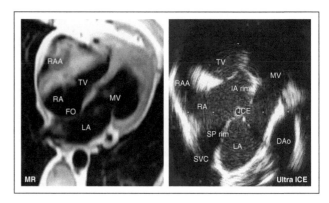

Figure 5.9
Long-axis four-chamber plane: the long-axis view is obtained with a 55° precurved introducer sheath advanced up to the end of the catheter and turned posterior and leftward, to longitudinally scan the atrial septum. On this plane, it is possible to visualize the right and left atria, right and left atrial auricles, tricuspid and mitral valves, and the descending aorta. Moreover, the atrial septum is longitudinally scanned and the fossa ovalis with its inferior–anterior and superior–posterior rims can be well appreciated. SVC, superior vena cava; RA, right atrium; RAA, right atrial auricle; FO, fossa ovalis; TV, tricuspid valve; MV, mitral valve; LA, left atrium; DAo, descending aorta; SP rim, superior–posterior rim; IA rim, inferior–anterior rim; ICE, intracardiac echocardiography probe.

Table 5.8	*Long-axis four-chamber parasagittal plane: interrogated structures*
Right and left atria	
Tricuspid and mitral valves	
Atrioventricular junction	
Interatrial septum:	
fossa ovalis	
inferior–anterior rim	
superior–posterior rim	

the fossa ovalis distances to the inlet of the inferior vena cava (inferior–posterior rim), as well as the coronary sinus or atrioventricular junction (inferior–anterior rim), may be measured accurately. Finally, abnormalities such as atrial septal aneurysm and lipomatous hypertrophy of the atrial septum may be readily detected on this section by Ultra ICE.

Current uses of Ultra ICE in the cardiac catheterization laboratory

The applications of Ultra ICE in the cardiac catheterization laboratory consist in monitoring and guiding catheter-based

Table 5.9 *Main applications of Ultra ICE consist in (a) monitoring and guiding catheter-based interventional procedures and (b) diagnosing associated atrial septal abnormalities*

Catheter-based interventional procedures
- Ostium secundum atrial septal defect
- Patent foramen ovale with/without atrial septal aneurysm

Associated atrial septal abnormalities
- Ostium primum atrial septal defect
- Sinus venosus defects
- Right-sided partial anomalous pulmonary venous drainage
- Lipomatous hypertrophy of the atrial septum

closure of atrial septal defect and patent foramen ovale with or without atrial septal aneurysm as well as in diagnosing associated atrial septal abnormalities (Table 5.9).

The pivotal roles of Ultra ICE during catheter-based procedures are the following:

1. Ultra ICE can distinguish between the septum primum (low echo signal intensity) and the septum secundum (high signal intensity), whereas on transesophageal ultrasound these structures are of similar echogenicity
2. it can be helpful to confirm the presence of additional structural anomalies such as partial anomalous drainage of pulmonary veins
3. it can be used to evaluate the spatial relationship of the atrial septal defect with other structures such as the aorta, superior and inferior caval veins, coronary sinus, mitral and tricuspid valves
4. it allows morphometric evaluation of the atrial septal defect directly rather than using indirect measurements of a balloon catheter.

The most accepted and frequently used methods for selection of the atrial septal defect occluder and its deployment are the balloon-sizing maneuver[13,14] and transesophageal echocardiographic monitoring.[15] Although transesophageal echocardiography and balloon sizing have been shown to represent important requirements for a successful procedure, their positive predictive accuracy and specificity are low.[16–18] Moreover, both these methods have drawbacks: in particular, balloon sizing can give inaccurate measurements causing possible over- or underestimation of occluder size; it can also cause septum primum membrane damage, eventually enlarging the defect.[19] Transesophageal echocardiography usually requires general anesthesia with/without endotracheal intubation. Furthermore, aspiration, airway obstruction, esophageal perforation, and vocal cord dysfunction have been reported, although infrequently.[20,21] Finally, the esophageal probe is usually not well tolerated by the patient.

On the other hand, Ultra ICE facilitates the monitoring and guiding of catheter closure of atrial septal defect and

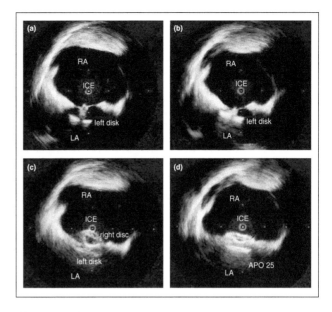

Figure 5.10
Ultra ICE permits an optimal monitoring of the different steps of patent foramen ovale catheter closure in the *parasagittal* view on the four-chamber plane. (a) Left disk opening of the Amplazter PFO occluder 25 mm (APO 25); (b) left disk of APO toward the atrial septum; (c) right disk opening of APO 25; (d) device correctly implanted. RA, right atrium; LA, left atrium; ICE, intracardiac echocardiography probe.

patent foramen ovale (Figure 5.10), thus eliminating the cumbersome balloon-sizing maneuver and the need for general anesthesia or deep sedation during transesophageal echocardiographic monitoring.

Indeed, in the cardiac catheterization laboratory Ultra ICE permits a proper measurement of the septal defect size (major and minor axis of the fossa ovalis, rim length) and an appropriately sized device selection, simply using two standardized orthogonal views (the *axial* view on the aortic valve plane and the *parasagittal* view on the four-chamber plane) (Table 5.6 and 5.8, Figure 5.11). Finally, the selection of the appropriate size of the Amplatzer Septal Occluder™ (ASO) device can be easily achieved using a mathematical formula available in a simple software program.[22] In all patients of our series with atrial septal defects, we were able to obtain high quality images of the atrial septum, which allowed us to measure the size of the defect and to visualize more clearly the occluder during the different stages of the closure procedure[23] (Figure 5.12).

To sum up briefly, the main advantages of Ultra ICE during catheter-based procedures are:

1. appropriate selection of type and size of the device, avoiding the balloon-sizing maneuver
2. optimal monitoring of device deployment, mainly because of its ability to provide images at 360° reconstruction

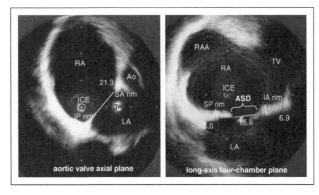

Figure 5.11
Two standardized orthogonal views, the *axial* view on the aortic valve plane and the *parasagittal* view on the four-chamber plane, are used during catheter atrial septal defect (ASD) closure to provide quantitative and qualitative information for proper occluder device size selection. RA, right atrium; TV, tricuspid valve; LA, left atrium; Ao, aortic valve; SA rim, superior–anterior rim; IP rim, inferior–posterior rim; SP rim, superior–posterior rim; IA rim, inferior–anterior rim; RAA, right atrial auricle; ICE, intracardiac echocardiography probe.

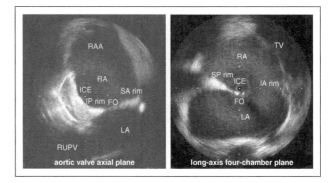

Figure 5.13
Ultra ICE can properly document the *ostium primum atrial septal defect* in the presence of developmental deficiency of the inferior–anterior rim on the long-axis four-chamber plane. RA, right atrium; RAA, right atrial auricle; FO, fossa ovalis; TV, tricuspid valve; LA, left atrium; RUPV, right upper pulmonary vein; SP rim, superior–posterior rim; IA rim, inferior–anterior rim; SA rim, superior–anterior rim; IP rim, inferior–posterior rim; ICE, intracardiac echocardiography probe.

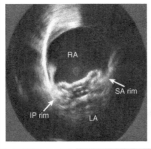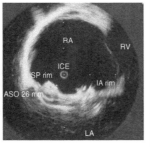

Figure 5.12
Ultra ICE is able to clearly visualize an Amplatzer Septal Occluder (ASO) device implanted. The occluder device is seen in both orthogonal views: on the left, the *axial* view on the aortic valve plane, and on the right, the *parasagittal* view on the four-chamber plane. RA, right atrium; LA, left atrium; RV, right ventricle; SP rim, superior–posterior rim; IA rim, inferior–anterior rim; SA rim, superior–anterior rim; IP rim, inferior–posterior rim; ICE, intracardiac echocardiography probe.

3. good tolerance by the patient for a relatively prolonged time period
4. ease of performance (single operator)
5. limited fluoroscopic exposure time.

The major drawbacks are:

1. no color-Doppler capability
2. additional costs (dedicated review stations and disposable catheter).

Moreover, mechanical interrogation of intracardiac structures can be useful in diagnosing other atrial septal abnormalities that represent contraindications to interventional procedures.

Atrial septal aneurysm (ASA) is a well-recognized cardiac abnormality of uncertain clinical significance. It is rarely present as an isolated lesion (so-called 'lone' ASA),[24] whereas it is usually associated with congenital or acquired heart disease.[25] The ICE definition of ASA agrees entirely with transthoracic (TT) and transesophageal echocardiographic (TEE) criteria previously published by Hanley et al:[26] diameter of the base of the aneurysmal portion of the atrial septum measuring ≥ 15 mm, bulging of the atrial septum or fossa ovalis ≥ 15 mm, and phasic excursion of the atrial septum or fossa ovalis during the cardiorespiratory cycle ≥ 15 mm in total amplitude. The major advantages of ICE over TEE are the larger field view and the superior soft-tissue contrast, allowing for an easy and precise evaluation of ASA.

The *ostium primum atrial septal defect* can be clearly identified in the presence of developmental deficiency of the inferior–anterior rim on the long-axis four-chamber plane, that underlines that this malformation involves the atrio-ventricular canal (Figure 5.13).

The superior and inferior vena cava types of *sinus venosus defect* are shown unequivocally by Ultra ICE; in fact, mechanical ultrasound interrogation may clearly underline that the interatrial communications are outside the confines of the fossa ovalis, with the mouths of the superior or inferior vena cava having biatrial connection and overriding the intact superior–posterior or inferior–posterior muscular borders of the fossa ovalis, respectively.

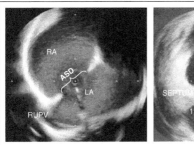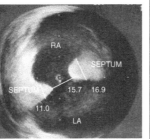

Figure 5.14

Ultra ICE can identify massive fatty deposits in the secundum atrial septum and a septum secundum ≥ 15 mm thick. On the left, an atrial septal defect (ASD) with normal septum secundum; on the right, a case of lipomatous hypertrophy of the atrial septum. RA, right atrium; RUPV, right upper pulmonary vein; LA, left atrium.

Moreover, the *right-sided partial anomalous pulmonary venous drainage* can be diagnosed as a 'drop-out' (high connection pattern) or a 'tear-drop' (low connection pattern) appearance of the superior vena cava on the great vessels plane or on the superior vena cava–right atrial junction plane, respectively.

Finally, the *lipomatous hypertrophy of the atrial septum*, characterized by massive fatty deposits in the secundum atrial septum and a septum secundum ≥ 15 mm thick, can be differentiated from myxoma, thrombus, or tumors[27] (Figure 5.14).

When this condition is associated with atrial septal defect, it must be considered a contraindication to all catheter-based closure procedures due to the impossibility of achieving a correct device deployment, independent of the closure systems. Lesser degrees of atrial septal hypertrophy, between 6 and 14 mm, represent a more common condition, especially in patients with high blood pressure, and in obese and elderly female patients, and are relative contraindications.

Other applications of Ultra ICE

Other current applications of Ultra ICE involve interventional electrophysiologic procedures, cardiac biopsy, assessment of procedural complications, transseptal puncture, and monitoring of endovascular thoracic and abdominal aortic aneurysm repair (Table 5.10).

The following *electrophysiologic procedures* are clearly monitored by Ultra ICE:

- radiofrequency catheter ablation of the superior portion of the sinus junction in inappropriate sinus tachycardia[6]

Table 5.10 *Other current applications of Ultra ICE*
• Interventional electrophysiology
• Cardiac biopsy
• Transseptal puncture
• Procedural complications assessment
• Thoracic and abdominal aortic endoprosthetic procedures monitoring

- radiofrequency catheter ablation of the slow posterior pathway in atrioventricular nodal reentrant tachycardia[28]
- radiofrequency catheter ablation of the crista terminalis in ectopic right atrial tachycardia[29]
- radiofrequency catheter ablation of the cavo-tricuspid isthmus in atrial flutter.

The most useful Ultra ICE plane during radiofrequency ablation procedures is the axial cavo-tricuspid isthmus plane, because it allows anatomic details to be obtained in order to perform catheterization of the coronary sinus and to identify the location and the boundaries of the Koch's triangle.

Cardiac biopsy, particularly in high risk cases in which abnormal tissue is adjacent to thin walls or delicate structures, can be facilitated using Ultra ICE guidance. It allows exact delineation of tumor tissue, enabling the operator to guide the bioptome and avoiding inadvertent damage to thin atrial or ventricular walls or valve apparatus.

Another useful application of Ultra ICE is in safely and effectively assisting *transseptal puncture* of the septum primum, showing the tip of Mullins transseptal sheath and the Brockenbrough needle seated against the middle of the fossa ovalis, causing a slight 'tenting effect'.

Moreover, Ultra ICE permits early recognition of *procedural complications* by continuous monitoring of the pericardial space, allowing diagnosis and treatment of cardiac perforation and tamponade. In fact, both acquired and iatrogenic pericardial effusion may be detected as an echo-free space outside the right atrial free wall, whereas the bright parietal echo signal may be seen intermittently, depending on the size of the effusion (Figure 5.15).

Finally, during *vascular endoprosthesis implantation* at the thoracic or subrenal aortic level, the mechanical probe may be used to provide an exact evaluation of the lesion and to ensure that the expansion of the endograft is complete and symmetric. The echographic examination with a mechanical transducer is particularly useful for two main reasons: first, to confirm the aortic pathology and the previous morphometric evaluation obtained by computed tomography or magnetic resonance; secondly, to determine the complete and symmetric expansion of the

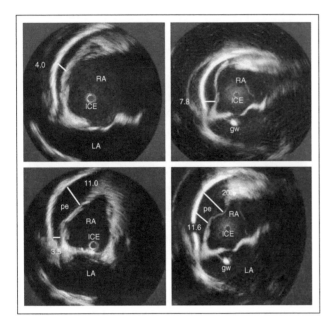

Figure 5.15
Ultra ICE permits continuous monitoring of the pericardial space, allowing diagnosis of cardiac perforation and tamponade. The pericardial effusion may be detected as an echo-free space outside the right atrial free wall. RA, right atrium; LA, left atrium; pe, pericardial effusion; gw, guidewire; ICE, intracardiac echocardiography probe.

endoprosthesis struts, in order to reduce the risk of acute and subacute graft occlusion.[30]

Conclusions

Two-dimensional ICE is the newest advance in ultrasound technologies and we believe that the important question is not whether conventional echocardiography, cardiac MR imaging, or ICE is the globally superior technique for imaging analysis, but rather how to best utilize imaging technologies to provide optimal benefit in specific clinical situations.

The major effects of Ultra ICE technology are:

1. a 100% duty cycle combining imaging of cardiac anatomy and interventional systems, in the sense that images are continuously available during all the stages of catheter-based procedures, allowing not only immediate pre- and post-imaging of the procedure, but also vision-guided and sophisticated monitoring of the interventions
2. a high spatial resolution, no acoustic barriers or interference from irregular cardiac and respiratory cycles
3. excellent soft tissue contrasting capabilities and the ability to image cardiac structures deep within the heart

4. ease of obtaining specific tomographic views, generally less operator dependent and considerably less operator dexterity related than transthoracic or transesophageal echocardiography, and
5. effective manipulation of the Ultra ICE catheter by means of a precurved long sheath and rotation of the transducer to critically optimize an image-specific orientation.

These advantages are governed by a short distance of interrogated tissue from the transducer and a relatively homogeneous fluid path due to the uniform, omni-directional backscatter of the red cells. This image quality and wealth of information dramatically reduce examination time and render Ultra ICE a valuable tool, not only for diagnosis but also for *in-vivo* morphometry. However, a thorough understanding of the tomographic imaging from the inner confines of the right atrium and great veins requires anatomic and radiologic identification and validation for a rapid feedback and a reliable study.

Limitations which still exist and features which may limit the optimal use of a mechanical array technology include:

1. relatively large delivering Ultra ICE catheter
2. potentially overall increased cost of interventional procedures due to the need for a dedicated system and disposable catheter
3. abrupt transitions from the transverse to the longitudinal plane
4. lack of Doppler hemodynamic and parametric capabilities, and
5. inadequate depth penetration for imaging the pulmonary artery trunk and the ventricles with the catheter positioned in the right atrium.

The major clinical application of the Ultra ICE, in our opinion, is facilitating the catheter-based interventional procedures, and Ultra ICE should contribute to the pediatric and adult cardiology arsenal for both diagnostic and therapeutic procedures, because the catheter can remain in place for the entire procedure with excellent patient tolerance, discovering a new imaging modality (seeing and treating) to sophisticated interventions.

Obviously, the minimum requirements for the performance and interpretation of intracardiac ultrasound should satisfy the general principles of the American College of Cardiology/American Heart Association clinical competence statement on echocardiography,[31] that include:

1. skills in inserting and manipulating the catheter to obtain the required views
2. knowledge of the physical principles of the echocardiographic image and instrument settings, and finally
3. knowledge of the anatomy, physiology, and pathology of the heart and great vessels.

References

1. Mitchel JF, Gillam LD, Sanzobrino BW et al. Intracardiac ultrasound imaging during transseptal catheterization. Chest 1995; 108: 104–8.
2. Epstein LM, Smith I, Tenhoff H. Non fluoroscopic transseptal catheterization: safety and efficacy of intacardiac echocardiographic guidance. J Cardiovasc Electrophysiol 1998; 9: 625–30.
3. Mangrum JM, Mounsey JP, Kok LC et al. Intracardiac echocardiography-guided, anatomically based radiofrequency ablation of focal atrial fibrillation originating from pulmonary veins. J Am Coll Cardiol 2002; 39: 1964–72.
4. Johnson SB, Seward JB, Packer DL. Phased–array intracardiac echocardiography for guiding transseptal catheter placement: utility and learning curve. Pacing Clin Electrophysiol 2002; 25: 402–7.
5. Hung JS, Fu M, Yeh KH et al. Usefulness of intracardiac echocardiography in complex trans-septal catheterization during percutaneous transvenous mitral commissurotomy. Mayo Clin Proc 1996; 71: 134–40.
6. Chu E, Kalman JM, Kwasman MA et al. Intracardiac echocardiography during radiofrequency catheter ablation of cardiac arrythmias in humans. J Am Coll Cardiol 1994; 24: 1351–7.
7. Kalman JM, Olgin JE, Karch MR, Lesh MD. Use of intracardiac echocardiography in interventional electrophysiology. Pacing Clin Electrophysiol 1997; 20: 2248–62.
8. Olgin JE, Kalman JM, Chin M et al. Electrophysiological effects of long, linear atrial lesions placed under intracardiac ultrasound guidance. Circulation 1997; 96: 2715–21.
9. Hijazi ZM, Wang Z, Cao Q et al. Transcatheter closure of atrial septal defects and patent foramen ovale under intracardiac echocardiographic guidance: feasibility and comparison with transesophageal echocardiography. Cathet Cardiovasc Interven 2001; 52: 194–9.
10. Jan SL, Hwang B, Lee PC et al. Intracardiac ultrasound assessment of atrial septal defect: comparison with transthoracic echocardiographic, angiocardiographic, and balloon-sizing measurements. Cardiovasc Interven Radiol 2001; 24: 84–9.
11. Zanchetta M, Pedon L, Rigatelli G et al. Intracardiac echocardiography evaluation in secundum atrial septal defect transcatheter closure. Cardiovasc Interven Radiol 2003; 26: 52–7.
12. Zanchetta M, Rigatelli G, Onorato E. Intracardiac echocardiography and transcranial Doppler ultrasound to guide closure of patent foramen ovale. J Invas Cardiol 2003; 15: 93–6.
13. King TD, Thompson SL, Mills NL. Measurements of the atrial septal defect during cardiac catheterization. Experimental and clinical results. Am J Cardiol 1978; 41: 41–2.
14. Hijazi ZM, Cao Q, Patel HT et al. Transesophageal echocardiographic results of catheter closure of atrial septal defect in children and adults using the Amplatzer devices. Am J Cardiol 2000; 85: 1387–90.
15. Masura J, Gavora P, Formanek A, Hijazi ZM. Transcatheter closure of secundum atrial septal defects using the new self-centering Amplatzer Septal Occluder. Cathet Cardiovasc Diagn 1997; 42: 388–93.
16. Hellenbrand WE, Fahey JT, McGowan FX et al. Transe sophageal echocardiographic guidance of transcatheter closure of atrial septal defect. Am J Cardiol 1990; 66: 207–13.
17. Metha RH, Helmcke F, Nanda NC et al. Uses and limitations of transthoracic echocardiography in the assessment of atrial septal defect in the adult. Am J Cardiol 1991; 67: 288–94.
18. Godart F, Rey C, Francart C et al. Two-dimensional echocardiographic and color Doppler measurements of atrial septal defect, and comparison with the balloon-stretched diameter. Am J Cardiol 1993; 72: 1095–7.
19. Lee CH, Kwok OH, Chow WH. Pittfalls of atrial septal defect using medictech sizing balloon. Cathet Cardiovasc Interven 2001; 53: 94–5.
20. Daniel WG, Erbel R, Kasper QW et al. Safety of transesophageal echocardiography. A multicenter survey of 10 419 examinations. Circulation 1991; 83: 817–21.
21. Urbanowicz JH, Kernoff RS, Oppenheim G et al. Transesophageal echocardiography and its potential for esophageal damage. Anesthesiology 1990; 72: 40–3.
22. Zanchetta M, Onorato E, Rigatelli G et al. Intracardiac echocardiography-guided transcatheter closure of secundum atrial septal defect. A new efficient device selection method. J Am Coll Cardiol 2003; 42: 1677–82.
23. Zanchetta M, Rigatelli G, Pedon L et al. Transcatheter atrial septal defect closure assisted by intracardiac echocardiography: 3-year follow-up. J Interv Cardiol 2004; 17(2): 95–8.
24. Lazar AV, Pechacek LW, Mihalick MJ et al. Aneurysm of the interatrial septum occurring as an isolated anomaly. Cathet Cardiovasc Diagn 1983; 9: 167–73.
25. Mugge A, Daniel WG, Angermann C et al. Atrial septal aneurysm in adult patients. A multicenter study using transthoracic and transesophageal echocardiography. Circulation 1995; 91: 2785–92.
26. Hanley PC, Tajik AJ, Hynes JK et al. Diagnosis and classification of atrial septal aneurysm by two-dimensional echocardiography: report of 80 consecutive cases. J Am Coll Cardiol 1985; 6: 1370–82.
27. Levine RA, Weyman AE, Dinsmore RE et al. Non-invasive tissue characterization: diagnosis of lipomatous hypertrophy of the atrial septum by nuclear magnetic resonance imaging. J Am Coll Cardiol 1986; 7: 688–92.
28. Fisher WG, Pelini MA, Bacon ME. Adjunctive intracardiac echocardiography to guide slow pathway ablation in human atrioventricular nodal reentrant tachycardia: anatomic insights. Circulation 1997; 96: 3021–9.
29. Kalman JM, Olgin JE, Karch MR et al. Crystal tachycardias: origin of right atrial tachycardias from the crista terminalis identified by intracardiac echocardiography. J Am Coll Cardiol 1998; 31: 451–9.
30. Zanchetta M, Rigatelli GL, Pedon L et al. IVUS guidance of thoracic and complex abdominal aortic aneurysm stent-graft repairs using an intracardiac echocardiography probe: preliminary report. J Endovasc Ther 2003; 10: 218–26.
31. Quinones MA, Douglas PS, Foster E et al. ACC/AHA clinical competence statement on echocardiography: a report of the American College of Cardiology/American Heart Association/American College of Physicians–American Society of Internal Medicine Task Force on clinical competence. J Am Soc Echocardiogr 2003; 16: 379–402.

6

Three-dimensional echocardiography: present and future applications in the catheterization laboratory

Gerald R Marx, Wayne Tworetzky, and Audrey Marshall

Introduction

Certainly, more than two decades of successful diagnostic interventional cardiology have been experienced in catheterization laboratories throughout the world. Imaging for such procedures has been based on two-dimensional (2D) views, often in a singular plane, be it fluoroscopy, angiography, or echocardiography. Hence, one might maintain that three-dimensional (3D) imaging would provide little additional information to aid the interventionalist. On the other hand, one might argue that additional information might be very important for the more difficult or unusual cases. Additionally, in as much as interventional catheterization occurs in a 3D space, the associated imaging should provide a 3D perspective for the interventional cardiologist. Hence, 3D imaging might reduce the time of the procedure, the time for fluoroscopy, and the occurrence of unexpected deleterious outcomes. Furthermore, 3D imaging might provide important additional information to determine the outcomes of the interventional procedure, either for the individual or for large population studies.

Although reports on the clinical application of 3D echocardiography for cardiac catheterization or interventional procedures have been written,[1–9] to date such imaging has not been widely accepted in most catheterization laboratories. However, with very significant recent improvements in technology, 3D echocardiography will become more widely applied for interventional cardiology. This will include pre-selection of patients for interventional procedures, imaging during the intervention, and follow-up and assessment of the procedure itself.

Instrumentation

Perhaps the major impediment to the application of 3D echocardiography to cardiac catheterization was the significant time required to acquire the 3D images, post-process, and then render the digital data information into a usable 3D display. Several years ago, one of the most widely employed 3D echocardiographic methods employed the sequential acquisition of 2D images, with gating for spatial and temporal alignment.[1] Depending on the patient's heart rate, the acquisition time was from 3 to 5 minutes. Most acquisitions were done with a rotational transesophageal echocardiographic probe.[1] Once the images were acquired over a 180° arc, they had to be post-processed into a volume digital data set. This would require a minimum of 3 to 5 minutes. Last, the data sets could then be segmented, rotated, and cropped to obtain the required views. However, this rendering did not provide for on-line feedback of the ultimate 3D images, and hence would again require significant additional time. These limitations were quite obvious for the person performing the cardiac catheterization. Although excellent images could be obtained, the use of the transesophageal approach naturally limited the application. Although transthoracic rotational probes were developed, obviating a transesophageal approach, such image acquisition was limited by less than optimal image quality. Despite the inherent difficulties with this mode of 3D echocardiographic acquisition, this set the framework for 3D echocardiography for catheterization based echocardiographic procedures.

The development of a matrix array transducer, together with the increased sophistication and power of computer technology, has now allowed for 'real-time' 3D echocardiographic

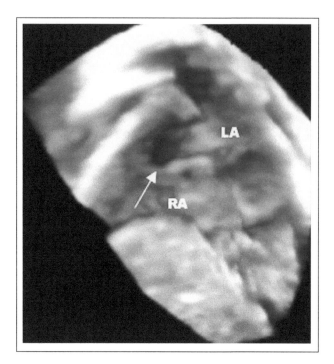

Figure 6.1
Live three-dimensional echocardiogram immediately after balloon atrial septostomy in a newborn with transposition of the great arteries, d-TGA. The arrow shows the enlarged atrial septal defect from a right atrial *en-face* view. LA, left atrium; RA, right atrium.

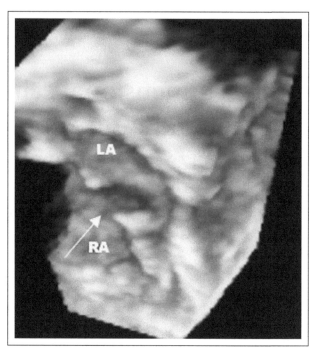

Figure 6.2
Live three-dimensional echocardiogram immediately after balloon atrial septostomy in same newborn as Figure 6.1 with d-TGA. The arrow again shows the enlarged atrial septal defect from the left atrial *en-face* view. LA, left atrium; RA, right atrium.

imaging.[10] The matrix array probe has up to 3000 crystal elements, each individually wired. With parallel processing, and extremely fast computer 'number crunching', a real-time 3D imaging can be obtained immediately (Figure 6.1). This image can be rotated with a track ball, enhancing the 3D echocardiographic effect. The only drawback is that the image display is in a more narrowed sector angle, reducing the 3D echocardiographic field of view. However, this approach can be utilized for immediate 3D display and has been used in our laboratory for such procedures as a balloon atrial septostomy in the cardiac catheterization laboratory (Figures 6.1 and 6.2).

In a different modality using the matrix array transducer, a full digital volume can be acquired by gating over four cardiac cycles. This full volume digital data set can be readily segmented, and the images cropped and rotated with instantaneous feedback, allowing for excellent 3D echocardiographic display (Figure 6.3). Similarly, a 3D echocardiographic color flow jet can be acquired over seven cardiac cycles (Figure 6.4). This new technology has significantly enhanced the application of 3D echocardiography in day-to-day clinical practice. However, to date the matrix array probe is large, with low transmit frequencies, and lower resolution than with standard pediatric transthoracic probes. Additionally, transthoracic imaging is an impediment to standard use in the catheterization laboratory. None-the-less, this modality is increasingly being used for pre-selection of patients, and to evaluate the outcome of patients who have undergone an

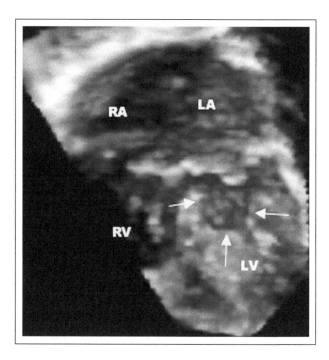

Figure 6.3
Full volume acquired three-dimensional echocardiogram from the left ventricular septal surface demonstrating a very large inlet muscular ventricular septal defect (arrows) in a 3-month-old infant. LA, left atrium; RA, right atrium. LV, left ventricle; RV right ventricle.

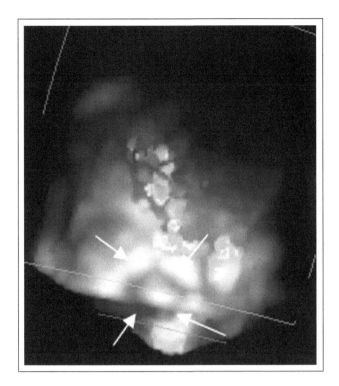

Figure 6.4
Three-dimensional color flow echocardiogram in a 41-year-old woman with a paravalvar leak. The arrows depict the annulus of the prosthetic mitral valve. The specific position of two paravalvar leaks is seen outside the prosthetic mitral valve annulus. (See also color plate section.)

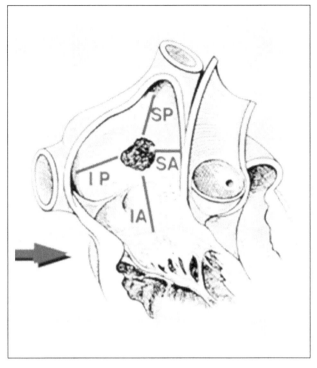

Figure 6.5
Schematic diagram of the atrial septum and rims surrounding a secundum atrial septal defect as seem from a three-dimensional echocardiographic *en-face* view. IA, inferior anterior; IP, inferior posterior; SA, superior anterior; SP, superior posterior.

interventional catheterization procedure. Examples of these applications, including some examples of use during the catheterization procedure, will be discussed below.

Application of three-dimensional echocardiography for selection of patients for catheterization interventions

Two-dimensional echocardiography has been the mainstay in the evaluation of patients prior to device closure of an atrial septal defect. However, despite optimal 2D imaging, selection of certain patients may sometimes be challenging. Three-dimensional imaging provides the opportunity to more fully comprehend the relationship of the atrial septal defect to the other cardiac structures, and better evaluate the surrounding rim tissue necessary to anchor the atrial septal defect device. [1–4,11] Moreover, 3D echocardiographic views provide for a description of such defects as would be best described by an anatomist, as if looking directly at a

heart specimen. Such imaging planes can be obtained either from the left or right atrium. As a frame of reference, the various rims of tissue surrounding the defect can more readily be categorized (Figure 6.5). For example, from a right atrial *en-face* view, the superior–anterior rim is from the defect to the aorta, whereas the inferior–anterior rim would be the distance from the rim towards the tricuspid valve. The superior–posterior rim would be the region from the defect to the superior vena cava, whereas the posterior–inferior rim would be the atrial wall towards the inferior vena caval (IVC) entrance. Such anatomic delineation would help in the communication between the echocardiographers and cardiac interventionalist.

Perhaps the most enigmatic aspect to closing a secundum atrial septal defect is the determination of sufficient rim tissue to anchor the device. This can be difficult to ascertain in 2D planes, since only one discrete region can be visualized at a time. However, 3D imaging can provide a more comprehensive delineation of the entire rim in a single volume data set. Multiple cut planes and projections demonstrate in a comprehensive format the size and shape of the atrial septal defect, the relationship of the defect to various anatomic structures, and the relative size and shape of the right and left atria (Figure 6.6a,b). Another factor that makes device

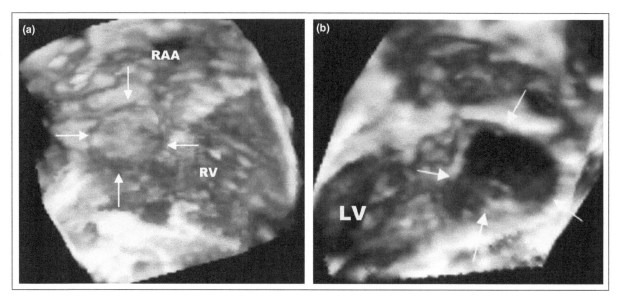

Figure 6.6 (a) and (b)
Three-dimensional echocardiogram in an 18-month-old infant with a large secundum atrial septal defect. Panel (a) shows the exact circumference of the atrial septal deflect (arrows) from a right atrial *en-face* view, and panel (b) is from a left atrial *en-face* view. RAA, right atrial appendage; RV, right ventricle; LV, left ventricle.

closure more challenging is the number and size of additional fenestrations. This can often be difficult to see with standard 2D imaging, even if using color flow Doppler in orthogonal views. Overlapping defects are obscured by large defects in the more proximal imaging plane. Three-dimensional *en-face* views will delineate contiguous defects, that would otherwise be obscured in 2D imaging projections (Figure 6.7).

Similar to atrial septal defects, 3D echocardiography can provide additional anatomic information for patients with muscular ventricular septal defects that are being considered for device closure. Perhaps the most important aspect is that 3D *en-face* planes from the left ventricular side of the interventricular septum can be obtained[12] (Figure 6.3). This will provide a much more comprehensive analysis of muscular ventricular septal defects that, from the right ventricular side, might be hidden behind either tricuspid valve tissue or papillary muscles of the tricuspid valve or by heavy right ventricular trabeculations. Muscular ventricular septal defects are not hidden by either heavy trabeculations or atrio-ventricular valve tissue from the left ventricular *en-face* plane. Furthermore, muscular ventricular septal defects are much easier to delineate against the smooth left ventricular septal wall surface. Although 2D imaging provides excellent imaging of the membranous ventricular septal defect, 3D imaging can provide direct *en-face* views to delineate more precisely the anatomic relationship of the ventricular septal defect to the aorta. Another major consideration for closure of ventricular septal defects is associated prolapse of the aortic valve leaflets. Unique 3D echocardiographic cut planes and projections can provide visualization of a prolapsing valve leaflet that may be difficult to appreciate with standard 2D echocardiography.

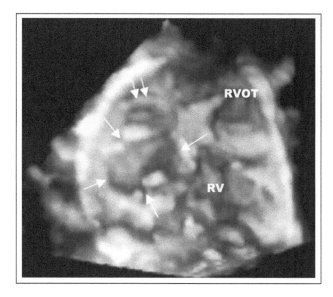

Figure 6.7
Three-dimensional echocardiogram in a 4-year-old child with a large secundum atrial septal defect (single arrows), and an additional small fenestration (double arrows). RV, right ventricle; RVOT, right ventricular outflow tract.

Again, another major subset of patients in whom 3D echocardiography would provide important additional information is those being considered for cardiac catheterization balloon dilation valvuloplasty. Again, similar to closure of atrial and ventricular septal defects, 2D imaging has been very adept in the pre-selection of patients for balloon dilation angioplasties. None-the-less, despite appropriate standard catheterization techniques, the valvar

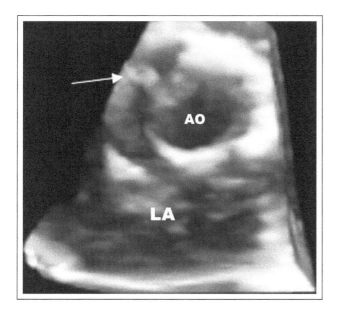

Figure 6.8
Three-dimensional echocardiogram from an 8-year-old boy with
severe aortic stenosis, prior to successful balloon dilation. This
is an *en-face* view from above, during diastole, showing the
thickened raphe (arrow) between the rudimentary right and
non-coronary cusp. AO, aorta; LA, left atrium.

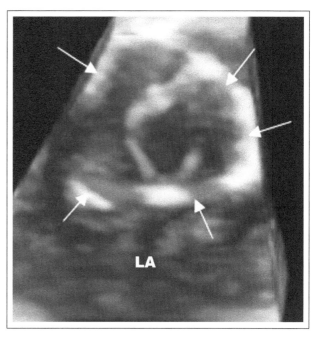

Figure 6.9
Three-dimensional echocardiogram from the same patient as in
Figure 6.8. Again, an image taken from above now during systole,
showing the reduced effective orifice area from the bicommissural
aortic valve. The arrows depict the annulus. LA, left atrium.

gradient may not be reduced despite optimal balloon
dilation. Furthermore, balloon dilation valvuloplasty has
an important associated incidence of development of
regurgitation. Three-dimensional echocardiography may
help in the pre-selection of the appropriate patient, but
more importantly may be utilized to comprehend, in a
global sense, the anatomic characteristics of the valve that
will be amenable to significant gradient reduction, without
causing significant regurgitation.

More specifically, direct *en-face* views of the valve being
considered for dilation can be obtained from both the inferior and superior surfaces.[13–14] Most importantly, 3D imaging
allows depiction of the entire surface area of the leaflets. In
comparison, 2D imaging shows the valve leaflet edges. Again,
with 3D imaging, the areas and not surfaces of coaptation
can be fully assessed in dynamic motion. Regions of commissural fusion can be well depicted (Figure 6.8). Three-dimensional imaging will allow for direct planimetry of the effective
stenotic orifice area[8,15–17] (Figure 6.9). From the orthogonal
cut planes, the crop plane can be placed precisely at the distal
regions of the valve tips, allowing for accurate determination
of the smallest flow area. Three-dimensional color flow
Doppler can be applied for confirmation of the stenotic orifice area. Equally important, 3D imaging allows much more
robust images of color flow valvar regurgitation, prior to consideration for an angioplasty procedure. The true shape and
size of the regurgitant jet widths and vena contracta can be
imaged, again allowing for direct planimetry.

In patients with vessel stenosis undergoing balloon
dilation valvuloplasty, the diameters of the stenotic region
can be depicted from orthogonal 2D imaging planes. With
3D imaging the precise region of stenosis can be placed
within the crop plane, allowing for visualization and subsequent planimetry of the true stenotic circumference. This
advantage of 3D imaging has obvious implications when
the stenotic region has an abnormal shape, and hence the
true circumference cannot be ascertained in a singular or
even dual 2D plane.

Closure of paravalvar leaks has become an extremely
important and successful procedure in the catheterization
laboratory. None-the-less, 2D imaging, either by echocardiography or angiography, can be confusing in analysis of
the relationship of the paravalvar leak to the corresponding
prosthetic valve. Three-dimensional color flow imaging can
provide an anatomic map detailing the paravalvar leak to
the more precise region of the involved valve (Figure 6.4).
Direct *en-face* views can be shown of the valve from the dorsal or ventral surface. The position of the paravalvar leak
can be described in relationship to 360° around a circle, or
hours around a clock face. This is extremely important, in
that often the prosthetic valves are surgically placed in
unconventional positions that do not readily correspond
to the various anatomic planes of the heart. Thus with 3D
echocardiographic imaging, an anatomic 'road map' can
be constructed prior to the catheterization, detailing the
potential catheter course and ultimate device placement,

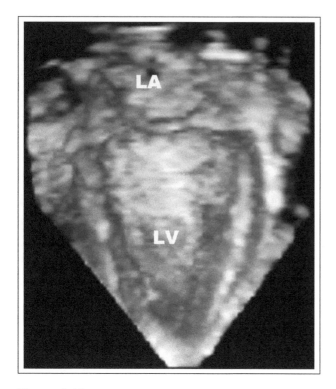

Figure 6.10
Three-dimensional full volume echocardiogram of the left atrium and left ventricle. LA, left atrium; LV, left ventricle.

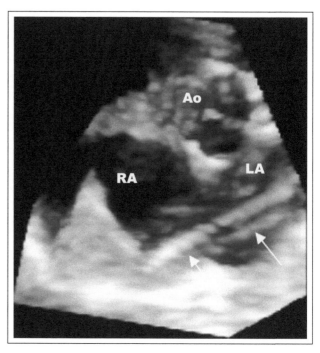

Figure 6.11
Live three-dimensional echocardiogram during deployment of an Amplatzer device for closure of a secundum atrial septal defect. The anatomic position of the sheath (arrows) can be seen in relation to the left atrium. Ao, aorta; LA, left atrium; RA, right atrium.

giving the relationship of the paravalvar leak to the valve itself. To date we have applied 3D echocardiography to a few patients with paravalvar leak, and have found the 3D color flow imaging aided in device closure. Most importantly, such imaging enhanced detailed discussion between the echocardiographers and interventionalist.

In the consideration of pre-selection of patients for interventional procedures and to evaluate the results of the procedure, evaluation of corresponding atrial and ventricular size and function is essential. To date, atrial and ventricular volume analysis has relied on 2D imaging. Obviously, measurements based on 2D imaging relied on assumptions of geometry to which mathematical models were applied. Such assumptions were tenuous for dilated and distorted left ventricles, and even more tenuous for right or single ventricles. Three-dimensional echocardiography has been shown to provide reliable determination of ventricular volumes, mass, and ejection fraction, both in laboratory experiments and clinical studies in human subjects.[18–27] As discussed above, the older technology was laborious, time consuming, and expensive. However, with present day matrix array scanning good results have been obtained comparing left ventricular volume determinations with magnetic resonance imaging studies (Figure 6.10). Adult centers have demonstrated the reliability of matrix array scanning 3D echocardiography to measure left ventricular volumes. Our experience has shown the clinical applicability of 3D echocardiographic analysis of left, right,

and single ventricle volumes and mass in pediatric patients. Preliminary results comparing 3D echocardiographic ventricular volumes to magnetic resonance angiography have show an excellent correlation, with good limits of agreement.

Three-dimensional echocardiography to guide interventional procedures

In a tank model, standard surgical texts were performed faster, and with more precision, with 3D echocardiographic guidance as compared to 2D imaging.[28] This has profound implications for both catheterization and surgical procedures. However, to date, the application of 3D echocardiography during catheter procedures has been limited. In part, this is related to use of the rather large matrix array probe, which can only be applied in the subcostal or transthoracic position, thus potentially interfering with the procedure itself. None-the-less we have had considerable success using real-time 3D echocardiographic imaging to guide balloon atrial septostomy in newborn infants with transposition of the great arteries (Figures 6.1 and 6.2). Visualizing the septostomy balloon in relationship to the left atrium and mitral valve apparatus provides a more comprehensive assessment of the safe position of the catheter prior to the 'pull-back'. Moreover, an

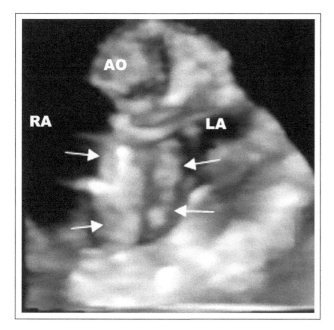

Figure 6.12
Live three-dimensional echocardiogram in the same patients as in Figure 6.11. The position of the left atrial disk to the left atrial septal surface is seen, before deployment of the right atrial disk. AO, aorta; LA, left atrium; RA, right atrium.

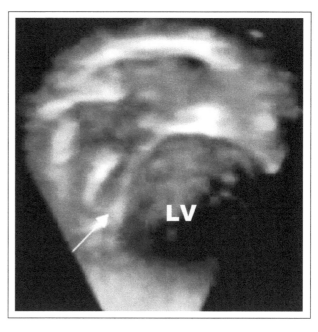

Figure 6.13
Three-dimensional echocardiogram showing the position and placement of a biopsy catheter in relation to the right ventricular free wall. LV, left ventricle.

immediate *en-face* view of the atrial septal defect is available to help determine the efficacy of the procedure.

Preliminary experience has shown the application of 3D echocardiography to guide atrial septal defect device closure at cardiac catheterization (Figure 6.11). A more comprehensive analysis of the spatial relationship of the left atrial disk to both the left atrium as well as the interatrial septum is readily appreciated (Figure 6.12). This may have important implications when choosing the device in a smaller patient with a smaller left atrium. (Obviously with large left to right atrial shunts the left atrium appears smaller with the corresponding larger right atrium.) Care must be taken that the device is not too large to either impinge on the pulmonary veins posteriorly, or the mitral valve anteriorly. In the same volume data set, the relationship of the left atrial disk to the roof of the left atrium can be discerned. This may have important relevance in avoiding the rare but reported incidence of erosion of the disk through the roof of the left atrium, months to years after placement. An appreciation of the spatial alignment of the left atrial disk to the atrial septum is also well appreciated with the live 3D imaging format. The 3D construct with rotation of the imaging plane in multiple projections allows for immediate depiction of the potential for protrusion of a portion of the disk across the atrial septum, before deployment of the right atrial disk. Certainly, 2D echocardiography has been used successfully for many years for this imaging analysis. However, this has required 2D imaging in several different orthogonal planes, with a mental

reconstruction in three dimensions. Although prospective randomized studies have not been performed to compare two- vs three-dimensional echocardiography for atrial septal defect device placement, the potential advantages are intuitively obvious.

Other centers employed 3D echocardiographic imaging to guide intra-endocardial biopsy procedures.[6] Again, with 3D echocardiographic imaging, advancement of the catheter or bioptome can be appreciated in the lateral, elevational, and most importantly the azthmuthal plane (Figure 6.13). Radiofrequency ablation therapy has been associated with development of pulmonary venous obstruction. Three-dimensional echocardiography allows for direct *en-face* imaging of pulmonary veins, and the true size and shape of the orifice can be seen (Figure 6.14). Under 3D echocardiographic guidance, the radiofrequency catheter should be directed away from this anatomic region.

Cardiac resynchronization therapy is becoming increasingly important for the modulation of ventricular shape and function. Three-dimensional echocardiography allows for assessment of simultaneous regional wall function (Figure 6.15). Investigators have reported the changes in regional wall function by 3D echocardiography before and after resynchronization therapy. An ongoing investigation is evaluating the optimal position of biventricular pacing electrodes, and the optimal timing from various pacemaker sites to optimize synchronization of global contraction. As the 3D echocardiographic assessment of regional function becomes more online, such analysis will become applicable

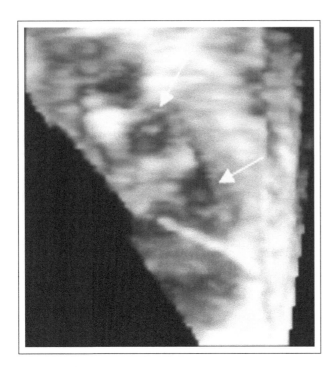

Figure 6.14
Live three-dimensional echocardiogram showing *en-face* views of the orifice of dilated pulmonary veins connecting to the left atrium.

during the procedure. Regardless, such analysis can be applied in pre-selection of patients for the procedure, and to analyze the results of the resynchronization therapy after it has been completed.

Cardiac perforation is an extremely rare event following endomyocardial biopsy. However, in patients who undergo multiple biopsies, damage to the tricuspid valve is becoming a more apparent problem. Again, with 3D echocardiographic imaging, direction of the bioptome away from the tricuspid apparatus should more readily be achieved.

Three-dimensional echocardiography in the evaluation of the interventional cardiac catheterization procedure

Magni et al reported on the use of 3D echocardiography to evaluate atrial septal defects, once they had been deployed.[1] Excellent cut planes and projections detailing the anatomic relationship of the devices to the left and right side of the septum were displayed. However, this technology used the sequential acquisition of 2D echocardiographic images. The time delay, in essence, obviated practical use in the catheterization laboratory. However, real-time 3D echocardiography

can provide excellent 3D images of various devices.[2–5] Images of the right and left sided disks to close various holes or communications can be imaged in a myriad of directions. The relationship of the device to the contiguous cardiac structures can be easily discerned. Moreover, this information can be available immediately in the live, but narrowed imaging format, or within 1 to 2 minutes in a wide, full volume sector format. However, to date, no studies have documented incremental information obtained with 3D echocardiographic imaging compared to standard catheterization fluoroscopy, angiography, or 2D imaging, yet the advantages of 3D imaging should be readily apparent. To date, perhaps the major deterrent to the application of 3D echocardiography to atrial or ventricular septal defect device closure in the catheterization laboratory has been the cumbersome transthoracic or subcostal placement of the imaging probe. With the development of either 3D transesophageal or 3D intracardiac echocardiography, application of such imaging will become standard clinical practice.

Three-dimensional echocardiography has aided in the pre- and post-catheterization assessment of adult patients undergoing cardiac catheterization balloon dilation angioplasty of stenotic rheumatic mitral valves.[8] In the pre-selection of patients, 3D imaging provides information as to the effective stenotic orifice area, the precise thickness of valve leaflets, and regions and magnitude of the commissural fusion. Moreover, 3D echocardiography provides important anatomic information as to the mechanism and hence results of the balloon dilation angioplasty. Specifically, the more precise regions of commissural 'splitting' or potential leaflet or chordae tear and disruption can be seen. Again, at our center we have only a few cases in which 3D imaging has aided in catheterization balloon dilation valvuloplasty of stenotic mitral valves. One such illustrative case was a young child who had surgery consisting of patch closure of a primum atrial septal defect, and suture closure of a cleft mitral valve. This patient had a forme-fruste of a parachute mitral valve deformity, with closely spaced papillary muscle. The pre-interventional 3D echocardiographic study demonstrated a markedly reduced effective orifice area, with a thickened somewhat immobile anterior leaflet (Figure 6.16a). The patient had a successful balloon dilation angioplasty with reduction of the pressure gradient. The 3D echocardiogram demonstrated a split anterior mitral valve leaflet, at the corresponding region of the previous cleft (Figure 6.16b). Three-dimensional echocardiographic color flow analysis showed that this was the precise region of increased effective antegrade flow across the mitral valve.

Another illustrative example was the application of 3D echocardiography in the balloon dilation of another young child with significant congenital mitral stenosis. Pre-catheterization 3D imaging confirmed a parachute mitral valve deformity, with markedly reduced interchordal space. Three-dimensional echocardiographic color flow analysis showed two distinct and separate inflow jets across the

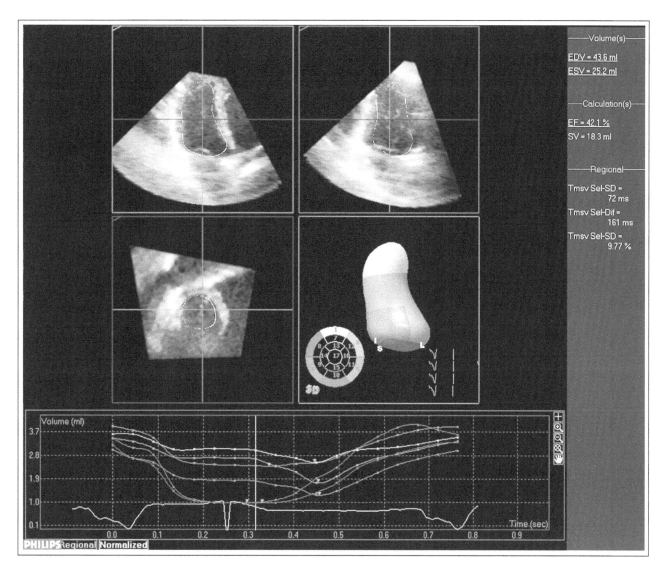

Figure 6.15
Three-dimensional echocardiogram showing regional wall motion as a function of time in a young girl with paradoxical motion of the interventricular septum. EDV, end-diastolic volume; ESV, end-systolic volume; EF, ejection fraction; SV, stroke volume. The indices of Tmsv SEL-SD, Tmsv Sel-diff and Tmsv Sel-SD are indices of synchronicity and indicate significant dysynchrony in this patient.

stenotic region of the chordal apparatus. The interventionalist expertly placed a catheter across the larger orifice and dilated this region. Again, catheterization documented a reduction in the mean inflow diastolic gradient. Three-dimensional echocardiography confirmed enlargement of the specific stenotic region without tear or disruption of the chordae or leaflets, and confirmed no significant change in mitral regurgitation after the procedure. Importantly, these are two illustrative case examples, and are not intended to imply that these results are expected in most pediatric patients undergoing such procedures. However, both examples do clearly document the potentially important clinical application of 3D echocardiographic imaging for interventional cardiac catheterization.

Application of three-dimensional echocardiography for fetal interventions

To date, 55 interventional cardiac catheterization procedures have been performed at Boston Children's Hospital. In particular, 35 fetal aortic and 8 pulmonary balloon dilation valvuloplasties have been undertaken. The selection criteria for dilation of the aortic valve have been the fetus with critical aortic stenosis and a normal to dilated left ventricle. Analysis of our database has documented that the natural history of

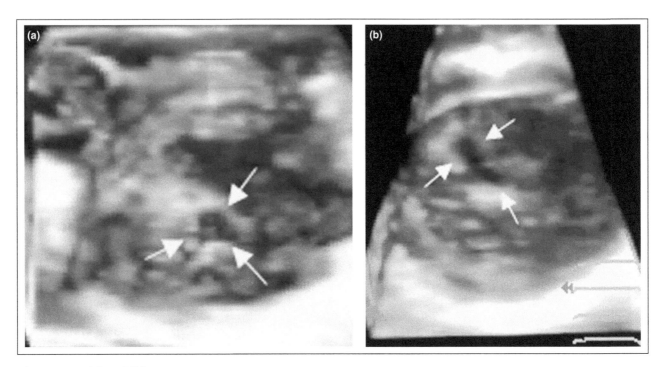

Figure 6.16 (a) and (b)
Three-dimensional echocardiogram in a young child with severe mitral stenosis after suture of a cleft mitral valve, with parachute deformity. Both (a) and (b) are *en-face* views as taken from the left ventricle apex directed superiorly towards the mitral valve. Panel (a) shows the markedly reduced mitral valve effective orifice prior to balloon dilation. The three arrows depict the distal edges of the severely stenotic mitral valve. Panel (b), after a successful dilation in the catheterization laboratory, the 3D echocardiogram shows the split in the prior sutured cleft (upper arrows); the lower arrow displays the mural leaflet.

such fetuses is progression to hypoplastic left heart syndrome requiring ultimate staged single ventricle operations.[29] Preliminary experience has shown that balloon dilation aortic valvuloplasty in selected fetuses has resulted in preservation of ventricular size, ultimately leading to two ventricular repairs. Certainly, the pre-selection of patients for this procedure is one of the most important issues. To date we have relied on the left ventricle to right ventricle length ratio. Many of these ventricles are spherical rather than elliptical, hence 2D echocardiographic analysis of ventricular volumes would be fraught with potential pitfalls. We have applied 3D echocardiographic analysis to measure ventricular volumes in the fetus with critical valvar aortic stenosis. With experience, using the matrix array scanner, the entire left ventricle can be acquired and aligned in a 3D echocardiographic data set, allowing for analysis of left ventricular diastolic volume (Figure 6.17). To validate our procedure, we measured very small ventricular volumes, 1–5 ml, in a tank model study, from displacement of fluid from a spherical balloon. Excellent agreement was found between these very small ventricular volumes and measurements obtained with the matrix array probe. Now that the application has been tested, we are applying this technology in the pre-selection and serial evaluation of these *in-utero* patients. We have demonstrated the feasibility of measuring these left ventricular volumes in the fetus with critical valvar aortic stenosis at various gestational

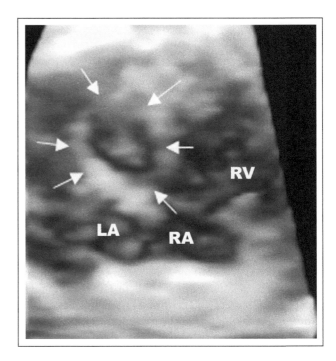

Figure 6.17
Three-dimensional echocardiogram in a fetus with a hypoplastic left heart (arrows) syndrome at 24 weeks' gestation prior to *in-utero* aortic balloon dilation. LA, left atrium RA, right atrium; RV, right ventricle.

ages. Along with our tank model study, which showed good agreement between 3D echocardiographic assessment of ventricular volumes and actual displacement of fluid from the balloon model, we are applying this to the serial evaluation of the fetus after balloon dilation to determine efficacy of the intervention.

With increasing volume, the catheterization interventional procedures are becoming increasingly successful. That is to say, the interventionalists, working closely with the obstetricians, have become extremely adept at crossing and dilating the aortic or pulmonary valve. Immediately following the procedure, a much larger antegrade jet can be seen traversing the stenotic valve. Additionally, regurgitant jets are also seen, further attesting to the dilation of the valve. The future will necessitate evaluation of the outcome of such patients, hence necessitating a reliable and repeatable method to evaluate corresponding atrial and ventricular size and function. Assessment of ventricular volume size and function will help guide decision-making as to the gestational timing of intervention, whether to repeat the balloon dilation procedure, and most importantly to determine whether performing an aortic balloon dilation valvuloplasty in the fetus with critical aortic stenosis prevents the progression to hypoplastic left heart syndrome, culminating in staged single ventricle surgery.

The future

As discussed above, 3D echocardiography has a very bright future for application for imaging in the cardiac catheterization laboratory. Despite the significant progress, in such a short period of time, certain improvements should greatly aid the application of this technology in the cardiac catheterization laboratory.

In comparison to standard transthoracic echocardiography probes, the matrix array scanner is rather large and cumbersome. As such, manipulating the probe between the ribs often results in imaging artifacts. Moreover, this present day probe's transmit frequency is low and hence has lower resolution. Additionally the frame rate is rather low, often at 20 to 25 frames/s. Such low frame rates certainly affect the imaging of fast moving structures such as valve motion. The frame rates associated with Doppler color flow imaging are even lower, often at 8 to 12 frames/s. This also affects the ability to choose the specific frame to measure the vena contracta of stenotic or regurgitant jets.

'Live' 3D echocardiography allows for immediate imaging in a 3D space. Such imaging certainly has inherent advantages and, with experience, scanning in 3D real-time echocardiography has become possible. However, the present disadvantage is that scanning in real time is done in a rather small sector format. This has inherent disadvantages for following a catheter course, or obtaining a large imaging road map of the anatomy involved. The full volume does allow for obtaining a much larger sector 'volume' format, but requires acquisition over four beats, with respiratory gating.

Importantly, although obtained in a 3D volume data set, the images are ultimately displayed on a conventional 2D screen. Although various gradations of gray scale are shown to enhance depth perception, an improved modality to display the structures in three dimensions would be desirable. Many imaging research institutes are working on 3D displays such as holography, or enhancing the 3D effects with stereoscopic imaging, the latter accomplished with lenses incorporated into glasses for the observer, or on the computer monitor itself.

Even if transthoracic 3D echocardiographic imaging were to improve, such technology would not be ideal in a complex catheterization or surgical arena. Echocardiographic imaging that will not invade the sterile space or impede the interventionalist's manipulations is essential. Transesophageal or intracardiac echocardiography 3D echocardiographic[30] imaging would certainly aid in this endeavor. Transesophageal echocardiography should be able to provide a much larger 3D sector angle. Similar to standard 2D echocardiographic transesophageal imaging, higher transmit frequencies should be able to be applied. However, for more refined, higher resolution imaging intracardiac ultrasound could be used. This may be at a much smaller sector angle, yet may provide the exquisite 3D imaging necessary for placement of sutures or affixing mitral valve leaflets such as for a catheterization based procedure to reduce mitral regurgitation. Furthermore, offline 3D echocardiographic analysis of ventricular volumes could be implemented as part of the portable echocardiographic machine. With improvements in semi to completely automated border detection, 3D echocardiographic ventricular volume size and function could expeditiously be undertaken to guide clinical decision-making.

Summary

This chapter has detailed the important applications of 3D echocardiography to cardiac catheterization. Similar to the development of 3D echocardiography, the application to cardiac catheterization is a work in progress. As detailed above, significant technological improvements need to continue and evolve. Regardless, the conceptualization of 3D imaging to better pre-select patients, guide the catheterization procedure, and ascertain clinical outcomes certainly has a strong foundation. Much of what has been presented in this chapter constitutes the important collaborative efforts between pioneers in cardiac catheterization and echocardiography. This type of collaborative effort is essential to continue and explore the frontiers of interventional cardiac catheterization procedures, and the best means to provide the best imaging for the interventionalist. As stated above, much of the efforts to date using matrix array or real-time imaging are preliminary. Although specific examples have been shown, this imaging format has not yet been shown to influence outcome, as compared to more standard modalities. However, similar to cardiac interventional procedures, today 3D echocardiographic imaging can be undertaken with good technical success. The future is to determine the clinical outcome of such procedures using 3D echocardiographic imaging.

References

1. Magni G, Hijazi ZM, Delabays A et al. Two and three-dimensional transesophageal echocardiography in patient selection and assessment of atrial septal defect closure by the new DAS-Angel Wings device. Circulation 1997; 96: 1722–8.

2. Zhu W, Cao QL, Hijazi ZM. Transcatheter closure of a large residual shunt after deployment of the Das-Angel device using the Amplatzer Septal Occluder. Cathet Cardiovasc Interven 1999; 48: 184–7.

3. Acar P. Three-dimensional echocardiography in transcatheter closure of atrial septal defects. Cardiol Young 2000; 10: 484–92.

4. Zhu W, Cao QL, Rhodes J, Hijazi ZM. Measurement of atrial septal defect size: a comparative study between three-dimensional echocardiography and the standard balloon sizing methods. Pediatr Cardiol 2000; 21: 465–9.

5. Acar P, Saliba Z, Bonhoeffer Z, Sidi D, Kachaner J. Assessment of the geometric profile of the Amplatzer and Cardioseal occluders by three-dimensional echocardiography. Heart 2001; 85: 451–3.

6. McCreery CJ, McCulloch M, Ahmad M, deFilippi CR. Real-time 3-dimensional echocardiography imaging for right ventricular endomyocardial biopsy: a Comparison with Fluoroscopy. J Am Soc Echocardiogr 2001; 14: 927–33.

7. Pepi M, Tamborini G, Bartorelli AL et al. Usefulness of three-dimensional echocardiographic reconstruction of the Amplatzer Septal Occluder in patients undergoing atrial septal closure. Am J Cardiol 2004; 94: 1343–7.

8. Zamorano J, Perez DL, Sugeng L et al. Non-invasive assessment of mitral valve area during percutaneous balloon mitral valvuloplasty: role of real-time 3D echocardiography. Eur Heart J 2004; 25: 2086–91.

9. Daimon M, Shiota T, Gillinov M et al. Percutaneous mitral valve repair for chronic ischemic mitral regurgitation. A real-time three-dimensional echocardiographic study in an ovine model. Circulation 2005; 111: 2183–9.

10. Sugeng L, Weinert L, Thiele K, Lang RM. Real-time three-dimensional echocardiography using a novel matrix array transducer. Echocardiography 2003; 20(7): 623–35.

11. Marx G, Fulton D, Pandian NG et al. Delineation of site, relative size and dynamic geometry of atrial septal defects by real-time three-dimensional echocardiography. J Am Coll Cardiol 1995; 25: 482–90.

12. Kardon RE, Cao QL, Masani N et al. New insights and observations in three-dimensional echocardiographic visualization of ventricular septal defects: experimental and clinical studies. Circulation 1998; 98: 1307–14.

13. Acar P, Laskari C, Rhodes J et al. Three-dimensional echocadiographic analysis of valve anatomy as a determinant of mitral regurgitation after surgery for atrioventricular septal defects. Am J Cardiol 1999; 83: 745–9.

14. Barrea C, Levasseur S, Roman K et al. Three-dimensional echocardiography improves the understanding of left atrioventricular valve morphology and function in atrioventricular septal defects undergoing patch augmentation. J Thorac Cardiovasc Surg 2005; 129: 746–53.

15. Chen Q, Nosir YE, Vletter WB et al. Accurate assessment of mitral valve area in patients with mitral stenosis by three-dimensional echocardiography. J Am Soc Echocardiogr 1997; 10: 133–40.

16. Mohr-Kahaly S, Menzel T, Kupfewasser I, Schlosser A, von Bardeleben S. Three-dimensional echocardiographic evaluation of aortic and mitral stenosis. Echocardiography 1999; 16: 723–30.

17. Sebag IA, Morgan JG, Handschumacher MD et al. Usefulness of three-dimensionally guided assessment of mitral stenosis using matrix-array ultrasound. Am J Cardiol 2005; 96: 1151–6.

18. Handschumacher MD, Lethor JP, Siu S et al. A new integrated system for three-dimensional echocardiographic reconstruction: development and validation for ventricular volume with application in human subjects. J Am Coll Cardiol 1993; 3: 743–53.

19. Gopal AS, Keller AM, Shen Z et al. Three-dimensional echocardiography: in vitro and in vivo validation of left ventricular mass and comparison with conventional echocardiographic methods. J Am Coll Cardiol 1994; 24: 504–13.

20. Gopal AS, Schnellbaecher MJ, Shen Z et al. Freehand three-dimensional echocardiography for determination of left ventricular volume and mass in patients with abnormal ventricles: comparison with magnetic resonance imaging. J Am Soc Echocardiogr 1997; 10: 853–61.

21. Ota T, Fleishman CE, Strub M et al. Real-time, three-dimensional echocardiography: feasibility of dynamic right ventricular volume measurement with saline contrast. Am Heart J 1999; 137: 958–66.

22. Shiota T, Jones M, Chikada M et al. Real-time three-dimensional echocardiography for determining right ventricular stroke volume in an animal model of chronic right ventricular volume overload. Circulation 1998; 97: 1897–1900.

23. Schmidt MA, Ohazama CJ, Kwabena OA et al. Real-time three-dimensional echocardiography for measurement of left ventricular volumes. Am J Cardiol 1999; 84: 1434–9.

24. Schroder KM, Sapin PM, King DL, Smith MD, DeMaria AN. Three-dimensional echocardiographic volume computation: in vitro comparison to standard two-dimensional echocardiography. J Am Soc Echocardiogr 1993; 6: 467–75.

25. Acar P, Maunoury C, Antonietti T et al. Left ventricular ejection fraction in children measured by three-dimensional echocardiography using a new transthoracic integrated 3D-probe. Eur Heart J 1998; 19: 1583–8.

26. Acar P, Marx GR, Saliba Z, Sidi D, Kachaner J. Three-dimensional echocardiographic measurement of left ventricular stroke volume in children: comparison with Doppler method. Pediatr Cardiol 2001; 22: 116–20.

27. Poutanen T, Ikonen A, Vainio P et al. Left atrial volume assessed by transthoracic three-dimensional echocardiography and magnetic resonance imaging: dynamic changes during the heart cycle in children. Heart 2000; 83: 537–42.

28. Cannon JW, Stoll JA, Salgo IS et al. Real time 3-dimensional ultrasound for guiding surgical tasks. Comput Aided Surg 2003; 8(2): 82–90.

29. Tworetzky W, Wilkins-Haug L, Jennings RW et al. Balloon dilation of severe aortic stenosis in the fetus: potential for prevention of hypoplastic left heart syndrome. Candidate selection, technique, and results of successful intervention. Circulation 2004; 110: 2125–31.

30. Roelandt JR, di Mario C, Pandian NG et al. Three-dimensional reconstruction of intracoronary ultrasound images. Rationale, approaches, problems, and directions. Circulation 1994; 90: 1044–55.

7

Cardiac computed tomography in the cath lab

Carlos E Ruiz, Vladimir Jelnin, and Sibyl C Medie

Introduction

The mathematical basis of X-ray image reconstruction dates back to 1917, when Radon,[1] an Austrian mathematician, published an analytic solution to the problem of reconstructing an object from multiple projections. The actual application of mathematical image reconstruction techniques of radiographic medical imaging was first reported in 1961 by Oldendorf,[2] and the first clinical computerized tomography was developed by the Nobel laureate, Sir Godfrey N Hounsfield. He applied the early mathematical theories to reconstruct the internal structure of the body from a number of different X-ray measurements, using a translate/rotate process, that was repeated until the entire circumference of the body was scanned.[3–5] Since then, computed tomography (CT) has become one of the most important imaging technologies using X-rays.

The use of CT as a cardiac diagnostic modality has been hindered primarily by limitations of temporal resolution. This was improved with the introduction of electron beam CT (EBCT) in the mid-1980s, resulting in the birth of cardiac CT technology. Conventional CT evolved with the introduction of spiral (helical) technology in the mid-1990s and stimulated new interest in cardiac CT imaging.

Principles of cardiac computed tomography

One of the primary objectives in imaging a fast moving organ (i.e. the heart) with CT is the *speed* in which a single transaxial image is acquired (temporal resolution). In the 1970s, 250 seconds were required to perform one full rotation of the X-ray tube around the body of the patient. The data collected from this rotation were used to reconstruct a single transaxial image. Currently, the time has been reduced to less than 0.4 s/image, and data from a half rotation may now be used for one slice reconstruction, further reducing the image acquisition time to 0.2 s/image.

Since its advent, EBCT has been the gold standard for cardiac CT, with an acquisition time of 100 ms/image or less, capable of freezing cardiac motion and producing clear cross-sectional images of the heart. The latest generation of EBCT (e-Speed) can further enhance the temporal resolution up to 33 ms. However, further increase in rotational speed of the multirow detector CT (MDCT) scanners is still being pursued, although the rotational force of the gantry components, which increases as the square of the rotational speed, poses a serious mechanical handicap.

Another crucial factor in obtaining high quality cardiac CT angiography is to acquire images with *high spatial resolution*. Spatial resolution is dependent upon the resolution in three planes, x, y, and z. x–y imaging planes are related to the matrix size, which is similar for both EBCT and MDCT (512×512 pixels), and the field of view (FOV) (the diameter of the area being reconstructed for visualization). Smaller pixel size offers higher quality axial two-dimensional (2D) images. Pixel size can be calculated by the formula:

$$\text{size} = \text{FOV/matrix size}$$

For example, a pixel size for a FOV of 26 cm, which is common for EBCT scanning, will be 0.26 mm^2 and for a FOV of 30 cm will give 0.33 mm^2 pixel size. The z plane is determined by the slice thickness or collimation. MDCT has the absolute advantage in z plane resolution when compared to EBCT. The submillimeter slice thickness demonstrated by the latest 64 slice MDCT creates sharp, high quality images far superior to the EBCT images, which routinely uses 1.5 to 3 mm slice thickness for cardiac imaging. The maximum in plane resolution at 33 ms acquisition time for the newer EBCT is 7 line pairs (lp)/cm, and at 100 ms is 13 lp/cm. The voxel is the basic unit of volume, based on the parameters of the x, y, and z planes. A smaller voxel size results in a higher quality of post-processed images.

ECG triggering is another fundamental principle in cardiac CT. Its necessity is based on obtaining multiple images of the moving heart at the same phase of the cardiac cycle. If cross-sectional images were to be acquired at different phases, a considerable amount of information would be lost.

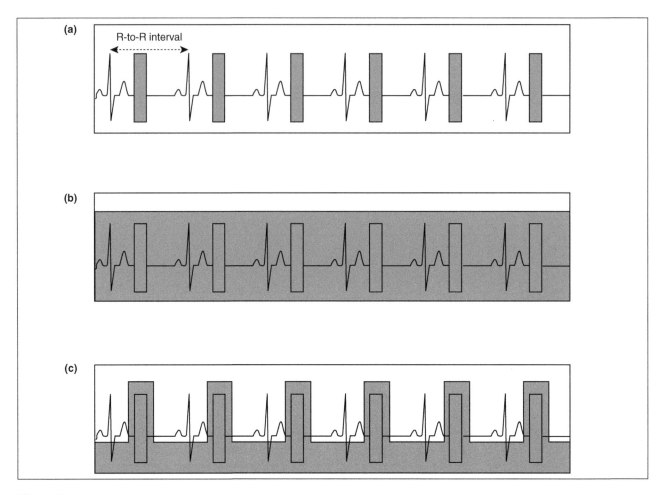

Figure 7.1
(Shading represents radiation exposure during cardiac cycle) (a) Prospective ECG triggering utilized by EBCT. The patient is exposed to X-rays only during pre-selected times (100 ms) of the cardiac cycle, routinely at 40% of the R–R interval, at the moment of minimum heart velocity. (b) Retrospective ECG triggering utilized by MDCT. X-rays produced continuously and data acquired during all phases of the cardiac cycle together with ECG recording. Same phase images are reconstructed using retrospective ECG gating. The reconstruction window can be positioned at any phase of the cardiac cycle. (c) Prospective triggering of X-ray tube output modulation by MDCT. The output of X-ray tube is at nominal exposure only at the phase which is used for image reconstruction and is decreased during the cardiac phase, which is not used for image reconstruction. ('pulse' X-ray tube modulation). (See also color plate section.)

Two types of ECG triggering exist, prospective and retrospective. Prospective triggering occurs when X-ray radiation is produced at pre-selected points within the cardiac cycle. All raw data from this exposure are used for image reconstruction. This method is the one utilized by EBCT.

Retrospective triggering is in actuality a retrospective ECG-gated image reconstruction. It involves acquiring data during the entire cardiac cycle, but only processes the part that occurs at the appropriate time during the cardiac cycle. A novel achievement in cardiac CT is ECG-gated X-ray tube output modulation. Frequently referred to as prospective ECG triggering for MDCT, this mode is specifically designed to reduce radiation exposure.[6]

Radiation dose is closely related to the type of ECG triggering (Figure 7.1). Cardiac CT, an X-ray based diagnostic modality, requires exposure of the patient to potentially harmful radiation doses. There have been a number of publications on the radiation exposure of cardiac CT.[7–9] Radiation exposure is much higher with MDCT in comparison to EBCT.[10,11] The effective radiation dose of four-slice spatial CT coronary angiography is between 9.3 and 11.3 mSv. The dose of an angiographic EBCT study using standard 3 mm slice thickness varies between 1.1 and 2.0 mSv. The dose is much lower because it is applied only during a short period of time using prospective ECG triggering. When retrospective ECG gating is used by MDCT, patients are exposed to radiation for the duration of data acquisition. In comparison, the yearly exposure from natural sources is approximately 3.6 mSv. During a routine coronary angiography procedure, the radiation dose varies between 3 and 10 mSv.

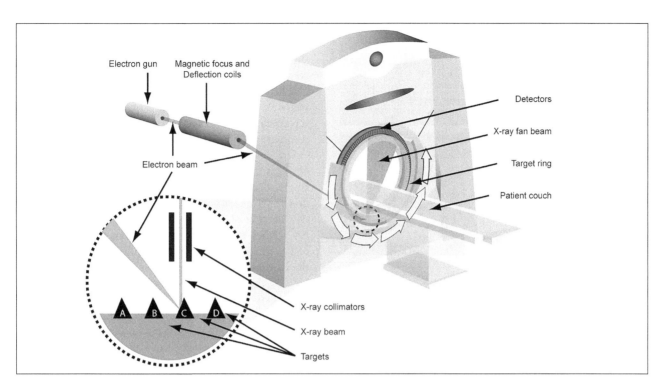

Figure 7.2
Electron beam computed tomography (EBCT) data acquisition. The electron gun generates an electron beam. Magnetic coils focus and direct the electron beam through the tungsten target rings. The electrons bombard the target, starting at the upper left, and are circularly scanned over 210°. Targets produce an X-ray fan beam (30°), which, after collimation, pass through the patient's body and attenuated radiation is collected by the opposing ring of detectors. After each image acquisition the patient couch is moved 2–3 mm to the next position to obtain the next slice.

Careful consideration of the risk/benefit ratio should be made in each case before the procedure. The high radiation dose could be acceptable when cardiac CT is used as an alternative to other X-ray based technologies such as a cardiac catheterization and angiography. The radiation dose should be significantly lower when using cardiac CT as a screening tool for silent coronary artery disease. The ultimate goal is to have another powerful imaging modality, preferably with lower radiation exposure. Therefore, the EBCT has definite advantages compared with MDCT by offering higher temporal resolution and much lower radiation dose, albeit at a lower spatial resolution. However, the lower spatial resolution is of the magnitude of 5× and the radiation dose is of the magnitude of 10×.

Technology

Electron beam computed tomography

EBCT was first developed by Douglas P Boyd and colleagues in 1983. The main technologic advantage of the EBCT is the absence of a moving (mechanically rotating) X-ray source, resulting in a higher temporal resolution

producing clear, motion-free cross-sectional images.[12] Instead, an electron generator fires electrons that are electromagnetically deflected to sweep four tungsten target rings located in the gantry beneath the patient. The X-rays generated by the electron sweep traverse the patient and are collected by fixed detectors located in the opposite side of the gantry. This is currently the technique with the fastest temporal resolution available[13] (Figure 7.2).

Modes of operation

Multislice mode. EBCT multilevel acquisition is an impressive achievement in CT technology. The four tungsten target rings and two detector arrays are used to acquire between two and eight slices of the heart without movement of the patient table. The number of slices may be increased, by moving the table to a new position. Two slices corresponding to the same target ring could be acquired in 50 ms. An 8 ms delay is necessary between acquisitions of the next two levels corresponding to the next target ring. Image scan width in this mode is 7 mm, with a 5 mm gap between each of two slices from the same target ring and 8 mm between each consecutive ring.

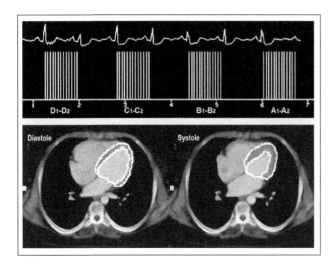

Figure 7.3
Top: each sequence of vertical lines demonstrates the point in time when a pair of images (slices) is acquired. Eight-level movie mode (above) uses image data from all four target rings to create image pairs (D_1–D_2, C_1–C_2, B_1–B_2, A_1–A_2). Data from the lowest target ring D are acquired first, creating levels 7 and 8. Consecutive usage of targets C, B, and A creates subsequent pairs of levels (6–5, 4–3, 2–1), without table movement.
Bottom: representative image of diastole and systole, within one sequence.

Single-slice mode. This mode uses only one of four tungsten targets and the high resolution detector ring. Images are acquired during continuous table movement. Slice thickness may be chosen from 1.5 mm, 3 mm, 6 mm, and 10 mm.

Preview and localization modes. These modes are used for visualization of anatomic structures to be scanned, in preparation for the actual scan. Two anteroposterior and sagittal views of the body are acquired in order to determine the first and last levels and number of slices needed. Similarly, the purpose of the localization study usually precedes the multislice mode study. Multiple cross-sectional images through the area of interest are acquired to localize the anatomy and to choose the table position.

Scanning protocols

The single-slice and multislice modes are both used for cardiac evaluation, depending on the clinical application.

Volume study. This protocol uses the single-slice mode. The acquisition sequence acquires cross-sectional images at various levels throughout a volume of anatomy in a manner similar to conventional CT. Contiguous scans are acquired when the table increments equal the image width. Routinely, one slice of the heart is acquired at a certain point of the cardiac cycle; the table moves to the next

location for the next slice acquisition at the same phase of the cardiac cycle. When ECG triggering is not necessary (imaging of motionless chest structures), the next slice could be taken at any cardiac phase. This scanning protocol is called 'continuous volume scan'. ECG-triggered volume study is the primary protocol for coronary calcium screening (CAS) and for cardiac CT angiography with 3D reconstruction.

Movie study. Movie studies may be performed in both single-slice and multislice modes. In multislice mode, the first scans are triggered at the R wave of the ECG signal, and two heart levels are scanned at the maximum rate (50 ms per frame) throughout the entire cardiac cycle. Playback of the image data displays the motion of the slice during the cardiac cycle. The sequence is repeated for each pair. Usually the entire ventricle can be imaged within a few heartbeats using an eight-level movie protocol. The same principle – movie study protocols – could be utilized in the high resolution single-slice mode. Only one slice may be assessed and this protocol is not used routinely. The 'movie' study protocol is often used for evaluation of ventricular (left and right) function (Figure 7.3).

Flow study. This scan sequence is used to track the characteristics of flowing contrast media through vascular anatomy. The initial scan is commenced manually and subsequent images of the same anatomic level or levels (depending on the use of single- or multislice mode) are acquired at ECG triggered time intervals, or simply at fixed time intervals (Figure 7.4).

Multirow detector CT

Instead of obtaining transaxial images by an X-ray tube rotating around the body, the X-ray follows a spiral or helical path around the body while the table moves through the gantry. Collected volumetric data are then reconstructed in a single transaxial plane an using an interpolation algorithm[14–16] (Figure 7.5).

In the early 1990s, helical CT (spiral) started using multirow detectors (MDCT) currently capable of generating up to 64 slices of varying thickness with each gantry rotation. Instead of one detector row, multiple parallel detector rows acquire data, allowing for much faster scan time (Figure 7.6).

Though previously unable to gate ECG, and with acquisition times greater than one second, helical technology has undergone a drastic revolution. The latest generation of scanners are capable of gating ECG retrospectively as well as prospectively – the so-called pulsed gating, which is different from prospective triggering used by EBCT.[6] Prospective pulsed gating consists simply of an attenuation of the mA output, significantly decreasing the radiation dose to a lesser degree than true prospective ECG triggering

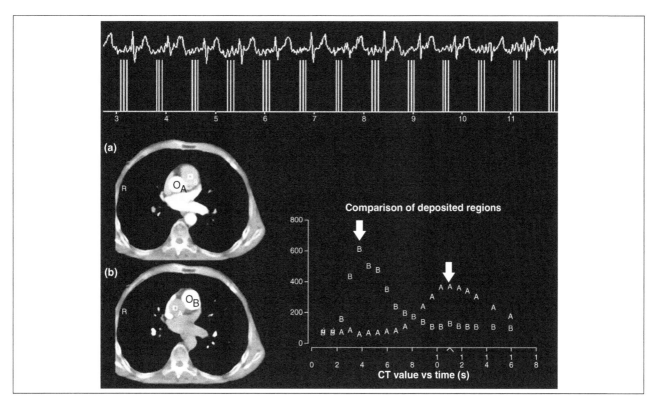

Figure 7.4

ECG triggered scan applied in 'flow' mode. Pairs of parallel tomograms at the same anatomic level are continually acquired during the same phase of the cardiac cycle. This mode is most frequently used to get contrast transit time from the injection site to the region of interest. A time/density curve can reliably establish the 'delay time', which is important for the CTA study. Tomograms were taken at the peak of contrast concentration in the aorta (A) and pulmonary artery (B). Arrows on the graph indicate the peak of contrast concentration for both the aorta (curve A) and pulmonary artery (curve B).

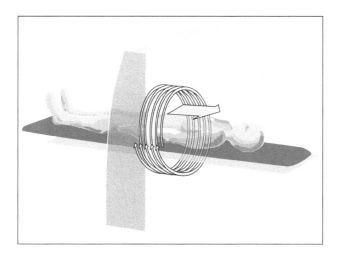

Figure 7.5

Spiral scanner acquires data continuously while the table moves through the gantry, therefore X-rays follow a helical path along the patient's body. The resulting projection data do not lie in any single transaxial plane, as does EBCT. Use of interpolation algorithms is necessary for the transaxial image reconstruction.

(Figure 7.1). X-ray tube rotation time decreased to under 400 ms/rotation and using a partial scan reconstruction algorithm, image acquisition (temporal resolution) dropped to under 200 ms. MDCT scanners are now capable of performing similar cardiac examinations which were previously available only by EBCT.

Spatial resolution also experienced significant improvements. MDCT scanners can produce submillimeter resolution, with 64-slice systems demonstrating spatial resolution as low as 0.35 mm, which is much higher than any EBCT system can produce. Furthermore, spatial resolution in the MDCT can also be improved by advanced beam hardening and by metal artifact reduction algorithms, especially when imaging cardiac stents. However, increasing z axis resolution (thinner slices) requires a higher radiation dose in order to maintain a high contrast-to-noise ratio. This has significantly changed the role of MDCT technology in cardiac scanning and has resulted in new excitement in this field. However, there is concern regarding the radiation dose that the patient receives during an MDCT angiography scan, which may be as high as 10 times that of an EBCT scan.

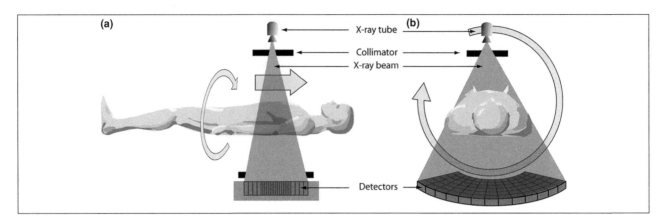

Figure 7.6
Multislice spiral CT scanners have several parallel detector rows, which allow simultaneous acquisition of several slices. As a result, larger sections can be scanned in a shorter time. (a) Lateral view; (b) coronal view.

Image post-processing

Three-dimensional computer reconstruction techniques are relatively new in medical imaging. There are obvious advantages to the visualization of human organs in three dimensions, with the possibility of manipulating the image and making precise measurements. There is no need to use imagination to build 3D mental images of the organ from biplane fluoroscopic images in the catheterization laboratory, or to do the same in reviewing X-ray or CT images in planning cardiac intervention. This task can be easily replaced by 3D manipulation in real time.

Three-dimensional workstations arrived in the early 1990s. Currently, all major CT manufacturing companies (GE, Siemens, Toshiba, Philips) can deliver their own dedicated 3D workstation with each scanner. Previously, 3D image reconstruction and image analysis was very time-consuming, but today real-time reconstruction is available. Choosing the right workstation depends on the needs of the user. Software packages are constantly being improved and updated, and most of them have similar functionality and tools.

All existing techniques use the original cross-sectional CT images as the source. The quality of the final 3D reconstructed images is directly related to the spatial resolution of the source image (voxel size). Combining all voxels of the data set and using specified reconstruction techniques (post-processing) allows the visualization of the anatomy in 3D views. There are a number of post-processing techniques available and the following section briefly discusses a few of the major techniques.

Post-processing techniques
Maximum intensity projection (MIP)

The resulting reconstruction is similar to the fluoroscopic view observed in the catheterization laboratory. It is a 2D projection image of the highest intensity voxels from the 3D data volume. Superimposing high density anatomic structures over the low density structures causes certain limitations of this technique. This may be reduced by thinning the 'slab' image or rotation of the image. This technique may be used for a fast review of the region of interest in the whole volume of data (Figure 7.7a).

Surface rendering technique

Surface rendering (Figure 7.7b) is one of the oldest 3D techniques used in post-processing. This reconstruction recreates the 3D image of the surface of the anatomic structures and is based on the selected threshold density of the voxels. Only selected voxels within a chosen range are visualized in the image, creating the 'surface' view. Usually only a limited portion of the volumetric data is used. An advantage of this method is the high speed of image manipulation allowed by the small size of the data. The disadvantage is the low level of anatomy size reproducibility due to the dependence on user defined reconstruction settings. Surface rendering has now been replaced by the volume rendering technique.

Volume rendering (VR) technique

Volume rendering is both the most impressive and most powerful 3D reconstruction method. All voxels of the volume available in the source images can be used for reconstruction and visualization. The main principle of this method is based on assigning specific color and opacity to the voxels, depending on their density. Standard color and opacity pre-sets are usually available in the majority of 3D workstations (Figure 7.7c).

By changing the opacity of the voxel values corresponding to the specific tissues, it is possible to make those tissues

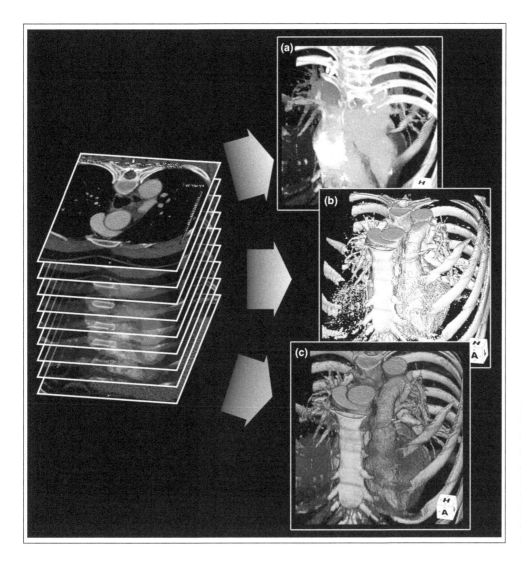

Figure 7.7
Different techniques used for image reconstruction from source tomograms (shown on the left). (a) Maximum intensity projection technique (MIP). (b) Surface rendering or shaded surface display (SSD). (c) Volume rendering (VR).

appear transparent or opaque depending on the anatomic structure which has to be examined. Flexibility in changing the color scheme and opacity can fully satisfy the operator's demands (Figure 7.8).

Other post-processing techniques and image manipulation

There are several other methods used in post-processing. Multiplanar reconstruction (MPR) allows the observer to change the plane of view from axial to sagittal, coronal, or oblique views, which is the standard method used for basic CT.

The curved multiplanar reconstruction (CMPR) method is widely used for vessel visualization and analysis. In this case, the cut plane is not flat but curved and is defined by the operator to follow the curvature of the vessel. The resulting image is a flattened representation (reformation) of the curved plane (Figure 7.9).

Image manipulations allow the application of different tasks on the already reconstructed 3D image. This includes image zooming, rotation, applying 'cut planes' to the 3D image, and changing volume rendering reconstruction parameters. The technique to use in a given situation remains the operator's choice. It is based mainly on individual experience, the techniques available on the workstation, and the time needed to obtain the desired results.

Understanding and minimizing motion artifacts

Motion artifacts are a source of diminished image quality. They can be divided into two subgroups: those related to the patient and those related to the CT equipment. Patient-related motion artifacts include body movement on the scanner table during image acquisition, breathing movements, and artifacts related to the heart motion itself. There are several ways to reduce movement of the patient during

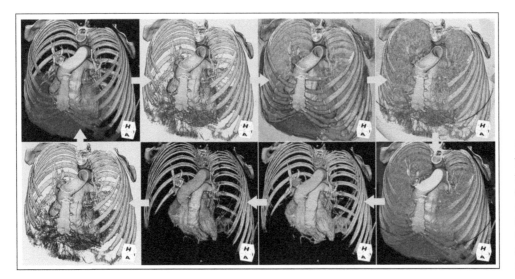

Figure 7.8
The volume rendering technique allows extensive color and opacity manipulation, which can be effectively used by the operator to view specific anatomic structures. (See also color plate section.)

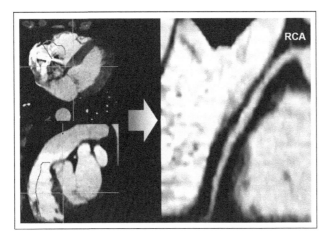

Figure 7.9
The blue line drawn follows the path of the right coronary artery (RCA) on the axial cross-sectional images (top, left) or sagittal images (bottom, left), creating the curved plane. The image on the right is a flattened view of this plane, showing the right coronary artery (RCA). (See also color plate section.)

the scan. Adult patients should be briefed in advance to avoid misinterpretation of the instructions given by the technologist during the scan. This information should include the scan time required and the time needed for breath hold, sensations caused by the contrast agent injection, and the importance of being motionless for the duration of image acquisition. This is not a big problem unless communication is impaired, as in patients with hearing problems, language barriers, infants, etc. With pediatric patients, there are different obstacles to overcome. At times verbal communication is simply impossible due to the age of the patients or their fear of the procedure. The need for appropriate sedation should be seriously considered to

minimize movement of the patient during data acquisition. Lack of attention to sedation may jeopardize the results of the CT examination and 3D reconstruction may not be of diagnostic quality.

Appropriate breath hold is also very important. With each respiratory cycle, the heart can move as much as 20 mm in the z axis within the chest cavity for any given tomographic level (Figure 7.10). Motion artifacts due to both body movement and breathing motion make 3D reconstructed images look unrealistic and may reduce diagnostic accuracy (Figure 7.11).

The prevention of motion artifacts due to heart motion independent of breathing motion is of primary importance in cardiac CT. The rapid perpetual motion of the heart makes its imaging difficult to obtain compared with imaging still organs. To eliminate heart motion artifacts during image acquisition, temporal resolution combined with ECG triggering becomes one of the fundamental considerations. An integral way of reducing this type of motion artifact depends on scanner characteristics such as gantry rotation time and reconstruction algorithms that affect temporal resolution for MDCT. Hypothetically, partial scan reconstruction can reduce effective temporal resolution up to 12.5% of the rotation time of the scanner. Unfortunately, at present the best temporal resolution demonstrated by MDCT scanners is around 200 ms. The relative temporal resolution can be improved by slowing down the moving object. In order to obtain sufficient image quality with the absence of motion artifacts, a heart rate below 70 bpm is recommended for MDCT. To achieve this rate, certain patients should be pre-medicated with beta blockers. This by itself poses a problem for small children, and more so for neonates, in whom this low heart rate would be unsafe.

EBCT does not have the option of partial scan reconstruction. However, with a fixed temporal resolution of

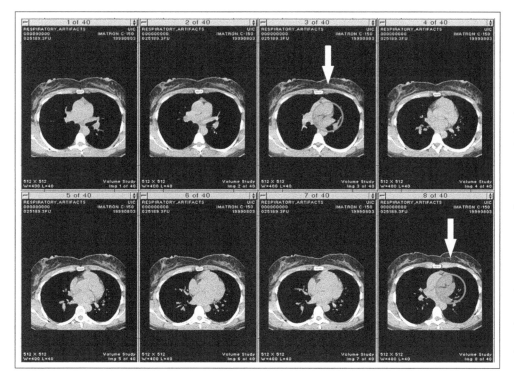

Figure 7.10
The figure shows eight contiguous slices of transaxial tomograms of the heart. Slice thickness is 3 mm, with 3 mm table increments between image acquisition by EBCT. Arrows pointing at image 3 and 8 display similar anatomic levels, however due to breathing motion, the image of slice 8 moved to the level of image 3, resulting in a motion amplitude of 15 mm between inspiration and expiration. (See also color plate section.)

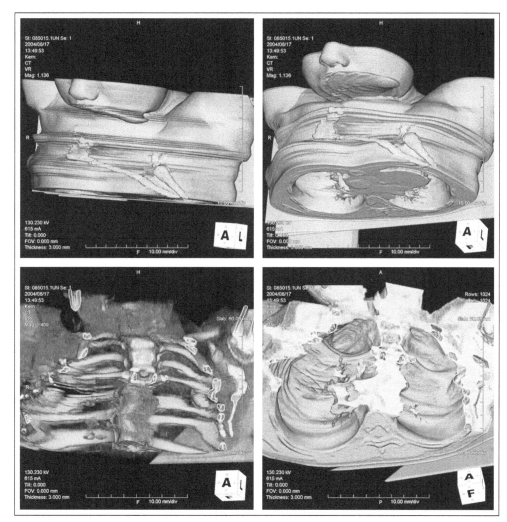

Figure 7.11
Body motion artifacts as a result of breathing motion and body movement.

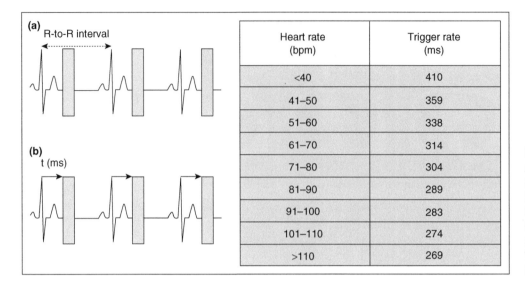

Heart rate (bpm)	Trigger rate (ms)
<40	410
41–50	359
51–60	338
61–70	314
71–80	304
81–90	289
91–100	283
101–110	274
>110	269

Figure 7.12
Algorithms for prospective ECG triggering. (a) Percentage of the distance between consecutive R-waves. (b) Absolute time distance after the R-wave. The table on the right shows heart rate vs trigger rate.[20]

50 ms, special reconstruction algorithms to achieve motion-free heart images are not essential. This temporal resolution permits handling a heart rate of about 120 bpm without noticeable motion artifacts.

Prospective triggering utilizes the ECG signal of the patient to determine when to generate X-rays for image acquisition. The most recognizable wave from the ECG, the R-wave, is used as the reference point. Scanning should occur during diastole, when the heart is at minimal motion. Published research has determined the minimal velocity to be 40–70% of the R–R interval. Image acquisition at the lowest heart velocity is an important principle in reducing heart motion artifacts. There are two types of prospective ECG triggering methods that may be applied. The first uses a percentage of the distance between consecutive R waves. The second involves choosing a triggering point at an absolute time distance after the R wave. The time of image acquisition depends on the heart rate (Figure 7.12). The second method has definite advantages for cases in whom certain disturbances in the cardiac rhythm are present, such as atrial fibrillation, frequent PVCs, etc.[17–20] The same rules apply to retrospective ECG gating – image acquisition at the lowest heart velocity. The reconstruction window can be positioned as a percentage of the distance between R–R waves or at the absolute time distance after an R-wave.

Cardiac CT applications and utility for the cath lab

Screening for coronary calcification

Screening for coronary calcification is the most well established type of examination in cardiac CT. Since the introduction of EBCT over 20 years ago, hundreds of publications have appeared, mostly in the last few years. The most authoritative data for this test relate to its ability to predict future coronary events in both symptomatic and asymptomatic individuals.[21–27] The most difficult part of this test is the prolonged breath hold by the patient. Usually 30–40 transaxial images 3 mm thick are obtained to image the entire coronary tree. EBCT has been the gold standard for coronary artery calcium (CAC) scanning since the late 1980s. The latest models of MDCT allow the performance of similar scans; however their data have not been validated so far. This test has proven to be one of the most cost-effective screening tools available for the early detection of coronary artery disease.[28]

Functional cardiac studies

Evaluation of cardiac function using CT requires contrast enhancement to visualize the heart chambers. Cross-sectional images are taken through the same level multiple times during the cardiac cycle. The playback of the image data displays the motion of the anatomic region of the heart during the cardiac cycle. This resulted in 'cine-CT' as one of the original names of the EBCT technology. Images of the heart acquired at different moments of the cardiac cycle are examined by means of computer software specifically designed to calculate important functional parameters, such as ventricular ejection fraction, ventricular volumes, stroke volumes, myocardial mass, etc. (Figure 7.13).

To achieve the same goals, MDCT uses the retrospective ECG-gated algorithms to reconstruct multiple frames from the raw data during a heart beat of the same anatomic level. The advantages of this technique in providing higher spatial resolution have been discussed previously. The main disadvantage of MDCT is the significant increase in radiation exposure for patients compared with EBCT.

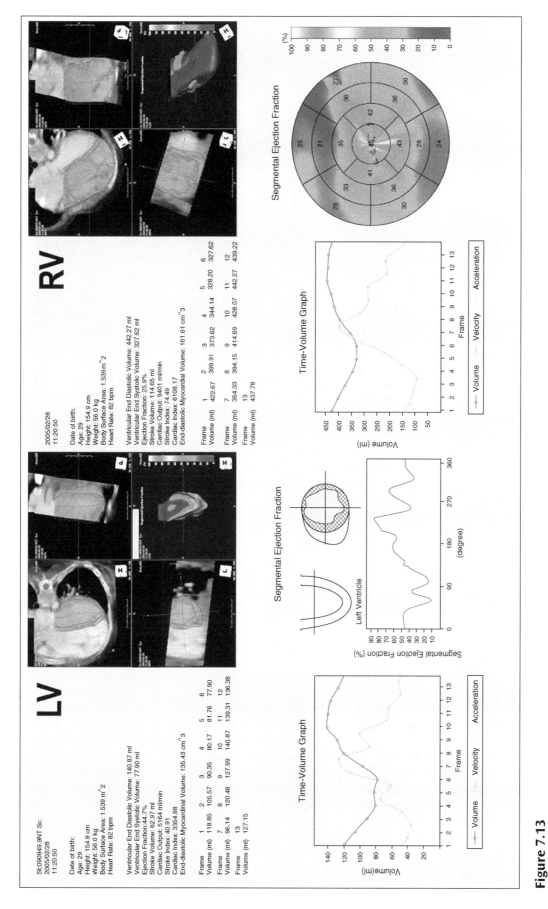

Figure 7.13

Contemporary computer software: 'Aquarius' workstation (TeraRecon, Inc, San Mateo, CA). Results of the functional cardiac analysis present all major function parameters as ejection fraction (EF), cardiac output, cardiac index, segmental EF, etc.

CT angiography with 3D image reconstruction

Cardiac CT angiography appeared in the clinical arena with the advent of 3D image reconstruction in the late 1990s.[29–32] The scanning protocol used for CT angiography is similar to that of coronary artery calcium screening. This is an ECG-triggered acquisition sequence through a volume of anatomy. The only difference is that cardiac CT angiography requires image enhancement through contrast injection.

Principles of contrast injection protocol

Cardiac CT angiography, like conventional angiography, involves the opacification of the blood vessels by intravascular injection of iodinated contrast agent. The injection site is less important when angiography is performed in patients with normal cardiac anatomy; however, for patients with different congenital malformations, the site of injection will need to be determined on a case-by-case basis, according to the anatomy and the area of interest. Central venous access is more invasive, but can be used, especially when the patient is scheduled for an interventional cardiac catheterization following the diagnostic CT. The size of the cannula to be used varies from 18 to 24 G. A mechanical injector is the most common way to administer contrast for CT angiography, whilst manual contrast injection makes the procedure more complex and less reliable. The main goal of contrast injection is to enhance density differences between blood vessels and surrounding soft tissues. This difference plays a significant role in cardiac CT 3D image post-processing. Without contrast enhancement, the diagnostic 3D reconstruction of the cardiovascular system is simply not possible. Based on our experience, the minimal level of blood enhancement needed for a reliable 3D imaging is at the density of 250 Hounsfield units (HU)[33] (Figure 7.14). The contrast injection protocol (i.e. injection rate, contrast volume, etc.) can be modified to take into account patient-related factors, substantially improving image enhancement and quality of 3D reconstruction. Parameters impacting the quality of image enhancement are numerous, all of equal importance and closely interrelated (Figure 7.15).

Volume of contrast media. The history of contrast allergy and renal function testing is important and should not differ from any other angiographic procedure, when iodine contrast is used. We try to limit contrast volume to 3 ml/kg. The amount of contrast used for routine coronary angiography is comparably smaller; however, we believe the benefits of 3D image reconstruction and manipulation of cardiac CT often outweigh the added risk. When the concentration of contrast is not sufficient to provide

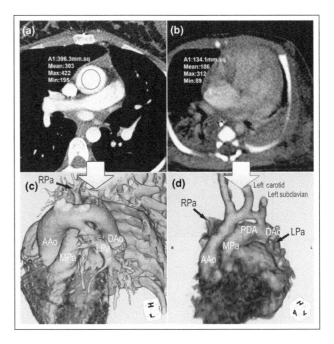

Figure 7.14
(a) A 23-year-old female with pulmonary artery anomaly – LPa originates from the aortic arch. Mean CT density in Pa: 303 HU. (b) A 4-day-old male with complex congenital heart disease (CHD) VSD, tricuspid atresia, transposition of great vessels. ... Mean CT density in the aorta: 189 HU. (c), (d) Three-dimensional computer reconstructed images from the source data, demonstrating quality differences depending on the level of contrast enhancement. AAo, ascending aorta; MPa, main pulmonary artery; LPa, left pulmonary artery; DAo, descending; aorta; PDA, patent ductus arteriosus; RPa, right pulmonary artery; HU, Hounsfield units. (See also color plate section.)

enough enhancement at the area of interest, the diagnostic accuracy is jeopardized (Figure 7.16). The volume of contrast is dependent on the injection rate and 'time factors', which include delay time, injection time, and scan time, which in turn are dependent on the heart rate and the levels of the scan (Figure 7.15). The higher volume of contrast allows more flexibility in choosing or correcting the scanning protocol for each individual situation.

Contrast injection rate. The rate of contrast injection is a crucial component of the protocol and special attention is paid to this. The speed at which a contrast agent mixes with blood dictates its concentration in the bloodstream and, accordingly, the level of X-ray attenuation. Injection rates in adults have been well studied, and range from 3.0 to 5.0 ml/s.[34–37] These rates give reliable opacification of the cardiac structure and the great vessels, with quality enhancement sufficient for 3D reconstruction. In pediatric patients, however, injection rates can vary up to 10-fold,[38] and range from 0.3 to 3.0 ml/s, to attain necessary contrast attenuation for successful 3D reconstruction. The wider range of injection

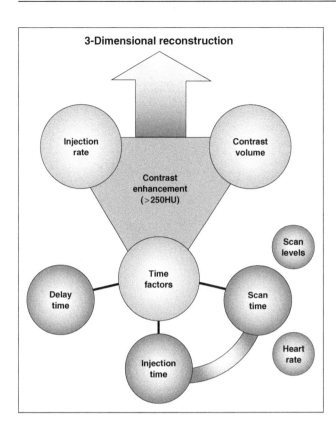

Figure 7.15
Intricate interactions of contrast protocol injections.

rates for pediatric patients is explained by the greater variability in the size of the patient and hemodynamic parameters such as heart rate, cardiac output, volume of circulating blood, etc. In practical terms, the table developed after retrospective analysis of cardiac CT examinations performed at the University of Illinois at Chicago Medical Center has been used[33] (Figure 7.17). This table is a reliable guide to choosing appropriate injection rates in pediatric patients based on their weight.

Time factors. Timing of contrast administration and CT scanning must be carefully planned to optimize the highest density at the area of interest during image acquisition.

Delay time: This is the time difference between the moment when contrast injection starts and the initial moment of image acquisition. Depending on the intravenous site, the time needed for contrast to reach the desired anatomic structure will vary. Furthermore, this time depends on other factors such as the patient size, cardiac function, and individual anatomy. In patients with congenital heart disease, with the presence of native or surgically placed shunts, the dilution factor from the shunt has to be considered. The most reliable method to perform an accurate calculation of the delay time is through performing a 'flow study' (EBCT

terminology) or 'smart preparation' (MDCT terminology). During this study a small bolus of contrast (about 5–10% of the total volume) is injected at the same rate as will be used in the study, through the same access site. Image acquisition starts simultaneously with injection. Pictures are taken through the same area of the heart in timed intervals (seconds or ECG triggered). Time/density software analysis allows the calculation of the transit time (Figure 7.4) in different cardiac structures with precise accuracy, even in complex congenital heart disease. Skipping the flow study is possible if the CT team has experience in performing angiography studies. It has been demonstrated that the average delay time for adults undergoing CT coronary angiography is standard and ranges between 18 and 25 s when the injection is made from an antecubital vein.[39]

Scan time: This component is dependent upon the distance to be covered and the specific characteristics of the scanner. With MDCT it will depend on the number of detectors, for example a 16 detector MDCT can cover 3 cm in 5 seconds at the pitch of 0.25 while a 64 detector scanner can cover 12.5 cm (average distance to cover the adult heart) in the same period of time at the same pitch. When using EBCT, the patient's heart rate will be an additional factor impacting the scan time. To cover an equivalent distance of 12.5 cm at a patient's heart rate of 60 bpm will take 40 s of scan time. The same distance at a heart rate of 90 bpm would take 27 s. The distance to cover is easily determined by performing a 'preview' study (scout image). Atropine is commonly used to increase the heart rate and to reduce the scan time, which is also important in preventing breathing motion artifacts.

Another important issue for EBCT users is the influence of faster heart rates in pediatric patients. The scanning protocol parameters require more modifications in pediatric patients than in adults. The higher heart rates seen in pediatric populations can result in doubling of the scan time, because the EBCT table is designed only to move with every heartbeat up to a maximum heart rate of 120 bpm. Above 120 bpm, the acquisition of images defaults to alternate heart beats. This will result in the need for larger volumes of contrast due to a prolonged injection time as a result of a longer scanning time.

Injection time: Injection time is dependent upon the scanning time and determines the volume of contrast needed for the study for a particular injection rate. Theoretically, injection time should be similar to the scanning time to maintain constant enhancement during acquisition. In reality, it may be shorter than the scan time due to certain characteristics of flow of contrast and dilution factors, so called 'bolus geometry' (Figure 7.18). In our experience, injection time should be at least 60% of the scanning time plus the delay time in order to obtain satisfactory enhancement contrast throughout the acquisition.

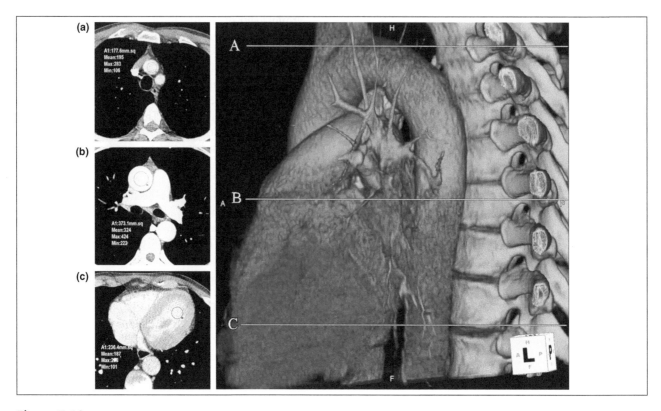

Figure 7.16

Illustration of 3D reconstruction with insufficient contrast volume. Injection stopped too early, which decreased opacification of the apical part of the heart while images were still being acquired. The image demonstrates differences in 3D quality depending on the contrast concentration. (a) Measurement of contrast enhancement taken from the ascending aorta above level A (on the right picture). Mean of density: 195 HU. (b) Measurement of contrast enhancement taken from the ascending aorta between levels A and B. Mean CT density: 324 HU.(c) Measurement taken close to level C, the apical part of the heart. Right ventricle mean density: 187 HU.

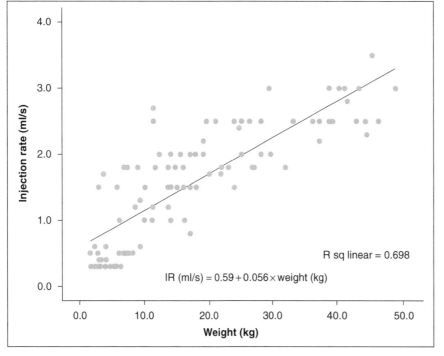

Figure 7.17

Correlation of injection rate with body weight ($\rho = 0.861$, $\rho < 0.01$).

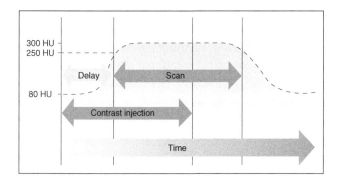

Figure 7.18
Time/density graph demonstrates the curve of the CT density in the ascending aorta and relations between contrast injection and scan in time. Base line density (without contrast enhancement) is taken around 80 HU (soft tissue density); 250 HU: minimal enhanced density necessary to start image acquisition.

Case reports

Case 1. A 34-year-old female referred to have a 4 mm PDA closed by percutaneous intervention. During the interventional procedure the wire crossed the PDA, but the delivery catheter was unable to cross. The EBCT angiogram was performed and revealed the presence of a double orifice ductus (Figure 7.19, see also color plate section). The wire was repositioned through the larger one and a 5 mm × 5 cm × 1.32 mm Gianturco coil (Cook Inc, Bloomington, IN, USA) (arrow, panel f) was deployed successfully, closing the PDA. PDA, patent ductus arteriosus; Ao, aorta; PA, pulmonary artery.

Case 2. A 17-year-old male with tetralogy of Fallot. The patient had a Blalock–Taussig shunt as an infant and a complete repair at age 5, with a take-down of the shunt and LPA enlargement. The patient presented at age 15 with absence of blood flow to the LPA. Pulmonary vein wedge angiograms revealed the presence of a 3 mm diameter distal LPA. After a unifocalization procedure with an 8 mm Gore-Tex (WL Gore & Assoc, Flagstaff, AZ, USA) graft for a period of 6 months, he underwent a take-down of the central shunt and a 10 mm Gore-Tex graft anastomosis of the rehabilitated distal LPA with the main PA. One month follow-up echo showed, again, absence of LPA flow. The patient underwent selective thrombolysis (red arrow indicates severe residual anastomotic stenosis post-thrombolysis) and stent placement at the distal and proximal anastomotic sites (yellow arrows) with 10 mm balloon expandable (Genesis, Johnson & Johnson, Warren, NJ, USA) stents (Figure 7.20, see also color plate section). Ao, aorta; PA, pulmonary artery; LPA, left pulmonary artery.

Case 3. A 3-day-old infant male with truncus arteriosus, in whom the arch was unable to be determined anatomically by 2D echocardiography. The EBCT angiography revealed the presence of a truncus arteriosus type III with interrupted aortic arch type B (Figure 7.21, see also color plate section). The patient underwent a successful single stage repair. CA, carotid arteries; Ao, aorta; PA, pulmonary artery; PDA, patent ductus arteriosus.

Case 4. A 7-year-old male with tetralogy of Fallot – pulmonary atresia – who underwent complete repair with a stented-valve conduit (Figure 7.22, see also color plate section). Arrows indicate the valve's stent. Ao, aorta; PA, pulmonary artery.

Case 5. A 72-year-old male with atypical chest pain. Coronary anomaly was reported by coronary angiography. Three-dimensional CT angiography was performed to establish the anatomic interrelations of the anomalous left coronary artery (Figure 7.23, see also color plate section). Exam showed a single coronary artery originated from right sinus of Valsalva. The RCA courses the usual path in the groove between the right atrium and right ventricle. The LM courses interiorly between the ascending aorta and the pulmonary artery. LM, left main coronary artery; RCA, right coronary artery; Ao, aorta; PA, pulmonary artery; LAD, left anterior descending coronary artery.

Case 6. A 20-year-old female with unrepaired DORV with 38 weeks' intrauterine pregnancy who underwent pulmonary artery banding of an isolated LPA from the descending aorta through a PDA. Figure 7.24 (a)–(d) Source tomograms. (e), (f) Three-dimensional images, see also color plate section. AA, aortic arch; DAo, descending aorta; LPA, left pulmonary artery; MPA, main pulmonary artery; Ao, ascending aorta; DORV, double outlet right ventricle; LPA, left pulmonary artery; PDA, patent ductus arteriosus.

Case 7. A 13-year-old female with single ventricle and status post lateral tunnel Fontan. The EBCT angiography reveals the presence of an unobstructed SVC–RPA connection, normal size pulmonary arteries without obstructions, and unobstructed IVC drainage (Figure 7.25, see also color plate section). SVC, superior vena cava; IVC, inferior vena cava; RPA, right pulmonary artery; LPA, left pulmonary artery; PV, pulmonary veins; Ao, aorta.

Case 8. A 63-year-old female. S/p CABG several years ago. Patient underwent transcatheter aortic valve (CoreValve, Irvine, CA, USA) placement. The stented valve can be seen proximal to the patent SVGs (Figure 7.26, see also color plate section). The native RCA is also visualized. The LIMA graft appears patent. SVG, saphenous vein graft; RCA, native right coronary artery; LIMA, left internal mammary artery.

Case 9. A 16-year-old male with a history of tetralogy of Fallot – pulmonary atresia with non-confluent pulmonary arteries. The patient had a bilateral unifocalization procedure; he now presented with severe progressive cyanosis. The EBCT

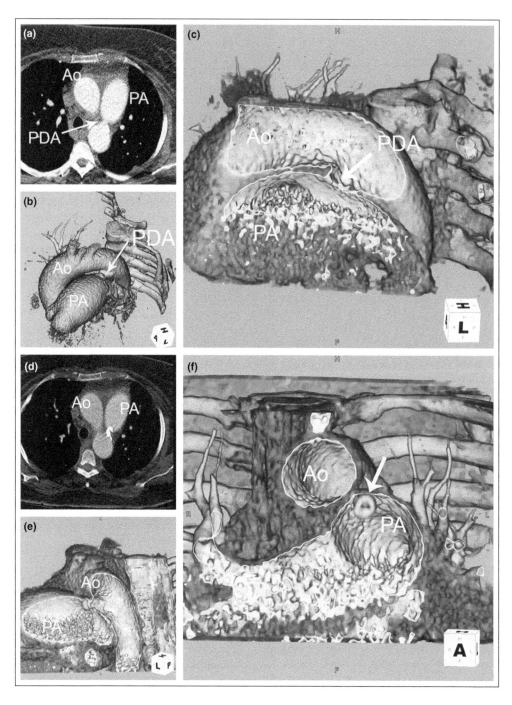

Figure 7.19
(See also color plate section.)

angiography confirmed the presence of levoacardia with situs solitus (Figure 7.27, see also color plate section). The intracardiac anatomy is consistent with a TOF-PA with a large aorta arising from the top of a large VSD. Both ventricles are of normal size. The aorta is left arch. There are no native pulmonary arteries. The left side unifocalization is connected to the left side of the transverse arch. There is a moderate degree of stenosis in the unifocalized vessel. The right side unifocalization is connected through a modified right Blalock–Taussig shunt. The wide arrows indicate the area of stenosis on the LPA. LPA, left pulmonary artery; Ao, aorta.

Case 10. A 24-year-old female with a very large secundum ASD underwent percutaneous closure with a 40 mm

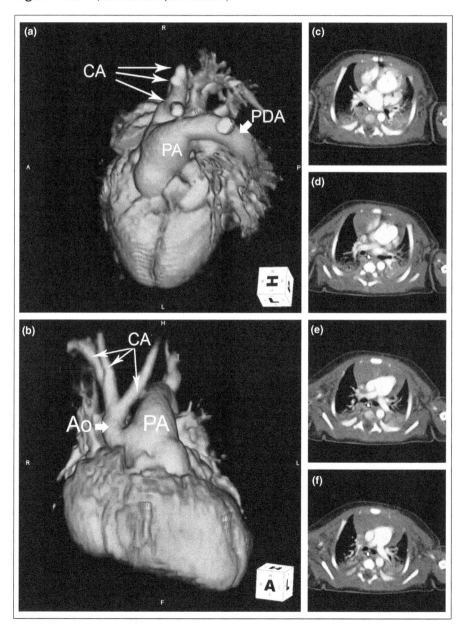

Figure 7.20 (See also color plate section.)

Figure 7.21
(See also color plate section.)

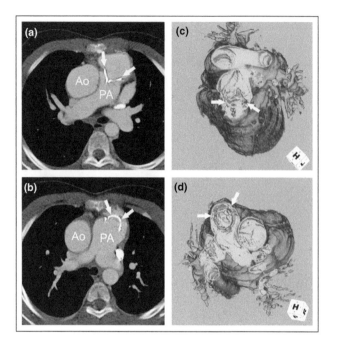

Figure 7.22   (See also color plate section.)

Figure 7.23   (See also color plate section.)

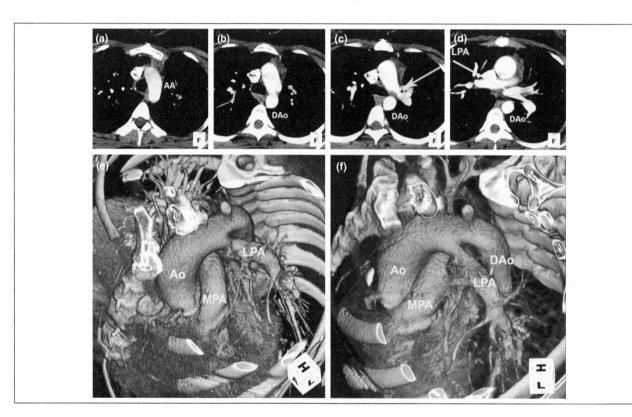

Figure 7.24   (See also color plate section.)

Amplatzer Atrial Septal Occluder (AGA, Minneapolis, MN, USA). The intracardiac as well as transthoracic echocardiograms were unable to determine the pulmonary venous drainage post-deployment because of severe echogenic interference from the device. The EBCT angiography confirmed that all pulmonary vein drainage was unobstructed, and the device was away from the mitral and tricuspid annulus, and of the coronary sinus drainage (Figure 7.28, see also color plate section.) PV, pulmonary veins; PA, pulmonary artery; LA, left atrium, LV, left ventricle, RV, right ventricle.

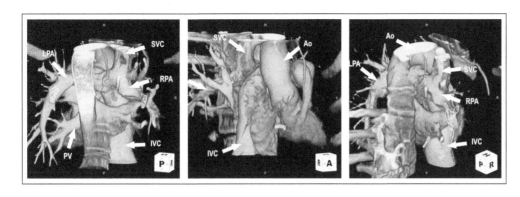

Figure 7.25
(See also color plate section.)

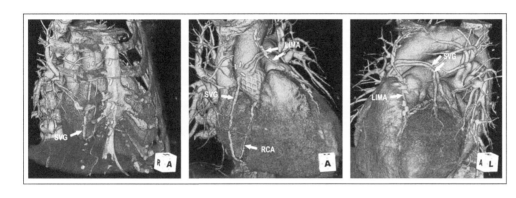

Figure 7.26
(See also color plate section.)

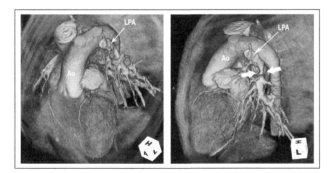

Figure 7.27
(See also color plate section.)

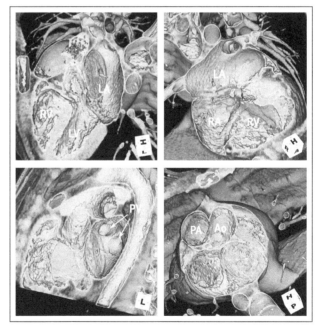

Figure 7.28
(See also color plate section)

Case 11. A 64-year-old female with severe aortic stenosis and moderate aortic regurgitation of rheumatic origin, who underwent transcatheter aortic valve placement with a CoreValve prosthesis (CoreValve, Irvine, CA, USA). The first prosthesis was deployed too distal to the native aortic annulus and the patient required a second prosthesis, during the same procedure, that was successfully placed slightly proximal to the first one and successfully resolved the severe aortic regurgitation caused by the first device. The arrows point to the double shadow corresponding to one prosthesis inside the other (Figure 7.29, see also color plate section.) Ao, aorta; RV, right ventricle; LV, left ventricle; LA, left atrium.

Case 12. A 12-year-old female, s/p failed renal transplantation, on chronic hemodialysis who developed high output cardiac failure. The EBCT angiography revealed a well defined surgically created arterio-venous fistula;

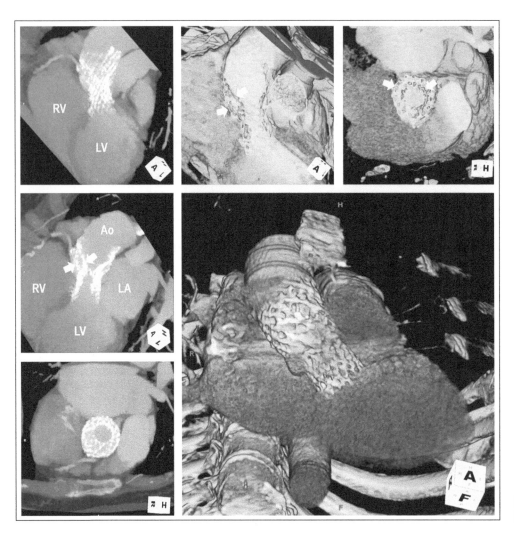

Figure 7.29
(See also color plate section.)

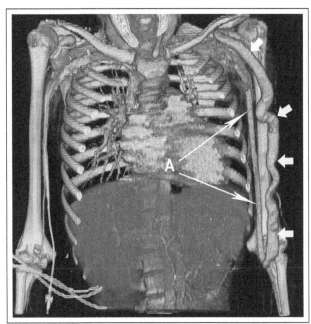

however there was a gigantic dilatation of the basilica vein (white arrows) approximating the size of the descending aorta (Figure 7.30, see also color plate section.). The intracardiac anatomy was normal, however there was severe biventricular dilatation. A, brachial artery.

Case 13. A 32-year-old male who sustained multiple gunshot wounds to the chest. On a follow-up study the patient was found to have progressive cardiomegaly. The EBCT angiography revealed the presence of a 'six-chambered heart' secondary to a large lobulated left ventricular pseudoaneurysm (arrows), that was successfully surgically treated (Figure 7.31, see also color plate section.) RV, right ventricle; LV, left ventricle; A, lobulated pseudoaneurysm.

Case 14. A 56-year-old asymptomatic marathon runner who was found to have severe LVH on a routine ECG. The EBCT angiography reveals the presence of significant LVH and the presence of an apical LV diverticulum (arrow) (Figure 7.32, see also color plate section.) RA, right atrium; RV, right ventricle; LA, left atrium; LV, left ventricle.

Figure 7.30
(See also color plate section.)

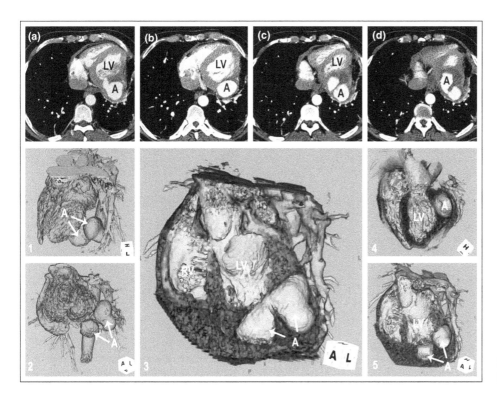

Figure 7.31
(See also color plate section.)

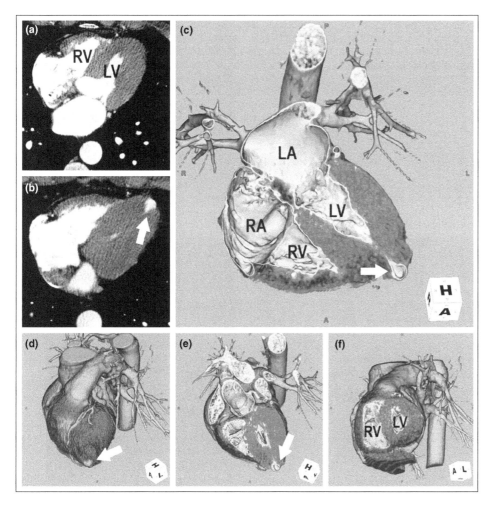

Figure 7.32
(See also color plate section.)

Acknowledgments

The authors are grateful to Mr Maxim Tsireshkin for the illustrations.

References

1. Radon J. Uber die Bestimmung von Funktionen durch ihre Integralwerte langs gewisser Manningfaltigkeiten. Bu Succss Akad Wiss 1917; 69: 262.

2. Oldendorf WH. Isolated flying spot detection of radio-density discontinuities displaying the internal structural pattern of a complex object. IRE Trans Bio Med Elect BME 1961; 8: 68–72.

3. Hounsfield GN. Computed medical imaging: Nobel Lecture, December 8, 1979. J Comput Assist Tomogr 1980; 4: 665–74.

4. Hounsfield GN. Computerized transverse axial scanning (tomography): I. Description of system. Br J Radiol 1973; 46: 1016–22.

5. Hounsfield GN. Picture quality of computed tomography. AJR 1976; 127: 3–9.

6. Jakobs TF, Becker CR, Ohnesorge B et al. Multislice helical CT of the heart with retrospective ECG gating: reduction of radiation exposure by ECG-controlled tube current modulation. Eur Radiol 2002; 12: 1081–6.

7. Morin RL, Gerber TC, McCollough CH. Radiation dose in computed tomography of the heart. Circulation 2003; 107: 917–22.

8. McCollough CH, Zink FE, Morin RL. Radiation dosimetry for electron-beam CT. Radiology 1994; 192: 637–43.

9. Cohen M, Poll L, Pittmann C et al. Radiation exposure in multi-slice CT of the heart. Foetshr Rontgenstr 2001; 178: 295–9.

10. Hidajat N, Wolfe M, Rademaker J et al. Radiation dose in CT of the heart for coronary artery disease and CT of lung for pulmonary embolism: comparison between single-slice detector CT, multislice detector CT and EBT. Radiology 2000; 217: 74–8.

11. Knollman FD, Hidajat N, Felix R. CTA of the coronary arteries: comparison of radiation exposure with EBCT and multi-slice detector CT. Radiology 2000; 217: 364–5.

12. Boyd D. Computerized transmission tomography of the heart using scanning electron beams. In: Higgins CB, ed. CT of the Heart and the Great Vessels: Experimental Evaluation in the Clinical Application. Mt Kisco, New York: Futura, 1983: 45–60.

13. McCollough CH, Morin RL. The technical design and performance of ultrafast computed tomography. Radiol Clin North Am 1994; 32: 521–36.

14. Kalender WA, Seissler W, Klotz E et al. Spiral volumetric CT with single-breath-hold technique, continuous transport, and continuous scanner rotation. Radiology 1990; 176: 181–3.

15. Kalender WA, Polacin A. Physical performance characteristics of spiral CT scanning. Med Phys 1991; 18: 910–15.

16. Crawford CR, King KF. Computed tomography scanning with simultaneous patient translation. Med Phys 1990; 17: 967–82.

17. Lu B, Mao S, Zhuang N et al. Coronary artery motion during the cardiac cycle and optimal ECG triggering for coronary artery imaging. Invest Radiol 2001; 36(5): 250–6.

18. Lu B, Zhuang N, Mao SS et al. Baseline heart rate-adjusted electrocardiographic triggering for coronary artery electron-beam CT angiography. Radiology 2004; 233(2): 590–5.

19. Mao S, Budoff M, Bin L, Liu SC. Optimal ECG trigger point in electron-beam CT studies: three methods for minimizing motion artifacts. Acad Radiol 2001; 8(11): 1107–15.

20. Mao S, Lu B, Takasu J et al. Measurement of the RT interval on ECG records during electron-beam CT. Acad Radiol 2003; 10(6): 638–43.

21. Arad Y, Roth M, Newstein D et al. Coronary calcification, coronary risk factors, and atherosclerotic cardiovascular disease events. The St. Francis Heart Study. J Am Coll Cardiol 2003; 41: 6–7.

22. Arad Y, Spadaro L, Goodman K et al. Predictive value of electron beam computed tomography of the coronary arteries. Circulation 1996; 93: 1951–3.

23. Agatston AS, Janowitz W, Kaplan GS et al. Electron beam CT predicts future coronary events. Circulation 1996; 94(Suppl 1): I–360.

24. Raggi P, Cooil B, Callister TQ. Use of electron beam tomography data to develop models for prediction of hard coronary events. Am Heart J 2001; 141: 375–82.

25. Kondos GT, Hoff J, Sevrukov A et al. Electron-beam tomography coronary artery calcium and cardiac events: a 37-month follow-up of 5635 initially asymptomatic low- to intermediate-risk adults. Circulation 2003; 107: 2571–6.

26. Wexler L, Brundage B, Crouse J et al. Coronary artery calcification: pathophysiology, epidemiology, imaging methods, and clinical implications. A statement for health professionals from the American Heart Association. Writing Group. Circulation 1996; 94: 1175–92.

27. Rumberger JA, Brundage B, Rader DJ, Kondos G. Electron beam computed tomographic coronary calcium scanning: a review and guidelines for use in asymptomatic persons. Mayo Clin Proc 1999; 74(3): 243–52.

28. Rumberger JA, Behrenbeck T, Breen JF, Sheedy II PF. Coronary calcification by electron beam computed tomography and obstructive coronary artery disease: a model for costs and effectiveness of diagnosis as compared with conventional cardiac testing methods. J Am Coll Cardiol 1999; 33(2): 453–62.

29. Budoff MJ, Chen GP, Hunter CJ et al. Noninvasive coronary angiography using computed tomography. Expert Rev Cardiovasc Ther 2005; 3(1): 123–32.

30. Achenbach S. [Clinical Use of Multi-Slice CT Coronary Angiography]. Herz 2003; 28(2): 119–25.

31. Achenbach S, Hoffmann U, Ferencik M, Wicky S, Brady TJ. Tomographic coronary angiography by EBCT and MDCT. Prog Cardiovasc Dis 2003; 46(2): 185–95.

32. Achenbach S, Moshage W, Ropers D et al. Noninvasive, three-dimensional visualization of coronary artery bypass grafts by electron beam tomography. Am J Cardiol 1997; 79(7): 856–61.

33. Jelnin V, Co J, Muneer B et al. Three dimensional CT angiography for patients with congenital heart disease: scanning protocol for pediatric patients. CCI 2006; 67(1): 120–6.

34. Lu B, Jing BL, Bai H et al. Evaluation of coronary artery bypass graft patency using three-dimensional reconstruction and flow study on electron beam tomography. J Comput Assist Tomogr 2000; 24(5): 663–70.

35. Ropers D, Moshage W, Daniel WG et al. Visualization of coronary artery anomalies and their anatomic course by contrast-enhanced electron beam tomography and three-dimensional reconstruction. Am J Cardiol 2001; 87(2): 193–7.

36. Lu B, Bai H, He S et al. Evaluation of electron beam tomographic coronary arteriography with three-dimensional reconstruction in healthy subjects. Angiology 2000; 51(11): 895–904.

37. Leber AW, Knez A, Becker C et al. Non-invasive intravenous coronary angiography using electron beam tomography and multislice computed tomography. Heart 2003; 89: 591–4.

38. Westra SJ, Galindo A, McNitt-Gray MF et al. Cardiac electron-beam CT in children undergoing surgical repair for pulmonary atresia. Radiology 1999; 213: 502–12.

39. Cademartiri F, Nieman K. Contrast material injection techniques for CT angiography of the coronary arteries. In: CT of the Heart. Principles and Applications, 1st edn. M. U. Joseph Schoepef, ed. Totowa: Humana Press, 2005: 237–45.

Section III

Vascular access

8

Access from the common carotid artery

Grazyna Brzezinska-Rajszys

It is rare for access to be required from the carotid artery for the purposes of cardiac catheterization. Nowadays this approach is reserved mostly for balloon valvuloplasty in newborns with aortic valve stenosis. In experienced hands, it is a safe approach and simplifies crossing the stenosed aortic valve and reduces vascular complications associated with the femoral arterial approach in very small patients.[1–7] It also shortens the time of the procedure, which is especially important in sick neonates with critical aortic valve stenosis.[7] The carotid artery approach is also very useful for interventions, in which relatively large sheaths are required. The choice of access via the right or left common carotid artery depends on the planned interventional procedure and the anatomy of the aortic arch and its branches. For example, balloon aortic valvuloplasty in babies with left sided aortic arch may be performed more easily through the right carotid artery approach, whereas stent implantation into the abdominal aorta in a patient with left aortic arch may be more easily performed through the left carotid arterial approach.

Ultrasound assessment of the morphology and the flow through the carotid artery after neonatal surgical cutdown has shown that the carotid artery is well preserved in more than 95% of the patients,[4,6] although an asymptomatic obstruction may occasionally be present.[8]

The common carotid artery cutdown should be performed by a surgeon or a cardiologist trained in this technique and not by anyone else.

Technique

The carotid artery takes its course in the triangle formed by the clavicle and the sternal and clavicular bellies of the sternocleidomastoid muscle insertions entering the chest under the head of the clavicle.

The patient is placed in a supine position with a wedge placed under the back to elevate the shoulders, with the head slightly turned to the opposite side to expose the neck and keep the chin away from the operating field. Forceful neck extension or serious leftward rotation of the head should be avoided as it may change the cervical vascular anatomy. Careful positioning of the patient is important as it improves identification of surface landmarks.

Anatomic landmarks including the sternal notch, the clavicle, and the sternocleidomastoid muscle should be assessed before preparation and draping for the procedure. The carotid artery should be palpated and its course determinated. The common carotid artery lies lateral to the trachea, usually under the medial sternal head of sternocleidomastoid muscle. General anesthesia and controlled ventilation are important. The carotid artery cutdown should be a sterile procedure starting with aseptic hand washing. A mask, cap, sterile gloves, and gown must be used by the operator. The skin is cleaned widely from the earlobe to the clavicle and the sternal notch with an appropriate antiseptic lotion. The relevant anatomy is identified, particularly the course of the carotid artery.

A transverse skin incision (parallel to the clavicle) is made above the sternocleidomastoid muscle halfway between the jugular notch and the thyroid cartilage. After the skin incision, the platysma should be blunt dissected and the medial border of the sternocleidomastoid muscle exposed. The common carotid artery takes its course together with the internal jugular vein and the vagus nerve as a neurovascular bundle medial to the sternocleidomastoid muscle. The common carotid artery is identified, located medially and deeper than the jugular vein. The artery is exposed with blunt dissection and an adequate length of artery is mobilized to allow proximal and distal control with vascular loops of rubber or silk. A purse-string suture of 7-0 or 6-0 monofilament (Prolene) is placed between the vascular loops. Artery puncture is performed in the center of the purse-string. Gentle traction on both vascular loops helps to control the bleeding. The artery is entered with the needle and a guidewire is introduced through it (Figure 8.1). An appropriate sized sheath is introduced over the guidewire. It is important to check carefully

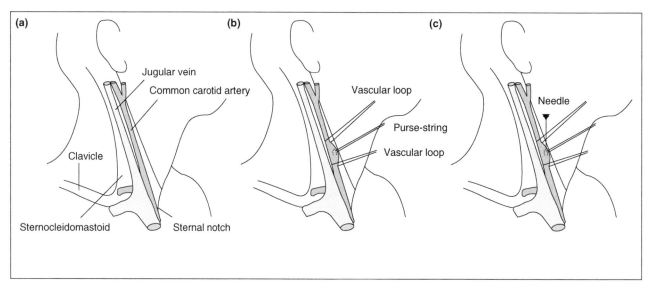

Figure 8.1
Technique for right carotid artery approach. Anatomic landmarks and carotid anatomy (a). Preparation of the carotid artery with vascular loops and purse-string (b). Artery puncture in the middle of the purse-string (c).

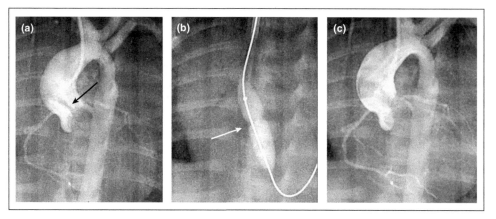

Figure 8.2
Right carotid artery access for aortic balloon valvuloplasty in neonate. Aortography before valvuloplasty with the jet of unopacified blood (arrow) (a). Balloon valvuloplasty catheter placed across the valve, indentation on the balloon reflects the level of the stenotic valve (arrow) (b). Aortography after successful balloon valvuloplasty (c).

the position of the end of the sheath under fluoroscopy as in neonates it can reach the aortic valve. If the balloon is then kept partially in the sheath during its inflation, it can cause serious damage to the sheath and may cause difficulties with its removal. The patient should be heparinized with 100 units/kg. In neonates, cerebral ultrasonography should be performed before the procedure to exclude cerebral hemorrhage, because this may influence heparinization.

Once the sheath is in place, intervention such as balloon dilation or stent implantation can be performed. After the procedure, whilst traction is maintained on both vascular loops, the sheath is removed, and the purse-string is tied to produce hemostasis. The vascular loops are then removed. The flow through the artery is checked by palpation and the wound is closed by a subcutaneous suture. The wound should be covered with a sterile dressing. Ultrasound scan with visualization of the carotid artery and Doppler examination with measurements of the blood velocity should be repeated before discharge from hospital.

Complications

With careful surgical technique, complications related to carotid access are very rare. Periprocedural complications such as arterial thrombosis or arterial damage treated with its ligation were reported in earlier series and should be

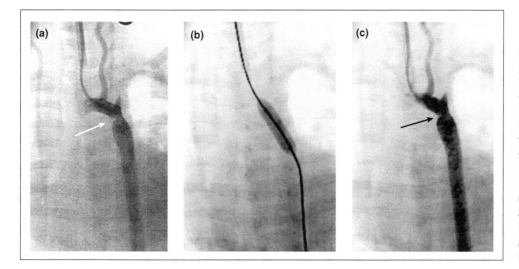

Figure 8.3
Right carotid artery access for balloon angioplasty of coarctation of the aorta in neonate. Procedure performed after aortic valvuloplasty during the same session. Aortography before angioplasty shows native coarctation of aorta (arrow) (a). Balloon angioplasty catheter placed in the isthmus (b). Aortography after successful balloon angioplasty (c).

Examples of applications

The carotid artery approach can be used for balloon valvuloplasty in neonates with isolated critical aortic valve stenosis (Figure 8.2). In patients with associated coarctation of the aorta, balloon angioplasty of coarctation can be performed through the carotid approach during the same session (Figure 8.3).[2,7] The carotid artery approach can be used for stent implantation into the aorta in small children (Figure 8.4),[9] for stent implantation into the pulmonary artery via Blalock–Taussig shunt in patients with complex congenital heart defects with pulmonary trunk atresia and pulmonary artery stenosis (Figure 8.5), and for occlusion of important aorto-pulmonary collaterals, mostly in neonates after surgery (for example after an arterial switch operation) (Figure 8.6).

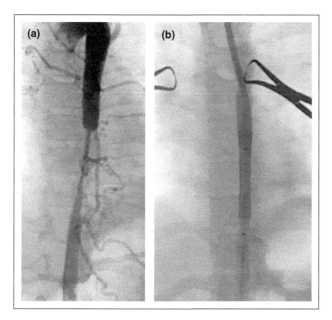

Figure 8.4
Stent implantation into the thoracic aorta for middle aortic syndrome by right carotid artery access. Angiogram shows severe narrowing of lower thoracic aorta (a). Stent implantation into the aorta (b).

treated individually.[6,8] Carotid artery stenosis is a potential complication of this approach, but seems to be exceptional.[6] In angiography performed 3 months after balloon aortic valvuloplasty, a normal right carotid artery was demonstrated.[3] In mid-term follow-up in some patients with ultrasound examination, the site of surgical incision could be identified without flow disturbances.[8] One of the main limitations of this procedure is the need for specialized training in the technique or the need for a surgeon to perform carotid arteriotomy.

Conclusion

The access from the common carotid artery performed carefully is safe and very helpful. The indications for this technique should be analyzed in detail before the planned interventional procedure, taking into consideration the vascular anatomy as well. Nowadays, with modern low profile balloon catheters, the role of common carotid artery access is diminishing, but in special circumstances it should still be considered. In low weight patients with critical aortic stenosis, this easy access seems to be very important, reducing both the time of the procedure and complications related to damage of the femoral artery.

Carotid access should be a technique available in pediatric catheterization laboratories. In centers familiar with this approach it is used more frequently for a variety of problems than aortic balloon valvuloplasty.

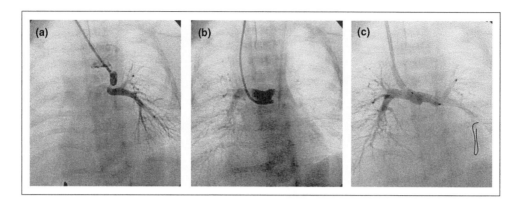

Figure 8.5
Right carotid artery access for stent implantation into the left pulmonary artery via right modified Blalock–Taussig shunt. Angiography in the arterial duct shows severe stenosis of the pulmonary artery end of the duct (a). Arteriography of pulmonary arteries with catheter placed through the Blalock–Taussig shunt shows severe stenosis of the left pulmonary artery (b). Arteriography through the sheath after stent implantation in the left pulmonary artery. Note that catheter and guidewire are still in the pulmonary artery (c).

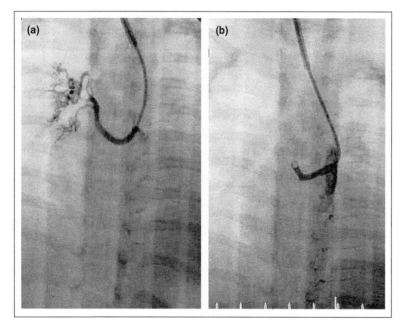

Figure 8.6
Right carotid artery access for embolization of major aorto-pulmonary collateral after switch operation for transposition of the great arteries in neonate. Selective angiography in collateral before (a) and after procedure (b).

References

1. Fischer DR, Ettedgui JA, Park SC et al. Carotid artery approach for balloon dilation of aortic valve stenosis in the neonate: a preliminary report. J Am Coll Cardiol 1990; 15: 1633–6.
2. Carminati M, Giusti S, Spadoni I et al. Balloon aortic valvuloplasty in the first year of life. J Interven Cardiol 1995; 8(6 Suppl): 759–66.
3. Maeno Y, Akagi T, Hashino K et al. Carotid artery approach to balloon aortic valvuloplasty in infants with critical aortic valve stenosis. Pediatr Cardiol 1997; 18: 288–91.
4. Weber HS, Mart CR, Kupferschmid J et al. Transcarotid balloon valvuloplasty with continuous transesophageal echocardiographic guidance for neonatal critical aortic valve stenosis: an alternative to surgical palliation. Pediatr Cardiol 1998; 19: 212–17.
5. Fagan TE, Ing FF, Edens RE et al. Balloon aortic valvuloplasty in a 1,600-gram infant. Cathet Cardiovasc Interven 2000; 50: 322–5.
6. Robinson BV, Brzezinska-Rajszys G, Weber HS et al. Balloon aortic valvotomy through a carotid cutdown in infants with severe aortic stenosis: results of the multi-centric registry. Cardiol Young 2000; 10: 225–32.
7. Pedra CA, Pedra SR, Braga SL et al. Short- and midterm follow-up results of valvuloplasty with balloon catheter for congenital aortic stenosis. Arq Bras Cardiol 2003; 81: 120–8.
8. Borghi A, Agnoletti G, Poggiani C. Surgical cutdown of the right carotid artery for aortic balloon valvuloplasty in infancy: midterm follow-up. Pediatr Cardiol 2001; 22: 194–7.
9. Brzezinska-Rajszys G, Qureshi SA, Ksiazyk J et al. Middle aortic syndrome treated by stent implantation. Heart 1999; 81: 166–70.

9

Transhepatic access

Makram R Ebeid

Introduction

Currently, many children undergo multiple cardiac catheterizations and surgical interventions early in their life, requiring intensive care admission and central line placement frequently involving the femoral vessels. As a result, these vessels may become occluded (Figure 9.1). In the presence of occluded femoral vessels alternate routes are sought to perform cardiac catheterization and/or intervention. The internal jugular approach or subclavian approach may be appropriate in some instances. In other instances where the patient has undergone cavo-pulmonary anastomosis it may be impossible to reach the area of interest using this approach. Additionally, it may be difficult to manipulate the catheters from that approach in certain areas of the heart and can be met with significant challenges.

History

In the mid-1990s the transhepatic approach emerged as an alternative to the traditional femoral vein approach for cardiac catheterization and/or intervention.[1–5] A number of catheterizers have subsequently reported favorable experiences with varying degrees of success and applicability.[6–10] Some (including the author) have felt that it is the preferred approach to be utilized in certain instances even when alternative venous routes are available.[2,5] The youngest patient reported was 1 day old[1] and the lowest weight was 2.3 kg.[3] The increasing experience with this approach and the varying complexity of cardiac catheterizations and interventions make this approach attractive for selective cases. The knowledge and skills to perform this approach should be acquired by the experienced pediatric interventionalist, to be used when deemed appropriate. The approach is more favorable than neck approaches for some interventions (personal experience), and for catheter manipulations, and may be even more attractive than the traditional femoral approach in some cases, as will be discussed.

Physiologic anatomy

The liver contributes about 2% of the total body weight. It contains 50 000–100 000 lobules, constructed around a central vein connecting to the hepatic vein and into the inferior vena cava.[11] Surrounding the hepatic lobule is the portal triad (Figure 9.2), formed from the tributaries of the bile

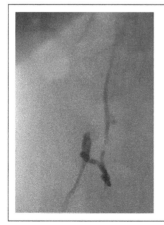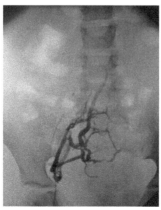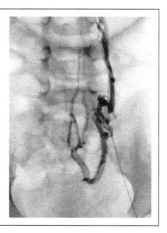

Figure 9.1
Angiograms outlining occluded femoral veins in three patients.

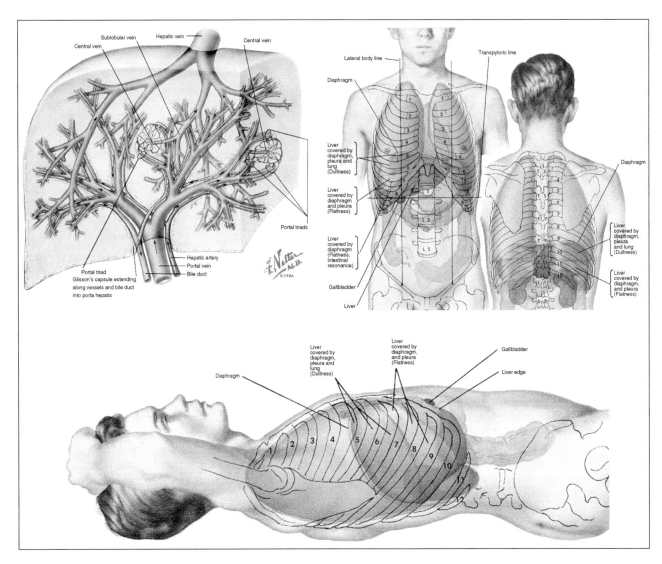

Figure 9.2
Diagrammatic representation of the hepatic lobule and the portal triad shown in the top left. The surface anatomy of the liver in the erect (top right) and supine positions (bottom) is outlined (reproduced with permission from Ciba).

duct, the portal vein, and the hepatic artery.[12] It receives its blood supply from two sources: the portal vein (75%) and the hepatic artery (25%). Most of the liver is covered by peritoneum.[12] Approximately 10% of the total blood volume is stored in the liver at any given time.[11] This volume can increase 2- to 3-fold in cases of elevated right atrial pressure. The liver lies close to the abdominal wall on its right and lateral anterior surface.[13] Its diaphragmatic surface (superior, right, and anterior borders) forms the convex surface of the liver lying beneath the diaphragm and is separated from its visceral (inferior) border by a sharp narrow inferior border. The gall bladder is located in the inferior surface approximately 4–5 cm to the right of the mid-line.[13] The projections of the liver on the body surface have acquired added significance in the performance of a transhepatic approach. The projections vary depending upon the position of the individual as well as the body build, particularly the configuration of the thorax. In the erect position (Figure 9.2) the liver extends downward to the 10th or 11th rib in the right mid-axillary line. Here, the pleura projects downward to the 10th rib and the lung to the 8th. The inferior margin of the liver crosses the costal arch in the right lateral body line, approximately at the level of the pylorus (transpyloric line). In the horizontal position (Figure 9.2) the projection of the liver moves a little upwards.[12]

Pre-catheter planning

Careful history taking to exclude underlying liver disease and to elicit a history of anticoagulation and antiplatelet regimens is very important in the planning. We generally like to avoid antithrombin but not necessarily antiplatelet medications prior to the transhepatic catheterization. The latter would usually favor closing the tract post-procedure (see later). When indicated, lab work to evaluate the bleeding and liver function should be considered. In patients with complex congenital heart disease and suspected heterotaxy it is mandatory to evaluate the liver location prior to the procedure. Ultrasound should be performed if not previously done. A history indicative of elevated central venous pressure (as in Fontan patients or patients with right sided lesions) is important to plan for pre- and post-management of the patients, though in itself is not a contraindication to this approach.

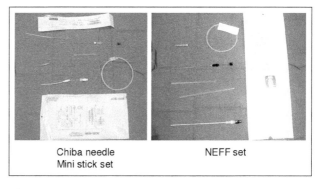

Figure 9.3
Transhepatic set. On the left is shown the Chiba needle with Mini stick™ kit, on the right is the NEFF set.

Technique

The procedure can be performed under conscious sedation or general anesthesia. In cases of conscious sedation, the area of entry should be well anesthetized and that includes the subcutaneous tissue as well as deep into the subcapsular area and the hepatic parenchyma, since the needle entry and sheath placement can be painful. It is important to monitor the blood pressure during the procedure and this is usually done using an indwelling arterial catheter. A long needle (21 or 22 gauge) with or without an obturator, such as the Chiba needle or the NEFF set (Cook, Bloomington, IN), is usually used (Figure 9.3). A 018 inch wire with a floppy end needs to be introduced through the needle. A transitional/coaxial sheath which allows the wire to be upsized will facilitate the placing of the required dilator and sheath to perform the procedure. It is part of the NEFF set, or can be obtained in separate kits as the Mini-stick™ kit (Boston Scientific, Glens Falls, NY). The needle is introduced under fluoroscopy with antero-posterior and lateral projection capability in the mid to anterior axillary line below the costal margin, angled superiorly, posteriorly, and medially towards the patient's left shoulder (Figure 9.4). Alternative approaches include introducing the needle mid-way between the xiphoid sternum and the right mid-axillary line, directing the needle to the right atrium at an angle of 20–30°[9] or to the mid-liver in the intercostal spaces, below the diaphragm, as guided by fluoroscopy (Z Hijazi, personal communication).

The needle most commonly used is 15 cm long. The needle and obturator are introduced until they are 1 cm from the mid-line. A 'pop' may be felt when the needle is in a large vein. The obturator is removed and a contrast filled syringe is applied to the needle. Gentle aspiration is performed while withdrawing the needle until blood is obtained. Once blood is obtained, the needle is held steady and a small contrast injection is performed while the image is acquired on antero-posterior and lateral projections to outline the hepatic vein. The distinction between the hepatic and portal veins is made by noting the direction of flow of the blood

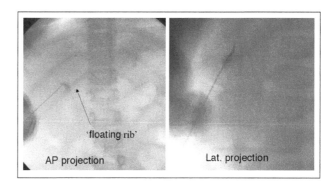

Figure 9.4
The needle orientation in the antero-posterior and lateral projections.

(Figure 9.5a). Occasionally, despite outlining a hepatic vein, the vein is seen to be very tortuous with a sharp curve, which makes it more difficult to use for the catheterization (Figure 9.5b). The needle may have to be readjusted slightly or pulled further while small injections are performed to outline a useful hepatic vein. Once a suitable hepatic vein has been identified (Figure 9.5c,d) the syringe is removed and the wire is inserted under fluoroscopy guidance. The wire should go smoothly and easily to the right atrium and preferably positioned in the superior vena cava or in the pulmonary veins if there is an atrial septal defect. Alternatively, the wire is maintained in the right atrium or the right ventricle. We attempt to maintain the stiffer part of the wire along the transhepatic tract.

Depending on the sheath size, multiple dilators may be used to dilate the hepatic tract and allow for insertion of the required sheath. Frequently, a transitional sheath such as the Mini-stick™ kit or Neff set is used. By the use of this sheath, the 0.018 inch wire can be upsized to a larger and stiffer wire (0.035–0.038 inch). Alternatively, a second 0.018 inch wire can be placed side by side, especially if there is concern about premature removal of the initially placed wire. This will provide a

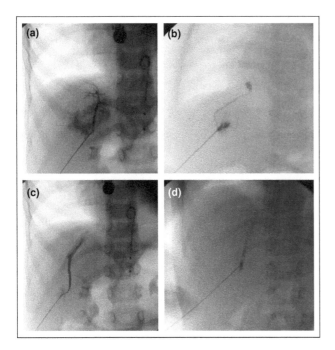

Figure 9.5
(a) Angiogram outlines a portal vein. Note the direction of blood flow. (b) A tortuous hepatic vein is seen. Its course would make it difficult to introduce the wire/sheath. (c) and (d) Two favorable hepatic veins useful for placing the sheath and performing the cardiac catheterization.

larger effective wire caliber which can be used to advance stiffer dilators/sheaths (Figure 9.6). Rarely, despite placing the wire, it may be difficult or impossible to advance the required sheaths and dilators. This may happen because of the sharp angle the floppy wire may take when it curves in the capsular space/liver parenchyma while entering the hepatic vein. In these rare instances, when the sheath and the dilator will not

follow, the procedure may have to be repeated, entering a higher intercostal space (Figure 9.7). Preferably, the entry point should be the subcostal area, though, depending on the hepatic position, one or two intercostal spaces above can also be used, allowing a straighter wire/sheath course. Ultrasound has been used as an adjunct to[9] or instead of fluoroscopy to identify a suitable hepatic vein and obtain transhepatic access.[14] The use of heparin is based on the planned procedure, arterial line placement, and operator preference. If heparin is used, it is administered after access has been obtained. The decision to reverse heparin before removal of the sheath is guided by the activated clotting time, heparin dose, time elapsed from heparin administration, and the procedure performed. We prefer to avoid heparin reversal, if possible, in cases of atrial septal device placement.

Catheter manipulations

After transhepatic access has been obtained and the appropriate sheath has been placed, catheter manipulations using that route can differ from catheter manipulations from other approaches. Most of the approaches from the transhepatic route need pre-shaped catheters with reasonably good torque, such as the Judkins right catheter and the Judkins left catheter (with the tip cut off), and occasionally some catheters with tight curves, such as the shepherd's hook or Simmons type (Merit Medical Systems, Inc, South Jordan, UT).

Right heart
Right and left superior vena cava

Entry to the superior vena cava is relatively simple by the aid of a guidewire and pre-shaped catheters. Entry to the coronary sinus and left superior vena cava is generally easier than

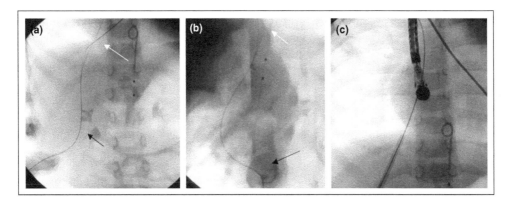

Figure 9.6
Antero-posterior (a) and lateral projections (b) of transhepatically placed wire making a sharp angle (black arrow). Notice two 0.018 inch caliber wires (white arrow) are placed side by side, which facilitated placing a large caliber dilator. (c) Subsequently, a super stiff wire was positioned in the innominate vein, allowing an 11 Fr sheath to be placed for atrial septal defect closure.

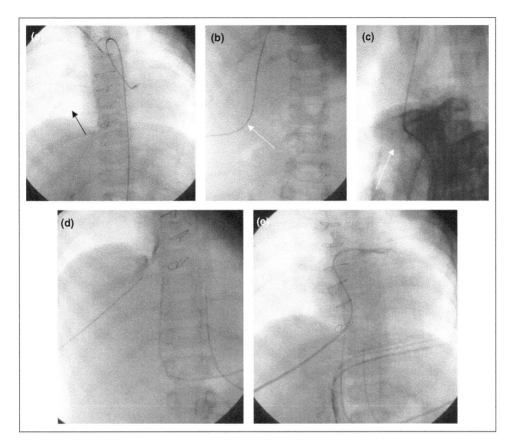

Figure 9.7
(a) A floppy wire was successfully placed in the right pulmonary vein using the subcostal approach. (b) Antero-posterior and lateral (c) projections of the wire show a sharp tight curve. Despite using multiple dilators it was not possible to place the required sheath. (d) A repeat hepatic puncture slightly higher avoided the sharp tight curve of the wire and allowed easy placement of the required sheath (e).

other approaches since the transhepatic route directs the catheter posteriorly towards the coronary sinus (Figure 9.8).

Inferior vena cava

Usually the entry to the inferior vena cava is straightforward. Occasionally, the wire needs to be directed from the right atrium to the inferior vena cava by a pre-shaped catheter as the Simmons or Cobra type curved catheters (Merit Medical Systems, Inc).

Right ventricle

Entry into the right ventricle involves slightly more manipulations since the transhepatic route carries the catheter, posteriorly and leftward. The wire should be directed by the aid of a pre-shaped catheter, anteriorly, to the right ventricle. This is carried out relatively simply by Judkins right

type catheters (Figure 9.9). Alternatively, a custom made, specially angulated transhepatic sheath can be used (Cook, Inc, Bloomington, IN) which may facilitate transhepatic catheter manipulations.

Pulmonary artery and branches (Figure 9.10)

Entry from the right ventricle to the main pulmonary artery is relatively simple and similar to entry from the femoral vessels (Figure 9.10a–c). The entry is facilitated by using pre-shaped catheters (or sheaths) and floppy wires. Directing the catheter/wire to the left pulmonary artery guides it into a relatively smooth curve (Figure 9.10f) when compared to the right pulmonary artery (Figure 9.10d,e). This lends itself well to interventions on the left pulmonary artery, whether to perform balloon angioplasty or stent placement. Intervention on the right pulmonary artery is also feasible, though it involves more curvature.

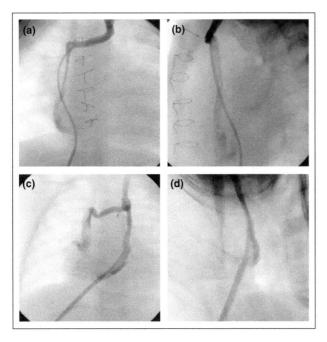

Figure 9.8
Entry to the right superior vena cava (a,b) and left superior vena cava (c,d). Note the straight entry to the coronary sinus and left superior vena cava.

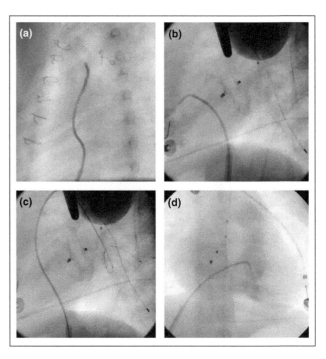

Figure 9.9
Right ventricle entry is facilitated by the use of pre-shaped curved catheters to allow redirecting the wire/catheter from the posterior leftward transhepatic orientation to the anterior/rightward direction towards the right ventricle. The catheter is shown in a left anterior oblique projection (a), lateral (b,c), and antero-posterior projections (d).

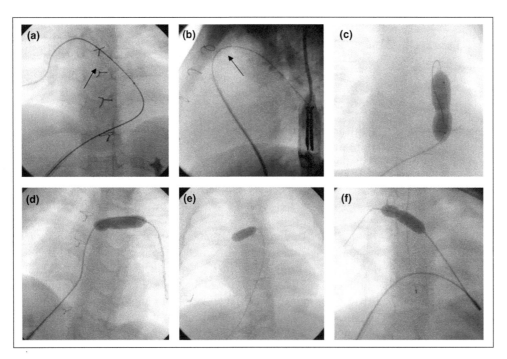

Figure 9.10
Transhepatic interventions in the pulmonary artery system. Antero-posterior (a) and lateral projections (b) of transhepatic stent placement (arrow) in a stenosed homograft. (c) Pulmonary balloon valvuloplasty. (d) Balloon angioplasty of the left and right pulmonary arteries (e,f). Notice the relatively smooth curve of the left pulmonary artery catheter as contrasted to the somewhat sharper curve of the right pulmonary artery catheter.

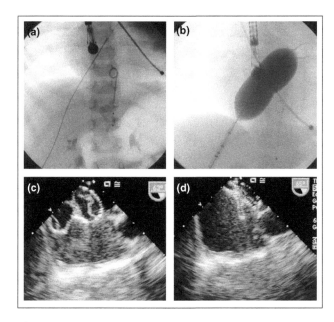

Figure 9.11
Crossing the atrial septal defect using this approach is simple. (a) Note the straight catheter course. (b) Balloon sizing shows the orientation of the atrial septum almost perpendicular to the transhepatic approach, which renders itself for easy placement of occluder devices. (c,d) Transesophageal imaging planes with (c) and without (d) tension on the cable. Note that even with applying tension the device is oriented parallel to the septum, and does not change with release of the tension.

Atrial septum and left heart structures

Atrial septum

The transhepatic approach directs the catheter leftward and posteriorly. It lends itself to direct access to the atrial septum and the left atrium. This feature is extremely helpful in closing atrial septal defects and placing devices, especially in cases of large atrial septal defects (especially with deficient rims). The sheath entry is almost perpendicular to the atrial septum, which aligns the device in plane parallel to the atrial septum (Figure 9.11).[15] Even when the femoral vein is not occluded, this approach will avoid other maneuvers described to align the atrial septal device, parallel to the septum, avoiding prolapse of any part of the device through the deficient rim.[16,17] This will also avoid the difficulties that might be encountered if the device were to be deployed using the internal jugular approach when the femoral vein is not accessible.[18]

Left atrium

Entry to the left atrium is facilitated by the transhepatic route. This route directs the catheter posteriorly and

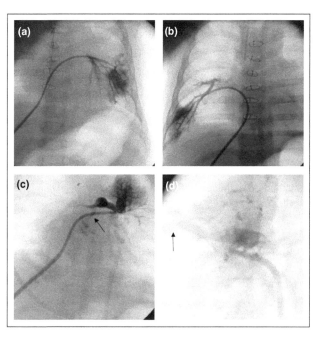

Figure 9.12
Left atrial entry is facilitated by this approach. Two patients are shown with occluded femoral vessels and hypoplastic left heart syndrome. It would have been more difficult to obtain these angiograms using the internal jugular approach. (a) and (b) Left and right pulmonary vein wedge angiograms outlining the distal pulmonary arteries in a patient with Norwood stage I. (c) and (d) Antero-posterior and lateral left pulmonary vein wedge angiograms outlining a Sano modification (arrow).

leftward towards the left atrium and to the pulmonary veins (especially the left) (Figure 9.12).

Left ventricle

Entry to the left ventricle will require turning the catheter anteriorly from its straight posterior approach. It can sometimes be accomplished with balloon directed catheters with or without the use of a tip deflector or pre-shaped wires. It may also be facilitated by the use of pre-curved catheters with a sharp curve, such as a Judkins left catheter with the tip cut off, allowing the placement of a wire in the left ventricle, and exchanging the catheter for a more flexible one with a smoother curve (Figure 9.13).

Central line placement

After transhepatic access has been established, a peal away sheath is positioned. Sufficient local anesthetic is infiltrated and a tunnel measuring a few centimeters is formed by the use of a hemostat extending from the entry site. A Broviac™ catheter (CR Bard, Inc, Salt Lake City, UT) is cut to the

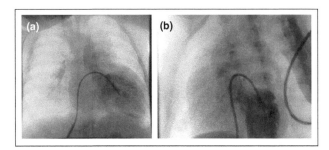

Figure 9.13
Right anterior oblique (a) and left anterior oblique (b) of a left ventriculogram using the transhepatic approach.

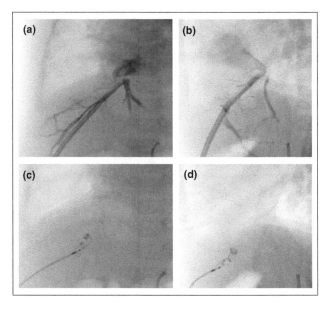

Figure 9.14
(a) and (b) Antero-posterior and lateral angiograms using the sheath side arm while slowly withdrawing the sheath outlines the position of the tract. (c) and (d) A flipper coil is shown placed in the transhepatic tract.

required length and introduced along the tunnel and into the peel away sheath. Once the catheter is in place the sheath is removed. The catheter and the entry sites are then sutured. Alternatively, an antibiotic treated catheter such as Cook Spectrum® or Cook Spectrum® Glide™ can be used which may not require tunneling (Cook, Inc, Bloomington, IN). The latter may be inserted through the peel away sheath or over a wire, or both, after being cut to the required length then sutured in place.

Closure of the tract

Closure of the transhepatic tract was suggested[1,2] using coils[1,2] or Gelfoam (Upjohn, Kalamazoo, MI)[5] to avoid retroperitoneal bleeding and liver hematoma. Others have felt that closure is not necessary and that no significant complications follow if this is not done.[9] Conservative management was successful in controlling the bleeding in two cases with significant retroperitoneal bleeding.[19] The decision to close the tract continues to be debatable. Our practice has been to consider closure in patients who are on antiplatelet treatment, requiring relatively large sheaths, in younger patients, or in those with elevated right atrial pressure. Using this approach we had one hematoma in a patient in whom a central line smaller than the sheath size was left in position. This patient was managed conservatively by removal of the smaller catheter and administration of blood products.

In order to outline the tract a catheter smaller than the sheath size is left in position. This catheter (4 or 5 Fr) will be used to deliver the occlusion coil. The sheath is slowly withdrawn while small hand injections are performed using the side arm of the sheath (J Cheatham, personal communication). This identifies the tract well (Figure 9.14) and avoids premature sheath withdrawal from the tract, especially in instances where the liver may have shifted because of unrecognized intraperitoneal or capsular bleeding.[2,19] We generally use detachable coils for closure which allows accurate placement and avoids the potential of coil embolization. Alternatively, an Amplatzer vascular plug (AGA Medical,

Golden Valley, MN) which allows for controlled deployment can be used. Gelfoam has been used,[9] though its radiolucency makes it less attractive.

Post-removal of the sheath, extra attention to the entry site while obtaining hemostasis is necessary, whether the tract is closed or not. Absence of blood oozing from the skin site does not mean that hemostasis has been achieved inside the liver parenchyma. The entry site should be held firmly against the liver parenchyma for at least 10 minutes, even if visible skin hemostasis has been achieved prior to that.

Post-catheterization care

This is similar to the regular cardiac catheterization. We have not routinely performed an ultrasound, blood count, or liver profile. The need for care and its impact on management should be assessed on a case-by-case basis. Most patients are transferred to the regular floor and discharged the following day, unless otherwise indicated.

Complications

The potential complications may include intra/retroperitoneal bleeding, hemobilia, pneumothorax, pleural effusions, perforation of the gall bladder, portal vein thrombosis, and liver abscess/peritonitis. Fortunately, serious complications are infrequent and account for <5%, with the majority being managed conservatively. The complication rate can be minimized by careful attention to detail, administering antibiotics when necessary, and coil closure when indicated. The most common reported complication is retroperitoneal bleeding, with an estimated incidence of clinically detected bleeding of <5%.[19] It is likely that in all these patients some degree of self-limiting insignificant intra/retroperitoneal bleeding occurs. Though there are rare reports of mortality as a result of retroperitoneal bleeding,[20,21] most of these patients, even with clinically detectable intraperitoneal bleeding, can be managed with a conservative approach.[19] The latter approach has been advocated for managing even some traumatic liver injuries,[22–25] which have been traditionally addressed surgically. Transient elevation in liver function tests has also been reported,[20] and responded to removal of an indwelling central line.

Conclusion

The transhepatic cardiac approach has lent itself to the arena of cardiac catheterizations and interventions. In the absence of other venous routes it may be the only available approach. In other instances it may be the preferred approach for accessing certain areas of the heart and for the successful performance of the planned catheterization or intervention.

References

1. Shim D, Lloyd TR, Cho KJ et al. Transhepatic cardiac catheterization in children: evaluation of efficacy and safety. Circulation 1995; 92: 1526–30.
2. Shim D, Lloyd TR, Beekman RH. Transhepatic therapeutic cardiac catheterization: a new option for the pediatric interventionalist. Cathet Cardiovasc Interven 1999; 47: 41–5.
3. Sommer RJ, Golinko RJ, Mitty HA. Initial experience with percutaneous transhepatic cardiac catheterization in infants and children. Am J Cardiol 1995; 75: 1289–91.
4. Johnson JL, Fellows KE, Murphy JD. Transhepatic central venous access for cardiac catheterization and radiologic intervention. Cathet Cardiovasc Diagn 1995; 35: 168–71.
5. Wallace MJ, Hovsepian DM, Balzer DT. Transhepatic venous access for diagnostic and interventional cardiovascular procedures. Vasc Interven Radiol 1996; 7: 579–82.
6. Book WM, Raviele AA, Vincent RN. Repetitive percutaneous transhepatic access for myocardial biopsy in pediatric cardiac transplant recipients. Cathet Cardiovasc Diagn 1998; 45(2): 167–9.

7. Fischbach P, Campbell RM, Hulse E et al. Transhepatic access to the atrioventricular ring for delivery of radiofrequency energy. J Cardiovasc Electrophysiol 1997; 8(5): 512–6.
8. Sommer RJ. New approaches for catheterization and vascular access: the transhepatic technique. Progr Pediatr Cardiol 1996; 6: 95–104.
9. McLeod KA, Houston AB, Richens T, Wilson N. Transhepatic approach for cardiac catheterization in children: initial experience. Heart 1999; 82(6): 694–6.
10. Ebeid MR. Trans-hepatic cardiac interventions. A single operator experience. Cathet Cardiovasc Intereven 2005; 66: 112 (abstract).
11. Guyton AC, Hall JE. The liver as an organ. In: Textbook of Medical Physiology, 11th edn. Philadelphia, PA Elsevier Saunders, 2006: 859–60.
12. Netter FH. Part III liver, biliary tract and pancreas. In: Oppenheimer E, ed. The Ciba Collection of Medical Illustrations, Volume 3, A Compilation of Paintings on the Normal and Pathological Anatomy of the Digestive System, 2nd edn. Ciba: Summit, NJ, 1967: 4–6.
13. Healy JC, Borley NR. Abdomen and pelvis. In: Standring S, ed. Gray's Anatomy. The Anatomical Basis of Clinical Practice, 39th edn. Philadelphia, PA Elsevier, Churchill Livingstone, 2005: 1214.
14. Johnston TA, Donnelly LF, Frush DP, O'Laughlin MP. Transhepatic catheterization using ultrasound-guided access. Pediatr Cardiol 2003; 24(4): 393–6.
15. Ebeid MR, Joransen JA, Gaymes CH. Transhepatic closure of atrial septal defect and assisted closure of modified Blalock/Taussig shunt. Cathet Cardiovasc Interven 2006; 67: 674–8.
16. Wahab H, Bairam AR, Cao Q, Hijazi ZM. Novel technique to prevent prolapse of the Amplatzer Septal Occluder through large atrial septal defect. Cathet Cardiovasc Interven 2003; 60: 543–5.
17. Varma C, Benson LN, Silversides C et al. Outcomes and alternative techniques for device closure of the large secundum atrial septal defect. Cathet Cardiovasc Interven 2004; 61: 131–9.
18. Sullebarger JT, Sayad D, Gerber L et al. Percutaneous closure of atrial septal defect via transjugular approach with the Amplatzer Septal Occluder after unsuccessful attempt using the CardioSEAL device. Cathet Cardiovasc Interven 2004; 62: 262–5.
19. Erenberg FG, Shim D, Beekman RH III. Intraperitoneal hemorrhage associated with transhepatic cardiac catheterization: a report of two cases [see comment]. Cathet Cardiovasc Diagn 1998; 43(2): 177–8.
20. Kadir S. Transhepatic cholangiography and biliary drainage. In: Kadir S, ed. Current Practice of Interventional Radiology. Philadelphia, PA Decker, 1991: 497–511.
21. Book WM, Raviele AA, Vincent RN. Transhepatic access in pediatric cardiology patients: an effective alternative in patients with limited venous access (abstract). Pediatrics 1998; 102: 674–5.
22. Andersson R, Bengemanrk S: Conservative treatment of liver trauma. World J Surg 1990; 14: 483–6.
23. McConnel DB, Trunkey DD. Nonoperative management of abdominal trauma. Surg Clin N Am 1990; 70: 677–88.
24. Uranus S, Mischinger HJ, Pfeifer J et al. Hemostatic methods for the management of spleen and liver injuries. World J Surg 1996; 20: 1107–12.
25. Demetriades D, Rabinowitz B, Sofianos C. Non-operative management of penetrating liver injuries: a prospective study. Br J Surg 1986; 73: 736–7.

10

Recanalization methods for post-catheter vessel occlusion

Frank F Ing

Background

It is not an uncommon experience for a cardiologist to take a patient with congenital heart disease (CHD) to the catheterization laboratory and spend excessive time to gain vascular access for a diagnostic or interventional procedure. A typical scenario is for the operator to encounter difficulty threading a wire into the femoral vein in spite of excellent blood return from the percutaneous needle. After many attempts, the operator may give up and assume the femoral vein to be occluded. Alternatively, some may inject a small amount of contrast into the needle to evaluate the vein and, if occlusion is discovered, the contralateral femoral vein is attempted. If both veins are occluded or multiple venous access is necessary for a complicated intervention, alternative venous access (jugular, transhepatic, etc.) is used. While alternative venous access is helpful, the direct femoral venous access is best for a majority of cardiac catheterization procedures. Unfortunately, CHD patients who have had multiple cardiac catheterizations or multiple surgeries, especially as an infant, or who have had chronic indwelling lines placed in the femoral vein are the most susceptible to femoral vein occlusions. These same patients are also the ones who require femoral vein access the most. The current chapter will review some techniques to evaluate the occluded femoral vein and recannulize these vessels.

Clinical presentation, anatomy, and pathophysiology

For the most part, CHD patients who develop femoral vein occlusions remain asymptomatic. Most commonly, the occlusion develops at a very young age and venous collaterals to the paravertebral venous system develop and, together with the deep femoral venous system, maintain adequate venous return from the leg. Occasionally, the occlusion is a long segment and involves the iliac vein and even the distal inferior vena cava (IVC). In that case, the paravertebral venous system will channel blood to the contralateral iliofemoral venous system and eventually back to the IVC, usually at the level of the renal veins. The pathophysiology of this type of venous obstruction is different from the adult who presents with IVC obstruction due to abdominal and pelvic malignancies. IVC syndrome (leg pain, edema, venous ulcerations) from the latter cause is most likely due to acute obstruction and inadequate development of collateral venous channels.

History of the procedure

While there are many reports of stenting of the obstructed IVC and iliofemoral vein in adults,[1-5] there is only scant literature on stenting of obstructed veins in children or patients with congenital heart disease.[6,7] Ing et al first reported a series in which stents were used to recannulize severely stenotic or occluded iliofemoral veins or IVC in CHD patients for the purpose of re-establishing vascular access for future repetitive cardiac catheterizations or surgery.[6] In that series, 24 patients received 85 stents in 22 iliofemoral veins and 6 IVCs. Thirteen of the 28 vessels were completely occluded and various techniques were used to cross the occlusion for stent implantation. The fact that 85 stents were necessary suggested that most of these occlusions were long segments and multiple overlapping stents were used.

Technique of recannulization

Due to the lack of signs or symptoms of the occluded iliofemoral venous system in CHD patients undergoing cardiac catheterization, the operator must have a high index of suspicion and be prepared to handle an occlusion, especially if the patient has a history of multiple vascular access as an infant. When excellent blood return from a needle is not met with successful passage of a guidewire into the femoral vein, one should make a small hand injection into the needle to evaluate the vessel rather than simply remove the needle to start again. If the femoral vein is occluded, contrast will enter into venous collaterals that commonly circulate into the paravertebral venous system and eventually exit into a more proximal patent iliac system or IVC or contralateral iliofemoral venous system. An angiogram should be performed in both antero-posterior (AP) and lateral projections to evaluate these vessels. Special attention should be paid at the beginning of the injection to look for the 'beak' of the remnant superficial femoral vein (Figure 10.1) before superimposition by contrast in the venous collaterals. Even when the angiogram is taken at 30 to 60 frames per second, only 1–2 frames may show this 'beak'. Sometimes, the beak is obvious and, at other times, it can be very subtle, as shown in two patients in Figures 10.2 and 10.3. The lateral projection is particularly helpful because of the anterior course of the superficial femoral vein remnant in contrast to the venous collateral flow, which takes a more posterior course into the paravertebral venous system.

When this 'beak' is identified, there is a high likelihood for a successful recannulization. First, a small (0.014–0.018 inch) guidewire is passed into the tip of the 'beak' under fluoroscopic guidance. The needle is replaced with a cannula to secure the initial access. Occasionally, an angled

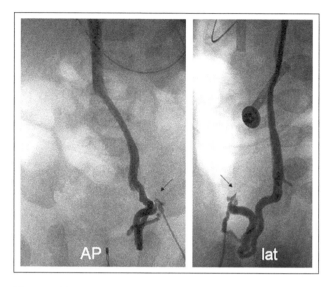

Figure 10.1
'Beak' (arrows) of occluded left superficial femoral vein shown in AP and lateral projection.

guidewire is all that is needed to push past the 'beak' and up the occluded vessel. More commonly, the wire will simply buckle. The cannula should be exchanged for a 4–5 Fr dilator, which prevents the wire from buckling during its advancement. With support from the dilator, which is pushed up to the tip of the 'beak', the angled guidewire is advanced. If the front end of the wire is too soft, then the stiffer back end of the wire can be used. The wire is advanced in small

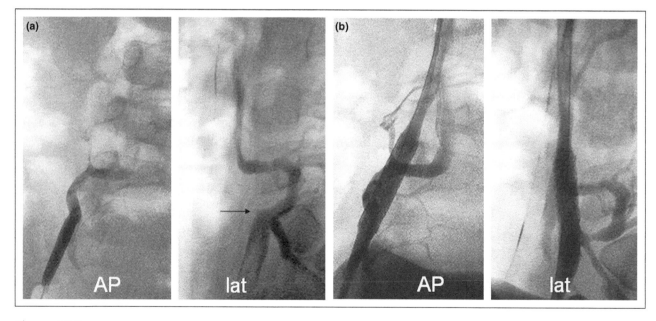

Figure 10.2
(a) In this patient, the 'beak' of the occluded right femoral vein is superimposed by the posterior paravertebral venous collateral and is not seen in the AP projection. It is very subtle (arrow) in the lateral projection and could be easily missed. (b) Wide patency of vessel after stent implantation.

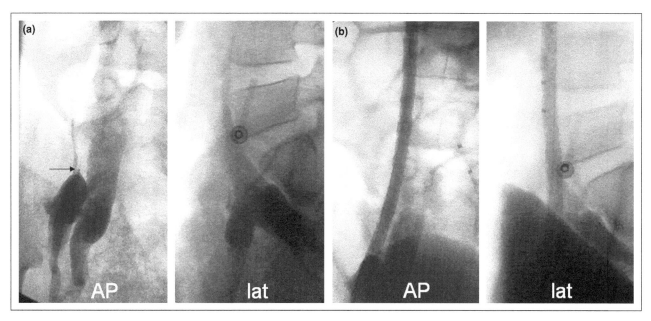

Figure 10.3
(a) In this patient, the remnant 'beak' (arrow) of the occluded right femoral vein is only subtly visible in the AP projection and is obscured by the venous collateral vessel on the lateral projection. (b) Femoral vein access is re-established after implantation of three overlapping stents.

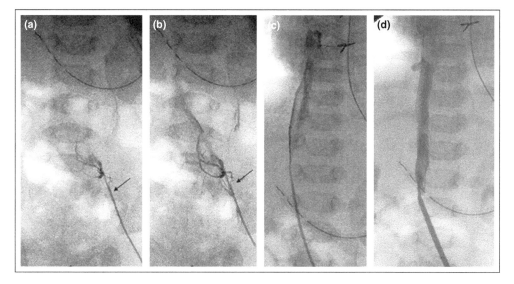

Figure 10.4
(a) and (b) An angled guidewire or the stiff end of a 0.014–0.018 inch wire through a 4–5 Fr dilator is advanced in small increments through the occluded vein. Small hand injections are taken through the dilator (arrows) to evaluate the occluded vessel course. Contrast stains the occluded segment or enters into smaller collateral. (c) When the patent IVC is entered, contrast flows freely into the right atrium. (d) The dilator is exchanged for a long sheath.

increments (mm), followed by advancement of the dilator. The wire is removed and repeated small hand injections are made to evaluate the course (Figure 10.4a, b). Contrast may stain the lumen of the thrombosed vessel. This sequence is repeated until contrast is seen flowing freely in the proximal patent vessel, which could be the iliac vein if the occluded segment is short, or even as far as the IVC if there is a long segment

occlusion (Figure 10.4c, d). It is important to note the anterior course of this vessel and to assess for extravasation (Figure 10.5a–c).

Once the wire is passed into the patent segment, the occluded segment can be serially dilated with either progressively larger dilators or dilation balloons until it is large enough to accommodate a sheath. It is advisable to use a

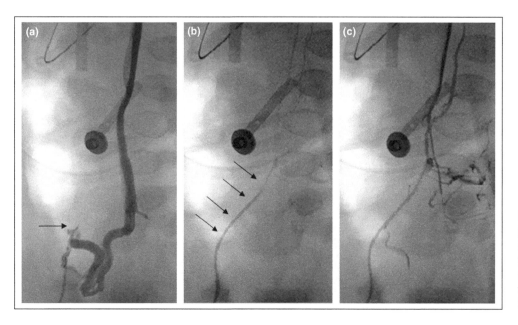

Figure 10.5
(a)–(c) The anterior course of the femoral and iliac veins (arrows) is noted during advancement of the wire and dilator in the lateral projection.

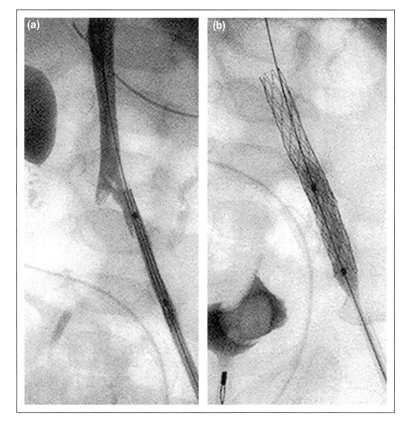

Figure 10.6
(a) Stent and balloon are positioned across the most proximal segment of the occluded left iliac vein. (b) A second stent is implanted more distally in the occluded superficial femoral vein segment and telescoped into the first stent.

long sheath (such as a Cook Mullins© sheath) to secure a long segment occlusion for the cardiac catheterization. The planned procedure should be performed first and the vessel should be stented at the end of the planned procedure. An angiogram of the entire length of the iliofemoral venous system and IVC should be performed in order to assess the diameters for proper stent and balloon size selection. When a single stent is inadequate to cover the entire length of the occluded segment, multiple overlapping stents should be used, starting from the most cranial end (Figure 10.6a,b).

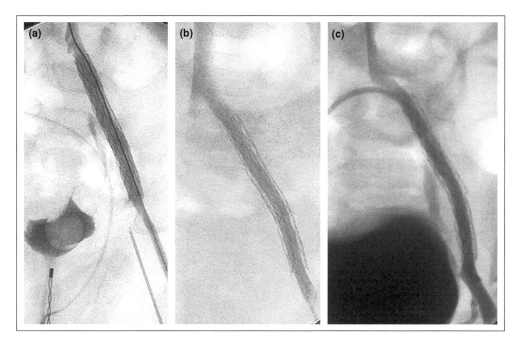

Figure 10.7
(a) Follow-up angiogram after stent implantation indicates successful recannulization of the occluded left iliac and femoral vein. (b) and (c) Follow-up cardiac catheterization (for other interventions) 4 months (b) and 18 months (c) later show patency of the stented segment. A thin layer of intima is noted within the stents.

When the occlusion involves the IVC, patency is often seen at the level of the renal veins, most likely due to the high flow of these veins back into the IVC. Presently, only balloon expandable stents are used in growing children to accommodate future further dilation as the child grows. The Genesis© stent is a good choice for these vessels. Balloon size selection should be based on the normal caliber of the adjacent patent vessel.

During stent implantation, a clamp is placed on the inguinal ligament to define the caudal limit for stent positioning. A needle is usually placed on the groin, parallel to the femoral vein course, to help determine the level at which the tip of the needle can enter the stent. By positioning the stent such that the most caudal edge can be entered by the percutaneous needle, future access into the stent is ensured even if the stent becomes re-occluded. However, it must be kept in mind that, on the lateral projection, the stent should not be positioned too anteriorly so that flexion of the hips will distort the stent. In general, if the stent is positioned such that its most caudal edge is in the mid-portion of the bladder, it is safe from hip flexion. At the end of the procedure, the hips can be flexed under lateral fluoroscopy to ensure stent positioning. A follow-up angiogram should be taken to evaluate inflow (Figure 10.7a–c). If the distal femoral vein is small or the inflow into the stent appears inadequate, there is a possibility of stent re-occlusion. This should not pose a hemodynamic problem since the vein was occluded in the first place prior

to recannulization. However, by having the stent in place, future catheterizations can still be performed even if the stent occludes. By using bi-plane fluoroscopic guidance, a needle can be directed into the lumen of the radio-opaque stent and advanced further into the patent vessel distally. As long as the needle remains inside the stent, extravasation is avoided.

As shown in Figures 10.8 and 10.9, multiple catheterizations were performed for cardiac biopsies in a transplant patient in whom an occluded femoral vein was stented and became re-occluded due to poor inflow. As the child grew, longer (Chiba©) needles were needed to reach the stent edge but, once there, a wire was easily advanced through the thrombosed stent and finally into the more cranial patent segment of the femoral vein. Following stent implantation in a systemic vein, lifetime antiplatelet therapy with low dose aspirin was prescribed. Occasionally, the occluded venous segments can be quite extensive, requiring multiple stents involving bilateral femoral and iliac veins as well as the IVC, as shown in Figures 10.10–10.13.

Follow-up data

There are few data on the long term results of stented peripheral systemic veins in patients with coronary heart disease. Mid-term follow-up data were available in the

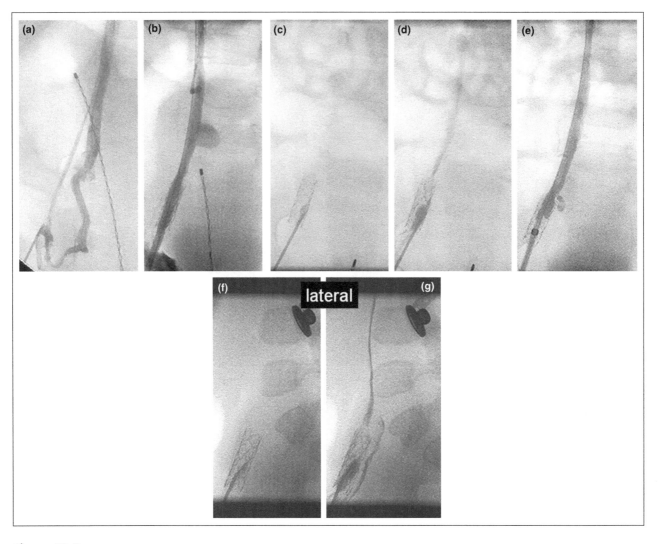

Figure 10.8
(a) Right femoral vein occlusion was found in this 3-month-old infant after orthotopic heart transplant rendering cardiac biopsy difficult due to vascular access. (b) A stent was implanted initially. (c) Due to poor distal venous inflow, the stent was found to be re-occluded at follow-up cardiac catheterization. (d) However, using the radio-opaque stent as a target, a needle can be introduced back into the stent. (e) The occluded stent and vessel can be recanulated. (f) and (g) Lateral projection of the same patient. Using both AP and lateral views, the needle can be easily guided back into the occluded stent to regain vascular access of the femoral vein.

paper by Ing et al, which reported a patency rate of 87% for 12 patients (15 vessels).[6] Two stented veins were found to be occluded due to poor inflow, but were easily recannulated and redilated for successful cardiac catheterization. In another (unpublished) series of 27 patients in whom 53 stents were implanted, follow-up catheterization was performed in 12 patients at a mean of 2.2 years showing a stent patency rate of 83% (10/12 vessels), while intimal hyperplasia was found in 25% (3/12 vessels) (Ing, unpublished

results). Two occluded stents were easily recannulized. Longer term follow-up is warranted.

Summary

In summary, patients with congenital heart disease who have undergone multiple cardiac catheterizations or surgery during infancy may develop occlusions of the

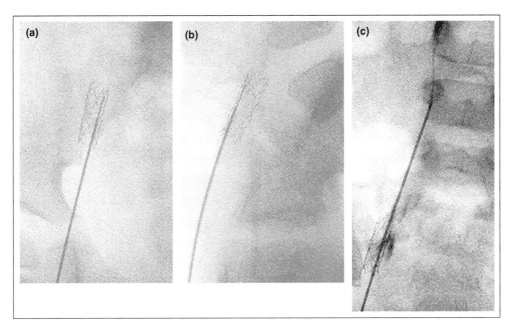

Figure 10.9
(a)–(c) This transplanted patient has had multiple follow-up catheterizations over 5 years. As the child grew, the stent shifted further cranially. A longer (Chiba) needle is needed to gain access into the occluded stent using the AP (a) and lateral (b) views. Free flow of contrast into the IVC is noted in (c).

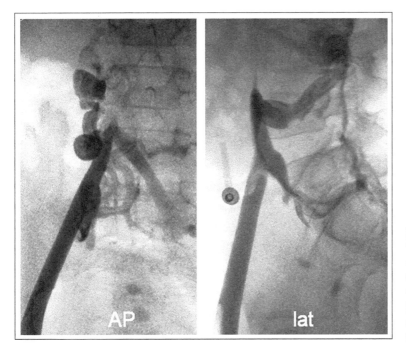

Figure 10.10
This patient with complex congenital heart disease was found to have significant distal IVC occlusion at the level of the iliac bifurcation. Bifurcating stents will be needed to recanalize the distal IVC without jailing either iliac vein. Note the extension venous collaterization into the paravertebral venous system.

iliofemoral venous system in spite of the lack of signs or symptoms. Recannulization and stenting of these occluded vessels is possible if the cardiologist can identify the remnant superficial femoral vein 'beak' during angiography.

Preservation of femoral vein access with this technique may avoid more complicated alternative venous access routes and simplify future diagnostic or interventional cardiac catheterizations.

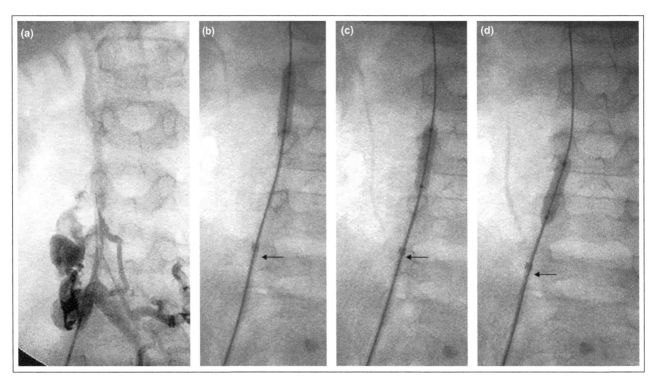

Figure 10.11
(a) Angiogram after wire and dilator was advanced past the IVC occlusion. (b)–(d) Initial balloon dilation of the occluded distal IVC and right iliac vein was performed to permit passage of the sheath (arrow) into the IVC.

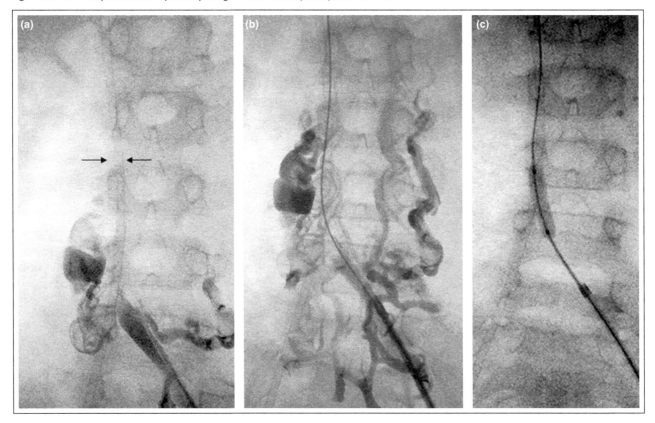

Figure 10.12
(a) A Mullins sheath (arrows) is advanced from the right femoral vein into the IVC. (b) A wire is advanced from the left femoral vein to cross the occluded IVC segment. (c) Balloon dilation is carried out at the junction of the distal IVC and left iliac bifurcation.

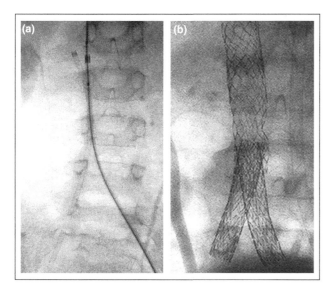

Figure 10.13
(a) Bilateral sheaths are placed from the femoral veins into the
IVC for stent implantation. (b) Two overlapping stents are
implanted in the distal IVC and two bifurcating stents in bilateral
iliac veins.

References

1. Charnsangavej C, Carrasco CH, Wallace S et al. Stenosis of the vena cava: preliminary assessment of treatment with expandable metallic stents. Radiology 1986; 161: 295–8.
2. Nazarian GK, Bjarnason H, Dietz CA et al. Iliofemoral venous stenosis: effectiveness of treatment with metallic envdovascular stents. Radiology 1996; 200: 193–9.
3. Fletcher WS, Lakin PC, Pommier RF, Wilmarth T. Results of treatment of inferior vena cava syndrome with expandable metallic stents. Arch Surg 1998; 133: 935–8.
4. Change TC, Zaleski GX, Funaki B, Leaf J. Treatment of inferior vena cava obstruction in hemodialysis patient using Wallstents: early and intermediate results. Am J Radiol 1998; 171: 125–8.
5. Funagi B, Szymski GX, Leef JA et al. Treatment of venous outflow stenoses in thigh grafts with Wallstents. Am J Roentgenol 1999; 172: 1591–6.
6. Ing FF, Fagan TE, Grifka RG et al. Reconstruction of stenotic or occluded iliofemoral veins and inferior vena cava using intravascular stents: re-establishing access for future cardiac catheterization and cardiac surgery. JACC 2001; 37: 251–7.
7. Ward CJB, Mullins CE, Nihill MR et al. Use of intravascular stents in systemic venous and systemic venous baffle obstructions: short-term follow-up results. Circulation 1995; 91: 2948–54.

11

Transseptal left heart catheterization

Igor F Palacios

Transseptal left heart catheterization

Transseptal catheterization, which allows access to the left atrium, is the first step of several interventional procedures and one of the most crucial. Transseptal left heart catheterization was introduced independently in 1959 by Ross and Cope, and later modified by Brockenbrough and Mullins.[1–4] The procedure was introduced as an alternative to the methods available at that time, such as directly measuring left atrial and left ventricular pressures using either the transbronchial or transthoracic approaches.[5] The developments of the flotation pulmonary artery catheter in 1970 by Swan and Ganz[6] and retrograde cardiac catheterization of the left ventricle led to a significant decline in utilization of the transseptal technique. Furthermore, with fewer patients with valvular disease and improved echocardiography, a smaller number of cardiologists were trained to perform the procedure.[7,8] With fewer procedures came fewer qualified personnel, and, because of concern over potentially grave complications and associated mortality, the procedure attained an 'aura of danger and intrigue'.[9] With the introduction of interventional procedures such as percutaneous mitral valvuloplasty, antegrade percutaneous aortic valvuloplasty, and now radiofrequency ablation of left-sided bypass tracts, there has been an increased demand for, and rekindled interest in, transseptal catheterization.[10,11] We will describe the technique, indications, and complications of transseptal left heart catheterization.

Technique

The physician performing a transseptal catheterization must be aware of the indications and contraindications of this technique and should be well familiarized with the anatomy of the interatrial septum. Transseptal catheterization is performed using the percutaneous technique only from the right femoral vein. Although the right subclavian and the right jugular veins have been used occasionally, they are not standard techniques. Transseptal catheterization is also possible from the left femoral vein, but it is more painful to the patient due to the sharp angulation between the left iliac vein and the inferior vena cava. Biplane fluoroscopy, if available, is the ideal imaging system. However, a single plane 'C' arm fluoroscope, which can be rotated from the antero-posterior (AP) to lateral position, may also be used.

There are two different transseptal needles: the Ross needle and the Brockenbrough. The Ross needle is a 17 gauge needle, has a more pronounced curve, and is typically used with the Brockenbrough catheter. The Brockenbrough needle is more frequently utilized. It is an 18 gauge needle which tapers at the distal tip to a 21 gauge and is typically used with the Mullins sheath.

Prior to attempted puncture of the interatrial septum, full familiarity with the transseptal apparatus (Mullins sheath and dilator, Brockenbrough needle and stylet, and the Palacios transseptal kit (Cooks Inc. Bloomington, IN, USA)) is essential. The Mullins transseptal introducer (Medtronic, Minneapolis, Minesota, USA and Cooks Inc. Bloomington, IN, USA) is composed of a 59 cm sheath and a 67 cm dilator. The distance the dilator protrudes from the sheath should be noted prior to the procedure. The Brockenbrough needle is 71 cm in length. The flange of the needle has an arrow that points to the position of the tip of the needle. Before use, the operator should be sure that the needle is straight and that the arrow of the flange is perfectly aligned with the needle tip. This arrow will allow the operator to know exactly where the distal tip of the needle is pointing. When the needle tip lies just within the dilator there is approximately 1.5–2 cm distance between the dilator hub and the needle flange. This measurement also should be noted.

Once satisfied with the spatial relationship of the components of the transseptal system, a 0.032–0.035 inch J wire is positioned at the junction of the superior vena cava and left innominate vein from the right femoral vein. Venipuncture must be as horizontal as possible to facilitate manipulation of the transseptal system and permit maximal transmission of pulsations. Tactile as well as visual clues are important in

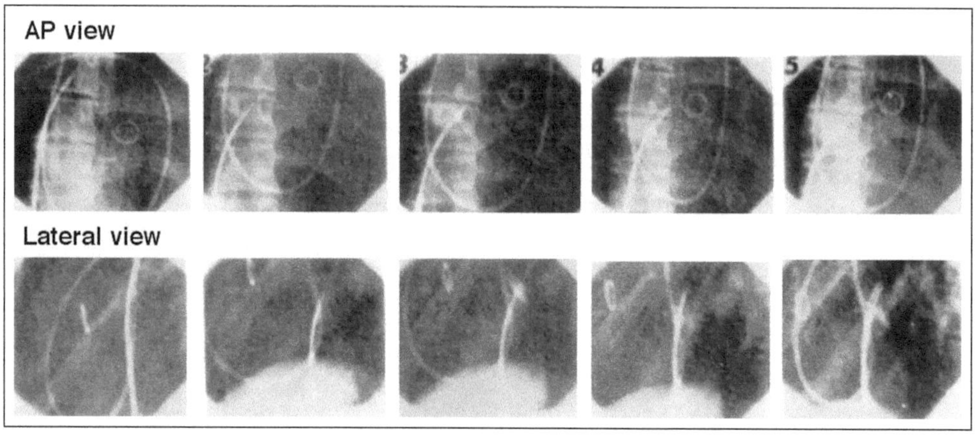

Figure 11.1

Simultaneous AP and lateral views during transseptal left heart catheterization. A pigtail catheter is positioned retrogradely in the right coronary sinus to correctly identify the aorta with the use of biplane fluoroscopy. Under antero-posterior fluoroscopy, the entire system is then withdrawn across three sequential landmark 'bumps,' or leftward movements of the needle. These landmark 'bumps' represent movement of the apparatus (1) as it enters the right atrium/superior vena cava junction, (2) as it moves over the ascending aorta where the tactile sensation of aortic pulsations aids in localization, and (3) as it passes over the limbus to intrude into the fossa ovalis. On a lateral view, the correct position for puncture of the apparatus is posterior and inferior to the aorta.

properly identifying the puncture site. To ease insertion of the Mullins sheath, pre-dilatation with an 8 Fr dilator is recommended. A pigtail catheter is positioned retrogradely in the right coronary sinus. To correctly identify the aorta with the use of the pigtail catheter and biplane fluoroscopy, the spatial relationship of the ascending aorta and its surrounding structures should be known. The pigtail catheter must be flushed with heparinized saline every 3 minutes to prevent clot formation and embolic complications.

Before proceeding, the right and left heart borders and apical pulsations are surveyed under fluoroscopy. Under fluoroscopic guidance, the Mullins sheath and dilator are advanced over the J wire into the superior vena cava/left innominate vein junction. The sheath must never be advanced without the wire as the stiff dilator can readily perforate the inferior vena cava, superior vena cava, or right atrium. Once the Mullins sheath is properly placed, the wire is removed. The Brockenbrough needle is then advanced to lie just inside the dilator, using the predetermined distance between the needle flange and dilator as a guide. When advancing the needle to this position, it must rotate freely within the dilator and not be forcibly turned to prevent damage to the needle tip or dilator. Occasionally there is some resistance as the transseptal needle is advanced through the iliac vein or the inferior vena cava, particularly at the pelvic brim. Under these circumstances the needle should not be forcibly advanced, instead the needle with its stylet inside and the Mullins sheath should be advanced as a unit through the areas of resistance.

Once properly advanced to the tip of the Mullins dilator, the Brockenbrough needle is double flushed and pressure

tubing is connected. To avoid confusion, we recommend displaying only this single pressure tracing, and on a 40–50 mmHg scale. At this point, proper orientation of the assembly is critical. The side arm of the sheath and needle flange should always have the same orientation. Initially, they point horizontally and to the patient's left. This directs the tip of the apparatus medially in the antero-posterior fluoroscopic view. The entire system is then rotated clockwise until the needle flange arrow and sheath side arm are positioned at 4 o'clock (with the patient's forehead representing 12 o'clock and the patient's occipital 6 o'clock). This directs the assembly to the left and slightly posterior.

Under antero-posterior fluoroscopy, the entire system is then withdrawn across three sequential landmark 'bumps,' or leftward movements of the needle. These landmark 'bumps' represent movement of the apparatus (1) as it enters the right atrium/superior vena cava junction, (2) as it moves over the ascending aorta where the tactile sensation of aortic pulsations aids in localization, and (3) as it passes over the limbus to intrude into the fossa ovalis. On a lateral view, the correct position for puncture of the apparatus is posterior and inferior to the aorta (marked by the pigtail catheter) (Figures 11.1 and 11.2).

The system is advanced (needle within the dilator) until further movement is limited by the limbus. In approximately 10% of cases, the foramen ovale is patent and the apparatus directly enters the left atrium. In the remainder, the tip of the Brockenbrough needle is advanced into the left atrium under continuous fluoroscopic and pressure monitoring. Care should be taken to advance only the tip of

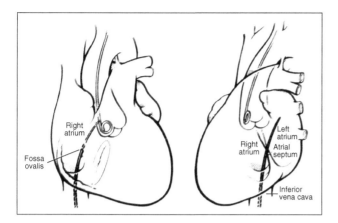

Figure 11.2
Under antero-posterior fluoroscopy, the entire system is then withdrawn across three sequential landmark 'bumps,' or leftward movements of the needle (right panel). On a lateral view, the correct position for puncture of the apparatus is posterior and inferior to the aorta (left panel). The proper orientation of the Mullins sheath/dilator in the left atrium after successful puncture of the interatrial septum: in the antero-posterior view (left), the sheath lies at the mid-portion of the right atrial silhouette. In the lateral view (right), it is located posterior and inferior to the aortic valve plane (demarcated by the pigtail catheter).

the needle and not the entire apparatus. Successful penetration of the septum is heralded by a change from right atrial to left atrial pressure waveform, accompanied by a small but definite lateral movement of the needle tip on fluoroscopy. A palpable 'pop' may occur with septal penetration, confirmed by injecting contrast, which should flow freely into the left atrium. If the pressure tracing is damped, injection of contrast will aid in localizing the puncture site. If there is staining of the interatrial septum, the needle must be advanced further. A stained septum must not be interpreted as failure and, in fact, the tattoo septum may indeed be used as a guide for future attempts. If the left atrium cannot be entered, the entire system must be withdrawn to the inferior vena cava/right atrial junction, the needle removed, and the J wire advanced through the Mullins system and repositioned in the superior vena cava for a second attempt. If there is aortic or pericardial staining, or the presence of an aortic pressure tracing, the tip of the needle must be removed and the patient re-evaluated prior to a second attempt. If the procedure is being performed in preparation for percutaneous mitral balloon valvuloplasty or antegrade aortic balloon valvuloplasty, we generally postpone a second attempt for another day because the patient would need systemic anticoagulation. If the aorta or pericardium has been entered only with the tip of the needle and the procedure is only being performed in the course of diagnostic catheterization, the procedure may be attempted again.

The proper positioning of the needle after successful puncture is at the mid-portion of the right atrial silhouette in the antero-posterior view. In the lateral view, it lies posterior and inferior to the aortic valve plane, as demarcated by the pigtail catheter (Figures 11.1 and 11.2). Slight variations in the technique may be required in the presence of abnormal atrial or aortic anatomy and with different interventional procedures. In patients with left atrial enlargement, the septum lies more horizontally. The site of puncture is more posterior and inferior. In aortic valve disease accompanied by a dilated aorta, the septum is more vertical. The fossa ovalis and the puncture site are therefore more superior and slightly anterior. With right atrial enlargement, the transseptal apparatus may not reach to the septum. A gentle curve placed on the needle 10–15 cm from the distal tip may allow engagement of the fossa ovalis. During double balloon percutaneous mitral balloon valvuloplasty, PMV, or with antegrade percutaneous aortic ballon valvuloplasty, PAV, a low puncture site in the middle posterior third of the septum provides a straight pathway to the mitral orifice and apex of the left ventricle to facilitate manipulation of guidewires and catheters. A slightly higher puncture is preferred when using a single Inoue balloon to allow the straightest course for the flow-directed distal balloon through the mitral valve (Figure 11.3).

After successful interatrial puncture, the entire system is rotated counterclockwise to 3 o'clock and carefully advanced under fluoroscopic and hemodynamic guidance until it is certain the dilator lies within the left atrium. The needle is withdrawn into the dilator. The sheath is then advanced into the left atrium, keeping the needle within the sheath to avoid puncturing the left atrium. The needle and dilator are then removed, and the sheath double flushed prior to being connected to pressure tubing. If the sheath has entered an inferior pulmonary vein, it must be withdrawn slightly with counterclockwise rotation to position it in the left atrium. Care should be taken after entering the left atrium with the needle. Perforation of the left atrial wall could occur if the system is advanced without careful pressure and fluoroscopic monitoring. If the left atrial pressure becomes damped, the apparatus may be against the left atrial wall and further advancement of the system could result in perforation and tamponade. Immediately after completion of transseptal left heart catheterization heparin, 5000 units, is administered intravenously.

Indications

In the past, in the majority of cases, transseptal catheterization was performed for diagnostic purposes. However, today interventional procedures requiring access to the left atrium comprise a large group of patients in need of the transseptal technique.[10,11]

Transseptal left heart catheterization should be performed whenever direct measurement of left atrial pressure is needed (when the accuracy of pulmonary capillary wedge

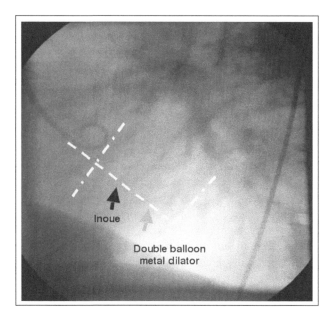

Inoue

Double balloon
metal dilator

Figure 11.3
Transseptal puncture site according with planed procedure. The interatrial septum below the aortic knob identified by the pigtail in the right coronary cusp is divided into three. The upper third is preferentially used for the Inoue technique, the middle third for the double balloon technique of PMV and for antegrade aortic balloon valvuloplasty, while the lower third is preferentially used for the Cribier metallic dilator technique of PMV.

pressure is questionable) or retrograde access to the left ventricle is unobtainable or dangerous. In patients with mitral stenosis and pulmonary artery hypertension, the true capillary wedge may be unobtainable or inaccurate[5,10–13] and there is a slightly higher incidence of pulmonary artery perforation with balloon flotation in the pulmonary arteries. In patients with prosthetic mitral valves the pulmonary capillary wedge pressure may overestimate the diastolic gradient across the valve.[12] A false mitral gradient could be the result of the presence of pulmonary hypertension and/or a phase delay in the pulmonary wedge 'v' waves resulting in a higher mean diastolic gradient compared to the left atrial pressure obtained by transseptal catheterization (Figure 11.4). This may lead to the calculation of an erroneously small prosthetic mitral valve area and unnecessary repeat mitral valve surgery.[12] In mitral regurgitation, the regurgitant fraction can be quantified by injecting indocyanine green dye into the left ventricle and obtaining dye curves by sampling the left atrium and femoral artery.[13]

Aortic valvular disease or aortic valve replacement may preclude safe retrograde left ventricular catheterization. In patients with mechanical aortic valves retrograde catheterization is not possible. Many cardiologists prefer the transseptal technique in patients with bioprosthetic aortic valves or native aortic stenosis to avoid damaging the valve

during catheterization. In critical aortic stenosis the transaortic gradient is more reliable when left ventricular and ascending aortic pressures are measured simultaneously via transseptal puncture. When the valve area is 0.6 cm^2 or less, the catheter itself may significantly obstruct the orifice and falsely increase the recorded gradient[14] or result in transient hemodynamic deterioration. In heavily calcified valves, transseptal catheterization may avert possible dislodgement and embolization of calcium.[7] Transseptal left heart catheterization should be performed in patients with aortic valve replacements in whom evaluation of the aortic gradient or ventriculography is needed.

Other diagnostic uses for transseptal catheterization include aortic valve endocarditis where crossing the valve could be deleterious, the evaluation of dynamic left ventricular outflow obstruction, in allowing simultaneous recording of both left ventricular and aortic pressures, and in distinguishing dynamic outflow obstruction from catheter entrapment. Transseptal catheterization allows direct measurement of left atrial pressure in mitral regurgitation, cor triatriatum, and pulmonary hypertension, and provides access for pulmonary vein angiography in the evaluation of pulmonary atresia and pulmonary veno-occlusive disease.[13]

The resurgence of interest in transseptal catheterization is a direct result of its role in interventional procedures. Transseptal catheterization is a prerequisite in percutaneous mitral valvuloplasty[15] and antegrade percutaneous aortic valvuloplasty (Figure 11.5).[16] Likewise, in the pediatric population, balloon atrioseptostomy in the treatment of transposition of the great arteries, pulmonary atresia with intact ventricular septum, total anomalous pulmonary venous return, and tricuspid atresia requires transseptal catheterization.[17]

Currently, the vast majority of radiofrequency ablations of left-sided bypass tracts are performed via retrograde left ventricular catheterization. However, successful ablation of left free wall, posteroseptal, and septal bypass tracts have been reported using a transseptal approach.[18] A transseptal approach may allow for the ablation of otherwise inaccessible pathways and, perhaps, may facilitate the procedure in some patients, reducing both their discomfort and radiation exposure.

Contraindications

Contraindications to transseptal catheterization include:

1. obstruction of the inferior vena cava (e.g., by tumor, thrombus, therapeutic ligation, or filter placement)
2. systemic anticoagulation
3. bleeding diathesis
4. anatomic deformity such as severe kyphoscoliosis or patients with previous pneumonectomy resulting in severe rotation of the heart

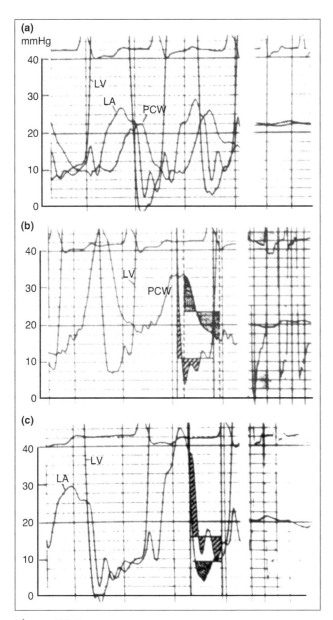

Figure 11.4

In patients with prosthetic mitral valves the pulmonary capillary wedge pressure may overestimate the diastolic gradient across the valve. A false mitral gradient could be the result of the presence of pulmonary hypertension and/or a phase delay in the pulmonary wedge 'v' waves resulting in a higher mean diastolic gradient compared to the left atrial pressure obtained by transseptal catheterization. This may lead to the calculation of an erroneously small prosthetic mitral valve area and unnecessary repeat mitral valve surgery.

5. congenital deformities resulting in obscured landmarks of the atrial septum
6. thrombus in the right or the left atrium documented by echocardiography; patients with previous clinical emboli can have transseptal catheterization if they have been adequately anticoagulated with Coumadin and the

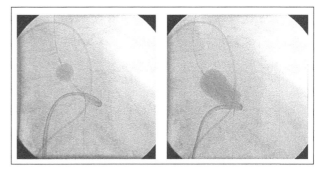

Figure 11.5

Antegrade aortic balloon valvuloplasty using the Inoue balloon catheter.

left atrium is free of thrombus by transesophageal echocardiography
7. presence of atrial myxoma
8. patients with a large right atrium represent a particular problem because of the flattening of the septum and sometimes the inability of the needle to touch the interatrial septum.

Complications

In part, the decline in the frequency of transseptal catheterization can be ascribed to concern over potentially lethal complications. Penetration of the inferior vena cava, atria, or aorta can occur and may lead to tamponade and/or death.[19–22] Earlier studies utilized a single antero-posterior fluoroscopic view and, in some series, used larger gauge needles than today. Lateral fluoroscopy allows the visualization of the needle to place it posterior and inferior to the aortic valve plane, thus avoiding penetration of the aorta and an extreme posterior needle position, which risks left atrial perforation. Today transseptal catheterization can be performed safely with a low incidence of complication[5,7,10,11,13] and reflects operator experience and perhaps the addition of biplane fluoroscopy. Others, however, have reported low complication rates utilizing single plane fluoroscopy.[23,24] The transseptal 'needle tip only' can inadvertently puncture the atria or the aorta. However, adverse sequelae do not develop, provided that this inadvertent puncture is immediately recognized before the apparatus is advanced further. In a series utilizing biplane fluoroscopy, inadvertent pericardial puncture occurred in 3/217 patients (1.4%) and none resulted in tamponade.[25] Several series have noted that at surgery following uneventful transseptal catheterizations, blood-stained pericardial fluid is not infrequently present, implying unnoticed atrial puncture during the procedure.[3,20,26] Cardiac tamponade occurs with advancement of the larger dilator and not with inadvertent needle puncture. Cardiac tamponade occurs less frequently in patients with prior cardiac surgery, making transseptal catheterization safer in postoperative patients. Tamponade is less likely to occur because of the obliteration of the pericardial space by adhesions.[27]

Two-dimensional transthoracic, transesophageal echocardiography and intravascular echocardiography have been used as an adjunct to fluoroscopy to avoid such complications. The interatrial septum and aorta are best visualized in the apical four-chamber view and saline contrast allows localization of the needle before and after septal puncture.[28] Needle tip punctures are not eliminated, and occurred in 1 of 13 transseptal catheterizations (with no adverse sequelae).[26] Thus, concomitant echocardiography adds little to biplane fluoroscopy and may be impractical in many catheterization laboratories.

Systemic embolization is another grave complication of transseptal catheterization. Cerebral emboli are most frequently reported, but emboli to coronary, splanchnic, renal, and femoral arteries have occurred.[19–30] We do not routinely order echocardiograms prior to diagnostic transseptal catheterization unless the patient is at high risk for an atrial thrombus (e.g., atrial fibrillation, mitral stenosis). As part of the evaluation for percutaneous mitral valvuloplasty, patients have an echocardiogram to visualize the atrial appendage and the presence of thrombus, as well as to be ranked by echo score.[31] Transseptal catheterization in the presence of a non-echogenic atrial myxoma has resulted in tamponade.[32] It is also conceivable that not all thrombi are visible by echo. In addition to thrombus, embolization of air to the coronary and cerebral vessels has occurred,[32] as well as embolization of a perforated guide catheter, later discovered in the left popliteal artery.[29] Bleeding and vasovagal reactions occur more frequently but are more easily managed.

Early studies utilized a single antero-posterior view, accounting for higher morbidity and mortality than occurs today. Lateral fluoroscopy allows orientation of the catheter posterior and inferior to the aorta and reduces inadvertent penetration of the aorta and left atrium. A high success rate has been reported using modified single plane fluoroscopy. A right anterior oblique (40–50°) view provides an end face view of the atrial septum and defines the inferior, posterior, and superior borders of the right atrium. A pigtail in the aorta demarcates its posterior wall and the level of the aortic valve. The recommended point of puncture lies mid-way between the posterior borders of the right atrium and aorta, and 1–3 cm below the aortic valve.[23] Using this technique, atrial puncture occurred in 2/118 (1.7%) and cardiac tamponade in 1/106 (0.9%), for an overall inadvertent puncture rate of 1.3%.[6,7] This suggests a marked improvement over previous series relying solely on antero-posterior fluoroscopy, but higher numbers are needed before definite conclusions can be drawn. The modified technique offers no advantage over biplane fluoroscopy, although it has been suggested that it may be more appropriate for less experienced 'low volume' operators because it provides a greater margin of safety in terms of locating the area of septal puncture.[23]

Several authors have suggested that there is a 'learning curve' for transseptal catheterization, and that the majority of complications occur in the first 25–50 procedures.[13,33,34] Even at a leading academic catheterization laboratory, the technique had to be 're-learned' for percutaneous mitral valvuloplasty, resulting in a 2/61 (3.3%) incidence of tamponade resulting from transseptal catheterization.[35] A higher rate of complications has been noted when the procedure is not regularly performed.[36]

The rate of unsuccessful attempts at transseptal catheterizations also varies with operator experience. Inability to engage the septum in up to 1.4–7% of attempts has been reported, varying with different patient populations.[25,26,37]

Recently, intracardiac echocardiography (ICE) has emerged as a useful tool in the cardiac catheterization and electrophysiology laboratories for guiding transseptal left heart catheterizations. ICE is a useful tool for guiding transseptal puncture. During atrial septal puncture ICE is able to locate the needle tip position precisely and provides a clear visualization of the 'tenting effect' on the fossa ovalis. Finally, successful entry of the left atrium can be demonstrated by contrast echocardiography following the injection of agitated saline solution through the transseptal needle.

In conclusion, transseptal left heart catheterization remains an important skill of the interventional cardiologist. Although for diagnostic purposes the technique is less requested than in the past, it remains a necessity in percutaneous mitral valvuloplasty, antegrade percutaneous aortic valvuloplasty, and atrioseptostomy, and may offer advantages in radiofrequency ablation of left-sided pathways. In the proper hands, and with the proper equipment, there is little additional risk over routine left heart catheterization. Experienced operators are essential to assure low morbidity and mortality.

REFERENCES

1. Ross J Jr, Braunwald E, Morrow AG. Transseptal left atrial puncture: new technique for the measurement of left atrial pressure in man. Am J Cardiol 1959; 3: 653–5.
2. Cope C. Technique for transseptal catheterization of the left atrium: preliminary report. J Thorac Surg 1959; 37: 482–6.
3. Brockenbrough EC, Braunwald E, Ross J Jr. Transseptal left heart catheterization: a review of 450 studies and description of an improved technic. Circulation 1962; 25: 15–21.
4. Mullins CE. Transseptal left heart catheterization: expeience with a new technique in 520 pediatric and adult patients. Pediatr Cardiol 1983; 4: 239–46.
5. Dunn M. Is transseptal catheterization necessary? J Am Coll Cardiol 1985; S1393–4.
6. Swan HJC, Ganz W, Forrester J et al. Catheterization of the heart in man with use of a flow directed balloon-tipped catheter. N Engl J Med 1970; 283: 447–51.
7. Schoonmaker FW, Vijay NK, Jantz RD. Left atrial and ventricular transseptal catheterization review: Losing skills? Cathet Cardiovac Diagn 1987; 13: 233–8.

8. Lundovist CB, Olsson SB, Varnauskas E. Transseptal left heart catheterization: a review of 278 studies. Clin Cardiol 1986; 9: 21–6.

9. Baim DS, Grossman W. Percutaneous approach, including transseptal catheterization and apical left ventricular puncture in cardiac catheterization, angiography and intervention, 7th edition, 2006. Philadelphia, PA: Lippincott, Williams and Wilkins: 100–3.

10. Clugston R, Lau FYK, Ruiz C. Transseptal catheterization update 1992. Cathet Cardiovasc Diagn 1992; 26: 266–74.

11. Roelke M, Smith AJC, Palacios IF. The technique and safety of transseptal left heart catheterization. The Massachusetts General Hospital experience with 1,279 procedures. Cathet Cardiovasc Diagn 1994; 32: 332–9.

12. Schoenfield MH, Palacios IF, Jutter AM et al. Underestimation of prosthetic mitral valve areas: role of transseptal catheterization in avoiding unnecessary repeat mitral valve surgery. J Am Coll Cardiol 1985; 5: 1387–92.

13. O'Keefe JH, Vlietstra MB, Hanley PC, Seward JB. Revival of the transseptal aproach for catheterization of the left atrium and ventricle. Mayo Clin Proc 1985; 60: 790–5.

14. Carabello BA, Barry WH, Grossman W. Changes in arterial pressure during left heart pullback in patients with aortic stenosis: a sign of severe aortic stenosis. Am J Cardiol 1979; 44: 424–7.

15. Palacios IF. Techniques of balloon valvotomy for mitral stenosis. In: Robicsek F, ed. Cardiac Surgery: State of the Art Reviews. Philadelphia, PA: Hanley R Belfus, Inc, 1991: 229–38.

16. Block PC, Palacios I. Comparison of hemodynamic results of antegrade versus retrograde percutaneous balloon aortic valvuloplasty. Am J Cardiol 1987; 60: 659–62.

17. Rashkind WJ. Transcatheter treatment of congenital heart disease. Circulation 1983; 67: 711–16.

18. Saul JP, Hulse JE, Hulse E et al. Catheter ablation of accessory atrioventricular pathways in young patients: use of long vascular sheaths, the transseptal approach, and a retrograde left posterior parallel approach. J Am Coll Cardiol 1993; 21: 571–83.

19. Lindeneg O, Hansen AT. Complication in transseptal left heart catheterization. Acta Med Scand 1966; 180: 395–9.

20. Adrouny AZ, Sutherland DW, Griswold HE, Ritzman LW. Complications with transseptal left heart catheterization. Am Heart J 1963; 65: 327–33.

21. Braunwald E. Transseptal left heart catheterization. Circulation 1968; 37(Suppl III): 74–9.

22. Nixon PGF, Ikram H. Left heart catheterization with special reference of the transeptal method. Br Heart J 1965; 28: 835–41.

23. Croft CH, Lipscomb K. Modified technique of transseptal left heart catheterization. J Am Coll Cardiol 1985; 5: 904–10.

24. Doorey AJ, Goldenberg EM: Transseptal catheterization in adults: enhanced efficiency and safety by low-volume operators using a 'non-standard' technique. Cathet Cardiovasc Diagn 1991; 8: 535–42.

25. Ali Khan MA, Mulins CE, Bash SE et al. Transseptal left heart catheterisation in infants, children, and young adults. Cathet Cardiovasc Diagn 1989; 17: 198–201.

26. Singleton RT, Scherlis L. Transseptal catheterization of the left heart: observations in 56 patients. Am Heart J 1960; 60(6): 879–85.

27. Folland ED, Oprian C, Giancomini J et al. Complications of cardiac catheterization and angiography in patients with valvular heart disease. Cathet Cardiovasc Diagn 1989; 17: 15–21.

28. Kronzon I, Glassman E, Cohen M, Winer H. Use of two-dimensional echocardiography during transseptal cardiac catheterization. J Am Coll Cardiol 1984; 4(2): 425–8.

29. Libanoff AJ, Silver AW. Complications of transseptal left heart catheterization. Am J Cardiol 1965; 16: 390–3.

30. Peckham GB, Chrysohou A, Aldridge H, Wigle ED. Combined percutaneous retrograde aortic and transseptal left heart catheterization. Br Heart J 1964; 26: 460–8.

31. Wilkins GT, Weyman AE, Abascal VM et al. Percutaneous mitral valvotomy: an analysis of echocardiographic variables related to outcome and the mechanism of dilatation. Br Heart J 1988; 60: 299–308.

32. Henderson MA. Transseptal left atrial catheterization (letter). Cathet Cardiovasc Diagn 1990; 21: 63.

33. Laskey WK, Kusiak V, Unkreter WJ, Hirshfield JW Jr. Transseptal left heart catheterization: utility of a sheath technique. Cathet Cardiovasc Diagn 1982; 8: 535–42.

34. Weiner RI, Maranhao V. Development and application of transseptal left heart catheterization. Cathet Cardiovasc Diagn 1988; 15: 112–20.

35. Wyman RM, Safian RD, Portway V et al. Current complications of diagnostic and therapeutic cardiac catheterization. J Am Coll Cardiol 1988; 12: 1400–6.

36. Lew AS, Harper RW, Federman J et al. Recent experience with transseptal catheterization. Cathet Cardiovasc Diagn 1983; 9: 601.

37. Gordon JB, Folland ED. Analysis of aortic valve gradients by transseptal technique: implications for noninvasive evaluation. Cathet Cardiovasc Diagn 1989; 17: 144–51.

Section IV

12

Fetal cardiac interventions

Michael Tynan

Historic aspects

By the late 1980s it was possible to diagnose many congenital cardiac malformations in fetal life,[1] including valvar aortic stenosis with left ventricular dysfunction.[2] In this particular anomaly the Fetal and Paediatric Cardiology Units at Guy's Hospital in London found that of those patients going on to term there were no survivors of surgery or balloon valvoplasty. We therefore examined the possibility of balloon valvoplasty in the fetus. At the same time we were accumulating data on normal cardiac pressures in the normal fetus.[3] Our guidelines for intervention were: an echocardiographic diagnosis of aortic stenosis with left ventricular dysfunction and a high left ventricular pressure at the time of intervention. The interventions were performed with local anesthesia to the maternal skin and direct needle puncture of the fetal left ventricle via the uterus and the fetal chest wall.[4] In four fetuses five attempts were made; two achieved balloon dilation, of whom one is alive at age 15 years, following post-natal balloon valvoplasty on two occasions, at 3 days and 60 days of age.[5] Considerable technical difficulties were encountered in this early experience. Firstly ultrasound imaging of the fetal heart, with the transducer on the mother's abdomen, was less than ideal. The equipment was not ideal either; we used a wide bore 18 gauge needle for access and even with a custom made balloon it was difficult, nigh impossible, to withdraw the balloon after inflation and fragments of the catheter were sheared off in two cases, including the one long term survivor. Whilst this did not have a deleterious effect on the survivor it was deemed an unsatisfactory state of affairs. Furthermore, the ability to perform the procedure was heavily dependent on the fetal lie.

In the wake of this experience Kohl and his colleagues collected cases of fetal cardiac intervention worldwide and reported that of 14 fetuses where the procedure was attempted for various conditions, 8 of which were isolated aortic valve stenosis, there was only one long term survivor.[6] As Kohl and Gembruch have pointed out recently,[7] the poor outcomes were more due to poor results of post-natal treatment than to failure of the intrauterine interventions. In any event, this experience and improving outcomes of neonatal catheter and surgical interventions led to further attempts at fetal cardiac interventions being put 'on the back burner.' However, animal experimentation in the field continued.[8,9]

Current status

Current clinical work on fetal cardiac interventions centers on three major aspects. Firstly, although the treatment of fetal aortic stenosis still arouses interest, balloon aortic valvoplasty is being performed to investigate the possibility of preventing the development of hypoplastic left heart syndrome.[10] Secondly, the possible role of fetal atrial septostomy in improving the ultimate survival of fetuses with established hypoplastic left heart syndrome with intact or restrictive atrial septum is under study.[11] Finally, some groups are investigating the possible utility of intervention in fetuses with critical pulmonary stenosis or atresia with intact ventricular septum.[12]

Prevention of the hypoplastic left heart syndrome

In 2004 Tworetzky published a series of fetal balloon aortic valve dilations with the aim of preventing the evolution from aortic stenosis to the hypoplastc left heart syndrome.[10] The ultimate objective was to achieve a 'two ventricle circulation' in post-natal life.

Indications for intervention centered on four major issues:

- only mid-trimester fetuses were considered for inclusion
- the dominant lesion had to be aortic stenosis
- the left ventricle had to be salvageable
- the fetus had, most probably, to be going to progress to the hypoplastic left heart syndrome.

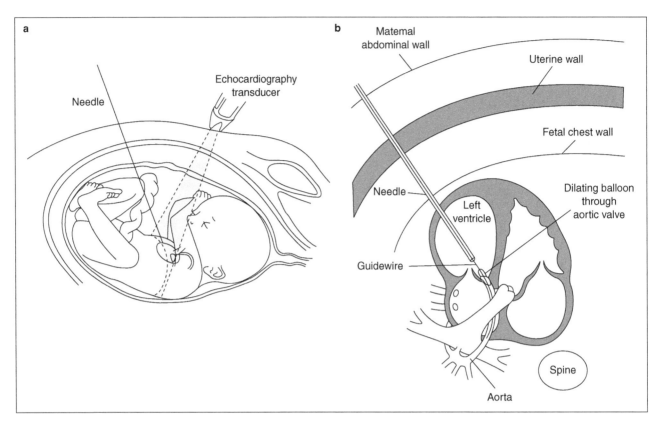

Figure 12.1
(a) The fetus is in the ideal position. The cannula and stylet are shown traversing the maternal abdomen, the uterus, and the anterior aspect of the fetal chest under ultrasound guidance. (b) The positions of the cannula in the left ventricle and the dilating balloon are shown.

These last two criteria could prove to be the most contentious. Salvageability was based on a left ventricular length not more that 2 standard deviations below the mean for gestational age and the likelihood of progressing to the hypoplastic left heart syndrome was based heavily on there being little forward flow through the aortic valve and thus, presumably, there being predominantly retrograde flow in the ascending aorta.

Once selected, the procedure was carried out with light general anesthesia to the mother and the fetus was paralyzed. The details of the anesthetic protocol are given in the publication.[10] The subsequent approach was initially similar to previous attempts (Figure 12.1). Using transabdominal ultrasound with the transducer on the maternal skin, access was achieved using a 19 gauge thin walled cannula and stylet manufactured by Cook Inc. The cannula and stylet were inserted through the maternal skin, passing through the uterine wall and puncturing the fetal thorax and left ventricle. A 0.014 coronary guidewire, with a gently pre-curved tip, was manipulated across the aortic valve. A coronary balloon with a high burst pressure (18 atmospheres), 10% smaller in diameter than the aortic root, was passed over the guidewire and, under transcutaneous ultrasound guidance, was inflated in the aortic root. At completion of the dilation

the deflated balloon was withdrawn into the cannula and removed and the cannula itself was then removed.

Early technical failures led to revisions in the procedure. Rather than rely on ultrasound imaging alone, the skin to aortic valve distances were measured and the wire and the catheter were marked so that no more than 4 cm of the wire and no more than the full length of the balloon were extruded from the cannula. A further modification, when the fetal position was unfavorable or the mother was obese, was that a 'mini laparotomy,' essentially a Pfananstiel incision, was made to expose the uterus. The fetus could then be manipulated to a better lie and the procedure performed via the uterine wall.

Since the publication of the paper[10] further fetuses have been treated. As of May 2005 (W Tworetzky, personal communication), 41 patients were considered as candidates, 6 declined the procedure, of these 2 elected for termination and 4 went to term and all 4 were born with the hypoplastic left heart syndrome. In 35 patients fetal balloon valvoplasty was attempted. In 7 it was unsuccessful and of these 1 died 24 hours after the procedure, 1 elected for termination, 4 developed the hypoplastic left heart syndrome and 1 was still *in utero* at the time of the report. Thus of the 13 who did not have valvoplasty all those who continued to term had developed the hypoplastic left heart syndrome. There were

28 in whom the valvoplasty was successful, 7 are alive with 'two ventricle circulation,' 12 were born with the hypoplastic left heart syndrome, and one was not yet born at the time of the report. The remainder died *in utero* or shortly after premature delivery. If the predictions of the echocardiographers who judged that these fetuses would all have evolved to the hypoplastic left heart syndrome were correct, then this shows a significant improvement over the natural history. Further experience is needed before we know the answer.

Atrial septostomy in fetuses with established hypoplastic left heart syndrome

Using a similar approach, and similar equipment, as for balloon aortic valvoplasty, the results of balloon atrial septostomy were reported in 2004.[11] The procedure was performed under maternal light general anesthesia or epidural anesthesia. The right atrium was perforated with a 19 gauge cannula and stylet, although in one case an 18 gauge cannula and stylet were used. The right atrial wall and the atrial septum were perforated, either with the cannula and stylet or, more commonly, with the stylet withdrawn, a 22 gauge Chiba needle (Cook Inc) was used. A 0.014 guidewire was passed through the needle or cannula and balloon dilation of the atrial septum with a high pressure coronary balloon was performed. Recent results (W Tworetzky, personal communication) demonstrate that of 11 attempts made, all percutaneously, technical success was achieved in 10. The failure was due to suboptimal fetal position and poor imaging. In the remaining 10 the interatrial communication was larger than before the procedure, with increased flow on color Doppler echocardiography. Six of the patients are alive, including the patient in whom the procedure was not achieved. One was not yet born at the time of the communication. However, an adequate atrial septal defect was only found in two patients at birth. Of the remainder, one suffered fetal death and three neonatal death. The fetus who died *in utero* was found to have a hemothorax and a small pericardial effusion. It may be significant that this fetus was the only one in which an 18 gauge cannula was used rather than one of 19 gauge. There were no maternal complications. Whilst these workers have demonstrated the feasibility of creating or enlarging an interatrial defect in the fetus it has yet to be determined whether this will improve post-natal outcome.

Pulmonary atresia or critical pulmonary stenosis with intact ventricular septum

Tulzer and coworkers were the first to publish on fetal interventions in pulmonary atresia/critical pulmonary stenosis with intact ventricular septum.[12] They reported two cases, one with pulmonary atresia and one with critical pulmonary stenosis. Interventions were performed at 28 and 30 weeks' gestation, respectively. The first was performed with light maternal general anesthesia and the second with local anesthesia to the mother. The second fetus was given fentanyl 0.04 mg/kg, pancuronium 0.1 mg/kg, and atropine 0.02 mg/kg to the intrahepatic vein. The right ventricle was perforated with a 16 gauge needle; this was also used to perforate the atretic valve. Over a guidewire which passed into the arterial duct the pulmonary valve was dilated using a 4 mm and a 3 mm coronary balloon, respectively. Both fetuses had pericardial effusions after the procedure which resolved spontaneously. Both babies survived to term. In the first the valve remained patent and a post-natal balloon pulmonary valvoplasty was successful. After initial improvement the second baby progressed to pulmonary atresia and required post-natal radiofrequency assisted balloon pulmonary valvoplasty. Interestingly, in both babies the right ventricle and tricuspid valve showed encouraging increases in size in fetal life.

Subsequently treatment has been attempted in three more similar cases (H Gardiner, personal communication). In one with pulmonary atresia, successful perforation and balloon dilation were achieved at 24 weeks but atresia recurred, so the procedure was repeated at 31 weeks. However, although the right ventricle had increased in size the tricuspid valve remained small; the Z score was −7.8 at birth. The post-natal treatment included a systemic to pulmonary artery shunt and later a one and a half ventricle repair. In the fourth case, at 29 weeks' gestation, the procedure was abandoned due to placental bleeding on puncture of the uterus. Fetal bradycardia unresponsive to atropine resulted in an emergency cesarean section; the child suffered a cerebral hemorrhage and treatment was withdrawn. In the fifth fetus the stenosed pulmonary valve could not be crossed and the procedure was abandoned. This work is a collaboration between Dr Tulzer's group in Linz, Austria, and that of Dr Gardiner in London, UK.

On the basis of this small series it is difficult to assess the utility of intervening in pulmonary valve atresia or valve stenosis.

At present there are technical limitations to be overcome. The equipment is not ideal and the imaging is still suboptimal. A novel approach to improving imaging has been researched and employed in the clinical setting by Dr Thomas Kohl and his colleagues.[13] Aortic stenosis was diagnosed in a fetus at 20 + 2 weeks' gestational age in whom the aortic annulus was deemed to be small for balloon aortic valvoplasty. Progression to aortic atresia and complete closure of the atrial septum was observed. At approximately 27 weeks a balloon atrial septostomy was performed by direct puncture of the right atrium and atrial septum under maternal abdominal ultrasound control. Although a hole was made it was observed to have closed after 3 days.

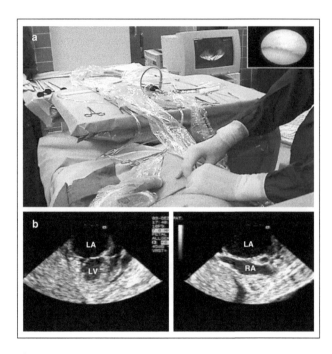

Figure 12.2
(a) The set up for fetal transesophageal echocardiography. (b) The two panes show the high quality of the images obtained in a fetus with aortic atresia and an intact atrial septum. I am grateful to Dr T Kohl for this picture.

A second procedure was therefore performed, but as maternal abdominal ultrasound imaging was suboptimal it was decided to use fetal transesophageal echocardiography. An 11 Fr sheath was placed transcutaneously in the amniotic cavity and, with the aid of fetoscopy, the tip of the sheath was placed in the fetal oropharynx. The fetoscope was removed and, through the sheath, a 10 Fr single plane intravascular ultrasound catheter, AcuNav (Acuson Corp.-A-Siemens Company), was advanced to the fetal esophagus and excellent images were obtained. Despite multiple punctures of the atrial septum no permanent hole could be made. This paper demonstrated the excellent images obtained using this approach. Figure 12.2 shows the basic set up and a fetal transesophageal echocardiogram.

It is apparent that the situation is not yet ideal for the wholesale employment of fetal cardiac interventions. However, there is a very strong case for units with the requisite equipment and expertise to continue to investigate this field. It can be considered another form of 'hybrid intervention.'

Not only is the participation of pediatric interventionists and specialists in fetal medicine and anesthesia required but, since complications are basically obstetric ones, the whole obstetric and neonatology departments must be involved.

Acknowledgments

I would like to thank Doctors W Tworetzky, H Gardiner, and T Kohl for giving me data, advice, and pictures.

References

1. Allan LD, Chita SK, Sharland GK et al. The accuracy of fetal echocardiography in the diagnosis of congenital heart disease. Int J Cardiol 1989; 25: 279–88.
2. Sharland GK, Chita SK, Fagg NL et al. Left ventricular dysfunction in the fetus: relation to aortic valve anomalies and endocardial fibroelastosis. Br Heart J 1991; 66: 419–24.
3. Johnson P, Maxwell DJ, Tynan MJ, Allan LD. Intracardiac pressures in the human fetus. Heart 2000; 84: 59–63.
4. Maxwell D, Allan L, Tynan MJ. Balloon dilatation of the aortic valve in the fetus: a report of two cases. Br Heart J 1991; 65: 256–8.
5. Allan LD, Maxwell DJ, Carminati M, Tynan MJ. Survival after fetal aortic balloon valvoplasty. Ultrasound Obstet Gynecol 1995; 5: 90–1.
6. Kohl T, Sharland G, Allan LD et al. World experience of percutaneous ultrasound-guided balloon valvuloplasty in human fetuses with severe aortic valve obstruction. Am J Cardiol 2000; 85: 1230–3.
7. Kohl T, Gembruch U. Author reply: In-utero intervention for hypoplastic left heart syndrome – a perinatologist's perspective. Ultrasound Obstet Gynecol 2006; 27: 332–3.
8. Kohl T, Szabo Z, Suda K et al. Fetoscopic and open transumbilical fetal cardiac catheterization in sheep. Potential approaches for human fetal cardiac intervention. Circulation 1997; 95: 1048–53.
9. Kohl T, Witteler R, Strumper D et al. Operative techniques and strategies for minimally invasive fetoscopic fetal cardiac interventions in sheep. Surg Endosc 2000; 14: 424–30.
10. Tworetzky W, Wilkins-Haug L, Jennings RW et al. Balloon dilation of severe aortic stenosis in the fetus: potential for prevention of hypoplastic left heart syndrome: candidate selection, technique, and results of successful intervention. Circulation 2004; 110: 2125–31.
11. Marshall AC, van der Velde ME, Tworetzky W et al. Creation of an atrial septal defect in utero for fetuses with hypoplastic left heart syndrome and intact or highly restrictive atrial septum. Circulation 2004; 110: 253–8.
12. Tulzer G, Arzt W, Franklin RCG et al. Fetal pulmonary valvoplasty for critical pulmonary stenosis or atresia with intact septum. Lancet 2002; 360: 1567–8.
13. Kohl T, Muller A, Tchatcheva k et al. Feta transesophageal echocardiography: clinical introduction as a monitoring tool during cardiac intervention in a human fetus. Ultrasound Obstet Gynecol 2005; 26: 780–5.

Section V

13

Special considerations in small infants and newborns

Martin BE Schneider

Introduction

Since Rashkind[1] introduced the balloon atrioseptostomy in the early 1960s, the number of different transcatheter interventions in newborns and small infants has increased dramatically. Today a broad variety of interventional procedures can be performed in very small patients on a routine basis. These interventional procedures include pre-operative palliations such as the 'Rashkind' maneuver, interventions as an alternative to surgical procedures like balloon dilations of pulmonary valve stenosis, and a wide spectrum of postoperative interventions to optimize surgical results.

The major limitation of transcatheter interventions in this age group is the size of the vessels in relation to the size of the catheter materials. Therefore the first part of this chapter will focus on different vascular access routes and catheter materials. The second part emphasizes technical aspects of interventions in small patients presented by selected acute or elective procedures. This part can only present a small overview on a wide spectrum of different interventional procedures and will be continued by other authors in some of the following chapters. Both materials and techniques play a key role in the success of interventional procedures in newborns, particularly as many of these interventions have to be performed in emergency situations.

Vascular access in small patients

In order to avoid damage to the arterial vessels, venous access is preferred. The femoral vein on the venous side is the most common access point, followed by the jugular vein. In newborns the umbilical vein offers an alternative access. As this vein enters the right atrium close to the foramina ovale, it appears to provide good access for transseptal interventions such as the Rashkind maneuver or the antegrade balloon dilation for critical aortic stenoses (Figure 13.1). In contrast, balloon dilation of pulmonary valve stenoses or other interventional procedures on the right ventricle are easier to perform via the femoral vein as the inferior caval vein runs into the right atrium close to the tricuspid valve. In cases where an arterial puncture is inevitable the femoral artery is the usual vascular access. For selected interventions a surgical cut down of the axillary artery (Figure 13.2) can be necessary.

These selected interventional procedures include occlusions of major aorto-pulmonary collateral arteries, dilation or stent implantation in renal artery stenoses, and stent implantation into modified Blalock–Taussig shunts or into the arterial duct in cases where the duct originates from the aortic arch (Figure 13.3).

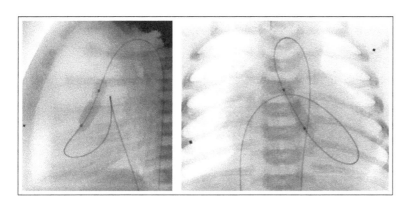

Figure 13.1
Antegrade balloon dilation of critical aortic stenoses in a newborn.

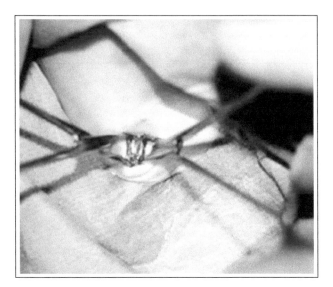

Figure 13.2
Tips for the surgical cut down of an axillary artery:
- use sharp instruments for the skin insertion
- anatomic preparation can be performed using two blunt bended clamps
- a bundle of nerves in this region looks like the axillary artery; pulsation is the best visible and perceptible identification
- after preparation the artery should be surrounded and held by two strings
- puncture the vessel by the 'Seldinger' technique while tightening the distal string.

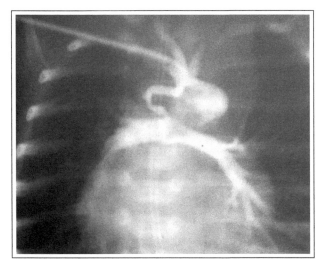

Figure 13.3
Right axillary artery as vascular access for implantation of a stent into an arterial duct which originates from the aortic arch.

Materials

Although the number of catheters particularly designed for very small infants is still limited, many companies now offer a broad spectrum of different catheter materials for adult patients. Therefore, pediatric interventionalists should take note of catalogs from catheter manufacturers aimed at cardiologists, urologists, radiologists, and especially neurologic-radiologists working with adult patients.

This chapter tries to give an overview on materials often used in small patients at our institution. This makes no claim to be exhaustive, but might give an impression of the difficulties accompanying the search for the right materials in this patient group.

Sheaths

In patients of body weight less than 3 kg, use of a sheath larger than 4 Fr at the arterial side or 7 Fr at the venous side should be avoided. Larger sheaths bear the risk of severe damage to the vessels. Terumo Radiofocus (Terumo Corporation) sheaths can be recommended, because of their smooth surface and a good relationship between a relatively large inner lumen and the small outer diameter.

Sheaths of size 3 Fr are available (Balt Company), but the 3 Fr catheter materials have some disadvantages. Most of these catheters, such as the Pigtail or the Cobra, are relatively rigid, leading to kinking of the catheter when it is maneuvered inside the vessels. On the other hand, the inner lumen of 3 Fr catheters appears to be too small for adequate contrast injection.

Guidewires

For diagnostic catheterization we use 0.018 inch and 0.035 inch Teflon coated wires (Cook company, THSF) virtually exclusively. The advantages of these guidewires are the very soft tip at one side and a stiff but flexible end at the other side. This stiff end can be easily pre-shaped by pulling it gently over the tip of the thumb. Depending on the individual anatomy, different wire shapes can be so created for maneuvering a catheter into difficult positions. We use the pre-shaped stiff end of the guidewires for most of the complex catheter maneuvers.

The following examples will help to demonstrate the use of individual shaped wires in different anatomic positions:

- A U shape of the 0.018 inch wire for positioning a 4 Fr wedge catheter on an antegrade route across the aortic valve (Figure 13.4).
- The same wire with an S shape is used to move the same catheter across the pulmonary valve (Figure 13.5). Alternatively, a mild C shape of a 0.035 inch wire can be used to guide a Cobra catheter into the same anatomic position (Figure 13.6).

The C-shaped guidewire supports the Cobra catheter on the tricuspidal level. To enter the right ventricular outflow tract and thereafter the pulmonary artery the bent tip of this catheter can be used by holding the wire in position

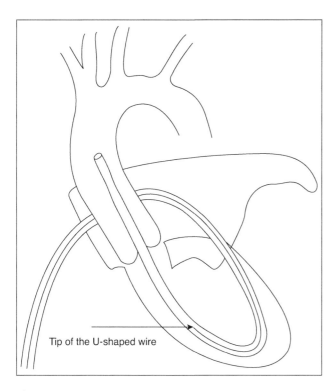

Figure 13.4
Antegrade positioning of a 4 Fr wedge catheter across the aortic valve (see also Figure 13.1). A U-shaped stiff end of a 0.018 inch Teflon coated guidewire is fixed with the cardiologist's right hand in the apex of the left ventricle while the left hand pushes the catheter over this railway towards the left ventricular outflow tract and across the aortic valve.

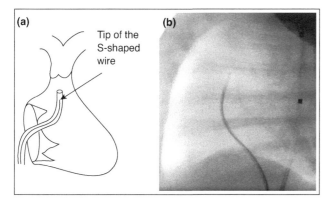

Figure 13.5
Entering the pulmonary artery using a 4 Fr wedge catheter and the stiff end of a 0.018 inch Teflon coated guidewire; (a) antero-posterior view, (b) right lateral view.

with its tip in the middle part of the right ventricle and pushing the catheter while twisting counter clockwise.

The 0.018 inch wire is used to guide the 4 and 5 Fr Berman angiographic and the Berma wedge catheters. With

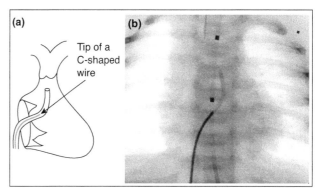

Figure 13.6
Entering the pulmonary artery using a 4 Fr 'Cobra' catheter and the stiff end of a 0.035 inch Teflon coated guidewire; (a) and (b) anteroposterior views.

the 0.035 inch wire, catheters such as the Cobra, Pigtail, and Judgins can be maneuvered.

Coronary guidewires can be useful for some interventional procedures, for example recanalization of obstructed vessels, interventional perforation in patients with pulmonary atresia, or dilations with coronary angioplasty balloons. For recanalization a stiff and sharp wire like the Cross It 400 XT Hi Torgue (Guidant Company) can be recommended. Floppy and soft tips (e.g. Wizdom™ 3 cm soft tip, Cordis Company, or Cross It Pilot 50, Guidant Company) are useful to sound out small distorted vessels. In this situation the Terumo™ wires can be used as an alternative.

Stent implantation should be performed with the support of stiff wires. The size of the wire depends on the inner lumen of the catheter of the stent/balloon ensemble. When a 0.035 inch guidewire fits into the inner lumen of the balloon catheter the 0.035 inch Teflon coated THSF wire from Cook Company can be recommended, even in small patients. If the inner lumen of the balloon catheter varies from 0.018 to 0.028 inch, the 0.18 inch SV 5™ Straight Wire (Cordis Company), with its short floppy tip, gives excellent support to the stent mounted on the balloon.

List of catheter materials often used in newborns and small patients

Diagnostic catheters

Angiographic catheters

- Berman angiographic catheter (Arrow) 4 and 5 Fr, 0.018 inch lumen
- Pigtail 4 Fr Terumo™, 0.038 inch lumen
- Pigtail catheters 4 and 5 Fr Cordis, 0.035 inch lumen
- Pigtail 3 Fr catheter BALT, 0.021 inch lumen
- Cobra with side holes, Cordis
- NIH Cordis catheter.

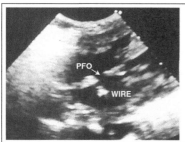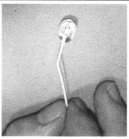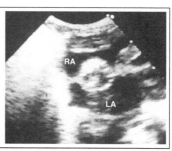

Figure 13.7
Balloon atrioseptostomy in a preterm baby with a bodyweight of 1180 g.

End-hole-catheters
- Bermann wedge catheter (Arrow), 4 and 5 Fr
- Cobra 4 and 5 Fr (Cordis), 0.035 inch lumen
- Judkins R and L (Cordis), 4 and 5 Fr different shapes, 0.035 inch lumen (note: Judkins catheters are quite long (> 100 cm) for small patients)
- Terumo™ catheters 4 Fr (Terumo™): Cobra, Non Taper Angle and Straight Taper, 0.038 inch lumen.

Interventional materials

Rashkind catheters. For regular Rashkind procedures in term babies the Miller balloon (Edwards Company Lifesciences) can be used. These catheters are labeled as 5 Fr, but at least a 6 Fr sheath is necessary to introduce the balloon with some effort, and it goes easily through a 7 Fr sheath.

In preterm babies the Z-5 atrioseptostomy catheter from Numed, with a 9.5 mm diameter non-compliant balloon and 1 ml maximum volume, can be recommended (Figure 13.7). This catheter needs a 5 Fr introducer and a 0.014 inch guidewire. The use of a guidewire is highly recommended as the surface of the non-inflated balloon has a marked edge, with a potential to damage intracardiac structures. Therefore the Rashkind maneuver should be performed under fluoroscopy with the guiding wire positioned in the left upper pulmonary vein.

Balloon catheters. The Numed Company produces balloon catheters specially designed for small patients. The Tyhak mini series, with a balloon diameter between 4 and 10 mm, need introducer sizes of only 3–4 Fr. However these balloons can only be guided by 0.014 inch wires! Alternatively, the Tyshak II balloons, 4–8 mm in diameter, fit into 4 Fr introducer sheaths and can be guided by 0.018 inch (maximum 0.021 inch) wires. These balloons are excellent for valvuloplasty maneuvers, particularly the antegrade dilation of aortic stenoses.

The Savvy balloons from Cordis Company (2–6 mm in diameter) are useful for dilation of narrow rigid stenoses. These balloons have a very low profile. The maximum inflation pressure goes up to 10 atmospheres; with a lumen of 0.018 inch they fit into a 4 Fr introducer.

Very often coronary angioplasty catheters are used in newborns. The pediatric cardiologists usually borrow coronary balloons from the adult cardiologist colleagues in their centers. Therefore the decision for special coronary balloon catheters usually orientates to the individual balloons the cardiologists prefer for percutaneous transluminary coronary angioplasty (PTCA). It is important to know that the vast majority of PTCA balloons work on a rapid exchange basis and on 0.014 inch guidewires only.

Stents. One of the greatest limitations from the 'material point of view' is the use of stents in newborns as they are not designed for a lifelong stay in patient bodies. Obviously the companies do not have a great interest in the development of new stent systems for pediatric patients, particularly newborns. On the contrary, one of the only short peripheral stents, the Palmaz P128 (Cordis Company), with the potential for re-dilation up to 19 mm diameter, was withdrawn from the market some years ago. This stent could be easily implanted into infant vessels and re-dilated according to patient growth. It was replaced by the Genesis PG 1910P stent with a minimum length of 19 mm – which in most small patients is simply too long.

According to this problem there are basically three different indications for stent implantation in newborns and small infants:

1. *Short term palliation* for a time period between weeks and 6 months. For example, the palliative stenting of critical coarctation or the stenting of the arterial duct. Because of the short period a re-dilation of those stents is not necessary. Therefore, the stents used for such indications are mainly pre-mounted coronary stent systems with a diameter of 3.5–4.5 mm and a length between 8 and 12 mm. The decision for the stent type most often depends on what the adult cardiologists have in stock, such as the coronary balloon catheters mentioned above. Although stents in the arterial duct can usually stay in place for a lifelong period because most of them will be closed due to intimal hyperplasia after some months, coronary stents in other anatomic locations do need to be removed by the surgeons. Thus,

implantation of coronary stents in newborns or small infants has to be discussed and planned together with the surgeons as part of an interdisciplinary therapeutic concept!

2. *Mid term stent strategies* for a time period between 6 months and 2 years followed by surgical removal. Balloon expandable peripheral stents with the potential of re-dilation from 4 mm up to 10–12 mm in diameter are required. These stents in general are pre-mounted stent–balloon ensembles and this is the major advantage. We often use Cordis Palmaz Genesis stents on Slalom balloons, Medium series. The balloon diameters used in small patients range from 4 to 8 mm and the stent length may be 12, 15, or 18 mm. All of them have a 0.018 inch lumen and need 5–6 Fr introducers. For example, in patients with hypoplastic pulmonary arteries and mayor aorto-pulmonary collateral arteries (MAPCAs) they can be implanted into the right ventricular outflow tract to increase an antegrade flow into the pulmonary artery to stimulate vessel growth. By re-dilation these stents can be adapted to the patient's growth during the first 1 or 2 years of life until the size of the pulmonary arteries has become sufficient for surgical therapies such as correction of tetralogy of Fallot instead of unifocalization.

3. *Long term stent treatment*: in a very few circumstances stents with the potential for re-dilation up to 19–20 mm can be used even in small infants. Today the shortest stent available for use in small patients is the Genesis PG1910P, which is 19 mm long and, together with a balloon, fits into at least a 7 Fr introducer. Therefore it can only be implanted in small patients via venous access. The Intra Maxi LD stents (EV3 Company) are shorter than 19 mm, but it is difficult to mount them on balloon catheters with a very low size and profile. Implantation into a central part of the systemic veins is one of the few options in small patients.

Miscellaneous. For transcatheter perforation of atretic valves in this age group stiff guidewires, laser catheters, or radiofrequency wires can be used. We only have experience with the radiofrequency method and use 1 Fr ablation wires from Osypka Company with a 0.25 mm tip. This wire fits together with a 0.014 inch floppy wire into an end hole catheter with an inner lumen of 0.035 or 0.038 inch (Figure 13.8). After successful perforation the ablation wire can be carefully removed by simultaneously pushing the floppy wire across the small hole created for further successive dilations of the valve.

Techniques

The rest of this chapter will give some examples of the technical aspects for transcatheter interventions in newborns and small infants. It will show cases where interventional procedures replaced surgery, prepared for or even made surgery possible, and optimized surgical results.

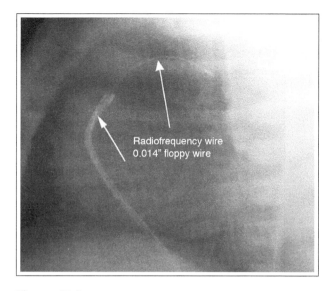

Figure 13.8
Successful perforation of an atretic pulmonary valve. The radiofrequency wire and a 0.014 inch floppy wire were together positioned with their ends at the tip of a 4 Fr Cobra catheter. After perforation the radiofrequency wire had to be pulled back and simultaneously, the floppy wire had to be pushed forward across the hole in the valve.

For each case, we will first illustrate the anatomic problem and then the interventional solution. Thereafter we will discuss the technical aspects of obtaining the interventional objectives.

Case 1: stent into the arterial duct. This case shows a 2-day-old boy with a body weight of 2.9 kg. He was born with a duct dependent congenital heart disease. He had a critical pulmonary valve stenosis with a hypoplastic right ventricle. Three interventional procedures were performed on his second, third, and sixth days of life (Figures 13.9 and 13.10).

Technical aspects

Intervention on the second day of life (Figure 13.11). A 4 Fr Cobra catheter was positioned in the right ventricular outflow tract with the help of the C-shaped stiff end of a 0.35 inch Teflon coated guidewire (see above). Thereafter the wire was exchanged for a 0.014 inch floppy Wizdom wire. The floppy wire was easily pushed across the stenotic valve and far into the peripheral pulmonary artery. Alternatively, one could try to push the wire across the duct far into the descending aorta. It is important to have the stiff part of the floppy wire at the level of the valve otherwise you will lose the wire position whilst you change the Cobra catheter for the balloon catheter.

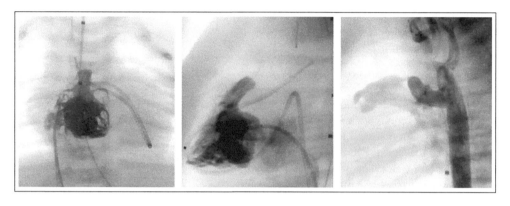

Figure 13.9
Case 1: anatomy before interventional treatment.

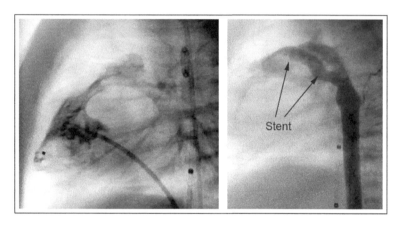

Figure 13.10
Case 1: interventional result.

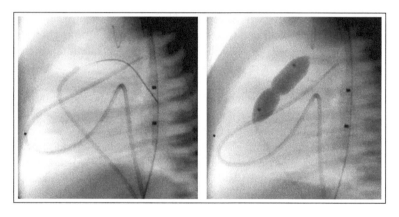

Figure 13.11
Case 1: intervention on the second day of life: dilatation of the pulmonary valve.

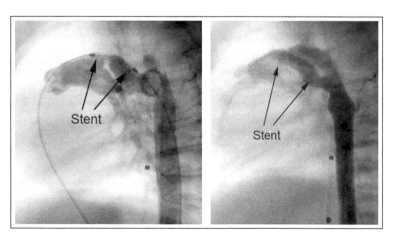

Figure 13.12
Case 1: intervention on the third day of life: stent implantation into the arterial duct.

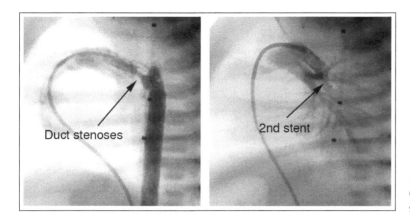

Figure 13.13
Case 1: intervention on the sixth day of life: second stent into the arterial duct.

Once the correct wire position had been achieved, the end-hole catheter had to be pulled back, pushing the wire at the same time, and then the balloon catheter was brought on the wire to the valve. In this patient we used a 6 mm diameter Tyshak mini balloon with a length of 2 cm. Note that there was a second catheter, which was placed ante-gradely into the ascending aorta, still in place. This catheter was used for a final angiogram to demonstrate the size and the shape of the arterial duct after balloon dilation of the pulmonary valve (Figure 13.11). The duct was shown to be wide open with a diameter greater than 5 mm. Therefore, an implantation of a coronary stent at this time was impossi-ble. The prostaglandin infusion was stopped and the patient was brought back to the neonatal ward.

After 24 hours the arterial oxygen saturation dropped down due to closure of the duct. The patient was re-admitted to the catheterization laboratory.

Intervention on the third day of life (Figure 13.12). For the stent implantation a 4 Fr Pigtail catheter was introduced via the femoral artery into the descending aorta. At the same time, a 4 Fr Cobra catheter was postioned into the pulmonary artery (see above) and a 0.18 inch SV 5 straight wire pushed through the narrowed duct far into the descending aorta. A pre-mounted 12 mm Cordis Genesis stent, 1240 PPS, on a 4 mm diameter Opta PRO balloon, was then positioned into the duct via the femoral vein. The stent was inflated at the narrow pulmonary duct segment. The aortic segment was shown to be still too wide for a secure stent placement (Figure 13.12).

Intervention on the sixth day of life (Figure 13.13). At this time the aortic segment of the duct was narrow enough for the secure implantation of a second stent. The same stent was implanted by the telescope technique, in the same way as the first, in order to cover the whole duct.

Case 2: palliative stenting of a hypoplastic aortic arch and a coarctation. The second case shows a 4-week-old preterm baby with a body weight of 1.8 kg. The child had a univentricular left heart with a rudimentary subaortic right ventricle, a severe obstructive ventricular septal defect, and a hypoplastic aortic arch with an additional coarctation. As well as his complex cardiac defect, this little boy had many additional problems due to his premature birth. During the first weeks of life he developed a septicemia and a necrotic col-itis followed by surgical resection of part of his bowel. In addi-tion he suffered from severe pulmonary hyperperfusion and infections of the lung. At this stage the cardiac surgeons refused to operate and a combined interventional/surgical strategy was developed (Figure 13.14). The plan was to stop the prostaglandin infusion after dilation of the narrow aortic arch by stent implantation and postpone the Norwood opera-tion till the patient is in good clinical condition and has reached a weight between 2500 and 3000g.

Technical aspects

Interventional catheterization at the age of 4 weeks: palliative stenting of the aortic arch and the coarctation (Figure 13.15). At the age of 4 weeks the patient was brought to the catheterization laboratory in a relatively stable clinical condition. After puncture of the femoral artery, a 3 Fr introducer was inserted. With a 3 Fr Cobra catheter, contrast medium was injected to visualize the aortic arch. A second 4 Fr Berman angiographic catheter was positioned into the ventricle in order to take angiograms during stent positioning, however due to the large left ventricle and the very large pulmonary arteries it was impossible to achieve a proper picture of the arch and this catheter was ineffective. We therefore used other extracardiac structures such as the tube or trachea as landmarks during the implantations.

Three pre-mounted coronary Cordis Velocity stents with a length of 8 mm and a balloon diameter of 4.5 mm were implanted by the telescope technique, starting with the proximal stent. To avoid damage to the artery the 3 Fr sheath was removed and the pre-mounted stents, on a 0.014 inch guidewire, were led directly through the skin. The first stent was positioned at the origin of the right subclavian artery, overlapping the right carotid artery. About 30% of

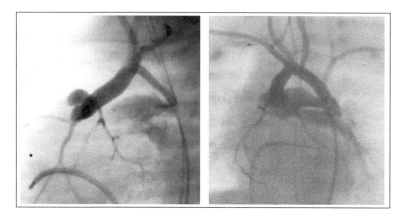

Figure 13.14
Case 2: anatomy before intervention (left) and interventional result (right).

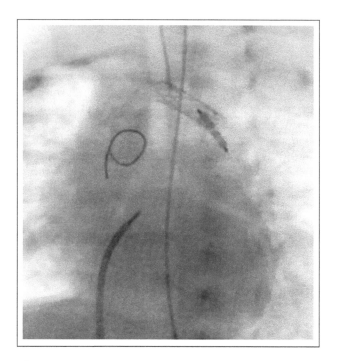

Figure 13.15
Stenting of hypoplastic aortic arch and coarctation.

the second stent's length was inserted into the first. This stent overlapped the left carotid artery and the last stent was put into the second, with its distal part at the duct level to overcome the coarctation (Figure 13.15).

The patient underwent a successful Norwood procedure 3 months later. During the operation one of the stents was removed and the other two stents were surgically cut and split in length direction.

Case 3: stenting of the right ventricular outflow tract in a patient with tetralogy of Fallot, hypoplastic pulmonary arteries, and major aorto-pulmonary collateral arteries (MAPCAs). The third case demonstrates a little girl at the

age of 3 days and a body weight of 2.7 kg. She had a severe tetralogy of Fallot with a critical right ventricular outflow tract and pulmonary valve stenosis, hypoplastic pulmonary arteries, and MAPCAs (Figures 13.16 and 13.17).

Technical aspects

First interventional catheterization at the age of 3 days. Balloon dilation and stent implantation into the right ventricular outflow tract were performed. The pulmonary artery was entered by a Cobra catheter. It was shown to be extremely narrow. In order to secure the access to the pulmonary artery, two floppy 0.014 inch guidewires were pushed into the distal part of the right upper lobe artery. A 4.5 mm diameter coronary balloon catheter ('over the wire system') was used for pre-dilation of the valve (Figure 13.18).

After pre-dilation a 4 Fr Cobra catheter was led on the two wires into the right pulmonary and the two wires exchanged with the stiff end of a C-shaped 0.035 inch Teflon coated guidewire. A 12 mm long Palmaz Genesis stent, pre-mounted on a 6 mm diameter Opta PRO balloon, could be easily positioned and implanted between the right ventricular outflow tract and the main pulmonary artery. This stent–balloon ensemble needs a 6 Fr introducer (Figure 13.19). When the stent was implanted we first recognized the left and right lower lobe pulmonary artery (Figure 13.20).

Second interventional catheterization at the age of 7 weeks. The child was re-catheterized electively for re-dilation of the stent. At this stage a severe stenosis of the main pulmonary artery distal to the stent was noted and a second stent implanted by the telescope technique. The technique of implantation and the stent we used were exactly the same as we used during the first intervention. After implantation of the second stent (Figure 13.21) the MAPCAs to the right side were closed in order to increase the growth of the right sided pulmonary artery by eliminating the competitive blood flow from the aorta (Figure 13.22). The left sided MAPCA was kept open because of an absent left upper lobe artery. After

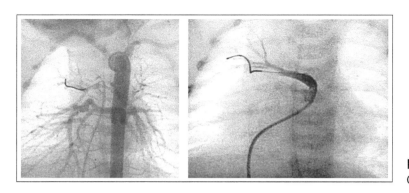

Figure 13.16
Case 3: anatomy before interventional treatment.

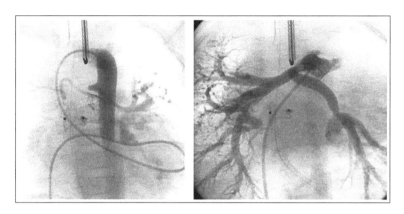

Figure 13.17
Case 3: interventional result after 6 months.

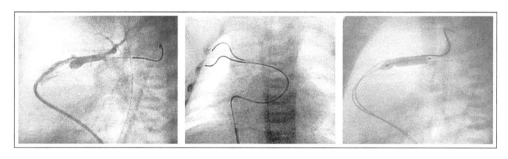

Figure 13.18
Balloon dilation of critical pulmonary valve stenosis.

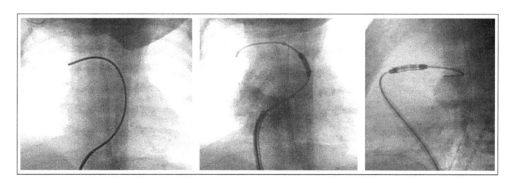

Figure 13.19
Stent implantation into the right ventricular outflow tract and main pulmonary stenosis.

another 4 months the stents were re-dilated up to 9 mm diameter and the patient underwent surgical correction of the tetralogy of Fallot instead of unifocalization at the age of 9 months.

Case 4: re-canalization of an obstructed modified Blalock-Taussig (BT) shunt 2 days after surgery. The patient with tetralogy of Fallot and hypoplastic pulmonary arteries was transferred from another center 2 days after a surgical shunt

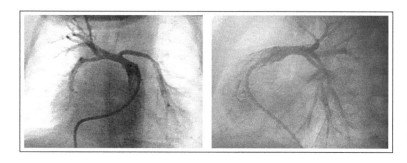

Figure 13.20
Interventional result after balloon dilation and stenting of the right ventricular outflow tract.

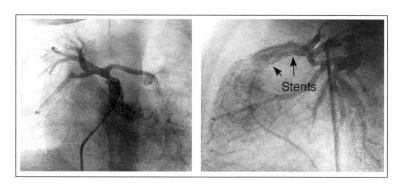

Figure 13.21
Follow up 1: second stent implantation into the main pulmonary artery and re-dilation of the two stents.

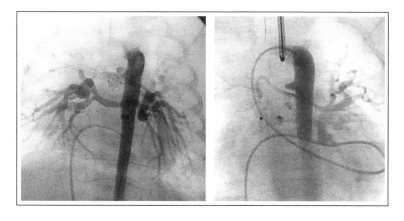

Figure 13.22
Follow up 2: interventional occlusion of major aorto-pulmonary collateral arteries (MAPCAs).

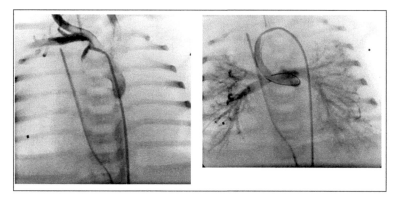

Figure 13.23
Case 4: anatomy before intervention (left) and interventional result (right).

operation from the right arterial trunk to the main pulmonary artery. The little boy had a severe cyanosis and was sent to our institute with an acute thrombosis of his shunt. After admission he was immediately catheterized at the age of 12 days and a body weight of 3.4 kg (Figure 13.23).

Technical aspects

Interventional catheterization was performed 2 days after the aorto-pulmonary shunt operation. A 4 Fr Cobra catheter was inserted via the femoral artery and hand injection of

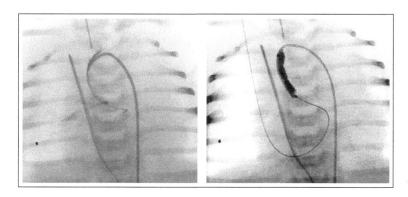

Figure 13.24
Balloon dilation of obstructed right sided Blalock-Taussig (BT) shunt.

contrast medium showed the BT shunt to be completely obstructed. The shunt was re-canalized by a 0.014 inch Cross It 400 XT Hi Torgue wire and dilated with a 2.5 mm SAVVY balloon followed by a 4 mm Tyshak II balloon (Figure 13.24).

To give the balloon catheter sufficient support on its sharp angled route the wire was pushed retrogradely across the pulmonary valve and, luckily, across the tricuspid valve into the superior caval vein. Initially the oxygen saturation increased from 48% to 75%, but decreased again after some minutes and an angiogram demonstrated again partial occlusion of the shunt, obviously due to repeat thrombosis (Figure 13.25).

At this point the decision for stent implantation was made. Using a 4 Fr Terumo™ Non-taper Angle catheter the 0.014 inch guidewire was exchanged with a 0.18 inch SV 5 straight wire, and the 4 Fr arterial introducer was exchanged with a 5 Fr one. A pre-mounted Palmaz Genesis stent PG1540PPS was implanted retrogradely via a short sheath in the femoral artery (Figure 13.26), resulting in a constant oxygen saturation of 80–83%. A high dose of heparin was administered at the same time.

In cases where stent implantation is necessary in a surgically inserted shunt, any coronary stent system can be used. In this situation the balloon catheter should be approximately 10% bigger than the fixed diameter of the shunt to give the stent enough support to avoid dislocation. Re-dilation is not necessary in an artificial shunt.

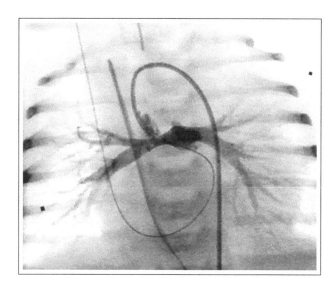

Figure 13.25
Result after shunt dilation.

Case 5: re-canalization of an obstructed superior caval vein (SVC) 5 days after surgical correction of a high positioned sinus venous defect with 'overriding' SVC. The last case describes another completely obstructed vessel. The patient had a sinus venous defect with 'overriding' SVC. He was surgically corrected in the neonatal period. During surgery the SVC had to be re-implanted because of its 'overriding' upon

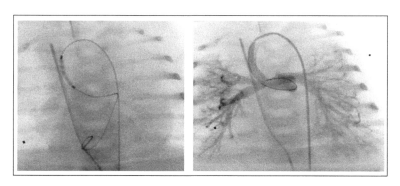

Figure 13.26
Stenting of right sided Blalock-Taussig (BT) shunt.

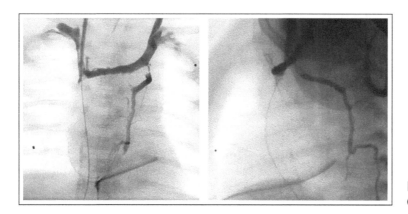

Figure 13.27
Case 5: anatomy before interventional treatment.

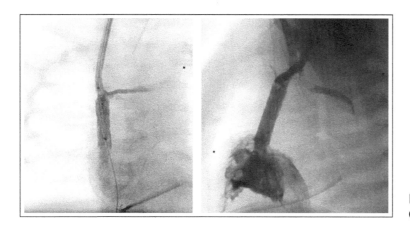

Figure 13.28
Case 5: interventional result.

the defect. Days after the operation the patient suffered from pleural effusion, and venous congestion at his head and neck was noted. Echocardiography showed the SVC to be complete obstructed. The patient was transferred to the catheterization laboratory 5 days after surgery at the age of 4 weeks and a body weight of 2.8 kg (Figures 13.27 and 13.28).

Technical aspects

The first angiogram was performed from a venous access in the right jugular vein. It showed a complete obstruction of the SVC. The SVC could be easily passed by a 0.014 inch soft floppy wire (Wizdom). The tip of the wire was pushed far into the IVC and snared out through an additional access in the right femoral vein by a 10 mm diameter snare, thus creating a stable railway. Then a 4 Fr straight Terumo™ catheter was inserted into the jugular sheath and pushed down over this wire to the femoral access, where it was led out of the sheath again. Across this catheter the 0.014 inch wire was exchanged for a 0.18 inch SV 5 straight wire. Balloon dilation with a 5 mm diameter Tyshak balloon (Figure 13.29) was unsuccessful because the vein collapsed

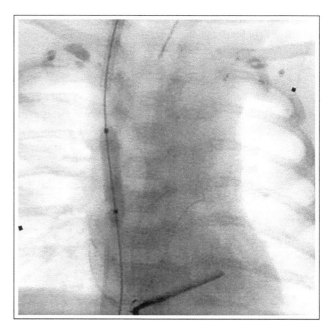

Figure 13.29
Balloon dilation of obstructed superior caval vein.

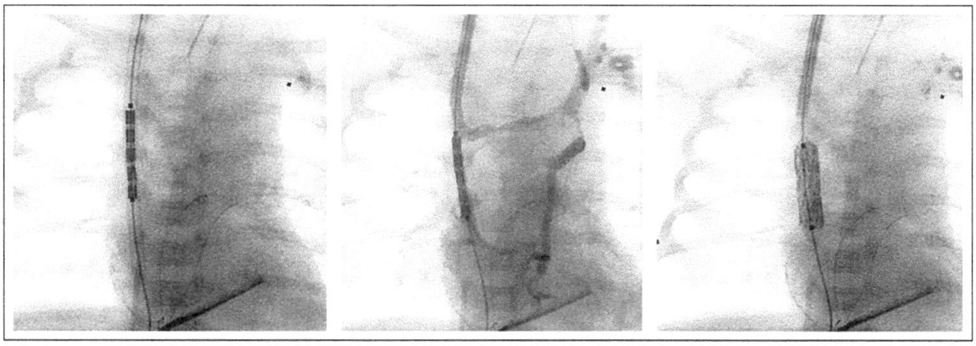

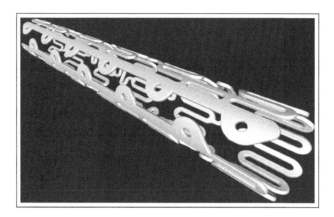

Figure 13.30
Stenting of superior caval vein.

again immediately after deflation. Obviously the reason for the obstruction was not a thrombosis at first hand. It was rather a stretching of the surgically re-inserted SVC, leading to a collapse of the vein and secondary to an additional mild thrombosis.

A stent implantation appeared to be the best solution for this problem. However, this time we had to choose a stent with a potential to stay in the SVC for a lifetime period because re-operation of a stented SVC appears to be a problem for the surgeon unrelated to the patient's age and size.

A Genesis PG 1910 P stent with the potential for re-dilation up to a diameter of 19 mm was manually mounted on a Tyshak II balloon catheter with a balloon length of 20 mm and a diameter of 5 mm. Due to the low profile of the balloon it was not possible to achieve an adequate fixation of the balloon. Usually a balloon loses its low profile when deflated after a first inflation. This results in a rough surface giving a manually mounted stent a better fixation. Therefore we used the same balloon we had before during the dilation. Additionally we inflated the balloon slightly whilst it was mounted and thirdly we 'glued' the stent on the balloon with some contrast medium. This stent–balloon ensemble was pushed through a 7 Fr sheath on a trial basis outside the patient's body.

When we recognized the stent on the balloon passing the 7 Fr sheath another 7 Fr short sheath was introduced from the jugular vein and positioned across the obstructed SVC, covering the stent during positioning as a long sheath would do in an older patient. When the stent was in position the sheath was slowly pulled back. Injection of contrast medium through the 7 Fr sheath revealed the stent to be in the right position. Finally the balloon was inflated and the stent implanted into the collapsed SVC (Figure 13.30).

Figure 13.31
A new stent concept: the breakable stent from Osypka Company, Germany.

this chapter. However, one can have only an imagination of the number of different procedures by the number of different congenital lesions. The use of materials from medical disciplines other than pediatric cardiology enables us to perform today many interventional procedures before or after surgical treatment, or even instead of surgery. Particularly on the stent field, new technology is required so that small patients may be treated by stent implantation without the necessity for later surgical removal. Bioabsorbable stents or breakable stents (Figure 13.31) could represent a solution to this problem in the near future.

Summary

By using a number of examples, the wide range of different and complex interventional procedures has been demonstrated in

Reference

1. Rashkind WJ, Miller WW. Creation of an atrial septal defect without thoracotomy. A Palliative Approach to Complete Transposition of the Great Arteries. JAMA 1966; 196: 991–2.

Section VI

Valves

14

Aortic valve, congenital stenosis

Oleg Reich

Anatomy

The aortic annulus is usually hypoplastic to some extent, the leaflets are thickened and the commissures are fused to varying degrees. Dysplastic or unicuspid valves (Figure 14.1a), often seen in newborns, are present in about 10% of infants and 3% of older children in whom the treatment is indicated. Tricuspid valves (Figure 14.1b) are seen in 25% of infants and in 40% of older patients who require treatment. The majority of the stenotic aortic valves are bicuspid.[1] There are two forms of bicuspid aortic valve: balanced or 'anatomically bicuspid' and unbalanced or 'functionally bicuspid.' The anatomically bicuspid valve is composed of two equally sized cusps with two sinuses of Valsalva (Figure 14.1c). The functionally bicuspid valve also opens as bicuspid, but it has three sinuses, two of them adjacent to a fused cusp which is actually formed by two unequal cusps conjoined by an unopened commissure. The fused cusp is larger than the opposite one, hence 'unbalanced bicuspid valve' (Figure 14.1d). This anatomic concept is important in regard to the prognosis of the valvuloplasty.[1] In the balanced bicuspid valves as well as in tricuspid stenotic valves, the orifices are usually enlarged by a splitting of the functioning commissures, whereas in the unbalanced bicuspid valves, the fused cusp is often torn aside from the rudimental commissure (Figure 14.2),[2] presumably due to unequal rigidity of the different sized cusps.

Pathophysiology

Aortic stenosis causes left ventricular pressure overload. Despite the high left ventricular pressure, the wall stress throughout the systole is usually not higher than normal because of an increased left ventricular wall thickness. Another compensatory mechanism is a lengthening of the ejection time at the expense of the diastole duration. Due to the adaptation, the systolic left ventricular function is

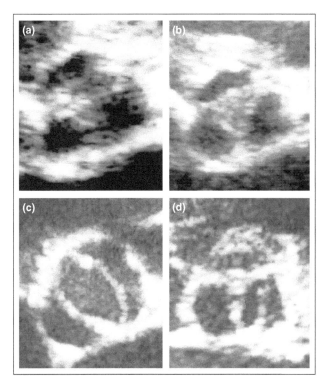

Figure 14.1
Anatomy of congenital aortic stenosis assessed by two-dimensional echocardiography in the parasternal short axis view. (a) Unicuspid valve; (b) tricuspid valve; (c) balanced bicuspid ('anatomically bicuspid') valve; (d) unbalanced bicuspid ('functionally bicuspid') valve.

usually well maintained over a long period of time. Diastolic function varies according to the severity of the left ventricular hypertrophy. In a pronounced hypertrophy, the compliance of the left ventricular wall is markedly decreased and the left ventricular end diastolic pressure is

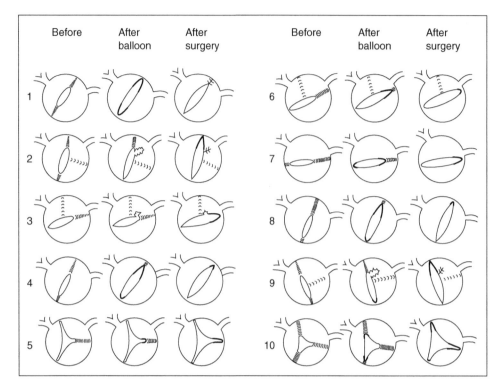

Figure 14.2
Schematic drawing of valves before intervention, after balloon dilation, and after surgical correction. Bold lines show the change obtained with each intervention. (Reproduced from Solymar et al.)

elevated. Elevated end diastolic pressure and a shortened diastole duration contribute to a limitation of the subendocardial coronary flow. In a severe stenosis, the restriction of the coronary flow causes subendocardial ischemia during exercise or even at rest. Acute myocardial ischemia during exercise may cause ventricular arrhythmias and a syncope or sudden death. Another sign of severe stenosis is the inability of the left ventricle to adequately increase cardiac output with exercise, which is reflected by an insufficient systolic pressure rise or even by a systolic pressure drop on exertion.

Clinical symptoms

Some infants present with congestive heart failure due to the left ventricular dysfunction. In some, subendocardial ischemia causes left ventricular endocardial fibroelastosis and fibrosis of the papillary muscles with mitral insufficiency. The majority of patients are asymptomatic and the disease is usually diagnosed by a murmur. Other most common signs are fatigue, exertional dyspnea, angina pectoris, and syncope. In a natural course, more than 70% of the patients with severe aortic stenosis die suddenly.[3]

Indications for treatment

The normal aortic valve area is approximately $2.0 \, cm^2/m^2$. Aortic stenosis is considered mild when the area is above $0.8 \, cm^2/m^2$, moderate with an area of 0.5 to $0.8 \, cm^2/m^2$, and severe with an area less than $0.5 \, cm^2/m^2$. In association with normal cardiac output, severe stenosis causes a peak systolic gradient over 75 mmHg. Severe aortic stenosis is an indication for treatment. Based on the clinical and echocardiographic criteria, treatment is indicated:

- in all patients with a Doppler peak systolic gradient ≥ 75 mmHg
- in patients with left ventricular strain on the ECG and a peak gradient ≥ 60 mmHg
- regardless of the gradient in all patients presenting with syncope, low cardiac output, or severe left ventricular dysfunction.

The gradient must be measured at rest and any factors that may increase the resting cardiac output, such as anemia, must be excluded. In borderline cases an exercise test is performed and, if subendocardial ischemia or a hypotensive reaction occurs, treatment is indicated. In patients with moderate to severe aortic regurgitation, surgical treatment is preferred to valvuloplasty.

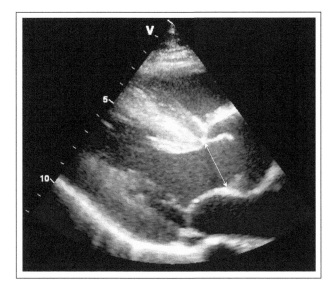

Figure 14.3
The aortic annulus diameter is measured between the hinge points of the valve leaflets in the two-dimensional parasternal long axis view. The annulus must be carefully and thoroughly scanned by transducer angulation so that the maximum possible diameter is obtained.

Alternatives

Studies that compared valvuloplasty with surgical valvotomy have had almost identical results for these methods.[4,5] Therefore in patients with aortic stenosis and zero to mild aortic regurgitation, balloon valvuloplasty is the method of choice. In patients with more significant than mild aortic regurgitation, the Ross procedure or valve replacement is indicated.

History of the procedure

Percutaneous balloon valvuloplasty was first described in 1983.[6] A year later, the effectiveness of the method in gradient reduction and the low incidence of re-stenosis shortly after the procedure was documented in children with congenital aortic stenosis.[7] In 1986, the first balloon valvuloplasty was performed in a newborn with critical aortic stenosis.[8]

Pre-catheter imaging

All the information needed for a valvuloplasty indication is gained by echocardiography. The aortic valve gradient is assessed by continuous wave Doppler from a subcostal, apical, jugular, and right subclavicular approach, and the highest gradient measured is considered. The peak gradient is calculated from maximum flow velocity and the mean gradient using a time–velocity integral. The morphology of the aortic valve is assessed by means of two-dimensional imaging from parasternal long and short axis views. The aortic annulus diameter is measured between the hinge points of the valve leaflets in the two-dimensional parasternal long axis view (Figure 14.3). The annulus must be carefully scanned through by transducer angulation so that the maximum possible diameter is obtained. With such a measurement, almost perfect agreement between the echocardiography and aortography is achieved in the annulus diameter measurements.[1] Aortic insufficiency is assessed by color flow mapping and pulsed Doppler.

Anesthesia

General anesthesia is used to avoid restlessness and agitation that can occur during the valve dilation due to severely impaired cardiac output or coronary pain. In patients in good clinical condition endotracheal intubation is not necessary. Anesthetics are chosen and administered so that adequate spontaneous ventilation is preserved. The most common medications are:

- intravenous ketamin 1%, 2.0 to 2.5 mg/kg, and midazolam 0.2 to 0.3 mg/kg, followed by a continuous infusion of ketamin in a 1 mg/kg per hour dosage
- in children older than 6 years propofol, 1.5 to 2.0 mg/kg, along with a slow injection of sufentanil, 1 to 2 μg/kg, followed by a continuous infusion of propofol in a dose of 100–200 μg/kg per minute.

Local anesthesia of the groin is supplementary to the general anesthesia. Oxygen is administered by mask prior to and during the dilation.

Access

Catheters are usually inserted through the femoral arteries. With a reliable echocardiographic measurement of the aortic annulus (see Pre-catheter imaging, above), a sheath of a diameter appropriate for the intended balloon catheter can be used from the beginning of the procedure. As the widest contemporary balloons can be inserted through 9 to 11 Fr sheaths, the limb perfusion is usually not at risk even in a long lasting procedure. If, however, any concern exists in this respect, a double-balloon technique (see below) should be considered.

Occasionally, it may be impossible to pass the guidewire from the retrograde approach to the left ventricle; in such cases the procedure can be completed from the femoral venous access. First, the foramen ovale patency is explored by a catheter inserted through a short sheath, which is then exchanged for an appropriate long sheath if a transseptal puncture is required.

Protocol of hemodynamic assessment

Pressure gradients

Crossing the stenotic aortic valve is often not easy and once the catheter is in the left ventricle it is not wise to pull it back. Therefore the gradient is usually measured by a simultaneous recording of the pressures in the left ventricle and behind the stenosis. Alternatively, the pull-back gradient measurement can be performed, by a catheter capable of the pressure transmission while wired, such as Multi-Track™ by NuMED, Canada.

The most accurate gradients are obtained by simultaneous or pull-back pressure recording in the left ventricle and in the ascending aorta. The simultaneous measurement can be obtained either by two catheters or by a special multiple-lumen catheter (see Brands available, below). Another option is to measure the distal pressure by a cannula in the femoral artery or by a sheath side port, provided that the diagnostic catheter is at least 1 Fr thinner than the sheath. However, with the use of a peripheral artery, the gradient is artificially reduced by the effect of pulse amplification.[9]

Catheter-measured gradients are usually lower than those measured by Doppler echocardiography. The reasons are numerous:

- Doppler measures instantaneous gradient whereas a catheter measures peak-to-peak gradient. The peak pressure in the aorta is somewhat delayed as compared to the left ventricular pressure[10] (Figure 14.4).
- Doppler tends to overestimate the gradients due to the pressure recovery effect.[11,12]
- If a peripheral artery is used, the gradient is reduced by the pulse amplification effect.
- During the catheterization, cardiac output is somewhat diminished due to the patient's anesthesia or sedation as compared to the echo measurements performed in a completely awake state. With a given valve area, less flow makes for less gradient.

Because of the last point, Doppler gradients are usually used for the valvuloplasty indication whereas a comparison of the catheter measured gradient prior to and after the valvuloplasty serves as an instant measure of its effectiveness.

Aortic valve area

The most accurate indication criterion as well as the most accurate assessment of valvuloplasty success is the calculation of the aortic valve area. The method requires correct simultaneous pressure recordings from the left ventricle and the ascending aorta along with correct measurement of cardiac output. Using the *Gorlin formula*, the

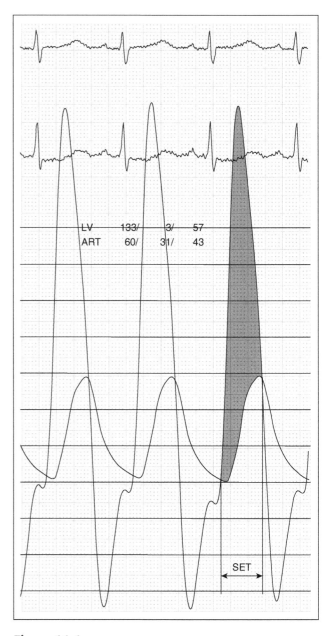

Figure 14.4

Simultaneous recording of pressures in the left ventricle (LV) and in the aorta (ART). The shaded area between the curves and the systolic ejection time (SET) is used for calculation of the aortic valve area.

aortic valve area (A_{AOV}) in cm^2 is calculated from the systemic flow (Q_s) in liters per minute, heart rate (HR) in beats per minute, systolic ejection time (SET) in seconds per heart cycle, and the mean systolic gradient (ΔP) in mmHg:

$$A_{AOV} = \frac{1000 \cdot Q_s}{44.3 \cdot HR \cdot SET \cdot \sqrt{\Delta P}}$$

If the systemic flow is indexed per m² of body surface area, the valve area is obtained in cm²/m². The actual routine is as follows:

1. In several consecutive heart cycles, the area between the left ventricular and aortic pressure curves and the SET is measured (Figure 14.4).
2. For each cycle, the area in mm² is divided by the SET in mm and the result is divided by the recorder excursion in mm per 1 mmHg. This way, the mean systolic pressure gradient in mmHg is obtained. The average mean systolic pressure gradient calculated from all the measured cycles is entered into the formula as the ΔP.
3. SET is converted from mm to seconds by dividing it by the recorder speed in mm/second and the average SET from all the measured cycles is entered into the formula.

Angiography

The biplane aortography with contrast media injection into the aortic root is performed to measure the valve annulus, assess the position of the aortic valve orifice, and exclude or document aortic valve incompetence. The aortic annulus diameter is measured between the leaflets' hinge points in the frontal projection. The aortography is also used to choose a balloon of the proper length (Figure 14.5).

Balloon

An ideal balloon catheter should have a low profile and fast inflation and deflation times. There is no need for high pressure balloons, but they should be non-compliant. Whereas in infants slim catheter shafts and introducers are necessary, in older patients thicker shafts capable of accommodating thicker guidewires are preferable as they can better support the balloon position during the left ventricular contraction. For proper balloon selection it is essential to have a wide spectrum of balloon sizes with the smallest possible balloon diameter increments instantly available.

Balloon diameter

The optimum valvuloplasty result would be maximum gradient relief with minimum valve incompetence caused. Such a result, however, is seldom attained and a reasonable goal should be to decrease the gradient below the indication level and at the same time to keep the valve incompetence to a minimum. Therefore a defensive balloon policy is employed:

* The balloon diameter should not exceed the diameter of the aortic annulus.[13,14]

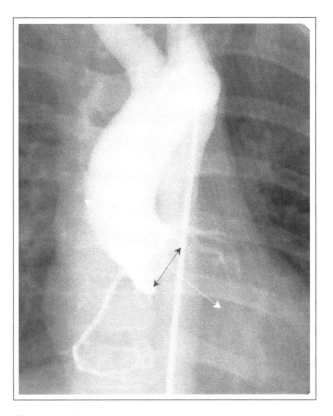

Figure 14.5
Aortography in the frontal projection. The aortic annulus diameter is measured between the leaflets' hinge points (black arrow) and the proper balloon length is assessed according to the measurement in the long axis of the left ventricular outflow tract and ascending aorta (white arrow).

* It is wise to start with a balloon diameter of about 90% of the aortic annulus and eventually increase its size by 1 mm if the gradient is not reduced sufficiently and the aortic valve remains competent.

Double-balloon technique

The aortic valve dilation can be performed by a simultaneous inflation of two balloons introduced into the valve from both the femoral arteries (Figure 14.6). The advantages of this double-balloon technique are as follows:

* In comparison to one big balloon, two smaller balloons usually require smaller introducers and accordingly the risk of a femoral artery injury is decreased.
* The two balloons' apposition is never complete and blood can vent between them; this reduces the forces expelling the balloons out of the valve during the left ventricular systole and avoids a severe aortic pressure drop during the dilation.[15]
* It is believed that, in bicuspid valves, the two balloons better comply with the valve anatomy and therefore are

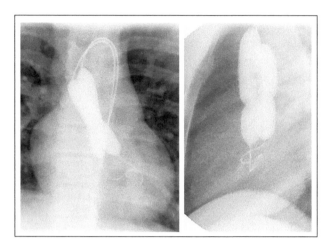

Figure 14.6
Double-balloon technique in frontal and lateral projections. The aortic valve dilation is performed by a simultaneous inflation of two balloons introduced into the valve from both the femoral arteries.

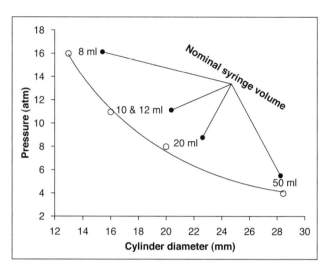

Figure 14.7
Maximum pressure attainable using different syringes.

less likely to cause a cusp disruption than a single balloon.[16]

- The double arterial access enables the most accurate measurement of the gradient and the valve area by a simultaneous pressure recording in the left ventricle and the ascending aorta (see Protocol of hemodynamic assessment, above).

A disadvantage of the double-balloon technique is the need for two guidewires to be passed through the aortic valve into the left ventricle, which may prolong the procedure. The *effective diameter* (D_{eff}) of a combination of two balloons with diameters D_1 and D_2 may be calculated from the following equation[17] (arccos is arcus cosinus):

Balloon burst pressures

Rated burst pressures of valvuloplasty balloons range from 5 to 8 atmospheres (atm) in the smallest diameters to 1.5 to 3 atm in the largest ones. The specified rated burst pressures should never be reached. The use of manometer equipped inflation syringes for valvuloplasty is impractical. Rather than watching the manometer dial, the operator should carefully observe the balloon position and the waist caused by the stenotic valve. Once the waist disappears, the inflating pressure should be released immediately. As a safety measure, syringes with different cylinder diameters (nominal volumes) can be used to reach different inflation pressures (Figure 14.7).

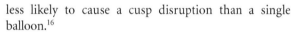

$$D_{eff} = \frac{D_1 \times \left(\pi - \arccos\left(\frac{D_1 - D_2}{D_1 + D_2} \right) \right) + D_2 \times \arccos\left(\frac{D_1 - D_2}{D_1 + D_2} \right) + 4 \times \sqrt{\frac{D_1 \times D_2}{4}}}{\pi}$$

or roughly but simply:

$$D_{eff} = \frac{D_1 + D_2}{1.22}$$

Balloon length

A balloon of the optimum length should safely straddle the aortic valve without overlapping the mitral valve chordae. The optimum ratio of the balloon length to the balloon diameter is ≥ 3 and it should never be < 2.

Brands available

Tyshak® and Tyshak II® (NuMED, Inc) are a good choice. They provide a wide range of balloon diameters from 4 to 30 mm with 1 mm increments up to 25 mm, with the exception of 21 and 24 mm which are not available. For

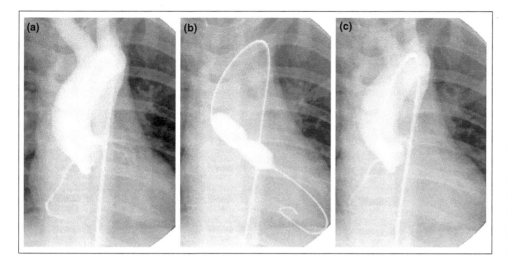

Figure 14.8
Aortic valvuloplasty from a retrograde approach. (a) On the aortogram prior to the procedure, doming of the aortic valve and the severely narrowed effective orifice is depicted by non-contrast blood; (b) waist on the balloon caused by the stenotic valve; (c) the effective orifice has been significantly enlarged by the valvuloplasty.

each diameter a sufficient range of balloon lengths is provided. The Tyshak® catheters as compared to the Tyshak II® catheters come with bigger shaft sizes capable of accommodating thicker guidewires, and they have slightly higher rated burst pressures. With the combination of thicker shaft and thicker wire, Tyshak® can better resist the left ventricular ejection power and therefore it is preferred in older children. On the other hand, Tyshak II® is preferable in infants in whom the lowest possible introducer profile is of paramount importance.

VACS II by Osypka, Germany is another low-profile balloon available in diameters 4 to 30 mm with 1 mm increments up to 18 mm, with the exception of 11 and 13 mm which are not available. Above the 18 mm diameter, the increments are 2 mm. Two to four different lengths are available per diameter, except for the 4, 5, and 6 mm diameters that come with the single length of 20 mm.

Another option is valvuloplasty balloons by Balt, available in balloon diameters from 8 to 40 mm with diameter increments of 2 to 3 mm up to 25 mm and 5 mm increments above that. Except for balloon diameters of 12 and 15 mm that come with two different balloon lengths, there is only a single balloon length per diameter. In comparison to Tyshak® and VACS II balloons, larger introducers are required and the thicker shafts along with the thicker wires used account for the higher overall system stiffness that may be an advantage in older patients.

Several catheters suitable for aortic valvuloplasty are produced by Boston Scientific (Cribier/Letac™, Pediatric, and Tripoly-AT™). They all are constructed with a double or triple lumen and with standard or pigtail tips. The triple lumen construction allows for simultaneous left ventricular and aortic pressure measurement and subsequent valvuloplasty without the need for catheter replacement. A drawback of the triple lumen construction is its big shaft size. The available balloon diameters range from 6 to 23 mm

with 2 to 3 mm increments. There is a single balloon length in all the diameters with the exception of the 8 and 10 mm diameters, for which two lengths are available.

Valvuloplasty

Heparin in a dose of 100 IU per kg of body weight is administered immediately after vascular access is established. Hemodynamic measurements and aortography are performed. A systolic frame of the aortography in which the position of the effective orifice is documented by a jet of non-contrast blood is used as a road map (Figure 14.8a). Angulated catheters such as the Cobra, right coronary, or left coronary bypass catheters or a pigtail catheter are used to guide a hydrophilic polymer coated wire (such as Radiofocus® by Terumo) through the valve orifice. The angle of attack is adjusted by two different kinds of movement: in the frontal plane by pushing or pulling the catheter and in the sagittal plane by catheter rotation. The wire is guided into the orifice by repeated gentle, yet sufficiently rapid stabs until it slides into the left ventricle. If the angle of attack is considered appropriate and the wire cannot cross the valve, a straight tip wire may be replaced for an angled tip one, and vice versa. If, however, the ideal angle of attack cannot be attained, the catheter is exchanged for one with a different angulation. In an extreme situation, the tip of a pigtail catheter may gradually be cut off to provide fine angle changes. Once the valve is crossed by the wire, the catheter is advanced to the left ventricle and the pressure gradient is measured. A J-shaped exchange wire is then inserted into the left ventricular apex and an appropriate balloon catheter is advanced over the wire. The exchange wire should aim to the apex rather than to the inflow portion of the left ventricle so that the mitral valve is not exposed to risk by the balloon inflation. In rare cases, it may

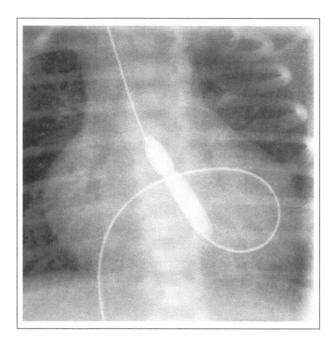

Figure 14.9
Prograde aortic valvuloplasty in an infant.

be impossible to pass the guidewire from the retrograde approach to the left ventricle. In such patients the procedure can usually be performed from a prograde approach using patent foramen ovale or a transseptal puncture (Figure 14.9). This way the catheter is introduced into the left ventricular inflow, and a J-shaped hydrophilic polymer coated guidewire is turned upward in the left ventricular apex into the aortic valve and advanced to the descending aorta. The catheter is then pushed over the wire to the descending aorta, the wire is exchanged, and an appropriate balloon catheter is advanced into the valve. During the dilation, care is taken to protect the anterior mitral leaflet and its chordae by keeping the loop in the left ventricle wide open and extended as far as possible into the apex.

To prevent air embolism due to a balloon rupture, the balloon is gently flushed with CO_2 before the insertion. It may be further degassed after the insertion by fluoroscopically controlled flushes with diluted contrast medium in the thoracic descending aorta. Using the balloon radiopaque markers and the road map, the balloon is then positioned to straddle the aortic valve and gradually inflated. Before the full inflation is reached, tiny position adjustments can be made if necessary. Once the waist caused by the stenotic valve (Figure 14.8b) has been abolished, the balloon is quickly deflated. During inflation, the balloon in the valve should remain as steady as possible. Displacement of the balloon prior to its full inflation prevents the effective valve dilation and to-and-fro movement of the inflated balloon may cause injury to the valve leaflets or surrounding tissues. There are four measures to minimize or prevent balloon movement during the dilation:

- *Rigid shaft–wire combination.* This can be achieved by using thicker shafts along with thicker wires (see Brands available, above) or by the usage of stiff exchange guidewires, such as Amplatz Extra Stiff by Cook. The diameters of these wires start at 0.025 inch, which is thin enough to be used even with the low profile balloon catheters (in Tyshak® from 4 mm balloons and in Tyshak II® and VACS II from 9 mm balloons).
- *Double-balloon technique.* During a simultaneous inflation of two balloons, the aortic orifice is never fully obstructed and thus presumably the forces responsible for the balloon displacement are weaker in comparison to the single-balloon technique.
- *Adenosine induced transient ventricular asystole.*[18] A 0.3 mg/kg dose of adenosine is introduced into an intravenous line and rapidly flushed. The cannula and the vein used should be wide enough to withstand the rapid injection. The femoral vein or the external jugular vein is a good choice. The subsequent asystole usually lasts for 5 to 10 seconds, a sufficient time to perform the dilation safely.
- *Rapid right ventricular pacing.*[19] A bipolar pacing catheter is introduced into the right ventricular apex. VVI pacing at a rate of 220 to 240 impulses per minute is started immediately before the balloon inflation and stopped immediately after its deflation. A standby defibrillator ready to terminate eventual sustained ventricular tachycardia or fibrillation must be within reach.

The adenosine administration and the rapid ventricular pacing are almost 100% effective in the prevention of balloon movement and one of the protocols should be used primarily or at least considered for a subsequent attempt whenever it is impossible to hold the balloon steady in the proper position. With the stable balloon position and the full obliteration of the balloon waist, a single balloon inflation will usually suffice to reduce the gradient provided that the balloon diameter was chosen properly.

Post-procedure protocol

After the valvuloplasty, the balloon catheter is replaced over the wire by a diagnostic catheter, the wire is removed, and the gradient is measured. If it is intended to calculate the aortic valve area after the dilation, the cardiac output must be measured again at this point. The aortography is then repeated to assess the widening of the effective orifice by a change in the jet diameter (Figure 14.8c) and to evaluate aortic insufficiency. A complete echocardiographic evaluation is performed on the following day.

Pitfalls, problems

Occasionally left anterior hemi-block or even a complete left bundle branch block is produced by compression of the conductive tissue caused by the balloon. The condition is always self-limiting and requires no treatment. Severe damage to the valve leaflets, myocardium, and the aortic wall can be prevented by avoiding oversized balloons and by keeping the inflated balloon stable in the aortic valve. A vessel injury may result from balloon rupture. Therefore, care is taken to operate always under the balloon rated burst pressure (see Balloon burst pressures, above). The mitral valve may be injured by the balloon inflation if the exchange wire is accidentally threaded through the anterior leaflet chordae. Therefore, a safe position of the wire tip in the ventricular apex and the wire course anterior to the mitral valve apparatus in the lateral view must be confirmed before each inflation. Proper access and hemostasis techniques along with the usage of low-profile balloons help to prevent vascular damage.

Post-catheter management

In children and young adults the sheaths are usually withdrawn in the catheterization lab at the end of the procedure. Before the removal, the activated clotting time should be shorter than 200 seconds. Thus in very short procedures, circulating heparin must be at least partially neutralized by protamine sulfate. Hemostasis is achieved by manual compression of the catheter entry site. A pulse oximeter is attached to a toe of the limb involved to measure the peripheral pulsation. The compression force should be balanced so that the distal pulses are still measurable while bleeding and hematoma formation are safely controlled. Only rarely, with the use of the widest sheaths, a vascular hemostatic device such as the Angio-Seal® (Quinton), VasoSeal™ (Datascope), or Duett™ (Vascular Solutions) is required to seal the artery. After hemostasis is achieved, the patient is transferred to an intensive care unit for further monitoring and is subsequently discharged 24 hours after the procedure if no complications have occurred.

Results

Good short term results have been demonstrated on a large cohort of children in a multi-centric study.[20] Mid-term results, however, have shown a substantial incidence of re-stenosis, severe aortic insufficiency, and re-interventions.[21,22] In our 189 patients treated with valvuloplasty at the age of 5 weeks to 23 years, with a median follow-up period of 7.5 years, the re-stenosis rate was 15% and severe aortic insufficiency developed in 20%. Similar rates have been observed by others.[23] While the re-stenosis may be successfully treated by a repeated valvuloplasty in the majority of cases,[24] aortic regurgitation is progressive in the long term perspective[1,25] and many patients require surgery during their childhood and early adulthood. The actuarial probability of survival 14 years after the valvuloplasty is 0.93 in infants and 0.98 in older patients, but the probability of surgery-free survival is only 0.52 in infants and 0.65 in older patients. The functionally bicuspid aortic valve has been documented to be an independent predictor of severe post-valvuloplasty aortic insufficiency and the need for surgery.[1]

References

1. Reich O, Tax P, Marek J et al. Long term results of percutaneous balloon valvoplasty of congenital aortic stenosis: independent predictors of outcome. Heart 2004; 90: 70–6.
2. Solymar L, Sudow G, Berggren H, Eriksson B. Balloon dilation of stenotic aortic valve in children. An intraoperative study. J Thorac Cardiovasc Surg 1992; 104: 1709–13.
3. Campbell M. The natural history of congenital aortic stenosis. Br Heart J 1968; 30: 514–26.
4. Gatzoulis MA, Rigby ML, Shinebourne EA, Redington AN. Contemporary results of balloon valvuloplasty and surgical valvotomy for congenital aortic stenosis. Arch Dis Child 1995; 73: 66–9.
5. Justo RN, McCrindle BW, Benson LN et al. Aortic valve regurgitation after surgical versus percutaneous balloon valvotomy for congenital aortic valve stenosis. Am J Cardiol 1996; 77: 1332–8.
6. Lababidi Z. Aortic balloon valvuloplasty. Am Heart J 1983; 106: 751–2.
7. Lababidi Z, Wu JR, Walls JT. Percutaneous balloon aortic valvuloplasty: results in 23 patients. Am J Cardiol 1984; 53: 194–7.
8. Lababidi Z, Weinhaus L. Successful balloon valvuloplasty for neonatal critical aortic stenosis. Am Heart J 1986; 112: 913–6.
9. Marshal HW. Physiologic consequences of congenital heart disease. In: Hamilton WF, Dow P, eds. Handbook of Physiology: Section 2. Circulation. Washington DC: American Physiologic Society 2005: 417.
10. Beekman RH, Rocchini AP, Gillon JH, Mancini GB. Hemodynamic determinants of the peak systolic left ventricular–aortic pressure gradient in children with valvar aortic stenosis. Am J Cardiol 1992; 69: 813–15.
11. Cape EG, Jones M, Yamada I et al. Turbulent/viscous interactions control Doppler/catheter pressure discrepancies in aortic stenosis. The role of the Reynolds number. Circulation 1996; 94: 2975–81.
12. Gjertsson P, Caidahl K, Svensson G et al. Important pressure recovery in patients with aortic stenosis and high Doppler gradients. Am J Cardiol 2001; 88: 139–44.
13. Helgason H, Keane JF, Fellows KE et al. Balloon dilation of the aortic valve: studies in normal lambs and in children with aortic stenosis. J Am Coll Cardiol 1987; 9: 816–22.
14. Phillips RR, Gerlis LM, Wilson N, Walker DR. Aortic valve damage caused by operative balloon dilatation of critical aortic valve stenosis. Br Heart J 1987; 57: 168–70.
15. Mullins CE, Nihill MR, Vick GW et al. Double balloon technique for dilation of valvular or vessel stenosis in congenital and acquired heart disease. J Am Coll Cardiol 1987; 10: 107–14.
16. Beekman RH, Rocchini AP, Crowley DC et al. Comparison of single and double balloon valvuloplasty in children with aortic stenosis. J Am Coll Cardiol 1988; 12: 480–5.
17. Yeager SB. Balloon selection for double balloon valvotomy. J Am Coll Cardiol 1987; 9: 467–8.

18. De Giovanni JV, Edgar RA, Cranston A. Adenosine induced transient cardiac standstill in catheter interventional procedures for congenital heart disease. Heart 1998; 80: 330–3.

19. Daehnert I, Rotzsch C, Wiener M, Schneider P. Rapid right ventricular pacing is an alternative to adenosine in catheter interventional procedures for congenital heart disease. Heart 2004; 90: 1047–50.

20. Rocchini AP, Beekman RH, Ben Shachar G et al. Balloon aortic valvuloplasty: results of the Valvuloplasty and Angioplasty of Congenital Anomalies Registry. Am J Cardiol 1990; 65: 784–9.

21. Moore P, Egito E, Mowrey H et al. Midterm results of balloon dilation of congenital aortic stenosis: predictors of success. J Am Coll Cardiol 1996; 27: 1257–63.

22. Galal O, Rao PS, Al Fadley F, Wilson AD. Follow-up results of balloon aortic valvuloplasty in children with special reference to causes of late aortic insufficiency. Am Heart J 1997; 133: 418–27.

23. Jindal RC, Saxena A, Juneja R et al. Long-term results of balloon aortic valvulotomy for congenital aortic stenosis in children and adolescents. J Heart Valve Dis 2000; 9 : 623–8.

24. Shim D, Lloyd TR, Beekman RH. Usefulness of repeat balloon aortic valvuloplasty in children. Am J Cardiol 1997; 79: 1141–3.

25. Balmer C, Beghetti M, Fasnacht M et al. Balloon aortic valvoplasty in paediatric patients: progressive aortic regurgitation is common. Heart 2004; 90: 77–81.

15

Aortic valve stenosis in neonates

Alejandro J Torres and William Hellenbrand

Introduction

Aortic valve stenosis (AS) occurs in 3–6% of patients with congenital heart disease.[1] The aortic valve may be of adequate size for the body surface area but morphologically stenotic and dysplastic, anatomically small and dysplastic, or morphologically normal but small. The anatomic types of aortic valvular stenosis include unicuspid, bicuspid, tricuspid, quadricuspid, and undifferentiated aortic valves. The most common malformation of the aortic valve seen in patients with AS is the bicuspid valve. In these patients, thickening and partial fusion of the leaflets can cause clinically severe valve stenosis, even in infancy. Unicuspid aortic valve is present when there is fusion of all three leaflets of the valve. Most newborns with severe or critical AS requiring intervention in the first month of life have either a unicuspid or a severely stenotic bicuspid aortic valve. The unicommissural valves have either no true commissure and a tiny central opening or a small eccentric slit-like opening extending to the annulus. Males are affected three to five times as often as females. In the neonate, critical AS is a complex disorder, frequently associated with varying degrees of left ventricular and annular hypoplasia, mitral valve anomalies, endomyocardial fibroelastosis, and myocardial ischemia. Other cardiovascular anomalies such as aortic coarctation, patent ductus arteriosus, and ventricular septal defect occur in 20% of the patients and should be evaluated before an invasive procedure is undertaken. Numerous studies have attempted to demonstrate a correlation between left-sided heart structure sizes or hemodynamic relations and survival of biventricular versus single ventricle repair in critical AS.[2–7] Neonates with critical AS suffer from low cardiac output and shock secondary to poor left ventricular function and/or mitral insufficiency. Outcome is usually fatal in most of these patients within the first weeks of life with medical treatment alone. Intervention in the first days of life is therefore required in these patients. Open or closed surgical valvotomy was the only technique available until the mid-1980s. The use of percutaneous balloon aortic valvuloplasty was first introduced in 1984 and has become the first-line treatment for critical aortic valve stenosis in neonates.[6,8–12]

Precatheterization assessment and management

Newborns with critical AS present with some degree of heart failure and not infrequently in cardiogenic shock. When the diagnosis is made prenatally, arrangements should be made so the baby is born in a surgical center in order to avoid treatment delays due to the transfer. These newborns should be mechanically ventilated and sedated soon after birth to decrease the oxygen demands. Patients who present in shock should be hemodynamically stabilized as much as possible, but intervention should not be postponed for this reason. Acid–base status, blood count, coagulation times, and electrolytes should be evaluated and corrected if necessary.[13] Prostaglandin (PGE1) is started to augment cardiac output in the setting of a failing and obstructed left ventricle. We recommend inserting both venous and arterial umbilical catheters since these catheters can later be used as vascular access during the catheterization. Inotropic support is commonly initiated to increase cardiac output. Agents with the least chronotropic effect, such as dopamine or dobutamine, are the most commonly used. Their effect on the heart rate should be carefully monitored because a decrease in the filling time of the left ventricle can further compromise cardiac output. Transthoracic echocardiography is the imaging method of choice to establish the morphology and function of the aortic valve, assess left ventricular function, and rule out other congenital cardiac anomalies in newborns. The number and morphology of the aortic valve cusps are best determined from the parasternal short-axis view at the base of the heart. The movement of the aortic valve leaflets should be carefully examined in a slow-motion playback mode to determine the number of valve cusps. In many cases, the leaflets are immobile and a systolic opening cannot be visualized. Although defining the details of the aortic valve anatomy is important, it does not modify the management plan for these patients. The annulus and proximal ascending aorta are better visualized from the parasternal long-axis view. The annulus is usually 5 to 8 mm in diameter and post-stenotic dilatation of the ascending aorta is commonly seen. Several studies have shown a correlation between various left-sided heart structure sizes or hemodynamic relations and survival of biventricular repair in critical AS. A multi-variate equation and a risk factor analysis to predict suitability of biventricular repair in critical AS have been described by Rhodes et al.[6] In this study, outcome was estimated by scoring the presence of three components measured by echocardiography: indexed aortic root diameter (3.5 cm/m^2 or less), indexed mitral valve area (4.74 cm^2/m^2 or less), and a left ventricular long axis to heart long axis ratio of 0.8 or less. Different studies have described other predictors of biventricular suitability in critical AS.[3,4,12] Medical centers taking care of these patients should develop and become familiar with their own decision algorithms.

Quantitative assessment of flow velocities to determine the severity of the aortic valve stenosis using Doppler recordings is best obtained from the apical, suprasternal, and high right parasternal views. Limitations associated with this technique are the following:

- The correlation between the peak instantaneous pressure gradient measured with Doppler and the peak-to-peak measured at cardiac catheterization is not nearly as close as it is in pulmonary valve stenosis.
- This measurement is flow-dependent.

Thus, in patients with poor left ventricular systolic function and low cardiac output, a low transvalvular peak velocity may be obtained, even in the presence of severe stenosis. These patients should be distinguished from those with primary cardiomyopathy and severe left ventricular dysfunction in whom the normal aortic valve motion is limited in systole. In these cases, the transvalvular peak velocity is low but the aortic valve has a normal appearance, and there is no post-stenotic dilatation of the ascending aorta. In conclusion, a low pressure gradient measured with Doppler is of less significance in newborns with AS than in older children and can mislead the diagnosis if other echocardiographic and clinical findings are not considered. There should be no delay between the diagnosis and therapeutic decision processes, since patients with critical aortic valve stenosis invariably worsen rapidly if no intervention is performed.

Catheterization

Aortic valve dilatation in the neonate is associated with a higher rate of complications than in older children and adults. In the catheterization laboratory, attention to detail

is of great importance since these infants are particularly labile to minimal changes in acid–base status. Warming lights, heating blankets, or other devices to avoid excessive thermal stress are important. Complete sedation and paralysis are preferable to decrease the cardiac output demands and facilitate the procedure. Mechanical cardiac support with extracorporeal membrane oxygenation (ECMO) should be considered prior to the procedure in patients who present with unmanageable cardiogenic shock to achieve adequate systemic perfusion and oxygenation and reduce myocardial ischemia. Newborns with critical AS and poor left ventricular systolic function are at high risk of developing cardiac arrest or life threatening arrhythmias when catheters or wires are manipulated within the left ventricle. Resuscitation equipment and intravenous drugs, including an external defibrillator, cross-matched blood, and inotropic and antiarrhythmic agents, should be available in the catheterization laboratory.[13]

Technique

The crossing of the aortic valve with a wire can be achieved either from the aorta (retrograde approach) or from the left ventricle (antegrade approach). Each of these approaches has its limitations and disadvantages.

Retrograde approach

Catheters can be advanced into the ascending aorta using the femoral artery, umbilical artery,[11,13–15] or the surgically exposed right common carotid artery[16–18] or right subscapular artery.[19] The umbilical artery is preferable when available. A 0.018–0.021 inch J-Rosen guidewire is advanced into the aorta through either a 3 Fr or 5 Fr umbilical catheter, which is then exchanged for a 4 Fr pigtail. It is important to remember that both umbilical arteries travel from the umbilicus toward the groin and catheters should be advanced in that direction when introduced and not upward, as with the umbilical vein. If the femoral artery is used instead, the procedure can be performed with a 3 Fr sheath and a 3 Fr thin-walled pigtail. The pigtail catheter is placed in the ascending aorta and a 5 Fr Berman angiographic catheter is advanced from the inferior vena cava through the patent foramen ovale into the left ventricle. The gradient across the aortic valve can be measured by simultaneous recording of the aortic and left ventricular pressure.

In hemodynamically unstable patients we do not perform an aortic angiogram and the aortic annulus diameter measured by echocardiography is used to choose the balloon diameter. In the presence of hypotension and poor LV function in an ischemic myocardium, even a small amount of contrast in the ascending aorta can trigger ventricular arrythmias and cardiac arrest. In more stable patients, an

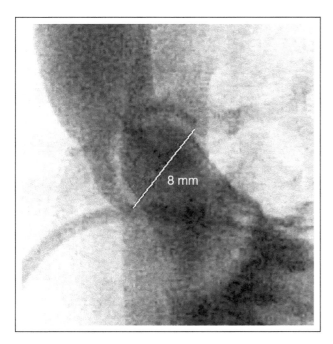

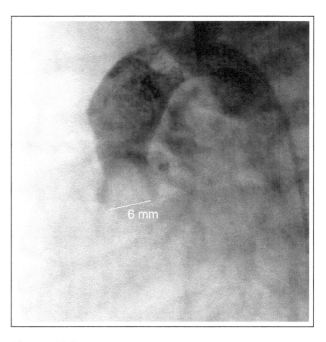

Figure 15.1
Measurement of the aortic annulus on the posterior-anterior projection. Left ventricular angiogram. An angiographic catheter was advanced from the venous side across a patent foramen ovale into the left ventricle.

Figure 15.2
Measurement of the aortic annulus on the lateral projection. Ascending aorta angiogram.

aortography is performed using the pigtail or a side hole catheter placed just above the aortic sinuses.

The straight posterior-anterior (PA) and lateral projections are usually adequate to profile the aortic valve annulus. The PA camera can be placed with a shallow left anterior oblique angulation to take the aortic valve off the spine and profile the aortic annulus. Post-stenotic dilatation of the ascending aorta is frequently noted and its absence would suggest subaortic stenosis. The stenotic aortic valve domes during systole and a jet of unopacified blood can be seen passing through the narrowed valve orifice. It is helpful to remember the orientation of the jet in both projections when attempting to cross the valve with a wire. The hinge points of the aortic valve are usually easy to identify. The diameter of the aortic annulus diameter is measured between the opposite hinge points on the projection where it is profiled the best (Figures 15.1 and 15.2). There is a fair correlation between the annulus angiographic diameter and the one measured by echocardiography on the long-axis parasternal view. We do not routinely perform a left ventricular angiogram unless it is necessary to assess the size of the ventricle or identify associated anomalies.

The pigtail catheter is then replaced with a 3 or 4 Fr JR1 or JR2 catheter, although the pigtail can also be used as a directional catheter. A soft straight or angled tipped 0.018 inch or 0.021 inch guidewire (torque control or glide wire) is used to cross the valve. It is useful to have reference images of the aortic angiogram in order to visualize the direction of the jet and the ostia of both coronary arteries. The commissure between the left and the non-coronary cusps is the most common area of opening of the valve and the guidewire–catheter system should be pointed in that direction, which is usually towards the left and posterior aspect of the aortic root. The guidewire is gently advanced and pulled into the catheter to avoid perforation of the valve or damage to the coronary arteries. Before advancing the catheter the position of the guidewire should be confirmed. A guidewire in the left coronary artery might occasionally be seen as being into the left ventricle, particularly on the postero-anterior projection. The guidewire position should then be compared with the two views of the left coronary artery in the aortic angiogram before advancing the catheter. Following crossing of the valve, the balloon dilatation catheter can be advanced over the same guidewire used to cross the valve if the internal diameter of the balloon catheter is the same size as the wire, and the wire is in a good position within the ventricle and has a stiff segment at the valve level. Otherwise, the guide-catheter can be advanced into the ventricle and the wire exchanged for a J-tipped wire with a diameter sized to the balloon catheter. The intraventricular pressure can be measured at this time if not done previously. A wide loop should be hand made on the J-tipped wire before advancing it into the ventricle to provide a better wire position (Figure 15.3). The wire is positioned in the left ventricular apex anterior to the mitral valve. A posterior position of the wire should be avoided

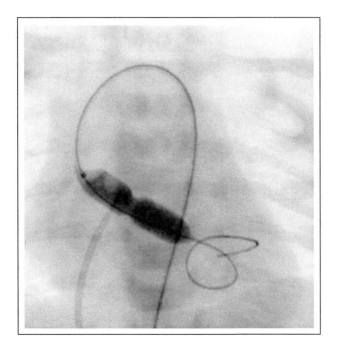

Figure 15.3
A wire is advanced from the ascending aorta into the left ventricle. During aortic balloon valvuloplasty a 'waist' is seen at the level of the aortic valve.

since it may result in mitral valve injury during balloon inflation if the wire is trapped in the mitral valve. Since the wire position can be somewhat unstable in a small ventricle, care should be taken not to accidentally pull the wire when the balloon is advanced in the aorta. If crossing of the valve has been unsuccessful within 20–30 minutes, the antegrade approach is considered.

This population has a higher risk of developing ventricular arrhythmias secondary to poor ventricular function, elevated intraventricular pressure, and myocardial ischemia. If severe ventricular tachycardia or fibrillation develops when the valve is crossed with the guidewire, it should not be pulled out of the ventricle, since the chances of performing a successful resuscitation in a patient in this hemodynamic situation are minimal. Instead, as resuscitation is initiated, the balloon should be quickly advanced and the valve should be balloon dilated. This will immediately decrease the intraventricular pressure and improve the myocardial ischemia.

A balloon with a diameter that is approximately 80–90% of the annulus is chosen. We use the Tyshak Mini and the Tyshak II (NuMED, Hopkinton, NY) for the 3 Fr and 4 Fr systems, respectively. The use of balloons with diameters of 100–110% of the valve annulus size has been associated with a higher incidence of significant valve insufficiency after balloon dilatation.[10–13,20] Balloon catheters of length 2 cm should be used to decrease the risk of mitral valve injury. If the wire is caught in the mitral valve apparatus, a

longer balloon may be inadvertently inflated within the mitral valve chordae.

The balloon is first placed in the descending aorta where it is carefully purged to remove all air from it. We usually purge the balloon using a stopcock device with one port attached to the balloon and the other two attached to two syringes, one with one-third contrast and two-thirds normal saline solution, and the other one empty. Then, on the stopcock, we open the balloon towards the empty syringe and, while aspirating, we switch the stopcock to open the contrast syringe towards the balloon. The balloon is then inflated under fluoroscopy; if air is noticed the procedure is repeated until no air remains in the system. This is usually achieved after two or three attempts. The balloon is then advanced until it straddles the aortic valve. Balloon inflation by hand is performed for a few seconds until the balloon is fully inflated or the waist in the balloon disappears. However, because a 'waist' (Figure 15.3) is not always seen during aortic balloon valvuloplasty in neonates and the balloon can move from the valve during inflation in patients with good cardiac output two inflations are performed to ensure that the balloon is properly positioned. Inflation–deflation cycles should last no more than 5–7 seconds (Figure 15.4). Since small increases in balloon diameter can be achieved by increasing pressure, inflation should be gentle to avoid rupture or a larger effective diameter, which may result in increased aortic insufficiency. The balloon is removed and hemodynamic measurements are repeated in a similar fashion to pre-dilation. When the procedure is performed with a 4 Fr system, another approach is to use a multi-track catheter that uses the wire as a monorail to allow pressure monitoring and pull-back gradient measurement without moving the wire. If the ductus arteriosus is not patent, a wide aortic differential pressure suggests significant residual aortic insufficiency. In order to avoid injury of the aortic or mitral valve, the wire is carefully pulled out with the catheter in the ventricle. In hemodynamically stable patients, an ascending aorta angiogram is repeated to assess aortic valve competence with the catheter positioned above the valve to avoid catheter induced valve insufficiency. Otherwise, residual aortic insufficiency is assessed only by echocardiography. Provided that there is no or trivial aortic valve regurgitation, a successful result has been achieved if the residual peak gradient has been reduced by more than 50% from the initial measurement. Other indirect signs of success are a fall in the left ventricular end diastolic pressure and an increase in oxygen saturation in the lower extremities in patients with an open ductus arteriosus. When a significant residual gradient is present and there is no significant residual aortic insufficiency, valvuloplasty can be repeated with the next larger balloon size, following the same sequence.

The right carotid artery approach to perform balloon aortic valvuloplasty was first described in 1990 and its use has been advocated by different centers.[17,18,21] The procedure is performed in the catheterization laboratory with the aid

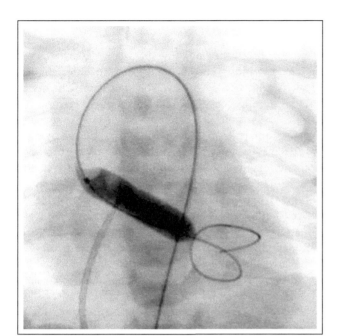

Figure 15.4
As in Figure 15.3. Fully expanded balloon during aortic valve valvuloplasty.

of a surgeon who exposes the right carotid artery. Access into the vessel is achieved by arteriotomy or with a 21 gauge needle. A 0.021 inch wire is introduced into the vessel and a 4 or 5 Fr pediatric sheath is advanced over the wire into the ascending aorta. The use of a sheath with a smaller catheter allows simultaneous pressure measurement of the aorta and the left ventricle. Full heparinization (100 U/kg) is usually administered. Pressure recording and an aortic angiogram are performed through the sheath. A catheter (e.g. multipurpose) is then advanced into the ascending aorta and a floppy-tipped 0.018 inch wire is used to cross the valve. Alternatively, the balloon catheter can be used as a guide catheter.[22,23] An advantage of carotid access is the direct angle of approach to the aortic valve, which makes crossing of the valve relatively easy. This procedure has been performed at the bedside using only transesophageal echocardiography for guidance.[24] The same floppy-tipped guidewire can be used to advance the catheter balloon or it can be exchanged for a stiffer Rosen with a tip hand-made loop. The position of the wire with respect to the mitral valve should be assessed before balloon dilatation. The balloon is then positioned across the valve and inflated for a few seconds. Evaluation of residual aortic valve gradient or insufficiency is performed as described with the other approaches. At the conclusion of the procedure, the sheath is removed and the carotid artery is primarily repaired. The risk of neurologic events during the procedure is low. Right carotid artery patency is well preserved after neonatal surgical cutdown. Patients with mild residual stenosis at the

site of the incision remain asymptomatic on mid-term follow-up.[21]

Antegrade approach

The aortic valve is crossed from the left ventricle after the left atrium has been entered via a patent foramen ovale. The main advantage of this approach is to reduce the risk of femoral arterial injury. Some authors have suggested that this approach also reduces the incidence of aortic insufficiency because the crossing of the aortic valve with a floppy-tipped guidewire from the left ventricle may decrease the risk of valve leaflet perforation. Disadvantages of this approach include the necessity of an atrial communication, the potential risk of mitral valve injury, and the risk of arrhythmias due to catheter manipulation within a compromised left ventricle.

A 5 Fr sheath is placed in a femoral vein or a 0.021 inch J-guidewire is advanced through the umbilical vein catheter into the right atrium and then the umbilical catheter is exchanged for a 5 Fr pediatric sheath. A small 3 Fr catheter can be placed in the femoral artery for monitoring of the blood pressure. This is not necessary if an umbilical artery catheter is in place. In patients in whom an ascending aortogram has not been performed, a 4 or 5 Fr Berman angiographic catheter is advanced into the left atrium through the patent foramen ovale. In patients with an intact atrial septum, transseptal puncture should be considered. The balloon is carefully inflated in the left atrium and advanced into the left ventricle. Care should be taken to avoid balloon inflation in the left atrial appendage or a pulmonary vein. Manipulation of the inflated balloon within a small left atrium to cross the mitral valve may be difficult. In order to point the tip of the catheter towards the mitral valve, we use the back (stiff end) of a 0.021 inch J-wire with a pre-shaped tight curve or a tip deflection wire. After measuring the left ventricular pressure, a low volume, low velocity angiogram is performed to assess the diameter of the aortic valve annulus. The Berman angiographic catheter is removed and a 4 or 5 Fr end hole catheter, preferably a balloon wedge catheter to avoid crossing the mitral valve through the chordae or the papillary muscle apparatus, is advanced in the left ventricular apex. Using again the curved back of the 0.021 inch J-wire or a tip-deflecting guidewire, the tip of the catheter is aimed towards the left ventricular outflow tract and advanced until it is positioned underneath the aortic valve. In patients in whom the catheter cannot be looped because of the small size of the left ventricle, a pigtail can be used to direct the guidewire. A soft-tipped wire (0.018 inch glide or torque wire) is used to cross the valve and advanced into the descending aorta. The catheter used to cross the valve is advanced and the 0.018 inch wire is exchanged for a Rosen guidewire that exactly matches the inner diameter of the balloon catheter. In this position, the wire leans on the

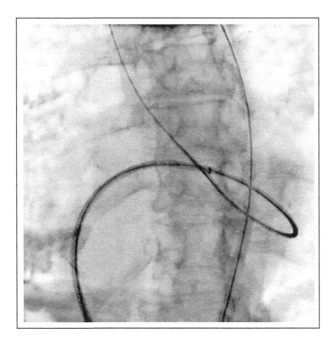

Figure 15.5
Antegrade approach. A loop is formed within the left ventricle in order to avoid mitral valve injury during inflation.

anterior leaflet of the mitral valve. In order to decrease the likelihood of mitral valve injury during balloon inflation,[25] a loop is formed with the wire within the left ventricle (Figure 15.5). The Rosen guidewire is hand shaped to allow for enough curve on the wire in the ventricular cavity. The appropriately sized balloon is advanced until it straddles the aortic valve and the dilation is performed. During inflation, left ventricular contraction may push the balloon forward into the aorta, particularly in patients with good systolic function. Care should be taken not to pull from the wire as an attempt to maintain balloon position, since this may straighten the wire within the ventricle and damage the mitral valve.

Combined approach

When the aortic valve cannot be crossed from the aortic side and a potential injury of the mitral valve is a concern, the aortic valve can be crossed as in the antegrade approach and the wire snared in the aorta. The wire is then gently pulled out through the femoral or umbilical artery. As the wire is pulled out, care should be taken to 'feed' enough wire from the venous side to avoid putting tension on the mitral valve. Then a pigtail or right coronary artery catheter is advanced through the aorta into the left ventricle and the wire is pulled out. As in the retrograde approach, a J-guidewire is advanced into the left ventricle and the catheter exchanged for a balloon catheter.

Complications

Catheter-based therapy of neonatal AS is associated with higher morbidity and mortality than in older children. Patients with a poor hemodynamic status have a higher risk of developing complications. In an early retrospective study,[10] a 9% mortality rate was related to left ventricular perforation, balloon dilation of a cusp followed by severe aortic insufficiency, and sepsis secondary to prolonged catheter manipulation through the umbilical artery. Other studies described similar complications.[15–27] However, many of these complications are now considered preventable with the current diagnostic tools and catheterization technology. In a recent large study,[28] 4% early mortality was reported and, among early survivors, a smaller left ventricle and a smaller aortic annulus were associated with decreased long term survival. In the same study, moderate or severe aortic insufficiency developed in 15% of the patients after balloon valvuloplasty and, as in other reports, a larger balloon–annulus ratio was associated with a higher risk of residual aortic insufficiency.[10,29–32] Some studies have also reported that an antegrade approach may be associated with a lower incidence of aortic insufficiency.[28,32]

A higher incidence of vascular complications remains a concern in newborns after aortic balloon valvuloplasty. Femoral artery access in neonates is followed by arterial injury and pulse loss in up to 30–39% of cases,[10,32–34] with thrombosis and potential growth retardation of the affected extremity.[35] Catheter manipulation in the umbilical artery has been associated with vessel disruption.[36] The transcarotid approach requires a cutdown and suture of the arteriotomy at the end of the procedure and carries the potential risk of residual stenosis of the right carotid artery.[16]

In general, we recommend the retrograde approach, preferably from the umbilical artery, as it is associated with the least number of complications.

Results and follow-up

Aortic valve stenosis is a lifelong disease and the parents of these patients should be informed about the palliative nature of the procedure. A gradient reduction of more than 50% is achieved in around 70% of the patients.[12–15] A low pre-dilation gradient and a small aortic annulus and aortic root have been identified as predictors of lower success rates. Most studies show that at 5-year follow-up, around 85% of patients are alive and 60% remain free of re-intervention.[12,15,28] The transvalvular gradient measured by Doppler is used to assess the residual severity and progression of AS. In most centers the recommendation is that in asymptomatic patients with a peak gradient of 70 mmHg or a mean gradient of 45 mmHg by Doppler, catheterization is indicated. Patients with symptoms or patients with moderate gradients by Doppler and progressive left ventricular hypertrophy on the electrocardiogram should also be sent to the catheterization laboratory for re-intervention.

References

1. Friedman WF. Aortic Stenosis. In: Adams FH, Emmnouilides GC, eds. Heart Disease in Infants, Children and Adolescents including the Fetus and Young Adult, 5th edn. Baltimore, MD: Williams & Wilkins, 1995.

2. Latson LA, Cheatham JP, Gutgesell HP. Relation of the echocardiographic estimate of left ventricular size to mortality in infants with severe left ventricular outflow obstruction. Am J Cardiol 1981; 48: 887–91.

3. Hammon JW, Flavian LM, Maples MD et al. Predictors of operative mortality in critical aortic stenosis presenting in infancy. Ann Thorac Surg 1988; 45: 537–40.

4. Parsons MK, Moreau GA, Graham TP et al. Echocardiographic estimation if critical left ventricular size in infants with isolated aortic valve stenosis. J Am Coll Cardiol 1991; 18: 1049–55.

5. Bu'Lock FA, Joffe HS, Jordan SC, Martin RP. Balloon dilatation (valvoplasty) as first line treatment for severe stenosis of the aortic valve in early infancy: medium term results and determinants of survival. Br Heart J 1993; 70: 546–53.

6. Rhodes LA, Colan SD, Perry SB et al. Predictors of survival in neonates with critical aortic stenosis. Circulation 1991; 84: 2325–35.

7. Zeevi B, Keane JF, Castaneda AR et al. Neonatal critical valvar stenosis: a comparison of surgical and balloon dilation therapy. Circulation 1989; 80: 831–9.

8. Rupprath G, Neuhaus KL. Percutaneous balloon valvuloplasty for aortic valve stenosis in infancy. Am J Cardiol 1985; 55: 1655–6.

9. Villalba Nogales J, Herraiz Sarachaga I, Bermudez-Canete Fernandez R et al. Balloon valvoplasty for critical aortic valve stenosis in neonates. An Esp Pediatr 2002; 57(5): 444–51.

10. Sholler GF, Keane JF, Perry SB et al. Balloon dilation of congenital aortic valve stenosis: results and influence of technical and morphological features on outcome. Circulation 1988; 78: 351–60.

11. Egito EST, Moore P, O'Sullivan J et al. Transvascular balloon dilation for neonatal critical aortic stenosis: early and midterm results. J Am Coll Cardiol 1997; 29: 442–7.

12. Huhta JC, Carpenter RJ Jr, Moise KJ Jr et al. Prenatal diagnosis and postnatal management of critical aortic stenosis. Circulation 1987; 75(3): 573–6.

13. Pass RH, Hellenbrand WE. Catheter intervention for critical aortic stenosis in the neonate. Cathet Cardiovasc Interven 2002; 55(1): 88–92.

14. Rao PS, Jureidini SB. Transumbilical venous, anterograde, snare-assisted balloon aortic valvuloplasty in a neonate with critical aortic stenosis. Cathet Cardiovasc Diagn 1998; 45(2): 144–8.

15. Beekman RH, Rocchini AP, Andes A. Balloon valvuloplasty for critical aortic stenosis in the newborn: influence of new catheter technology. J Am Coll Cardiol 1991; 17(5): 1172–6.

16. Weber HS, Mart CR, Kupferschmid J et al. Transcarotid balloon valvuloplasty with continuous transesophageal echocardiographic guidance for neonatal critical aortic valve stenosis: an alternative to surgical palliation. Pediatr Cardiol 1998; 19: 212–17.

17. Maeno Y, Akagi T, Hashino K et al. Carotid artery approach to balloon aortic valvuloplasty in infants with critical aortic valve stenosis. Pediatr Cardiol 1997; 18: 288–91.

18. Fischer DR, Ettedgui JA, Park SC et al. Carotid artery approach for balloon dilation of aortic valve stenosis in the neonate: a preliminary report. J Am Coll Cardiol 1990; 15: 1633–6.

19. Alekyan BG, Petrosyan YS, Coulson JD et al. Right subscapular artery catheterization for balloon valvuloplasty of critical aortic stenosis in infants. Am J Cardiol 1995; 76(14): 1049–52.

20. Helgason H, Keane JF, Fellows KE et al. Balloon dilation of the aortic valve: studies in normal lambs and in children with aortic stenosis. J Am Coll Cardiol 1987; 9(4): 816–22.

21. Borghi A, Agnoletti G, Poggiani C. Surgical cutdown of the right carotid artery for aortic balloon valvuloplasty in infancy: midterm follow-up. Pediatr Cardiol 2001; 22(3): 194–7.

22. Fagan TE, Ing FF, Edens RE et al. Balloon aortic valvuloplasty in a 1,600-gram infant. Cathet Cardiovasc Interven 2000; 50(3): 322–5.

23. Waight DJ, Hijazi ZM. Balloon aortic valvuloplasty: the single-wire technique. J Interven Cardiol 2004; 17(1): 21.

24. Weber HS, Mart CR, Myers JL. Transcarotid balloon valvuloplasty for critical aortic valve stenosis at the bedside via continuous transesophageal echocardiographic guidance. Cathet Cardiovasc Interven 2000; 50(3): 326–9.

25. Brierley JJ, Reddy TD, Rigby ML et al. Traumatic damage to the mitral valve during percutaneous balloon valvotomy for critical aortic stenosis. Heart 1998; 79(2): 200–2.

26. Kasten-Sportes CH, Piechaud JF, Sidi D, Kachaner J. Percutaneous balloon valvuloplasty in neonates with critical aortic stenosis. J Am Coll Cardiol 1989; 13(5): 1101–5.

27. Phillips RR, Gerlis LM, Wilson N, Walker DR. Aortic valve damage caused by operative balloon dilatation of critical aortic valve stenosis. Br Heart J 1987; 57(2): 168–70.

28. McElhinney DB, Lock JE, Keane JF et al. Left heart growth, function, and reintervention after balloon aortic valvuloplasty for neonatal aortic stenosis. Circulation 2005; 111(4): 451–8.

29. McCrindle BW, Jones TK, Morrow WR et al. Acute results of balloon angioplasty of native coarctation versus recurrent aortic obstruction are equivalent. Valvuloplasty and Angioplasty of Congenital Anomalies (VACA) Registry Investigators. J Am Coll Cardiol 1996; 28(7): 1810–17.

30. Hawkins JA, Minich LL, Shaddy RE et al. Aortic valve repair and replacement after balloon aortic valvuloplasty in children. Ann Thorac Surg 1996; 61(5): 1355–8.

31. Cowley CG, Dietrich M, Mosca RS et al. Balloon valvuloplasty versus transventricular dilation for neonatal critical aortic stenosis. Am J Cardiol 2001; 87(9): 1125–7, A10.

32. Magee AG, Nykanen D, McCrindle BW et al. Balloon dilation of severe aortic stenosis in the neonate: comparison of anterograde and retrograde catheter approaches. J Am Coll Cardiol 1997; 30(4): 10.

33. Wessel DL, Keane JF, Fellows KE et al. Fibrynolytic therapy for femoral arterial thrombosis after cardiac catheterization in infants and children. Am J Cardiol 1986; 58: 347–51.

34. Cassidy SC, Schmidt KG, VanHare GF et al. Complications of pediatric cardiac catheterization: a 3 year study. J Am Coll Cardiol 1992; 19: 1285–93.

35. Peuster M, Freihorst J, Hausdorf G. Images in cardiology. Defective limb growth after retrograde balloon valvuloplasty. Heart 2000; 84(1): 63.

36. Sasidharan P. Umbilical arterial rupture: a major complication of catheterization. Indiana Med 1985; 78(1): 34–5.

16

Balloon aortic valvuloplasty for aortic valve stenosis in the elderly

Alain Cribier, Helene Eltchaninoff, and Vasilis Babaliaros

Anatomy and pathophysiology

Degenerative disease of the aortic valve occurs with age. Areas of cusp flexion over time develop fibrosis and calcification, impeding valve excursion and creating obstruction to left ventricular outflow.[1] The degenerative process is often observed in those greater than 70 years of age, but patients with additional valve pathology (bicuspid aortic valves or rheumatic valvular disease) can present much earlier in life with deterioration of valve function and consequent symptoms.[2]

Balloon valvuloplasty has been shown to relieve obstruction of the stenotic aortic valve by three mechanisms: fracture of calcium deposits in the leaflets, separation of fused commissures, and stretching of the aortic annulus.[3,4] Calcium deposits are broken into separate fragments with balloon inflation, facilitating leaflet flexion and allowing better excursion during systole. Separation of commissures is quite effective by balloon aortic valvuloplasty (BAV), though commissural fusion (seen in rheumatic disease) is quite uncommon in the elderly patient. Stretching of the valve may explain the early gains by BAV, but valve recoil can occur within hours to days and, in this case, results of BAV will be fleeting. Late restenosis (after several months) probably results from progression of the original lesions that produced stenosis.

Clinical symptoms and indications for treatment

The development of symptoms can trail the onset of degeneration of the aortic valve by several decades.[5] When present, initial symptoms tend to be dyspnea on exertion and effort angina, though some patients may present with syncope or heart failure.[6] Once symptoms are detected, the prognosis is poor without intervention: patients are often dead within 5 years of angina, 3 years of syncope, and 2 years of heart failure.[7,8] Surgical valve replacement is currently the

standard of care for treatment of symptomatic patients with severe aortic stenosis (Class I indication). Asymptomatic patients, with severe aortic stenosis undergoing coronary artery bypass surgery, surgery on the aorta, or valve surgery, are also considered Class I indications for surgical valve replacement by present guidelines.

BAV has a special role in the elderly patient. In hemodynamically unstable patients who require a 'bridge' to high risk aortic valve replacement surgery, valvuloplasty is considered a Class IIa practice. Patients who require urgent non-cardiac surgery or patients without surgical options for valve replacement are considered Class IIb indications.[9]

History of the procedure

BAV was originally introduced in 1986[10] as the therapy of choice for patients with severe aortic stenosis who were considered either too old or a high risk for surgical valve replacement. By the 1990s, the scope of surgery had expanded to encompass many of these patients,[11–15] and the technique of BAV was largely abandoned because of the associated complication rate and the problem of valve restenosis.[16–22] Today, the BAV procedure is associated with a much lower incidence of complications because of improvements in technique and hardware. The problem of restenosis has been addressed by the advent of percutaneous aortic valve replacement.[23,24] Despite different surgical and percutaneous alternatives, BAV remains a valuable palliative procedure for the treatment of aortic stenosis in the elderly.

Pre-procedure evaluation

The evaluation of aortic stenosis begins with the patient history and the physical examination. Often, only transthoracic echocardiography (TTE) is used to quantify the degree of stenosis as retrograde catheterization has been associated with an increased risk of stroke.[25] If there is any discrepancy between the patient's presentation and echocardiographic results, retrograde catheterization should be performed to measure the simultaneous gradient across the aortic valve, as described below. In patients with low transvalvular gradient and low cardiac output, dobutamine infusion can aid in diagnosing patients with true aortic stenosis from those with 'flow-dependent' stenosis.[26–28] Assessment of concomitant coronary artery disease is important as coronary stenting should be done before BAV and can often be accomplished in the same session. Venous and arterial access sites should also be evaluated prior to the procedure.

BAV procedure

Vascular access, right heart catheterization, and supra-aortic angiography

The procedure begins with the administration of mild sedation and local anesthesia. The right common femoral artery and vein are cannulated with an 8 Fr sheath. If the right femoral artery is unavailable for access, the left femoral artery, the brachial artery, or an antegrade transseptal approach via the femoral vein can be used. In order to limit vascular complications in the arm, we recommend a cut down and maximum sheath size of 10 Fr. Heparin 5000 IU intravenously should be administered after vascular access. An 8 Fr Swan–Ganz catheter is advanced from the femoral vein and baseline right-sided pressures are recorded. Cardiac output measurements using either thermodilution or the Fick principle should wait until the aortic valve has been crossed to reduce the error in calculation of aortic valve area. A 6 Fr pigtail catheter is then advanced from the femoral artery and placed superior to the aortic valve. Aortic angiography is performed in the 40° LAO projection to define the details of the valve anatomy and assess the degree of insufficiency (Figure 16.1). Patients with ≥ grade 2 aortic regurgitation are in general not considered for BAV.

Crossing the native valve

With proper technique, crossing the stenotic valve should take 1 to 2 minutes. In our institution we use a 7 Fr Sones (B type) or Amplatz (AL) catheter and a straight 0.035 inch guidewire to cross the aortic valve (Figures 16.2 and 16.3). The starting position of the Sones catheter is in the left coronary cusp with the tip pointed superiorly, and the starting position of the Amplatz catheter should be with the tip pointed at the orifice between the left and right cusps. With either catheter, a slow pull back with clockwise rotation and careful probing with the guidewire should negotiate the stenotic orifice. The Amplatz catheter is more useful than

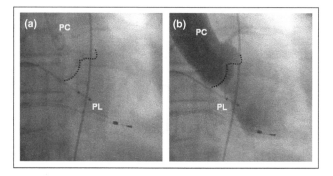

Figure 16.1
(a) The details of the aortic root and valve calcifications (dotted lines) are seen during supra-aortic angiography. (b) This patient had grade 2 aortic insufficiency and underwent dilatation without an increase in regurgitation. PC, pigtail catheter; PL, pacing lead.

the Sones catheter when the plane of the aortic valve is more vertical. The AL 2 catheter works well in a normal size aorta; an AL 1 is required for smaller patients. Once the valve has been crossed, the wire position is confirmed in the RAO projection and the crossing catheter is advanced into the left ventricle. Failure to cross the valve with the catheter usually means the wire has biased into a commissure. Repositioning the wire, which includes making a loop in the ventricle, may be required to move the wire more towards the central orifice. Exchanging for a smaller size catheter may also help. With the crossing catheter in place or exchanged for a pigtail catheter, the transvalvular gradient can be obtained, using the lateral arm of the sheath to record aortic pressure. Cardiac output should be measured at this time as well.

Guidewire and sheath exchanges

The straight guidewire is removed from the crossing catheter and replaced by a 0.035 inch, 260 cm stiff guidewire (Amplatz Extra Stiff, COOK, Bjaeverskov, DK). The flexible end of the guidewire is pre-shaped before use into an exaggerated pigtail curve using a standard hemostat. The curve in the distal wire decreases the risk of left ventricular trauma and the incidence of ventricular ectopy or tachycardia. The stiff wire is important to provide adequate support during advancing or inflating of the balloon catheter. The 8 Fr sheath is removed and replaced by a 12 Fr sheath.

The use of a 12 Fr arterial introducer (COOK) has markedly decreased the rate of local complications at the femoral puncture site. It is compatible with a 23 mm × 3 cm (diameter by length) or 20 mm × 3 cm ZMED balloon catheter (NuMED Canada, Inc, Cornwall, Canada). The 23 mm × 4.5 cm and 20 mm × 4.5 cm Cristal balloons (BALT Extrusion, Montmorency, France) are compatible with a 10 and 9 Fr sheath, respectively. Both 10 and 12 Fr sheaths can

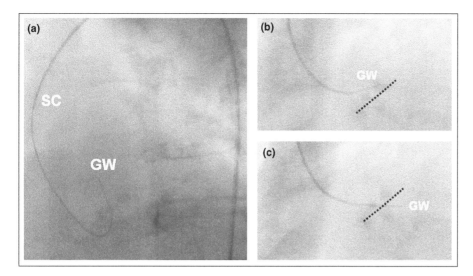

Figure 16.2
(a) The Sones catheter (SC) is advanced over a guidewire (GW) in the left coronary cusp in the left anterior oblique view. (b) The guidewire is used to probe the valve orifice (above the dotted line). (c) The guidewire has passed through the stenotic orifice (valve calcifications above the dotted line).

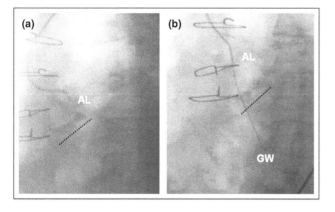

Figure 16.3
(a) The Amplatz catheter (AL) is directed towards the aortic orifice (valve calcifications above the dotted line). (b) The straight guidewire (GW) has passed through the stenotic orifice (valve calcifications above the dotted line).

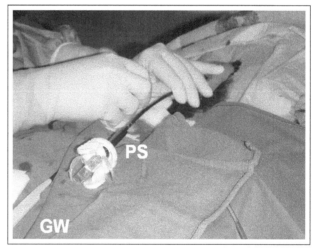

Figure 16.4
Prostar XL device (PS) inserted over the guidewire (GW) for closure of the arterial access site.

be closed percutaneously with a 10 Fr Prostar XL device (Abbott Vascular Devices, Redwood City, CA) without the need of pre-closure (Figure 16.4). The use of the Prostar XL device has further decreased the rate of bleeding complications after sheath removal.[29]

Balloon catheters

The balloon catheters used at our institution are the ZMED (NuMed Canada, Inc) and the Cristal (BALT Extrusion) balloons. The Cristal balloons are lower profile and tend not to dilate as well as the ZMED balloons, a characteristic which can be useful in certain cases. Both balloons are inserted over the stiff guidewire and purged of air in the descending aorta. We use a 30 ml syringe filled with 20 ml of a 10:90 mixture of contrast with saline to easily and completely inflate the valvuloplasty balloon. This dilution of contrast is adequate for visualization of the balloon under fluoroscopy and also decreases the time of deflation.

The balloon should pass the stenotic orifice without difficulty in most cases. If the balloon does not pass, the wire is probably biased into a commissure. In this situation, an empty 20 or 30 ml syringe can provide additional negative pressure to decrease the balloon profile. The wire position can also be changed by advancing the wire further into the ventricle or tracking the wire during balloon advancement. In special cases, we have purged the balloon of air after crossing the native valve in order to facilitate crossing. In most valvuloplasties, we begin with a 23 mm ZMED balloon; however, in patients with a small aortic annulus (<20 mm by TTE) or heavily calcified valve, sequential

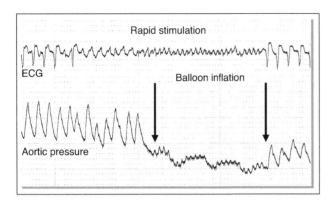

Figure 16.5
Aortic and ECG tracing during rapid stimulation depicts a predictable and abrupt decrease in cardiac output during which balloon valvuloplasty can be performed safely.

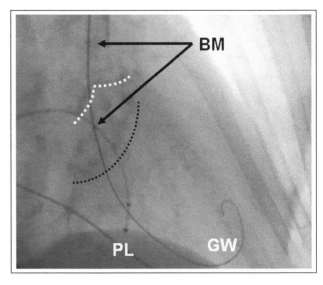

Figure 16.6
The balloon markers (BM) are centered around the aortic valve calcification (white dotted lines) prior to inflation. The guidewire tip (GW) has an exaggerated curve to prevent ventricular trauma or arrhythmia. PL, pacer lead; black dotted lines, mitral annulus calcification.

inflations with a 20 mm ZMED or a Cristal balloon are prudent. In these cases, progression to a larger size balloon is acceptable if the initial result is insufficient, the balloon size appears undersized, and there is no visible waist during inflation. We rarely inflate a balloon that is 30% larger than the aortic annulus size.

Rapid pacing and balloon inflation

Maintaining the position of the balloon catheter during inflation is critical for effective dilatation. This positioning is facilitated by rapidly pacing the right ventricle causing electrically induced arrest of the heart. From the femoral vein, we advance a 6 Fr pacing lead (Soloist, Medtronic, Inc, Minneapolis, MN) into the right ventricle. This lead should be connected to an external pulse generator that is capable of pacing at rates > 200 beats/min (Medtronic, Inc, Model 5348, Minneapolis, MN). Starting at 180 stimulations/minute, the minimal rate that causes a rapid and predictable decrease in systolic pressure to 30–40 mmHg should be found (Figure 16.5); typically a rate of 200–220 beats/min is needed. A back up rate of 80 beats/minute should be set to prevent episodes of bradycardia after dilatation.

With the markers of the balloon on either side of the valve calcification (Figure 16.6), rapid stimulation is started and coupled with cine-angiographic imaging and maximal balloon inflation. Normally, balloon deflation and arrest of stimulation are done simultaneously. If there is concern about the size of the aortic annulus (as when BAV is performed before percutaneous aortic valve implantation), stimulation can be stopped at maximal balloon inflation to see if the balloon moves freely within the valve or fits securely. Upon deflation, the balloon is quickly withdrawn from the valve orifice to promptly restore antegrade blood flow.

The valve is dilated in the same fashion once or twice more, depending on the quality of dilatation (adequate balloon size without movement at maximal inflation) (Figure 16.7). The goal of valvuloplasty should be a ≥ 50% decrease in the transvalvular gradient and a 100% increase in valve area. Even with suboptimal results, a larger balloon size (25 mm) is not often used in our practice to avoid the risk of aortic disruption.

Antegrade dilatation

If arterial access is not possible, the aortic valve can be dilated via the antegrade route (Figure 16.8). This approach requires venous access, transseptal catheterization, and a guidewire which is looped in the left ventricle and across the aortic valve. Though this method is not recommended for inexperienced operators because of potential damage to the atrial septum and mitral valve, we have performed this technique safely in patients under special circumstances. The antegrade approach is described in detail in the chapter on percutaneous aortic valve replacement (chapter 22).

Post-procedure evaluation and management

The transvalvular gradient and cardiac output should be measured as previously described. A final supra-aortic angiogram should define the degree of aortic regurgitation. The arterial access is closed percutaneously; in case of failure, manual compression is sufficient and protamine can also be administered to reverse the effects of heparin. When BAV is applied in the context of severely impaired left

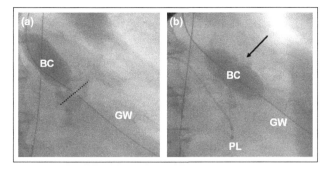

Figure 16.7
(a) Lack of rapid pacing results in movement of the balloon catheter (BC) distal to the aortic valve (dotted lines, aortic valve calcification) and inadequate dilatation. GW, guidewire. (b) Rapid pacing stabilizes the balloon during inflation, resulting in adequate valve dilatation. PL, pacing lead; arrow, aortic valve calcification.

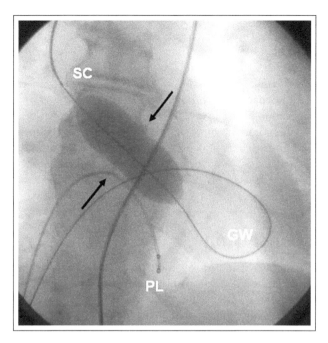

Figure 16.8
The guidewire (GW) is seen entering the heart from the right atrium, and then crosses the left atrium, mitral valve, left ventricle, and aortic valve. A balloon catheter is inflated in the aortic valve (arrows, valve calcification). A Sones catheter (SC) from the left femoral artery is used to stabilize the balloon during inflation, though this technique is not necessary for routine valvuloplasty. PL, pacing lead.

ventricular function or cardiogenic shock,[30] inotropic support may be transitorily required in the days following the procedure. If high degree atrioventricular block occurs, temporary pacing should be used for 24–48 hours; if there is no recovery of conduction, a permanent pacemaker should be considered. In other uncomplicated cases, the patients can be discharged after 2 days. Long term follow-up is sequentially assessed on clinical and echocardiographic evaluations. Only in patients in whom the recurrence of symptoms is delayed by 6 months or longer should repeat BAV be performed. In these cases, results are similar to initial BAV.[31]

Complications of BAV

Vascular injury

The complications associated with BAV have markedly decreased since that of the initial registries.[22] The incidence of vascular injury, traditionally the most common complication, has been markedly decreased by the use of lower profile arterial introducers and closure devices. In our institution, vascular complication has not required surgical repair in the last 3 years.

Massive aortic regurgitation

Massive aortic regurgitation after BAV can be a fatal complication. In patients with small stature or heavily calcified valves, sequential dilatation is useful to prevent this problem. Once massive aortic regurgitation occurs, surgical valve replacement is critical for those who develop hemodynamic compromise. In clinically stable patients, surgery can be postponed.

Embolic events

In our experience, the occurrence of clinically apparent cerebral events (<2%) is less common with BAV than reported with retrograde catheterization.[25] Heparin 5000 IU intravenously should be used at the beginning of the procedure, and the valve should be crossed with the minimal number of guidewire passes. Stroke can also occur during hypotension, induced by manipulation of the hardware across the diseased valve or balloon inflation, particularly in patients with vascular disease of the cerebral vessels or previous stroke. Short balloon inflation/deflation and stimulation time (<10 seconds) as well as hemodynamic support as needed are highly recommended. The development of neurologic changes should prompt urgent imaging and consultation with a neurologist.

Death

Procedural death (within 24 hours), the result of fatal arrhythmia, progressive heart failure, rupture of the aorta, or disruption of the aortic valve, can be seen in patients with severely depressed left ventricular function, cardiogenic shock, heavy calcification of the aortic valve, or porcelain aorta. If hypotension occurs during the procedure, the etiology should be sought immediately. Liberal use of echocardiography is invaluable, and pericardiocentesis can be lifesaving, particularly as a bridge to surgical therapy. Additional death (within 7 days) is usually a result of a complication from the initial procedure, which emphasizes the nature of intervening on this precarious group. Efforts to minimize contrast dye, procedure time and the number of interventions while being vigilant of all medical conditions are imperative.

Conclusion

In adult aortic stenosis, BAV is a palliative procedure that should be restricted to elderly patients with high operable risk. Most patients today are suitable for surgical valve replacement and, in these cases, BAV is in no way an adequate alternative. BAV is safe in experienced hands, and is a low-cost procedure that requires only a brief hospitalization and can temporarily relieve the symptoms of patients, even if repeated for restenosis (up to five times for some patients at our institution). In an era of percutaneous valve implantation, aortic valvuloplasty is a technique that interventional cardiologists should be comfortable performing.

References

1. Passik CS, Ackermann DM, Pluth JR, Edwards WD. Temporal changes in the causes of aortic stenosis: a surgical pathologic study of 646 cases. Mayo Clin Proc 1987; 62: 119.
2. Roberts WC. Valvular, subvalvular and supravalvular aortic stenosis. Morphologic features. Cardiovasc Clin 1973; 5: 97.
3. Safian RD, Mandell VS, Thurer RE et al. Postmortem and intraoperative balloon valvuloplasty of calcific aortic stenosis in elderly patients: mechanisms of successful dilation. J Am Coll Cardiol 1987; 9: 655.
4. Beatt KJ. Balloon dilatation of the aortic valve in adults: a physician's view. Br Heart J 1990; 63: 207.
5. Oakley CM. Management of valvular stenosis. Curr Opin Cardiol 1995; 10: 117.
6. Kennedy KD, Nishimura RA, Holmes DR et al. Natural history of moderate aortic stenosis. J Am Coll Cardiol 1991; 17: 313.
7. Ross J, Braunwald E. The influence of corrective operations on the natural history of aortic stenosis. Circulation 1968; 37(Suppl V): 61.
8. Frank S, Johnson A, Ross J. Natural history of valvular aortic stenosis. Br Heart J 1973; 35: 41.
9. ACC/AHA guidelines for the management of patients with valvular heart disease, a report from the American College of Cardiology/American Heart Association, Task Force on Practice Guidelines (Committee on Management of Patients with Valvular Disease). J Am Coll Cardiol 1998; 32: 1486–588.
10. Cribier A, Savin T, Saoudi N et al. Percutaneous transluminal valvuloplasty of acquired aortic stenosis in elderly patients: an alternative to valve replacement? Lancet 1986; 1(8472): 63–7.
11. Culliford AT, Galloway AC, Colvin SB et al. Aortic valve replacement for aortic stenosis in persons aged 80 years and over. Am J Cardiol 1991; 67(15): 1256–60.
12. Lytle BW, Cosgrove DM, Taylor PC et al. Primary isolated aortic valve replacement. Early and late results. J Thorac Cardiovasc Surg 1989; 97(5): 675–94.
13. Pereira JJ, Lauer MS, Bashir M et al. Survival after aortic valve replacement for severe aortic stenosis with low transvalvular gradients and severe left ventricular dysfunction. J Am Coll Cardiol 2002; 39(8): 1356–63.
14. Rothenburger M, Drebber K, Tjan TD et al. Aortic valve replacement for aortic regurgitation and stenosis, in patients with severe left ventricular dysfunction. Eur J Cardiothorac Surg 2003; 23(5): 703–9; discussion 9.
15. Sharony R, Grossi EA, Saunders PC et al. Aortic valve replacement in patients with impaired ventricular function. Ann Thorac Surg 2003; 75(6): 1808–14.
16. National Heart Lung and Blood Institute participants group. Percutaneous balloon aortic valvuloplasty. Acute and 30-day follow-up results in 674 patients from the NHLBI Balloon Valvuloplasty Registry. Circulation 1991; 84(6): 2383–97.
17. Cribier A, Letac B. Two years' experience of percutaneous balloon valvuloplasty in aortic stenosis. Herz 1988; 13(2): 110–18.
18. Cribier A, Letac B. Percutaneous balloon aortic valvuloplasty in adults with calcific aortic stenosis. Curr Opin Cardiol 1991; 6(2): 212–18.
19. Lieberman EB, Bashore TM, Hermiller JB et al. Balloon aortic valvuloplasty in adults: failure of procedure to improve long-term survival. J Am Coll Cardiol 1995; 26(6): 1522–8.
20. Otto CM, Mickel MC, Kennedy JW et al. Three-year outcome after balloon aortic valvuloplasty. Insights into prognosis of valvular aortic stenosis. Circulation 1994; 89(2): 642–50.
21. Safian RD, Berman AD, Diver DJ et al. Balloon aortic valvuloplasty in 170 consecutive patients. N Engl J Med 1988; 319(3): 125–30.
22. McKay RG. The Mansfield Scientific Aortic Valvuloplasty Registry: overview of acute hemodynamic results and procedural complications. J Am Coll Cardiol 1991; 17(2): 485–91.
23. Cribier A, Eltchaninoff H, Bash A et al. Percutaneous transcatheter implantation of an aortic valve prosthesis for calcific aortic stenosis: first human case description. Circulation 2002; 106(24): 3006–8.
24. Cribier A, Eltchaninoff H, Tron C et al. Early experience with percutaneous transcatheter implantation of heart valve prosthesis for the treatment of end-stage inoperable patients with calcific aortic stenosis. J Am Coll Cardiol 2004; 43(4): 698–703.
25. Omran H, Schmidt H, Hackenbroch M et al. Silent and apparent cerebral embolism after retrograde catheterisation of the aortic valve in valvular stenosis: a prospective, randomised study. Lancet 2003; 361(9365): 1241–6.
26. Bolognese L, Buonamici P, Cerisano G et al. Early dobutamine echocardiography predicts improvement in regional and global left ventricular function after reperfused acute myocardial infarction without residual stenosis of the infarct-related artery. Am Heart J 2000; 139(1 Pt 1): 153–63.
27. Carabello BA. Management of the elderly aortic stenosis patient with low gradient and low ejection fraction. Am J Geriatr Cardiol 2003; 12(3): 165–70; quiz 70–2.
28. Nishimura RA, Grantham JA, Connolly HM et al. Low-output, low-gradient aortic stenosis in patients with depressed left ventricular systolic function: the clinical utility of the dobutamine challenge in the catheterization laboratory. Circulation 2002; 106(7): 809–13.
29. Solomon LW, Fusman B, Jolly N et al. Percutaneous suture closure for management of large French size arterial puncture in aortic valvuloplasty. J Invasive Cardiol 2001; 13(8): 592–6.
30. Cribier A, Remadi F, Koning R et al. Emergency balloon valvuloplasty as initial treatment of patients with aortic stenosis and cardiogenic shock. N Engl J Med 1992; 326(9): 646.
31. Letac B, Cribier A, Eltchaninoff H et al. Evaluation of restenosis after balloon dilatation in adult aortic stenosis by repeat catheterization. Am Heart J 1991; 122(1 Pt 1): 55–60.

17

Percutaneous mitral balloon valvuloplasty

Igor F Palacios

Since its introduction in 1984 by Inoue et al,[1] percutaneous mitral balloon valvuloplasty (PMV) has been used successfully as an alternative to open or closed surgical mitral commissurotomy in the treatment of patients with symptomatic rheumatic mitral stenosis.[2–18] PMV produces good immediate hemodynamic outcome, low complication rate, and clinical improvement in the majority of patients with mitral stenosis.[2–18] PMV provides sustained clinical and hemodynamic improvement in patients with rheumatic mitral stenosis. The immediate and long term results appear to be similar to those of surgical mitral commissurotomy.[2–18] Today, PMV is the preferred form of therapy for relief of mitral stenosis for a selected group of patients with symptomatic mitral stenosis.

PMV patient selection

PMV is indicated for symptomatic patients (New York Heart Association (NYHA) functional class ≥ II) who have moderate or severe MS (mitral valve area (MVA) ≤ 1.5 cm^2) and a valve morphology that favors percutaneous intervention, with no thrombus in the left atrium or moderate or severe mitral regurgitation. PMV is not without risk and therefore should not be routinely indicated in asymptomatic patients. Exceptions to this rule are patients with severe mitral stenosis who require other major non-cardiac surgery, young women who wish to get pregnant, and patients at high risk for thromboembolism (former history of thromboembolic phenomena, dense spontaneous contrast in LA, recurring atrial fibrillation). Likewise, despite the good preliminary results, there is no consensus about the indication of such a procedure in patients with mild or moderate mitral stenosis, in an attempt to delay the progression of the disease, especially because those patients respond well to clinical treatment.

Patient selection is fundamental in predicting immediate outcome and follow-up results of PMV and requires a precise assessment of mitral valve morphology. The echocardiographic score is currently the most widely used method for the evaluation of the morphologic characteristics of the mitral valve apparatus. Because it is widely available and enables dynamic assessment of the mitral valve, allowing for pulmonary pressure estimation and for determining the concurrence of other valve disorders, the Doppler two-dimensional (2D) echocardiography is the diagnostic tool of choice for evaluation of a mitral stenosis patient. The interest in pre-valvuloplasty echocardiography derives from the significant previous surgical experience showing that the success of a surgical mitral commissurotomy is determined by valve morphology. Within this line of thought, in an attempt to find predictors for PMV immediate results, Wilkins et al.[19] described a morphologic score that graded morphologic changes of the mitral valve, including four characteristics: leaflet mobility, leaflet thickening, valve calcification, and involvement of the subvalvular apparatus – each of them classified in a 0–4 scale. The authors demonstrated with that paper that the only predictor of immediate results after PMV, regardless of any other clinical or hemodynamic variable, was the valve's total score. This score was validated by comparing echocardiographic findings with the anatomopathologic exam in a series of autopsies. The optimal combination point between sensitivity and specificity (72% and 73%, respectively) to forecast a good immediate PMV result was an echo score of ≤ 8.

Because it enables a quantitative assessment of how severely the mitral valve apparatus is affected by rheumatic disease, and because it predicts the immediate result of PMV, the Wilkins score became standard, providing the means to compare populations from different studies. Several limitations, however, were brought up about the score, including the fact that all its components have the same weight in the pathologic process. We have established that, among its components, the only one that correlates with an absolute change in MVA after valvuloplasty is thickening of the valve. This score does not take into account other factors that are important in predicting results, such as asymmetry of fused commissures and their degree of calcification, and it fails to predict severe mitral regurgitation. Therefore, other scores were devised, some addressing valve anatomy more thoroughly, others grading specific valve characteristics. None of them, however, has been shown to be better than others and, to different extents, all of them are limited in terms of reproducibility, underestimation of certain characteristics, and inability to predict mitral regurgitation development.

Finally, the immediate and long term outcome of patients undergoing PMV is multi-factorial. The use of the echocardiographic score in conjunction with other clinical and morphologic predictors of PMV outcome facilitates the identification of patients who will obtain the best outcome from PMV. We identified additional clinical and morphologic factors predicting immediate and long term results after PMV. They include pre-PMV variables such as mitral valve area, history of previous surgical commissurotomy, age, and mitral regurgitation, and post-PMV variables such as MR ≥ 3 Seller's grade and pulmonary artery pressure. The use of these factors in conjunction with the echocardiographic score allows optimal selection of patients for PMV.

Technique of PMV

PMV should be performed in the fasting state under mild sedation. Antibiotics (dicloxacillin 500 mg p.o. q/6 hours for four doses) are started before or cefalotin 1 g iv is given at the time of the procedure. Patients allergic to penicillin should receive vancomycin 1 gram iv at the time of the procedure.

All patients carefully chosen as candidates for mitral balloon valvuloplasty should undergo diagnostic right and left and transseptal left heart catheterization. Transseptal catheterization, which allows access to the left atrium, is the first step of the PMV procedure and one of the most crucial. Following transseptal left heart catheterization, systemic anticoagulation is achieved by the intravenous administration of 100 units/kg of heparin. In patients older than 40 years, coronary arteriography should also be performed.

Hemodynamic measurements, cardiac output, and cine left ventriculography are performed before and after PMV. Cardiac output is measured by thermodilution and Fick method techniques. Mitral valve calcification and angiographic severity of mitral regurgitation (Seller's classification) are graded qualitatively from 0 to 4, as previously described.[3] An oxygen diagnostic run is performed before and after PMV to determine the presence of left to right shunt after PMV.

There is no unique technique of percutaneous mitral balloon valvuloplasty. Most of the techniques of PMV require transseptal left heart catheterization and use of the antegrade approach. Antegrade PMV can be accomplished using a single[2,3,6] or a double balloon technique.[3–5,7] In the latter approach the two balloons can be placed through a single femoral vein and single transseptal punctures,[3,5,7] or through two femoral veins and two separate atrial septal punctures.[4]

In the retrograde technique of PMV the balloons dilating the catheters are advanced percutaneously through the right and left femoral arteries over guidewires that have been snared from the descending aorta.[19] These guidewires have been advanced transseptally from the right femoral vein into the left atrium, the left ventricle, and the ascending aorta. A retrograde non-transseptal technique of PMV has also been described.[20,21]

The antegrade double balloon technique

In performing PMV using the antegrade double balloon technique (Figure 17.1) a 7 Fr flow directed balloon catheter is advanced through the transseptal sheath across the mitral valve into the left ventricle.[22] The catheter is then advanced through the aortic valve into the ascending and then the descending aorta. A 0.035 or 0.038 inch, 260 cm long teflon coated exchange wire is then passed through the catheter. The sheath and the catheter are removed, leaving the wire behind. A 5 mm balloon dilating catheter is used to dilate the atrial septum. A second exchange guidewire is passed parallel to the first guidewire through the same femoral vein and atrial septum punctures using a double lumen catheter. The double lumen catheter is then removed, leaving the two guidewires across the mitral valve in the ascending and descending aorta. During these maneuvers care should be taken to maintain large and smooth loops of the guidewires in the left ventricular cavity to allow appropriate placement of the dilating balloons. If a second guidewire cannot be placed into the ascending and descending aorta, a 0.038 inch Amplatz type transfer guidewire with a preformed curlew at its tip can be placed at the left ventricular apex. In patients with an aortic valve prosthesis, both guidewires with pre-formed curlew tips should be placed at the left ventricular apex. When one or both guidewires are placed in the left ventricular apex, the balloons should be inflated sequentially. Care should be taken to avoid forward movement of the balloons and guidewires to prevent left ventricular perforation. Two balloon dilating catheters, chosen according to the patient's body surface area, are then advanced over each one of the guidewires and positioned across the mitral valve, parallel to the longitudinal axis of the left ventricle. The balloon valvuloplasty catheters are then inflated by hand until the indentation produced by the stenotic mitral valve is no longer seen. Generally one, but occasionally two or three inflations are performed. After complete deflation the balloons are removed sequentially. The double balloon technique of PMV is effective but demanding, and carries the risk of left ventricular perforation by the guidewires or the tip of the balloons. The multitrack system (Figure 17.2) introduced by Bonhoeffer shares the advantages of the traditional double balloon technique. It is safer, reducing the risk of accidental balloon displacement. The procedure is easier to perform as it only requires

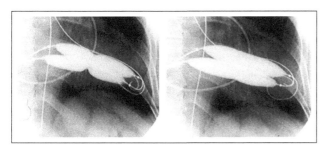

Figure 17.1
Double balloon technique of PMV. An indentation on the balloons is seen in the right side panel. Full inflation of the balloons is achieved in the left side panel. One of the guidewires is placed in the ascending and descending aorta and the second guidewire is placed in the left ventricular cavity with its curlew tip at the apex.

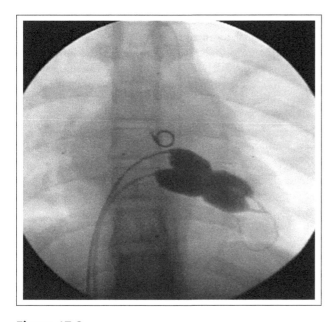

Figure 17.2
The multi-track technique of PMV is a modification of the double balloon technique. Two separate balloon catheters are positioned on a single guidewire. The first catheter, with only a distal guidewire lumen, is introduced into the vein and then advanced into the mitral orifice. Subsequently, a rapid exchange balloon catheter running on the same guidewire is inserted and lined up with the first catheter so the two are positioned side by side. Both balloons are then inflated simultaneously.

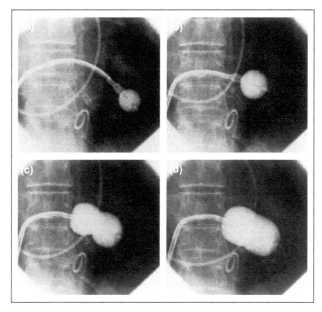

Figure 17.3
The Inoue balloon technique of PMV. Once the catheter is in the left ventricle, the partially inflated balloon is moved back and forth inside the left ventricle to assure that it is free of the chordae tendinae (a). The catheter is then gently pulled against the mitral plane until resistance is felt. The balloon is then rapidly inflated to its full capacity and then deflated quickly (b), (c) (d).

the presence of a single guidewire and therefore procedure time is reduced. The system is versatile and can be used in other indications. With this technique two separate balloon catheters are positioned on a single guidewire. The first catheter, with only a distal guidewire lumen, is introduced into the vein and then advanced into the mitral orifice. Subsequently, a rapid exchange balloon catheter running on the same guidewire is inserted and lined up with the

first catheter so the two are positioned side by side. Both balloons are then inflated simultaneously.

The Inoue technique of PMV

Nowadays PMV is more frequently performed using the Inoue technique (Figure 17.3).[1,15–17] The Inoue balloon is a 12 Fr shaft, coaxial, double lumen catheter. The balloon is made of a double layer of rubber tubing with a layer of synthetic micromesh in between.

Following transseptal catheterization, a stainless steel guidewire is advanced through the transseptal catheter and placed with its tip coiled into the left atrium and the transseptal catheter removed. A 14 Fr dilator is advanced over the guidewire and used to dilate the femoral vein and the atrial septum. A balloon catheter chosen according to the patient's height is advanced over the guidewire into the left atrium. The distal part of the balloon is inflated and advanced into the left ventricle with the help of the spring wire stylet, which has been inserted through the inner lumen of the catheter. After insertion of the stylet the catheter is advanced toward the mitral valve plane and, by using counterclockwise rotation of the stylet, facilitates entry into the left ventricle. Occasionally, and particularly in patients with a large left atrium or suboptimal transseptal puncture site, the above maneuver does not allow entry into the left ventricle. Under these conditions we rotate the stylet clockwise, allowing the catheter to initially rotate posterior in front of the pulmonary veins and then by advancing further the partially inflated balloon to the mitral plane, gentle movements of the stylet back and forth allow the balloon to enter the left ventricle. Once the catheter is in the left ventricle, the partially inflated balloon is moved back and forth inside the left ventricle to assure that it is free of the chordae tendinae. The catheter is then gently pulled against the mitral plane until resistance is felt. The balloon is then rapidly inflated to its full capacity and then deflated quickly. During inflation of the balloon an indentation should be seen in its mid-portion. The catheter is withdrawn into the left atrium and the mitral gradient and cardiac output measured. If further dilatations are required the stylet is introduced again and the sequence of steps described above repeated at a larger balloon volume. After each dilatation its effect should be assessed by pressure measurement, auscultation, and 2D echocardiography. If mitral regurgitation occurs, further dilation of the valve should not be performed. The Inoue technique has became the standard in most institutions. Unlike other techniques, PMV with the Inoue balloon does not require floating balloons or the placement of a guidewire in the left ventricle, and is therefore a simpler procedure with a substantially lower risk of perforating the LV. In addition, the balloon has a thinner profile, is shorter in length, easier to guide, and sturdily sets in the valve orifice during dilation, thanks to its hourglass shape. The technique's major limitation is the cost of the balloon.

Panels a–d in Figure 17.3 display the sequence of steps during an Inoue balloon mitral valvuloplasty. When performing PMV using the Inoue technique we use the stepwise technique under echocardiographic guidance. With this technique an initial balloon sizing 2 mm below the calculated reference balloon size is used. The optimal balloon size is calculated from an empirical formula based on the patient's height, which allows determination of the reference balloon size (maximum balloon volume = (patient's height in cm/10) + 10). This approach estimates reference balloon size, guides the selection of an appropriate balloon catheter that is nominally equal to or more frequently encompasses the reference balloon size, and serves as a guide to determine balloon size for the first inflation. Subsequently balloon size increments of 1 mm in both low and high pressure zones in low risk patients and of 0.5 mm in the high pressure zone in high risk scenarios (pre-existing MR or any suggestion of an increase in MR or severe subvalvular disease). The balloon high pressure zone refers to the last 2 mm range below an individual catheter balloon's nominal diameter (e.g., 26–28 mm in a 28 mm Inoue balloon catheter). Within these 2 mm the intraballoon pressure precipitously increases as the balloon diameter is increased from the low pressure zone. With the stepwise technique we use 2D or 3D echocardiography to assess changes in mitral regurgitation, commissure splitting, and changes in mitral valve area between balloon inflations. If mitral regurgitation is noted to increase after a balloon inflation, the procedure will be stopped even if less than an ideal result has been achieved.

Downsizing of the balloon catheter by switching to a catheter one size less than the calculated reference balloon size-matched size should be considered in the presence of balloon 'impasse.' This rare sign indicates that the catheter balloon, though deflated and properly aligned with the mitral orifice/apical axis, has been checked at the subvalvular lesion. This balloon impasse, in patients undergoing Inoue PMV, reflects severe obstructive subvalvular disease, even though echocardiographic evidence suggests otherwise, and portends severe mitral regurgitation if the usual balloon sizing method is used. Nevertheless, regardless of valve morphologic features, the initial balloon inflation is never performed within the high pressure zone.

Equally important during the Inoue PMV is the careful evaluation of the shape of the Inoue balloon in each of the balloon inflations. We should keep in mind that the Inoue balloon is associated with only 25% of bicommissural splitting. Therefore, if one of the balloon borders becomes flat during a given inflation it is likely that the balloon has successfully split one of the commissures and serious consideration should be given to stop the procedure then, as further increases in balloon volume more likely would result in damage of the mitral leaflets and the appearance of severe post-balloon mitral regurgitation (Figure 17.4). Our criteria for stopping the procedure are complete opening of at least one of the commissures with a valve area > 1 cm²/m² body surface area or > 1.5 cm², or the appearance of regurgitation or its increase by 25%.

Recently a technique of PMV using a newly designed metallic valvulotome was introduced (Figure 17.5). The device consists of a detachable metallic cylinder with two articulated bars screwed onto the distal end of a disposable catheter whose proximal end is connected to activating pliers. Squeezing the pliers opens the bars up to a maximum of 40 mm. The results with this device are at least comparable to those of the other balloon techniques of PMV. However, multiple uses after sterilization should markedly decrease procedural costs.

There is controversy as to whether the double balloon or Inoue technique of PMV provides superior immediate and long term results. We compared the immediate procedural and long term outcomes of patients undergoing PMV using the double balloon vs the Inoue techniques at the Massachusetts General Hospital. Seven hundred and thirty-four consecutive patients who underwent PMV using the double balloon ($n=621$) or Inoue technique ($n=113$) were studied. There were no statistically significant differences in baseline clinical and morphologic characteristics between the two groups of patients. The double balloon technique resulted in a superior immediate outcome, as reflected in a larger post-PMV mitral valve area (1.9 ± 0.7 vs 1.7 ± 0.6 cm²; $p=0.005$) and a lower incidence of 3+ mitral regurgitation post-PMV (5.4% vs 10.6%; $p=0.05$). This

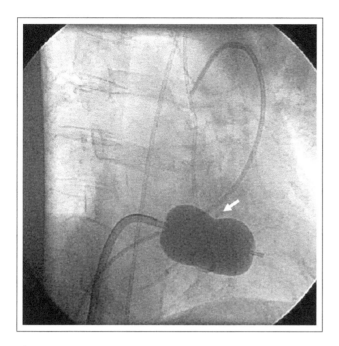

Figure 17.4
Full inflation of the Inoue balloon catheter shows a straight border inferiorly and an indentation in the upper border with commissural calcification. This image suggests that the postero-inferior commissure is open and the antero-lateral commissure is not. The procedure is completed as further attempt to open the antero-lateral commissure could result in severe mitral regurgitation.

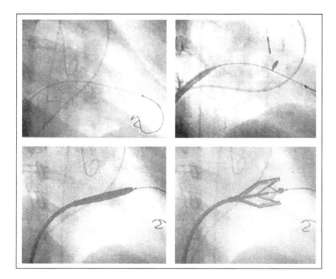

Figure 17.5
The Cribier metallic dilator technique. The device is advanced over a guidewire with its tip curlew in the ventricular apex. Squeezing the pliers opens the bars up to a maximum of 40 mm.

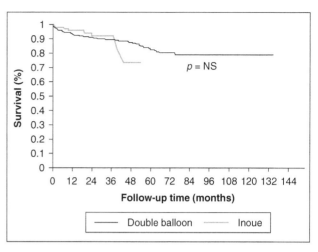

Figure 17.6
Kaplan–Meier survival curves of patients following percutaneous balloon mitral valvuloplasty with the double balloon and Inoue techniques.

superior immediate outcome of the double balloon technique was observed only in the group of patients with echocardiographic score ≤ 8 (post PMV mitral valve areas 2.1 ± 0.7 vs 1.8 ± 0.6; $p = 0.004$).

This early experience demonstrated that, compared with the Inoue technique, the double balloon technique resulted in a larger mitral valve area and a lesser degree of severe mitral regurgitation post-PMV. However, despite the difference in immediate outcome between both techniques, there were no significant differences in event-free survival at long term follow-up (Figures 17.6 and 17.7).

In a later study we analyzed the effect of the learning curve of the Inoue technique in the immediate and long term outcome of PMV. The learning curve of Inoue PMV was analyzed in 233 consecutive Inoue PMVs divided into two groups: 'early experience' ($n = 100$) and 'late experience' ($n = 133$). The results of the overall Inoue technique were compared with those of 659 PMVs performed with the double balloon technique. Baseline clinical and morphologic characteristics between early and late experience Inoue groups were similar. Post-PMV mitral valve area (1.9 ± 0.6 vs 1.7 ± 0.6; $p = 0.008$) and success rate (60% vs 75.9%; $p = 0.009$) were significantly higher in the late experience Inoue group. Furthermore, there was a trend for a lower incidence of severe post-PMV mitral regurgitation $\geq 3+$ in the late experience group (6.8% vs 12%; $p = 0.16$). Although the post-PMV mitral valve area was larger in the double balloon technique (1.94 ± 0.7 vs $1.81 \pm 0.6 \, \text{cm}^2$; $p = 0.01$), the success rate (71.3% vs 69.1%; $p = \text{NS}$), incidence of $\geq 3+$ mitral regurgitation (9% vs 9%), in-hospital complications, long-term survival, and event-free survival were similar with both techniques (Figures 17.5 and 17.6). We concluded that there is a significant learning curve for the Inoue technique of PMV and that both the Inoue and the double balloon techniques are equally effective techniques of PMV as they resulted in similar immediate success, in-hospital adverse events, long-term survival, and event-free survival.

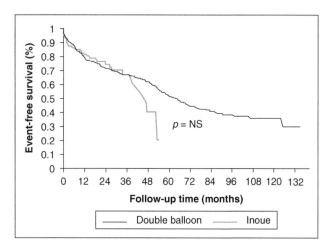

Figure 17.7
Kaplan–Meier event-free survival curves following percutaneous balloon mitral valvuloplasty with the double balloon and Inoue techniques.

In-hospital adverse events and complications

PMV complications are low and occur more frequently in patients with echocardiographic scores >8. Mortality and morbidity with PMV are low and similar to surgical commissurotomy. The failure rates of PMV range from 1 to 15%, and they reflect primarily the learning curve of the operators. The procedural mortality ranges from 0 to 3%. The incidence of hemopericardium varies from 0.5 to 12%. Embolism is encountered in 0.5 to 5% of cases. Severe mitral regurgitation is the most worrying complication. It occurs in 2 to 10% of patients and results from non-commissural leaflet tearing, primarily in cases with unfavorable anatomy, and even more so if there is a heterogeneous distribution of the morphologic abnormalities.[20–27] Surgery is often necessary later and can be conservative in cases with less severe valve deformity. Urgent surgery is seldom needed for complications (< 1% in experienced centers); it may be required for massive hemopericardium or, less frequently, for severe mitral regurgitation, leading to hemodynamic collapse or refractory pulmonary edema. Immediately after PMV, color Doppler echo shows small interatrial shunts in 40 to 80% of cases. The size of the defect is small as reflected in the pulmonary to systemic flow ratio of < 2:1 in the majority of patients. Older age, fluoroscopic evidence of mitral valve calcification, higher echocardiographic score, pre-PMV lower cardiac output, and higher NYHA class are the factors that predispose patients to develop left to right shunt post-PMV. Clinical, echocardiographic, surgical, and hemodynamic follow-up of patients with post-PMV left to right shunt demonstrated that the defect closed in 59%.

Persistent left to right shunt at follow-up is small (pulmonary to systemic flow ratio, QP/QS <2:1) and clinically well tolerated. In the series from the Massachusetts General Hospital there was one patient in whom the shunt remained significant at follow-up with evidence of hemodynamic compromise. This patient's residual atrial defect was closed with a clamshell device placed percutaneously using transcatheter techniques.

Clinical follow-up

We recently reported clinical follow-up information on 844 patients who underwent PMV at the Massachusetts General Hospital at a mean follow-up time of 4.2 ± 3.7 years. For the entire population, there were 110 deaths (25 non-cardiac), 234 mitral valve replacements, and 54 repeat PMV, accounting for a total of 398 patients with combined events (death, MVR, or redo PMV). Of the remaining 446 patients who were free of combined events, 418 (94%) were in NYHA class I or II. Follow-up events occurred less frequently in patients with an echo score ≤ 8 and included 51 deaths, 155 mitral valve replacements, and 39 redo PMV, accounting for a total of 245 patients with combined events at follow-up. Of the remaining 330 patients with an echo score equal to or less than 8 who were free of combined events, 312 (95%) were in NYHA class I or II. Follow-up events in patients with an echo score > 8 included 59 deaths, 79 mitral valve replacements, and 15 repeat PMV, accounting for a total of 153 patients with combined events at follow-up. Of the remaining 116 patients with echo score less than 8 who were free of any event, 105 (91%) were in NYHA class I or II.

Figure 17.8 shows estimated actuarial total survival curves for the overall population and for patients with an echo scores ≤ 8 and > 8. Actuarial survival rates throughout the follow-up period were significantly better in patients with an echo score ≤ 8. Survival rates were 82% for patients with an echo score ≤ 8 and 57% for patients with an echo score > 8 at a follow-up time of 12 years ($p < 0.001$). Survival rates were 82% and 56%, respectively, when only patients with successful PMV were included in the analysis. Figure 17.9 shows estimated actuarial total event free survival curves for the overall population and for patients with echo scores ≤ 8 and > 8. Event free survival (38% vs 22%; $p < 0.0001$) at 12 years' follow-up were also significantly higher for patients with an echo score ≤ 8. Event-free survival rates were 41% and 23%, respectively, when only patients with successful PMV were included in the analysis.

Cox regression analysis identified post-PMV MR $\geq 3+$, echo score > 8, age, prior commissurotomy, NYHA class IV, pre-PMV MR $\geq 2 +$, and post-PMV pulmonary artery pressure as independent predictors of combined events at long term follow-up.

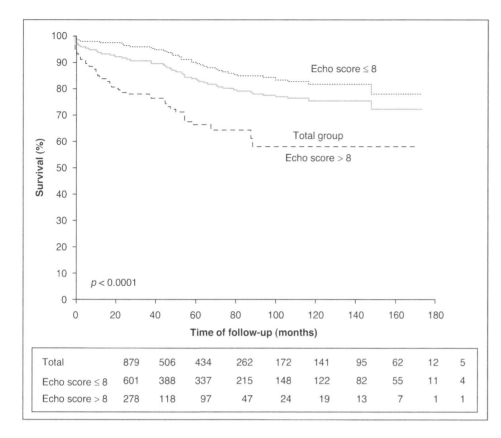

Figure 17.8
Kaplan–Meier survival estimates for all patients, and for patients with echo scores ≤8 and >8. Numbers at the bottom represent patients alive and uncensored at the end of each year of follow-up.

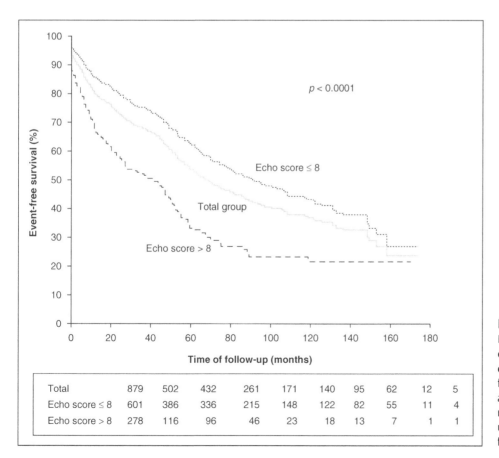

Figure 17.9
Kaplan–Meier event-free survival estimates (alive and free of MVR or redo PMV) for all patients, and for patients with echo scores ≤8 and >8. Numbers at the bottom represent patients alive and uncensored at each year of follow-up.

References

1. Inoue K, Owaki T, Nakamura T et al. Clinical application of transvenous mitral commissurotomy by a new balloon catheter. J Thorac Cardiovasc Surg 1984; 87: 394–402.

2. Lock JE, Kalilullah M, Shrivastava S et al. Percutaneous catheter commissurotomy in rheumatic mitral stenosis. N Engl J Med 1985; 313: 1515–18.

3. Palacios I, Block PC, Brandi S et al. Percutaneous balloon valvotomy for patients with severe mitral stenosis. Circulation 1987; 75: 778–84.

4. Al Zaibag M, Ribeiro PA, Al Kassab SA, Al Fagig MR. Percutaneous double balloon mitral valvotomy for rheumatic mitral stenosis. Lancet 1986; 1: 757–61.

5. Vahanian A, Michel PL, Cormier B et al. Results of percutaneous mitral commissurotomy in 200 patients. Am J Cardiol 1989; 63: 847–52.

6. McKay RG, Lock JE, Safian RD et al. Balloon dilatation of mitral stenosis in adults patients: postmortem and percutaneous mitral valvuloplasty studies: J Am Coll Cardiol 1987; 9: 723–31.

7. McKay CR, Kawanishi DT, Rahimtoola SH. Catheter balloon valvuloplasty of the mitral valve in adults using a double balloon technique. Early hemodynamic results. JAMA 1987; 257: 1753–61.

8. Abascal VM, O'Shea JP, Wilkins GT et al. Prediction of successful outcome in 130 patients undergoing percutaneous balloon mitral valvotomy. Circulation 1990; 82: 448–56.

9. Herrman HC, Wilkins GT, Abascal VM et al. Percutaneous balloon mitral valvotomy for patients with mitral stenosis: analysis of factors influencing early results. J Thorac Cardiovasc Surg 1988; 96: 33–8.

10. Rediker DE, Block PC, Abascal VM, Palacios IF. Mitral balloon valvuloplasty for mitral restenosis after surgical commissurotomy. J Am Coll Cardiol 1988; 2: 252–6.

11. Palacios IF, Block PC, Wilkins GT, Weyman AE. Follow-up of patients undergoing percutaneous mitral balloon valvotomy: analysis of factors determining restenosis. Circulation 1989; 79: 573–9.

12. Abascal VM, Wilkins GT, Choong CY et al. Echocardiographic evaluation of mitral valve structure and function in patients followed for at least 6 months after percutaneous balloon mitral valvuloplasty. J Am Coll Cardiol 1988; 12: 606–15.

13. Block PC, Palacios IF, Block EH et al. Late (two year) follow-up after percutaneous mitral balloon valvotomy. Am J Cardiol 1992; 69: 537–41.

14. Tuzcu EM, Block PC, Griffin BP et al. Immediate and long term outcome of percutaneous mitral valvotomy in patients 65 years and older. Circulation 1992; 85: 963–71.

15. Nobuyoshi M, Hamasaki N, Kimura T et al. Indications, complications, and short term clinical outcome of percutaneous transvenous mitral commissurotomy. Circulation 1989; 80: 782–92.

16. Chen CR, Cheng TO, Chen JY et al. Percutaneous mitral valvuloplasty with the Inoue balloon catheter. Am J Cardiol 1992; 70: 1455–8.

17. Hung JS, Chern MS, Wu JJ et al. Short and long term results of catheter balloon percutaneous transvenous mitral commissurotomy. Am J Cardiol 1991; 67: 854–62.

18. Cribier A, Eltchaninoff H, Koning R et al. Percutaneous mechanical mitral commissurotomy with a newly designed metalic valvulotome. Circulation 1999; 99: 793–9.

19. Wilkins GT, Weyman AE, Abascal VM et al. Percutaneous mitral valvotomy: an analysis of echocardiographic variables related to outcome and the mechanism of dilatation. Br Heart J 1988; 60: 299–308.

20. Palacios IF, Sanchez PL, Harrell LC et al. Which patients benefit from percutaneous mitral balloon valvuloplasty? Pre and post-valvuloplasty variables that predict 15 year outcome. Circulation 2002; 105(12): 1465–71.

21. Vahanian A, Palacios IF. Percutaneous approaches to valvular disease. Circulation 2004; 109(13): 1572–9.

22. Palacios IF. Techniques of ballon valvuloplasty for mitral strenosis. In: Robicsek F (ed). Cardiac Surgery: State of the art Reviews. Philadelphia, PA; Hanley R Belfus, Inc; 1991: 229–38.

23. Leon MN, Harrell LC, Simosa HF et al. Comparison of immediate and long-term results of mitral balloon valvotomy with the double balloon versus Inoue techniques. Am J Cardiol 1999; 83: 1356–63.

24. Sanchez PL, Harrell LC, Salas RE, Palacios IF. Learning curve of the Inoue technique of mitral balloon valvuloplasty. Am J Cardiol 2001; 88(6): 662–7.

25. Palacios IF. Farewell to surgical mitral commissurotomy for many patients. Circulation 1998; 97: 223–6.

26. Chen CR, Cheng TO, Chen JY et al. Long-term results of percutaneous mitral valvuloplasty for mitral stenosis. A follow-up study to 11 years in 202 patients. Cardiovasc Diagn 1966; 43: 132–9.

27. Hung JS, Lau KW, Lo PH et al. Complications of Inoue balloon mitral commissurotomy: impact of operators experience and evolving technique. Am Heart J 1999; 138: 114–21.

18

Pulmonary valve stenosis

P Syamasundar Rao

Introduction

Transcatheter therapy of valvar pulmonary stenosis is one of the first, if not the first, catheter interventions which have facilitated the application of catheter interventional technology to children, so that many children have benefited from less invasive treatment for structural congenital heart defects. In this chapter transcatheter management of pulmonary stenosis (PS) will be discussed.

Anatomy and pathophysiology

The pathologic features of the stenotic pulmonary valve vary;[1] the most commonly observed pathology is what is described as a 'dome-shaped' pulmonary valve. The fused pulmonary valve leaflets protrude from their attachment into the pulmonary artery as a conical, windsock-like structure. The size of the pulmonary valve orifice varies from a pinhole to several millimeters, most usually central in location, but can be eccentric. Raphae, presumably fused valve commissures, extend from the stenotic orifice to a variable distance down into the base of the dome-shaped valve. The number of the raphae may vary from zero to seven. Less common variants are unicuspid (unicommissural), bicuspid, and tricuspid valves. Thickening of the valve leaflets is seen, which may be due to an increase in valve spongeosa or due to excessive fibrous, collagenous, myxomatous, and elastic tissue. The valve annulus is abnormal in most cases with partial or complete lack of a fibrous backbone, thus a 'true' annulus may not be present.

Pulmonary valve ring hypoplasia and dysplastic pulmonary valves may be present in a small percentage of patients. Pulmonary valve dysplasia is characterized by thickened, nodular, and redundant valve leaflets with minimal or no commissural fusion, valve ring hypoplasia, and lack of post-stenotic dilatation of the pulmonary artery.[2] The obstruction is mainly related to thickened, myxomatous immobile pulmonary valve cusps and valve ring hypoplasia.

Changes secondary to pulmonary valve obstruction do occur, and include right ventricular muscle hypertrophy, proportional to the degree and duration of obstruction,[3] and dilatation of the main pulmonary artery, independent of the severity of obstruction, presumably related to a high velocity jet across the stenotic valve.[4]

Clinical features

The majority of children with valvar PS are asymptomatic and are detected because of a cardiac murmur heard on routine examination, although they can present with signs of systemic venous congestion (usually interpreted as congestive heart failure) due to severe right ventricular dysfunction or cyanosis because of right to left shunt across the atrial septum.

The right ventricular and the right ventricular outflow tract impulses are increased and a heave may be felt at the left lower and left upper sternal borders. A thrill may be felt at the left upper sternal border and/or in the suprasternal notch. The second heart sound is variable, depending upon the degree of obstruction. An ejection systolic click is heard in most cases of valvar stenosis. The click is heard best at the left lower, mid, and upper sternal borders and varies with respiration (decreases or disappears with inspiration). An ejection systolic murmur is heard best at the left upper sternal border and it radiates into the infraclavicular regions, axillae, and back. The intensity of the murmur may vary between grades II and V/VI; the intensity of the murmur is not necessarily related to the severity of the stenosis but rather its duration and time of peaking; the longer the murmur and the later it peaks, the more severe is the PS.

Indications for balloon pulmonary valvuloplasty

It is generally believed that indications for balloon pulmonary valvuloplasty are similar to those used for surgical pulmonary valvotomy, i.e., a moderate degree of pulmonary valve stenosis with a peak to peak gradient ≥ 50 mmHg with normal cardiac index.[5] Some workers use lesser gradients (gradient of 40 mmHg or right ventricular pressure of 50 mmHg) for intervention. Careful examination of all the available studies[5] suggested that there is only marginal reduction of right ventricular pressure if mild stenoses are dilated.[2] Natural history studies revealed that trivial and mild stenoses (< 50 mmHg gradient) are likely to remain mild at follow-up,[6] and an increase in gradient can easily be quantitated by echo Doppler studies at follow-up examination, and if an increase in gradient is documented, the patient could then undergo balloon dilatation. Based on these observations, I continue to advocate[7] that balloon dilatation should be performed only in patients with a peak to peak gradient > 50 mmHg.

Some workers have suggested that balloon dilatation should not be undertaken for very severe stenosis with right ventricular systolic pressure twice that in the left ventricle. In our own series,[8] 16 (23%) of 71 patients had right ventricular pressure twice that in the left ventricle and these children underwent successful balloon valvuloplasty. Therefore, it is believed that extreme stenosis is not a contraindication for balloon dilatation.

Pulmonary valve dysplasia has been considered by some workers as a relative contraindication for balloon dilatation. Based on our own experience[9] and that of others,[10] balloon valvuloplasty is the initial treatment of choice. Balloons that are 1.4 to 1.5 times the pulmonary valve annulus should probably be used in patients with dysplastic valves to achieve a good result.[9] But, more importantly, the determinant of a favorable result is the presence of commissural fusion.

In adult subjects with moderate to severe stenosis without symptoms, some authors were hesitant to recommend intervention.[11] However, based on poor response to exercise[12] and potential for development of myocardial fibrosis, I believe it is prudent to provide catheter-directed relief of the obstruction in all patients, including adults, with moderate to severe stenosis, irrespective of the symptoms.[13]

Surgical therapy

Until the early 1980s, surgical pulmonary valvotomy under cardiopulmonary bypass was the only treatment available, but at the present time relief of pulmonary valve obstruction can be accomplished by balloon pulmonary valvuloplasty. Indeed, at the present time balloon pulmonary valvuloplasty is the treatment of choice. Occasionally surgical intervention may become necessary when there is severe supravalvar stenosis, significant valve annulus hypoplasia, severely dysplastic pulmonary valves, or persistent and severe infundibular narrowing (most of this resolves spontaneously or with beta-blocker therapy[3,14]) despite successful balloon pulmonary valvuloplasty.

Historic aspects of balloon pulmonary valvuloplasty

The first attempt to relieve pulmonary valve obstruction by transcatheter methodology, to my knowledge, was in the early 1950s by Rubio-Alverez et al.[15,16] In 1979, Semb and his associates[17] employed a balloon-tipped angiographic (Berman) catheter to produce rupture of pulmonary valve commissures by rapidly withdrawing the inflated balloon across the pulmonary valve. More recently, Kan and her associates[18] applied the technique of Gruntzig et al[19] to relieve pulmonary valve obstruction by the radial forces of balloon inflation of a balloon catheter positioned across the pulmonic valve.

Technique

The diagnosis and assessment of pulmonary valve stenosis are made by the usual clinical, radiographic, electrocardiographic, and echo Doppler data. Once a moderate to severe obstruction is diagnosed, cardiac catheterization and cineangiography are performed percutaneously to confirm the clinical impression and to consider balloon dilatation of the pulmonary valve. It is important that a full explanation of the balloon dilatation procedure is given to the patients/parents, along with the potential complications. Such informed consent is essential, especially in view of the fact that acute complications can occur and long term results are limited. The technique of balloon pulmonary valvuloplasty involves positioning a balloon catheter across the stenotic valve, usually over an extra stiff exchange-length guidewire and inflating the balloon, thus producing valvotomy. Details of the technique will be discussed in the ensuing sections.

Pre-intervention non-invasive studies

Echo Doppler studies

Two-dimensional (2D) echocardiographic pre-cordial short and long axis and subcostal views are most useful in the evaluation of the pulmonary valve leaflets. Thickening and doming of the pulmonary valve leaflets can often be visualized.[20] Markedly thickened, nodular, and immobile pulmonary valve leaflets, suggestive of dysplastic pulmonary valves, may also be recognized. The pulmonary valve annulus can also be visualized and measured; the latter can be compared with normal values (or the Z score calculated) to determine whether the annulus is hypoplastic. Such measurements are also useful in the selection of balloon diameter during balloon valvuloplasty. Post-stenotic dilatation of the pulmonary artery can be imaged and the right ventricular size, wall thickness, and function can be evaluated by the 2D technique.

Pulsed, continuous wave, and color Doppler evaluation in conjunction with 2D echocardiography is most useful in confirming the clinical diagnosis and in quantitating the degree of obstruction. Pulsed Doppler interrogation of the right ventricular outflow tract with a sample volume moved across the pulmonary valve demonstrates an abrupt increase in peak Doppler flow velocity, suggesting pulmonary valve obstruction. In addition, the flow pattern in the main pulmonary artery is turbulent instead of being laminar. Color Doppler imaging will also show smooth, laminar subpulmonary flow (blue) with some flow acceleration (red) immediately beneath the pulmonary valve and turbulent (mosaic) flow beginning immediately distal to the pulmonary valve leaflets. Furthermore, a narrow jet of color flow disturbance can be visualized which should be used to align the continuous wave ultrasound beam to record maximum velocity. The angle of incidence between the ultrasound beam and color jet should be kept to a minimum. Two-dimensional and color flow directed continuous wave Doppler recordings from multiple transducer positions, including the pre-cordial short axis, high parasternal, and subcostal, should be performed for documenting the maximum velocity. Several studies have demonstrated the usefulness of peak Doppler velocities in predicting the catheter measured peak to peak gradients across the pulmonary valve. The peak instantaneous Doppler gradient may be calculated using a modified Bernoulli equation:

$$\Delta P = 4V^2$$

where, ΔP is the pressure gradient and V is the peak Doppler flow velocity in the main pulmonary artery.

Continuous wave and color Doppler interrogation for the tricuspid regurgitant jet is important to further confirm high right ventricular pressure. The right ventricular peak systolic pressure (RVP) may be estimated by using a modified Bernoulli equation:

$$RVP = 4V^2 + ERAP$$

where V is the peak tricuspid regurgitant jet velocity and ERAP is the estimated right atrial pressure (5 to 10 mmHg).

It is important that the Doppler study is performed when the patient is quiet and is in a resting state; young children and patients who are extremely anxious may have to be mildly sedated. It should be remembered that Doppler measurements represent peak instantaneous gradients whereas catheterization gradients are peak to peak gradients. It was initially thought that the peak instantaneous gradient is reflective of the peak to peak systolic gradient measured during cardiac catheterization; however, the peak instantaneous gradient overestimates the peak to peak gradient,

presumably related to a pressure recovery phenomenon.[21] In our experience, the catheter peak to peak gradient is somewhere in between the Doppler peak instantaneous and mean gradients.

Color Doppler and pulsed Doppler interrogation of the atrial septum is useful and may reveal a left to right or right to left shunt. Because of the high sensitivity of color Doppler, contrast echocardiography to document a right to left shunt is not routinely utilized.

Other non-invasive studies

Computed tomographic (CT) scan and magnetic resonance imaging (MRI) may demonstrate pulmonary valve stenosis, however the current state-of-the-art echo Doppler studies are more useful in diagnosing and quantitating pulmonary valve obstruction. Myocardial energy demands and perfusion may be evaluated by magnetic resonance spectroscopy and positron emission tomography, but at this time the clinical utility of these techniques in the management of pulmonic stenosis has not been established.

Sedation and anesthesia

I usually perform balloon pulmonary valvuloplasty with the patient sedated with a mixture of meperidine, promethazine, and chlorpromazine, given intramuscularly. If necessary, this is supplemented with intermittent doses of midazolam (versed) (0.05 to 0.1 mg/kg iv) and/or fentanyl (0.5 to 1.0 microgram/kg iv). General anesthesia with endotracheal ventilation is used in infants below the age of 3 months. Others use ketamine or general anesthesia for all interventional cases. However, institutional practices should be respected with regard to the type of sedation used and whether general anesthesia is employed.

Vascular access

The percutaneous femoral venous route is the most preferred entry site for balloon pulmonary valvuloplasty and should be used routinely. However, other sites such as the axillary,[22] jugular,[23] venous, or transhepatic[24] routes have been successfully used in the absence of femoral venous access. A 5 to 7 Fr sheath is inserted into the vein depending upon the age and size of the patient as well as the anticipated size of the balloon dilatation catheter. I usually use a 5 to 7 Fr Berman angiographic catheter to acquire the hemodynamic and angiographic data.

An arterial line (3 Fr in infants, 4 Fr in children, and 5 Fr in adolescents and adults) is inserted percutaneously into the femoral artery to continuously monitor the arterial blood pressure and to intermittently monitor oxygen saturation.

Hemodynamic assessment

Measurement of right ventricular and pulmonary artery pressures along with the peak to peak gradient across the pulmonary valve is performed. This peak to peak gradient is used to assess the severity of pulmonary valve obstruction. Calculation of the pulmonary valve area by the Gorlin formula has been advocated by some workers, but because of multiple assumptions that must be made during calculation and because of limitations in applying this formula to calculate the pulmonary valve area,[25] we do not routinely calculate it. Instead, we utilize peak to peak pulmonary valve gradients to assess the severity of obstruction after ensuring that the cardiac index is within the normal range.

If it is not possible to advance the Berman angiographic catheter into the pulmonary artery across the pulmonary valve, the catheter is exchanged with either a multi-purpose catheter or a right coronary artery catheter to obtain the pulmonary valvar gradients. Some cardiologists use a cobra catheter for this purpose. Whereas recording of pressure pullbacks is considered important, sometimes, when it is extremely difficult to cross the pulmonic valve, it may not be prudent to perform such a pullback tracing. In such instances, the separately recorded right ventricular and pulmonary arterial pressures are used to calculate the gradient.

Simultaneous recording of the right ventricular and femoral artery pressures is also undertaken. This also helps assess the severity of pulmonary valve obstruction; a right ventricular peak systolic pressure ≥ 75% of the peak systolic systemic pressure is considered significant.

Recordings of the heart rate, systemic pressure, and cardiac index are made to ensure that a change in the transpulmonary gradient is not related to a change in cardiac output, but is indeed related to balloon pulmonary valvuloplasty. During the initial phases of the development of this procedure we were diligent to record the cardiac index either by the thermodilution technique or by the Fick technique with measured oxygen consumption. We no longer undertake these, but rely on the Fick technique without measuring oxygen consumption.

Angiography

Biplane right ventricular cineangiograms in a sitting-up (antero-posterior camera tilted to 15° left anterior oblique, LAO, and 35° cranial) and lateral views (Figures 18.1a and 18.2a) are performed to confirm the site of obstruction, to evaluate the size and function of the right ventricle, and to measure the pulmonary valve annulus, preparatory to balloon pulmonary valvuloplasty. We use a Berman angiographic catheter for the right ventriculogram, with the inflated balloon positioned in the right ventricular apex.

Additional cineangiograms from other locations are not necessary unless the echocardiographic and hemodynamic

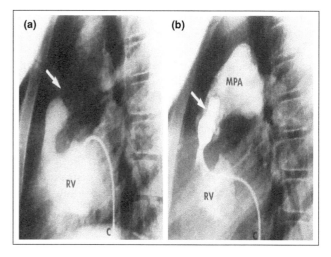

Figure 18.1
Selected frames from lateral views of right ventricular (RV) cineangiograms before (a) and after (b) balloon pulmonary valvuloplasty. Note extremely thin jet (arrow) prior to balloon dilatation (a), which increased to a much wider jet (arrow) after valvuloplasty (b), opacifying the main pulmonary artery (MPA). C, catheter. (Reproduced from Rao,[48] with permission from the publisher.)

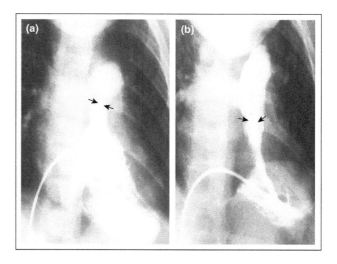

Figure 18.2
Selected cineangiographic frames from a 'sitting-up' view (15° left anterior oblique and 40° cranial) of a right ventricular angiogram prior to (a) and 15 minutes following (b) balloon pulmonary valvuloplasty. Note the thin jet of contrast material passing through the narrowed pulmonary valve (arrows in a) which has markedly increased after valvuloplasty (arrows in b). (Reproduced from Rao,[49] with permission from the publisher.)

data require exclusion of other abnormalities. Selective left ventricular angiography and coronary arteriography may be performed in patients older than 50 years, depending on the institutional policy, or in patients with suspected coronary artery disease.

Catheters/wires preparatory to balloon dilatation

Positioning a guide in the distal right or left pulmonary artery or in the descending aorta in neonates is a necessary prerequisite for undertaking balloon valvuloplasty. If the balloon angiographic (Berman) catheter easily crosses the pulmonary valve, we replace this catheter with the same French size balloon wedge catheter and advance it across the pulmonary valve. If the balloon angiographic (Berman) catheter is not easily advanced across the pulmonary valve, a 4 or 5 Fr multi-purpose (multi A2 – Cordis) catheter is positioned in the right ventricular outflow tract and a soft-tipped guidewire is used to cross the pulmonary valve. My personal preference is a 0.035 inch Benston straight guidewire (Cook). In neonates and young infants, a 0.014 inch coronary guidewire with a floppy end is used to cross the pulmonary valve. Instead of the multi-purpose catheter, a 4 or 5 Fr right coronary artery catheter, 4 Fr angled Glidecath catheter, or a cobra catheter may be used to cross the pulmonary valve. Once the guidewire is across the pulmonary valve the catheter is advanced into the distal right or left pulmonary artery or into the descending aorta via the patent ductus arteriosus. The catheter is then advanced over the guidewire, again into the distal right or left pulmonary artery or into the descending aorta. The catheter is left in place and the guidewire removed slowly and replaced with a guidewire that is suited to position the balloon dilatation catheter.

Balloon dilatation catheters

A variety of balloon angioplasty catheters have been used in the past. Initially balloon angioplasty catheters manufactured by Medi-Tech (Watertown, MA), Mansfield Scientific (Boston, MA), Surgimed (Oakland, NJ), Cook, Inc (Bloomington, IN), and Schneider-Medintag (Zurich, Switzerland) were utilized for balloon dilatation, depending on the availability at a given institution. Subsequently, specifically designed catheters such as XXL (Boston Scientific, Natick, MA), Ultrathin (Boston Scientific, Natick, MA), Diamond (Boston Scientific, Natick, MA), Marshal (Meditech, Watertown, MA), Maxi LD, Opta LP, and Opta Pro (Cordis Endovascular, Warren, NJ), PowerFlex (Cordis Endovascular, Warren, NJ), Tyshak I, II, Z-Med, Z-Med II, and Mullins catheters (NuMed, Hopkinton, NY), and others have been used. Currently, most cardiologists, including our group, use Tyshak II balloon angioplasty catheters for balloon pulmonary valvuloplasty because of their low profile, allowing their passage through small sized sheaths, and the ease with which they track over the guidewire. A number of other balloon dilatation catheters including Tyshak X, Z-Med X, Z-Med II X, and Mullins X (NuMed) have since been designed and are available commercially. The cited theoretic advantages of these catheters, however, have not been validated. The diameter and length of the balloon and number of balloons used for valvuloplasty are important and a discussion will follow.

Balloon diameter

The initial recommendations were to use a balloon that is 1.2 to 1.4 times the pulmonary valve annulus. These recommendations are formulated on the basis of immediate[26] and immediate as well as follow-up[27–29] results. Balloons larger than 1.5 times the pulmonary valve annulus should not be used because of the damage to the right ventricular outflow tract such large balloons may produce.[30] Furthermore, such large balloons do not have an advantage beyond that produced by balloons that are 1.2 to 1.4 times the annular size.[28,29] However, large balloons with a balloon/annulus ratio of 1.4 to 1.5 may be used when dilating dysplastic pulmonary valves.[9]

While the recommendation to use balloons 1.2 to 1.4 times the annulus is generally followed, recent reports of pulmonary insufficiency at late follow-up[31–35] raised concerns regarding the balloon size.[36–38] Based on detailed analysis of all the available data,[36–38] I recommended that we strive for a balloon/annulus ratio of 1.2 to 1.25 instead of the previously recommended 1.2 to 1.4. Such smaller balloons are likely to result in good relief of pulmonary valve obstruction while at the same time may help to prevent significant pulmonary insufficiency at late follow-up.

Balloon length

We generally use 20 mm long balloons in neonates and infants, 30 mm long balloons in children, and 40 mm long balloons in adolescents and adults. There are no data either from our own series or from the literature to assess whether a given length balloon is better than other lengths in producing a more successful relief of obstruction. With shorter balloons it is difficult to maintain the balloon center across the pulmonary valve annulus during balloon inflation. Longer balloons may impinge upon the tricuspid valve, causing tricuspid insufficiency,[39] or on the conduction system, causing heart block.[40] Consequently, use of 20, 30, and 40 mm long balloons for neonates and infants, children, and adolescents and adults, respectively, appears reasonable.

Number of balloons

When the pulmonary valve annulus is too large to dilate with a single balloon, valvuloplasty with simultaneous inflation of two balloons across the pulmonary valve (Figure 18.3) may be performed. When two balloons are

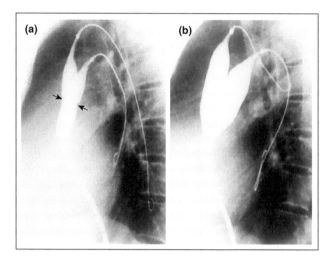

Figure 18.3
Selected cine frames of two balloon catheters placed across the pulmonary valve showing 'waisting' of the balloons (arrows in a) during the initial phases of balloon inflation which was completely abolished after complete inflation of the balloons (b). (Reproduced from Rao,[49] with permission from the publisher.)

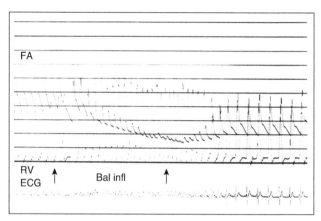

Figure 18.4
Simultaneous recording of the right ventricular (RV) and femoral artery (FA) pressures during balloon dilatation of the stenotic pulmonary valve. Note the marked increase in RV pressure, presumably related to complete obstruction of the RV. There is a simultaneous fall in FA pressure, again related to complete obstruction of the RV during balloon valvuloplasty. Following deflation of the balloon, the FA pressure returns towards normal. The 10 second period of balloon inflation (Bal infl) is marked with arrows. (Reproduced from Rao,[49] with permission from the publisher.)

utilized, the following formula may be used to calculate the effective balloon size:[27]

$$\frac{D_1 + D_2 + \pi \left(\dfrac{D_1}{2} + \dfrac{D_2}{2} \right)}{\pi}$$

where D_1 and D_2 are the diameters of the balloons used. This formula has been further simplified:[41]

$$\text{effective balloon diameter} = 0.82\,(D_1 + D_2)$$

Some cardiologists advocate the use of double balloon valvuloplasty instead of single balloon valvuloplasty,[42] especially for adult patients. We have compared the results of single balloon with double balloon valvuloplasty.[43] When equivalent balloon/valve annulus ratios are used, the results of double balloon valvuloplasty, though excellent, are comparable to, but not superior to those observed with single balloon valvuloplasty.[43,44] Furthermore, the double balloon technique does indeed prolong the procedure and involves an additional femoral venous site and the attendant potential complications. In addition, the availability of large diameter balloons carried on catheters with relatively small shaft sizes facilitates the use of a single balloon instead of two balloons.

Bifoil and trefoil balloons

Because of complete obstruction of the right ventricle with a single balloon during balloon inflation, there is necessarily systemic hypotension (Figure 18.4). However, during the double balloon procedure the right ventricular output may continue in between the balloons; this is one of the reasons for

recommending the double balloon technique in that it produces less hypotension.[42] Bifoil and trefoil balloon catheters[45–47] may serve this purpose in that they may allow (at least theoretically) right ventricular output during balloon inflation. But because of the fact that we use balloons larger than the pulmonary valve annulus, the theoretic advantage cited does not exist in that there is no space between the balloons and the pulmonary valve annulus. Furthermore, the bifoil and trefoil balloon catheter shafts are bulky, making it difficult to position the catheters across the pulmonary valve. In addition, our limited experience (Figure 18.5) suggests that the advantage of less hypotension during valvuloplasty is minimal.[44,48,49] Instead, we suggest short periods (5 seconds) of balloon inflation so that the hypotension is less severe and recovers faster (Figure 18.6).[48,49]

Pressure, number, and duration of balloon inflation

The recommendations for balloon inflation pressure (2.0 to 8.5 atm), number of inflations (one to four), and duration of inflation (5 to 60 seconds) varied from one investigator to the other, but without many data to support such contentions. We have examined these parameters from our study subjects.[44,48] The balloon inflation characteristics in the group with good results were compared with those with poor results. No significant differences were found, suggesting that the outcome of valvuloplasty is not related to the balloon

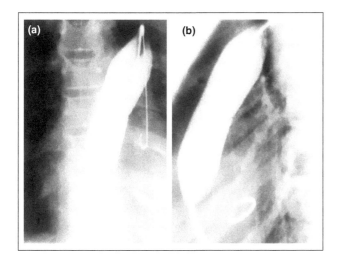

Figure 18.5
Trefoil balloon across the pulmonary valve in postero-anterior (a) and lateral views (b) is shown. Note the indentation of the balloon in the center produced by the pulmonary valve annulus. A guidewire in the left pulmonary artery in (a) and pigtail catheter in the left ventricle in (a) and (b) are shown. (Reproduced from Rao,[49] with permission from the publisher.)

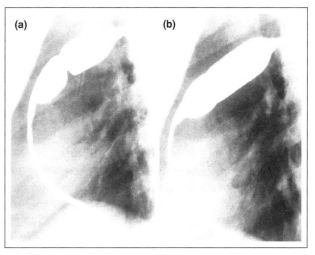

Figure 18.7
Selected cineradiographic frames of a balloon dilatation catheter placed across a stenotic pulmonary valve. Note 'waisting' of the balloon during the initial phases of the balloon inflation (a), which was almost completely abolished during the later phases of balloon inflation (b). (Reproduced from Rao,[49] with permission from the publisher.)

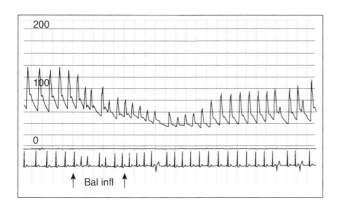

Figure 18.6
Femoral artery pressure during balloon inflation for pulmonary valvuloplasty in which a 5 second balloon inflation is used. Note the fall in femoral artery pressure, but the decrease in pressure is not as severe as with a 10 second inflation (Figure 18.4). Also, the return of pressure towards normal is not as slow as with 10 second inflation (Figure 18.4). The 5 second balloon inflation (Bal infl) is marked with arrows. (Reproduced from Rao,[49] with permission from the publisher.)

inflation characteristics. We have also scrutinized the data[44,48] with an arbitrary division of maximum pressure, number of balloon inflations, and duration of balloon inflation and determined that higher pressure, larger number of inflations, and longer duration of balloon inflation did not favorably influence residual gradients at follow-up, especially when the effect of the balloon/annulus ratio is removed.

Based on these and other considerations, we would recommend balloon inflation at or below the level of balloon burst pressure stated by the manufacturer, and will continue balloon inflation until the waisting of the balloon disappears (Figure 18.7). The duration of inflation is kept as short as possible, usually just until after the waisting disappears. Shorter balloon inflation cycles produce less hypotension and a more rapid return of pressures towards normal (Figures 18.4 and 18.6). We usually perform one additional balloon inflation after disappearance of waisting is demonstrated, to ensure adequate valvuloplasty.

Balloon valvuloplasty procedure (step by step)

1. Clinical and echocardiographic diagnosis of moderate to severe valvar pulmonary stenosis.
2. Informed consent.
3. Confirmation of the severity of the stenosis by hemodynamic measurements: gradients across the pulmonary valve and/or comparison of the right ventricular pressure with systemic pressure.
4. Right ventricular angiography in a sitting-up (15° LAO and 35° cranial) and straight lateral views.
5. Measurement of the pulmonary valve annulus is undertaken in both views and an average of these is calculated. If the valve annulus cannot be clearly identified, the echocardiographic measurement of the valve annulus may be used.

6. Selection of the balloon catheter to be used is made. An inflated diameter is selected such that it is 1.2 to 1.25 times the pulmonary valve annulus, as detailed in the preceding section. The length of the balloon should be 20 to 40 mm depending upon the patient's age and size, also as discussed in the preceding section.

7. If a femoral arterial line is not already in place, an arterial line is placed into the femoral artery (3 Fr in neonates and infants, 4 Fr in children, and 5 Fr in adolescents and adults) for monitoring of arterial pressure continuously. Heart rate, blood pressure, respirations, and pulse oximetry are also continuously monitored throughout the procedure.

8. We do not routinely administer heparin for pulmonary valve dilatations, but, if there is an intracardiac communication (patent foramen ovale or an atrial septal defect), we administer heparin (100 units/kg intravenously). If the procedure lasts for more than 30 minutes, activated clotting times (ACTs) are measured and maintained between 200 and 250 seconds.

9. A 4 to 6 Fr multi-purpose (multi A-2 [Cordis]) catheter is introduced into the femoral venous sheath and advanced across the pulmonary valve and the tip of the catheter is positioned in the distal left (preferable) or right pulmonary artery. In neonates and young infants the catheter may be positioned in the descending aorta via the ductus; this will increase the stability of the wire and may make it easier to pass the balloon catheter across the pulmonary valve. The type of catheter used for crossing the pulmonary valve varies – balloon wedge, right coronary artery catheter, cobra catheter, or other – dependent upon the operator's choice and the patient's anatomy. The use of soft-tipped guidewires to assist crossing the pulmonary valve was alluded to in the preceding section.

10. A 0.014 to 0.035 inch J-tipped, exchange length, extra stiff guidewire is passed through the catheter already in place and the catheter is removed. The selection of the wire diameter is dependent upon the selected balloon dilatation catheter. In difficult cases, a super stiff, short, soft-tipped Amplatzer guidewire (Meditech) may be used.

11. If the size of the sheath in the femoral vein does not accommodate the selected balloon angioplasty catheter, the sheath may be upsized to the appropriate size at this point. Alternatively, this may be undertaken prior to positioning the catheter across the pulmonary valve.

12. The selected balloon angioplasty catheter is advanced over the guidewire, but within the sheath, and positioned across the pulmonary valve. The bony landmarks, namely, ribs, sternum, or other fixed landmarks, are used for this purpose. A frozen video frame of the right ventricular cineangiogram displayed on the screen is helpful in this regard.

13. At times it may be difficult to position an appropriately sized balloon angioplasty catheter across the severely

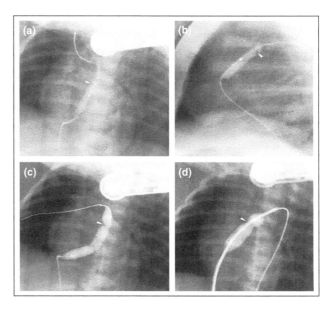

Figure 18.8
Selected cineradiographic frames demonstrating the use of progressively larger balloons in a 1-day-old infant with critical pulmonary stenosis. Initially, a 0.014 inch coronary guidewire was advanced into the pulmonary artery via a 5 Fr multi-A2 catheter (Cordis) positioned in the right ventricular outflow tract. A 3.5 Fr catheter carrying a 4 mm diameter balloon was positioned across the pulmonary valve. Postero–anterior (a) and lateral (b) view cine frames showing waisting (arrows) of the balloon during the initial phases of balloon inflation. After two balloon inflations, this balloon catheter was replaced with a 5 Fr catheter carrying a 6 mm diameter balloon (c) and finally a 5 Fr catheter (d) carrying an 8 mm diameter balloon. (Reproduced from Rao and Thapar,[53] with permission from the publisher.)

stenotic pulmonary valve, especially in neonates. In such instances we use smaller, 3 to 6 mm diameter balloon catheters initially to pre-dilate, then use larger, more appropriately sized balloon catheters (Figure 18.8).

14. The balloon is inflated with diluted contrast material (1 in 4) using any of the commercially available inflators, while monitoring the pressure of inflation. The inflation pressure is gradually increased up to the manufacturer's recommended pressure or until the balloon waist disappears. If the balloon is not appropriately centered across the pulmonary valve, the position of the catheter is re-adjusted and balloon inflation repeated. Once satisfactory balloon inflation is achieved, one more balloon inflation may be performed as per the operator's preference.

15. The balloon catheter is removed, leaving the guidewire in place.

Post-balloon protocol

Following balloon valvuloplasty, measurement of the pressure gradient across the pulmonary valve, pulmonary and femoral arterial oxygen saturations, and simultaneous femoral artery and right ventricular pressures are undertaken to assess the result of valvuloplasty. Either a multi-track catheter[50] or a Tuohy–Borst is used to record the pressure gradients across the pulmonary valve so that the guidewire is left in place across the pulmonary valve while the results of valvuloplasty are evaluated. If the result is not satisfactory (peak to peak valvar gradient in excess of 50 mmHg), a repeat dilatation with a larger balloon (2 mm larger than the first) is undertaken. Finally, the catheter and guidewire are removed, the Berman angiography catheter is repositioned in the right ventricular apex, and an angiogram is performed to evaluate the mobility of the pulmonary valve leaflets, to visualize the jet of contrast across the dilated pulmonary valve (Figures 18.1 and 18.2), to detect infundibular stenosis, and to discern any complications such as tricuspid insufficiency. We do not routinely perform echocardiography in the catheterization laboratory.

Pitfalls, problems and complications

Problems

The balloon may not be truly across the pulmonary valve during balloon inflation. It is important to ensure that the balloon is indeed across the valve. The waisting of the balloon may be produced by supravalvar stenosis or infundibular constriction. When in doubt, centering the balloon at various locations across the right ventricular outflow region may become necessary.

Acute complications

Complications during and immediately after balloon valvuloplasty have been remarkably minimal; the VACA registry reported a 0.24% death rate and 0.35% major complication rate[51] from the 822 balloon pulmonary valvuloplasty procedures from 26 institutions, attesting to the relative safety of the procedure. The study group involved the initial experience of many of the centers participating in the data collection and, with increasing experience, the complication rate should even be lower at the present time.

Transient bradycardia, premature beats, and a fall in systemic pressure during balloon inflation have been uniformly noted by all workers. These abnormalities return rapidly to normal following balloon deflation (Figures 18.4 and 18.6). Systemic hypotension may be minimal in the presence of a patent foramen ovale[52] because of a right to left shunt across it, filling the left ventricle. Use of the double balloon technique or use of bifoil or trefoil balloons has been suggested to circumvent this problem, but, as discussed in the preceding section, use of a short period of balloon inflation may help to reduce the degree and duration of hypotension.

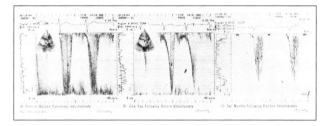

Figure 18.9
Doppler flow velocity recordings from the main pulmonary artery prior to (left), and 1 day (center), and 10 months (right) after successful balloon pulmonary valvuloplasty. Note that there is no significant fall in the peak flow velocity on the day after balloon procedure, but there is a characteristic triangular pattern, indicative of infundibular obstruction. At 10 month follow-up, the flow velocity decreased, suggesting resolution of infundibular obstruction. (Reproduced with permission from Thapar and Rao,[3] with permission from the publisher.)

Blood loss requiring transfusion has been reported, but with the better catheter/sheath systems that are currently available, the blood loss is minimal. Complete right bundle branch block, transient or permanent heart block, cerebrovascular accident, loss of consciousness, cardiac arrest, convulsions, balloon rupture at high balloon inflation pressures, rupture of tricuspid valve papillary muscle, and pulmonary artery tears, though rare, have been reported. Some of these complications may be unavoidable. However, meticulous attention to the technique, use of the appropriate diameter and length of the balloon, avoiding high balloon inflation pressures, and short inflation/deflation cycles may prevent or reduce the complications.

Development of severe infundibular obstruction has been reported. Infundibular gradients occur in nearly 30% of patients; the older the age and the higher the severity of obstruction, the greater is the prevalence of infundibular reaction.[3] When the residual infundibular gradient is ≥50 mmHg, beta-blockade therapy is generally recommended.[3,14] Infundibular obstruction regresses to a great degree at follow-up (Figures 18.9 and 18.10), just as has been demonstrated for infundibular reaction following surgical valvotomy, with a rare patient requiring surgical intervention. Issues related to the significance of infundibular obstruction and its management are discussed in greater detail elsewhere.[3,14,53]

Transient prolongation of the QTc and the development of premature ventricular contractions following balloon pulmonary valvuloplasty have been reported, causing concern that an R-on-T phenomenon may develop and produce ventricular arrhythmia. Rare cases of ventricular arrhythmia have been reported; however, none of the patients from our large series and many other studies were known to develop significant ventricular arrhythmia. Nonetheless, monitoring the patients following balloon valvuloplasty is warranted.

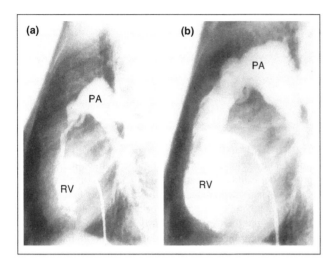

Figure 18.10
Selected frames from a lateral view of the right ventricular (RV) cineangiogram showing severe infundibular stenosis (a) immediately following balloon valvuloplasty (corresponding to Figure 18.9, center). At 10 months after balloon valvuloplasty the right ventricular outflow tract (b) is wide open and corresponds to Figure 18.9, right. Peak to peak pulmonary valve gradient was 20 mmHg and there was no infundibular gradient. PA, pulmonary artery. (Reproduced from Thapar and Rao,[3] with permission from the publisher.)

Complications at follow-up

Femoral venous occlusion and development of restenosis and pulmonary insufficiency have been noted. Between 7 and 19% of the patients may develop femoral venous obstruction;[54] the femoral venous obstruction is more likely in small infants. Recurrent pulmonary valve obstruction may occur in about 8% of patients and repeat balloon valvuloplasty may help relieve the residual or recurrent obstruction.[55] Causes of restenosis have been identified.[56] If the issues related to the technique are the reason for recurrence, repeat balloon valvuloplasty is useful. If the substrate (dysplastic valves without commissural fusion, supravalvar pulmonary artery stenosis, or severe fixed infundibular obstruction) is the problem, surgical intervention may become necessary. Long term follow-up data of balloon pulmonary valvuloplasty, reviewed in detail elsewhere,[32,36,38] indicate development of pulmonary insufficiency (PI); the frequency and severity of PI increase with time. From our study group, 70 of 80 (88%) had PI at long term follow-up, while only 10% had PI prior to balloon valvuloplasty.[31] Similar experiences documenting a high incidence of PI have been reported by other workers in the field.[32,38] Although none of our patients[31] or other patients reported by several other cardiologists[32,37] required pulmonary valve replacement for PI, 6% of patients followed by Berman et al.[33] developed severe PI, requiring (or requiring consideration for) pulmonary valve replacement. Development of

substantial PI at late follow-up is an important observation, and attempts to discern causes of late PI and devise methods to prevent such problems, as well as careful long term follow-up studies to confirm these observations, are warranted.

Post-catheter management

We usually perform an electrocardiogram and an echocardiogram on the morning following the procedure. Clinical, electrocardiographic, and echo Doppler evaluation at 1, 6, and 12 months after the procedure and yearly thereafter is generally recommended. Regression of right ventricular hypertrophy on the electrocardiogram following balloon dilatation has been well documented[57] and the electrocardiogram is a useful adjunct in the evaluation of follow-up results. However, electrocardiographic evidence for hemodynamic improvement does not become apparent until 6 months after valvuloplasty. The Doppler gradient is generally reflective of the residual obstruction and is a useful and reliable non-invasive monitoring tool.[13,31,48,49]

References

1. Gikonyo BM, Lucus RV, Edwards JE. Anatomic features of congenital pulmonary valvar stenosis. Pediatr Cardiol 1987; 8: 109–15.
2. Koretzky ED, Moller JH, Korns ME et al. Congenital pulmonary stenosis resulting from dysplasia of the valve. Circulation 1969; 60: 43–53.
3. Thapar MK, Rao PS. Significance of infundibular obstruction following balloon valvuloplasty for valvar pulmonic stenosis. Am Heart J 1989; 118: 99–103.
4. Rodbard S, Ikeda K, Montes M. Mechanisms of post-stenotic dilatation. Circulation 1963; 28: 791–8.
5. Rao PS. Indications for balloon pulmonary valvuloplasty. Am Heart J 1988; 116: 1661–2.
6. Nugent EW, Freedom RM, Nora JJ et al. Clinical course of pulmonic stenosis. Circulation 1977; 56 (Suppl I): I–18–47.
7. Rao PS. Balloon pulmonary valvuloplasty. Cathet Cardiovasc Diagn 1997; 40: 427–8.
8. Rao PS. Percutaneous balloon pulmonary valvuloplasty. In: Cheng T, ed. Percutaneous Balloon Valvuloplasty. New York: Igaku-Shion Med Publishers 1992: 365–420.
9. Rao PS. Balloon dilatation in infants and children with dysplastic pulmonary valves: short-term and intermediate-term results. Am Heart J 1988; 116: 1168–73.
10. Marantz PM, Huhta JC, Mullins CE et al. Results of balloon valvuloplasty in typical and dysplastic pulmonary valve stenosis: Doppler echocardiographic follow-up. J Am Coll Cardiol 1988; 12: 476–9.
11. Johnson LW, Grossman W, Dalen JE, Dexter L. Pulmonary stenosis in the adult: long-term follow-up results. New Engl J Med 1972; 287: 1159–63.
12. Krabill KA, Wang Y, Einzid S, Moller JH. Rest and exercise hemodynamics in pulmonary stenosis: comparison of children and adults. Am J Cardiol 1985; 36: 360–5.
13. Rao PS. Pulmonary valve disease. In: Alpert JS, Dalen JE, Rahimtoola S, eds. Valvular Heart Disease. 3rd edition. Philadelphia, PA: Lippincott Raven, 2000: 339–76.
14. Fontes VF, Esteves CA, Eduardo J et al. Regression of infundibular hypertrophy after pulmonary valvotomy for pulmonic stenosis. Am J Cardiol 1988; 62: 977–9.

15. Rubio-Alvarez V, Limon-Lason R, Soni J. Valvulotomias intracardiacas por medio de un cateter. Arch Inst Cordiol Mexico 1952; 23: 183–92.
16. Rubio-Alvarez V, Limon-Lason R. Treatment of pulmonary valvular stenosis and tricuspid stenosis using a modified catheter. Second World Congress of Cardiology. Washington, DC, program abstract, 1954: II: 205.
17. Semb BKH, Tijonneland S, Stake G et al. 'Balloon valvulotomy' of congenital pulmonary valve stenosis with tricuspid valve insufficiency. Cardiovasc Radiol 1979; 2: 239–41.
18. Kan JS, White RJ, Jr, Mitchell SE, Gardner TJ. Percutaneous balloon valvuloplasty: a new method for treating congenital pulmonary valve stenosis. New Engl J Med 1982; 307: 540–2.
19. Gruntzig AR, Senning A, Siegothaler WE. Non-operative dilatation of coronary artery stenosis: percutaneous transluminal coronary angioplasty. New Engl J Med 1979; 301: 61–8.
20. Weyman AE, Hurwitz RA, Girod DA. Cross-sectional echocardiographic visualization of the stenotic pulmonary valve. Circulation 1977; 56: 769–74.
21. Singh GK, Balfour IC, Chen S et al. Lesion specific pressure recovery phenomenon in pediatric patients: a simultaneous Doppler and catheter correlative study. J Am Coll Cardiol 2003; 41: 493A.
22. Sideris EB, Baay JE, Bradshaw RL et al. Axillary vein approach for pulmonary valvuloplasty in infants with iliac vein obstruction. Cathet Cardiovasc Diagn 1988; 15: 61–3.
23. Chaara A, Zniber L, Haitem NE et al. Percutaneous balloon valvuloplasty via the right internal jugular vein for valvar pulmonic stenosis with severe right ventricular failure. Am Heart J 1989; 117: 684–5.
24. Shim D, Lloyd TR, Cho KJ et al. Transhepatic cardiac catheterization in children: evaluation of efficacy and safety. Circulation 1995; 92: 1526–30.
25. Muster AJ, VanGrandelle A, Paul MH. Unequal pressures in central pulmonary arterial branches in patients with pulmonary stenosis: the influence of blood velocity and anatomy. Pediatr Cardiol 1982; 2: 7–14.
26. Radhke W, Keane JF, Fellows KE et al. Percutaneous balloon valvotomy of congenital pulmonary stenosis using oversized balloons. J Am Coll Cardiol 1986; 8: 909–15.
27. Rao PS. Influence of balloon size on short-term and long-term results of balloon pulmonary valvuloplasty. Texas Heart Institute J 1987; 14: 57–61.
28. Rao PS. How big a balloon and how many balloons for pulmonary valvuloplasty? Am Heart J 1988; 116: 577–80.
29. Rao PS. Further observations on the effect of balloon size on the short-term and intermediate-term results of balloon dilatation of the pulmonary valve. Br Heart J 1988; 60: 507–11.
30. Ring JC, Kulik TT, Burke BA et al. Morphologic changes induced by dilatation of pulmonary valve annulus with over-large balloons in normal newborn lamb. Am J Cardiol 1986; 52: 210–14.
31. Rao PS, Galal O, Patnana M et al. Results of three-to-ten-year follow-up of balloon dilatation of the pulmonary valve. Heart 1998; 80: 591–5.
32. Rao PS. Long-term follow-up results after balloon dilatation of pulmonic stenosis, aortic stenosis and coarctation of the aorta: a review. Progr Cardiovasc Dis 1999; 42: 59–74.
33. Berman W, Jr, Fripp RR, Raiser BD, Yabek SM. Significant pulmonary valve incompetence following oversize balloon pulmonary valvuloplasty in small infants: a long-term follow-up study. Cathet Cardiovasc Interven 1999; 48: 61–5.
34. Abu Haweleh A, Hakim F. Balloon pulmonary valvuloplasty in children: Jordanian experience. J Saudi Heart Assoc 2003; 15: 31–4.
35. Garty Y, Veldtman G, Lee K, Benson L. Late outcomes after pulmonary valve balloon dilatation in neonates, infants and children. J Invas Cardiol 2005; 17: 318–22.
36. Rao PS. Late pulmonary insufficiency after balloon dilatation of the pulmonary valve. Cathet Cardiovasc Interven 2000; 49: 118–19.
37. Rao PS. Balloon pulmonary valvuloplasty. J Saudi Heart Assoc 2003; 15: 1–4.
38. Rao PS. Balloon pulmonary valvuloplasty in children. J Invas Cardiol 2005; 17: 323–5.
39. Attia I, Weinhaus L, Walls JT, Lababidi Z. Rupture of tricuspid papillary muscle during balloon pulmonary valvuloplasty. Am Heart J 1987; 114: 1233–4.
40. Lo RNS, Lau KC, Leung MP. Complete heart block after balloon dilatation of congenital pulmonary stenosis. Br Heart J 1988; 59: 384–6.
41. Narang R, Das G, Dev V et al. Effect of the balloon–annulus ratio on the intermediate and follow-up results of pulmonary balloon valvuloplasty. Cardiology 1997; 88: 271–6.
42. Al Kasab S, Riberiro PA, Al Zaibag M et al. Percutaneous double balloon pulmonary valvotomy in adults: one-to-two year follow-up. Am J Cardiol 1988; 62: 822–5.
43. Rao PS, Fawzy ME. Double balloon technique for percutaneous balloon pulmonary valvuloplasty: comparison with single balloon technique. J Interven Cardiol 1988; 1: 257–62.
44. Rao PS. Balloon pulmonary valvuloplasty: a review. Clin Cardiol 1989; 12: 55–72.
45. Meier B, Friedli B, Oberhaensli I et al. Trefoil balloon for percutaneous valvuloplasty. Cathet Cardiovasc Diag 1986; 12: 277–81.
46. van den Berg EJM, Niemyeyer MG, Plokker TWM et al. New triple-lumen balloon catheter for percutaneous (pulmonary) valvuloplasty. Cathet Cardiovasc Diag 1986; 12: 352–6.
47. Meier B, Friedli L, von Segesser L. Valvuloplasty with trefoil and bifoil balloons and the long sheath technique. Herz 1988; 13: 1–13.
48. Rao PS. Balloon angioplasty and valvuloplasty in infants, children and adolescents. Current Problems in Cardiology. Chicago, IL: YearBook Medical Publishers, Inc, 1989; 14(8): 417–500.
49. Rao PS. Balloon pulmonary valvuloplasty for isolated pulmonic stenosis. In: Rao PS, ed. Transcatheter Therapy in Pediatric Cardiology. New York: Wiley-Liss, Inc, 1993: 59–104.
50. Bonnhoeffer P, Piechaud J, Stumper O et al. The multi-track angiography catheter: a new tool for complex catheterization in congenital heart disease. Heart 1996; 76: 173–7.
51. Stranger P, Cassidy SC, Girod DA et al. Balloon pulmonary valvuloplasty: results of the Valvuloplasty and Angioplasty of Congenital Anomalies Registry. Am J Cardiol 1990; 65: 775–83.
52. Shuck JW, McCormick DJ, Cohen IS et al. Percutaneous balloon valvuloplasty for pulmonary valve: role of right to left shunt through patent foramen ovale. J Am Coll Cardiol 1984; 4: 132–5.
53. Rao PS. Thapar MK. Balloon pulmonary valvuloplasty. Am Heart J 1991; 121: 1839.
54. Rao PS. Pulmonary valve in children. In: Sigwart U, Bertrand M, Serruys PW, eds. Handbook of Cardiovascular Interventions, New York: Churchill Livingstone, 1996: 273–310.
55. Rao PS, Galal O, Wilson AD. Feasibility and effectiveness of repeat balloon dilatation of restenosed obstructions following previous balloon valvuloplasty/angioplasty. Am Heart J 1996; 132: 403–7.
56. Rao PS, Thapar MK, Kutayli F. Causes of restenosis following balloon valvuloplasty for valvar pulmonic stenosis. Am J Cardiol 1988; 62: 979–82.
57. Rao PS, Solymar L. Electrocardiographic changes following balloon dilatation of valvar pulmonic stenosis. J Interven Cardiol 1988; 1: 189–97.

19

Pulmonary valve in cyanotic heart defects with pulmonary oligemia

P Syamasundar Rao

Cyanotic congenital heart defects, as a group, constitute up to 20 to 25% of all congenital heart defects. In cyanotic heart defects, the arterial oxygen desaturation is secondary to right to left shunting at the atrial, ventricular, or great artery level or because of transposition of the great arteries in which the deoxygenated blood recirculates through the body. In the latter group, balloon and/or blade atrial septostomy may be useful in augmenting admixture at the atrial level. These procedures have been described elsewhere in this book and will not be dealt with in this chapter. In the former group, obstruction to pulmonary blood flow by a stenotic or atretic pulmonary valve is an integral part of the cardiac malformation causing right to left shunt. The most common type of defect in this group is tetralogy of Fallot. Other defects include transposition of the great arteries, double outlet right (or left) ventricle, single ventricle, tricuspid atresia, ventricular inversion (corrected transposition of the great arteries), and other types of univentricular hearts, all with non-restrictive interventricular communication and severe pulmonary valve stenosis. These patients usually present with symptoms in the neonatal period or early in infancy. The degree of cyanosis and the level of hypoxemia determine the symptomatology. Physical findings and laboratory data (chest X-ray, electrocardiogram, and echocardiogram) depend upon the defect complex and are reasonably characteristic for each defect. The majority of cyanotic heart defects with pulmonary oligemia can be surgically treated. Total surgical correction may not be possible in some patients because of anatomic complexity. But yet, they may require palliation to augment pulmonary blood flow and to improve systemic arterial desaturation. Surgical aortopulmonary shunts have conventionally been utilized in these situations. Since the introduction of transluminal balloon dilatation techniques in children by Kan et al,[1] we and others[2–5] have utilized balloon pulmonary valvuloplasty to augment pulmonary blood flow instead of systemic to pulmonary artery shunt and successfully relieved pulmonary oligemia and systemic arterial hypoxemia.

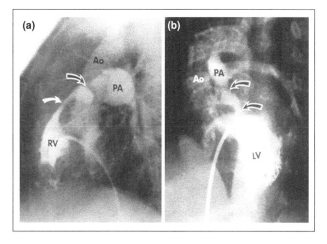

Figure 19.1
Selected cineangiographic frames from patients with tetralogy of Fallot (a) and dextro-transposition of the great arteries (b), demonstrating two sites of pulmonary outflow obstruction (two arrows). When the pulmonary valve obstruction is relieved by balloon valvuloplasty, the subvalvar obstruction remains and prevents flooding of the lungs. Ao, aorta; LV, left ventricle; PA, pulmonary artery; RV, right ventricle. (Reproduced from Rao et al,[6] with permission from the authors and publisher.)

The indications for balloon valvuloplasty that we have used[4,6] were cardiac defects not amenable to surgical correction at the age and size at the time of presentation, but nevertheless required palliation for pulmonary oligemia. Symptoms related to hypoxemia and erythrocytosis (polycythemia) are indications for intervention. Hypoplasia of the pulmonary valve ring, main, and/or branch pulmonary arteries is another indication, even if symptoms are not present. The presence of two or more sites of obstruction (Figure 19.1) is considered a prerequisite when employing balloon valvuloplasty,[4] because if valvar stenosis is the sole obstruction, relief from such an obstruction may result in a

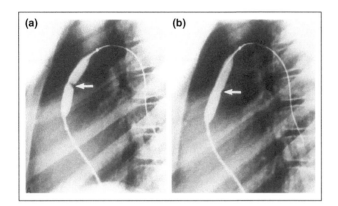

Figure 19.2
Selected cineradiographic frames of a balloon dilatation catheter placed across the pulmonic valve in an infant with tetralogy of Fallot. Note waisting (arrow) of the balloon during the initial phases of balloon inflation (a), which is almost completely abolished (arrow) during the later phases of balloon inflation (b). (Reproduced from Rao et al,[6] with permission from the authors and publisher.)

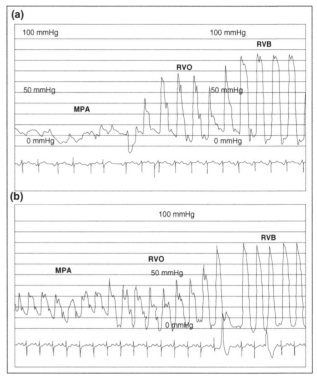

Figure 19.3
Pressure pullback tracings across the pulmonary valve and right ventricular outflow tract before (a) and 15 minutes after (b) balloon pulmonary valvuloplasty in a patient with tetralogy of Fallot. Note that the pulmonary valve gradient disappeared, whereas the infundibular gradient persisted after balloon pulmonary valvuloplasty. MPA, main pulmonary artery; RVO, right ventricular outflow tract; RVB, right ventricular body. (Reproduced from Rao and Brais with permission from the authors and publisher.)

marked increase in pulmonary blood flow and elevation of pulmonary artery pressure and resistance.

The technique of balloon pulmonary valvuloplasty is essentially similar to that used for isolated valvar pulmonary stenosis, described in the preceding chapter. Following the decision to go ahead with balloon valvuloplasty, a 4 or 5 Fr multi A-2 catheter (Cordis) is advanced across the pulmonary valve and positioned in the left or right pulmonary artery. An appropriately sized (0.014 to 0.035 inch) flexible tip J guidewire is positioned into the distal left or right pulmonary artery via the catheter already in place and the catheter is removed. A balloon angioplasty catheter is then positioned across the pulmonary valve and the balloon inflated (Figure 19.2). The diameter of the balloon is selected to be 1.2 to 1.25 times the pulmonary valve annulus, as discussed in the preceding chapter. One or more balloon inflations are usually performed. Between 10 and 15 minutes following valvuloplasty, systemic arterial saturation, oxygen saturation data to calculate systemic and pulmonary flow, pulmonary artery and/or right ventricular angiography, and pressure pullback across the pulmonary valve and infundibulum (Figure 19.3) are recorded.

Improvements in systemic arterial oxygen saturation, an increase in pulmonary blood flow and the pulmonary to systemic flow ratio (Qp:Qs), and a decrease in pulmonary valve gradients (while infundibular and total right ventricular outflow gradients remain unchanged) following balloon valvuloplasty have been observed.[4,6–8] Complications during and immediately after the procedure have been remarkably minimal. A transient fall in systemic arterial saturation while the balloon is inflated is seen, but improves rapidly following

balloon deflation. Hypotension during balloon inflation, so commonly seen in isolated pulmonary valve dilatations, is not seen in these patients, presumably related to the flow through the ventricular septal defect. Surprisingly, cyanotic spells following balloon valvuloplasty have not been a problem, presumably due to improvement of pulmonary blood flow following the procedure. However, an increase in cyanosis has been reported by some workers.[5]

An increase in the size of the pulmonary arteries (Figure 19.4) and of the left atrium/ventricle at follow-up occurred such that some patients who were thought to have uncorrectable defects became good risk candidates for surgical correction.[4–10] More recently, this technique has been extended[11] successfully to a group of children with truly diminutive pulmonary arteries. While most workers have favorable results, some investigators were unable to document the benefit. Battistessa and associates[12] examined the results of prior balloon valvuloplasty at the time of surgical correction of tetralogy of Fallot; they did not see evidence for significant growth of the pulmonary valve annulus in

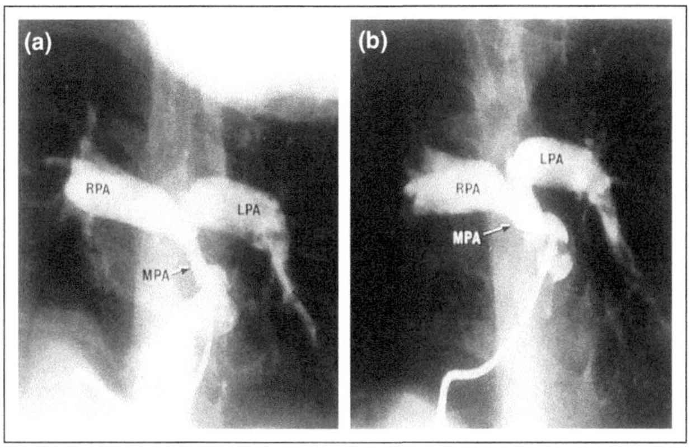

Figure 19.4
Selected frames from a pulmonary artery cineangiogram in a sitting-up view in a patient with tetralogy of Fallot patient prior to (a) and 12 months following (b) balloon pulmonary valvuloplasty. Note the significant improvement in the size of the valve annulus and main and branch pulmonary arteries at follow-up. LPA, left pulmonary artery; MPA, main pulmonary artery; RPA, right pulmonary artery. (Reproduced from Rao et al,[6] with permission from the authors and publisher.)

the 27 patients that they looked at. They also determined that the need for a transannular patch was not abolished at the time of intracardiac repair. Therefore, they were not supportive of balloon pulmonary valvuloplasty as a palliative procedure. However, it should be noted that 15 of the 27 patients who have previously been reported by Qureshi et al[5] were included in Battistessa's study. Also, Battistessa's patients form a subgroup of a larger experience reported by Sreeram at al.[10] These latter authors[5,10] indeed documented favorable results. The increase in the pulmonary artery annulus size is shown in the larger group of patients,[10] which included Battistessa's patients. Furthermore, the increased size ($p < 0.001$) of the pulmonary valve annulus was demonstrated in 24 patients who had also improved their systemic arterial oxygen saturation following balloon pulmonary valvuloplasty, and this increase in the size of the pulmonary valve annulus was greater ($p < 0.005$) than expected from normal growth.[10] The improvement in pulmonary artery size documented by several authors[3–10] is similar to that observed following the Brock procedure[13,14] and systemic to pulmonary artery shunts.[15–18]

In view of these varied observations as well as the current state of the art with the feasibility of surgical repair at a younger age, it would seem prudent that the balloon pulmonary valvuloplasty procedure be performed in selected patients with tetralogy of Fallot or other cyanotic defects. Not all cyanotic heart defect patients with pulmonary stenosis are candidates for balloon pulmonary valvuloplasty. Based on our experience and that reported by others, we[6,8,19] recommended this procedure be performed in selected patients. The selection criteria that I recommend are:

1. the infant/child requires palliation of pulmonary oligemia but is not a candidate for total surgical correction because of the size of the patient, the type of the defect or other anatomic aberrations
2. valvar obstruction is a significant component of the right ventricular outflow tract obstruction, and
3. multiple obstructions in series are present so that there is residual subvalvar obstruction after relief of pulmonary valvar obstruction such that flooding of the lungs is prevented.

Other indications are any type of contraindication for open heart surgery or refusal by parents/guardians for open heart surgical correction.

References

1. Kan JS, White RJ Jr, Mitchell SE, Gardner TJ. Percutaneous balloon valvuloplasty: a new method for treating congenital pulmonary valve stenosis. N Engl J Med 1982; 307: 540–2.
2. Rao PS. Balloon pulmonary valvuloplasty for complex cyanotic heart defects. Presented at the Pediatric Cardiology International Congress, Vienna, Austria, February 1987: 21–25.
3. Boucek MM, Webster HE, Orsmond GS, Ruttenberg HD. Balloon pulmonary valvotomy: palliation for cyanotic heart disease. Am Heart J 1988; 115: 318–22.
4. Rao PS, Brais M. Balloon pulmonary valvuloplasty for congenital cyanotic heart defects. Am Heart J 1988; 115: 1105–10.
5. Qureshi SA, Kirk CR, Lamb RK et al. Balloon dilatation of the pulmonary valve in the first year of life in patients with tetralogy of Fallot: a preliminary study. Br Heart J 1988; 60: 232–5.
6. Rao PS, Wilson AD, Thapar MK, Brais M. Balloon pulmonary valvuloplasty in the management of cyanotic congenital heart defects. Cathet Cardiovasc Diagn 1992; 25: 16–24.
7. Rao PS. Transcatheter management of cyanotic congenital heart defects: a review. Clin Cardiol 1992; 15: 483–96.
8. Rao PS. Role of balloon dilatation and other transcatheter methods in the treatment of cyanotic congenital heart defects. In: Rao PS, ed. Transcatheter Therapy in Pediatric Cardiology. New York: Wiley-Liss, 1993: 229–53.
9. Parsons JM, Laudusans EJ, Qureshi SA. Growth of pulmonary artery after neonatal balloon dilatation of the right ventricular outflow tract in an infant with tetralogy of Fallot and atrioventricular septal defect. Br Heart J 1989; 62: 65–8.
10. Sreeram N, Saleem M, Jackson M et al. Results of balloon pulmonary valvuloplasty as a palliative procedure in tetralogy of Fallot. J Am Coll Cardiol 1991; 8: 159–65.
11. Kreutzer J, Perry SB, Jonas RA et al. Tetralogy of Fallot with diminutive pulmonary arteries: preoperative pulmonary valve dilatation and transcatheter rehabilitation of pulmonary arteries. J Am Coll Cardiol 1996; 27: 1741–7.
12. Battistessa SA, Robles A, Jackson M et al. Operative findings after percutaneous pulmonary balloon dilatation of right ventricular outflow tract in Tetralogy of Fallot. Br Heart J 1990; 64: 321–4.
13. Brock RC. Late results of palliative operations for Fallot's tetralogy. J Thorac Cardiovasc Surg 1974; 67: 511–18.
14. Mathews HR, Belsey RHR. Indications for Brock's operation in the current treatment of tetralogy of Fallot. Thorax 1973; 28: 1–9.
15. Kirklin JW, Bargeron LM, Pacifico AD. The enlargement of small pulmonary arteries by preliminary palliative operations. Circulation 1977; 56: 612–17.

16. Gale AW, Arciniegas E, Green EW et al. Growth of pulmonary valve annulus and pulmonary arteries after the Blalock–Taussig shunt. J Thorac Cardiovasc Surg 1979; 77: 459–65.

17. Alfieri O, Blackstone EH, Parenzan L. Growth of pulmonary annulus and pulmonary arteries after the Waterston anastomosis. J Thorac Cardiovasc Surg 1979; 78: 440–4.

18. Guyton RA, Owens JE, Waumett JD et al. The Blalock–Taussig shunt: low risk effective palliation, and pulmonary artery growth. J Thorac Cardiovasc Surg 1983; 85: 917–22.

19. Rao PS. Interventional pediatric cardiology: state of the art and future directions. Pediatr Cardiol 1998; 19: 107–24.

20

Tricuspid valve stenosis

Ramesh Arora

Introduction

Tricuspid stenosis (TS) is a very uncommon valvular heart disease. It is almost always of rheumatic origin and virtually never occurs as an isolated lesion.[1] Its incidence may be underestimated because it is commonly overlooked, particularly when associated with mitral stenosis. Tricuspid valve pathology is present at autopsy in about 15% of patients with rheumatic heart disease and is of clinical significance in only about 5% of cases.[2] But organic tricuspid valve disease is more common in India than in the affluent countries and has been reported to occur in hearts of more than one-third of patients with rheumatic heart disease studied at autopsy in the subcontinent.[3] Other causes of obstruction to right atrial emptying are unusual – congenital, carcinoid syndrome, pericardial constriction, extracardiac tumors, and vegetations following infective endocarditis.

The anatomic changes of chronic rheumatic TS resemble those of mitral stenosis characterized by scarring and fibrosis of the valve leaflets, fusion of the leaflet commissures, and associated fibrosis, thickening and shortening of the chordae tendinae producing a diaphragm with a fixed central aperture.[4] When mitral disease is accompanied by TS, the mitral lesion is typically more severe and predominates clinically. Detection of concomitant TS is important, because a tricuspid lesion may lead to chronic elevation of right atrial pressure and low cardiac output despite surgical/ transcatheter relief of the left sided valvular disease.

The characteristic clinical features are of low cardiac output – fatigue, edematous feet, hepatomegaly, swelling of the abdomen, and anasarca out of proportion to the degree of dyspnea. The absence of symptoms due to pulmonary congestion (hemoptysis, paroxysmal nocturnal dyspnea, acute pulmonary edema) in a patient with obvious mitral stenosis should suggest the possibility of TS. The physical findings can be mistakenly attributed to mitral stenosis, therefore a high degree of suspicion is required to detect a tricuspid valve lesion. The main signs are a giant 'a' wave during sinus rhythm and a diminished rate of 'y' descent in the jugular venous pulse, the presence of tricuspid opening snap, and

a mid-diastolic murmur along the lower sternal border, increasing on inspiration. Moreover, electrocardiographic evidence of right atrial enlargement disproportionate to the degree of right ventricular hypertrophy and a roentgenogram showing a dilated right atrium without an enlarged pulmonary artery suggest TS.

The clinical diagnosis of TS is usually difficult and there is no perfect diagnostic method. Cardiac catheterization requires accurate simultaneous recording of right atrial and right ventricular pressures. Often the gradient is small and frequently tricuspid regurgitation is significant, reducing the accuracy of the method.[5] Joyner et al[6] suggested that a decreased diastolic slope (EF slope) of the tricuspid valve was a useful M-mode echocardiographic sign for the diagnosis of TS, while subsequent studies showed that a reduced EF slope may be present without TS. However, a reduced DE amplitude of < 10 mm associated with a decreased EF slope on the M-mode echocardiogram and diastolic doming of the tricuspid valve on the two-dimensional (2D) echo are useful signs in the diagnosis of TS.[7] The apical four-chamber view appears to be the most useful in diagnosing doming because motion of the entire tricuspid valve can be easily recorded. Although these findings are reported to be sensitive in detecting TS, it has not allowed quantification of the severity of the lesion. Doppler echocardiography provides an accurate non-invasive tool and compares very well to cardiac catheterization in the quantification of TS and the assessment of concomitant tricuspid regurgitation. Both mean tricuspid valve diastolic gradient and tricuspid valve area by Doppler pressure half time method can be easily obtained from the diastolic flow velocity profile. However, due to considerable respiratory variation, measurements should be on sufficient beats to cover at least one respiratory cycle for patients in sinus rhythm and two respiratory cycles for patients in atrial fibrillation. The constant of 190 for measurement of tricuspid valve area correlates more closely with cardiac catheterization than 220.[8]

Traditionally, stenotic valvular lesions were managed effectively by surgical valvotomy. After balloon valvuloplasty emerged as an alternative treatment to surgical valvotomy for patients with congenital or acquired pulmonic,[9] aortic,[10] or mitral stenosis,[11] an attempt was made to dilate the tricuspid valve concomitantly to obviate surgery.[12,13] The improvements in tricuspid valve area and symptoms were similar to those reported after surgical tricuspid valve commissurotomy.[14]

Balloon valvuloplasty

Patient selection

Patients with clinical features of intractable edematous feet, ascites, and hepatomegaly out of proportion to the degree of dyspnea on optimal diuretic therapy, as well as those with other valvular stenotic lesions who are being considered for intervention, should be carefully screened for tricuspid valve stenosis by detailed echocardiography (2D, Doppler, and color flow imaging). Apical four-chamber and parasternal long axis inlet right ventricular views are the most useful, as all three leaflets can be visualized by taking these two views. TS is diagnosed[8,15] when there is:

1. a reduced EF slope and reduced DE amplitude of less than 10 mm on the M-mode echocardiogram
2. doming of the anterior tricuspid valve leaflet in diastole, i.e., there is apparent restriction of leaflet tip motion with greater mobility of the body or belly of the leaflet
3. thickening and reduced excursion of the posterior septal leaflet or both
4. a reduction in the tricuspid orifice diameter of approximately 50% relative to the tricuspid annular diameter recorded in the same scan plane
5. a mean tricuspid valve diastolic gradient of 2 mm or more and a tricuspid valve orifice of 2.0 cm² or less.

Inclusion criteria

Patients taken up for balloon valvuloplasty are those with:

- an echocardiographic mean tricuspid valve diastolic gradient of 2 mm or more and a tricuspid valve area ≤ 2 cm²
- the presence of a grade I–II/III tricuspid regurgitation mean tricuspid valve diastolic gradient of 5 mm or more and a tricuspid valve orifice of ≤ 2 cm².

Procedure

Cardiac catheterization is performed under light sedation and local anesthesia. By the percutaneous Seldinger approach, the right femoral artery and femoral vein are cannulated with hemostatic sheaths. Either two separate

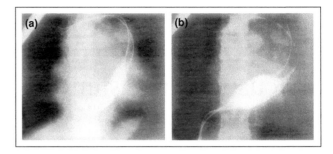

Figure 20.1
Double balloon technique over the wire. (a) Typical 'waist' at the stenotic tricuspid valve; (b) complete disappearance of the 'waist'.

venous punctures are performed or two ports are obtained from a single puncture. Unfractionated heparin 80–100 units/kg and antibiotic prophylaxis are given intravenously. Aortic pressure is monitored by placing a 5 Fr pigtail catheter in the descending aorta.

Double balloon technique

From the two right femoral vein hemostatic sheaths, 7 Fr tip hole balloon catheters (Swan–Ganz, Baxter, Health Care Corp, Edwards Division, California, USA) are placed one in the right atrium and the other in the right ventricle. The tricuspid valve gradient is measured by simultaneous recording of right ventricle and right atrial pressures. Cardiac output is measured by the Fick principle and the valve area is calculated using the Gorlin formula. A right atrial or right ventricular angiogram is performed in a shallow right anterior oblique (10°) projection to outline the position of the tricuspid valve (this can be omitted in very sick patients) using a 7 Fr pigtail catheter. The 7 Fr Swan–Ganz catheters from the two femoral vein hemostatic sheaths are advanced into the pulmonary artery. Two Teflon coated 0.038/0.035 inch 260 cm guidewires are then positioned distally into the pulmonary artery, one each through tip hole balloon catheters, which are then withdrawn. A Mansfield 15–20 mm diameter balloon catheter (Mansfield Scientific, Inc, Mass) is threaded over each guidewire and the balloons are positioned across the tricuspid valve (to obtain a cross-sectional area of 7–10 cm,² or the effective balloon diameter to annulus size is 90 to 110%).[16] Both balloons are inflated simultaneously to a maximum of 4 atm (Figure 20.1). The dilation balloons are then replaced by tip hole balloon catheters and the guidewires are withdrawn. The transtricuspid gradient is then repeated with simultaneous recording from one catheter in the right atrium and the other in the right ventricle, as well as withdrawal tracing from the right ventricle to the right atrium.

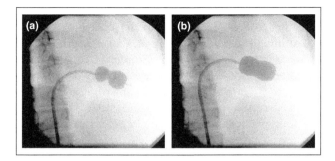

Figure 20.2
Inoue balloon – flotation technique (right anterior oblique projection). (a) 'Waist' at the stenotic tricuspid valve; (b) full inflation with disappearance of the 'waist'.

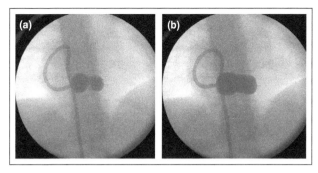

Figure 20.3
Inoue balloon special loop technique. (a) Balloon indentation during early inflation; (b) loss of balloon indentation after full inflation.

Inoue balloon over the wire technique[17]

A 0.025 inch exchange (260 cm) guidewire is positioned into the left lower lobe pulmonary artery branch or right ventricle through the Swan–Ganz catheter. Both the Swan–Ganz catheter and the hemostatic sheath are withdrawn. The Inoue balloon catheter, nearly 100% of the size of the annulus diameter, is inserted with the stretching tube through the right groin over the 0.025 inch exchange guidewire, so as to facilitate its entry percutaneously. After reaching the right atrium, the stretching steel tube is withdrawn, so as to direct the balloon catheter tip towards the tricuspid orifice. At this stage, withdrawal of the golden stylet up to the 2 inch mark helps in negotiating the balloon catheter over the wire into the right ventricle. The distal portion of the balloon is then inflated in the right ventricle and the catheter shaft is withdrawn until it straddles against the tricuspid valve. Rapid inflation and deflation of the balloon is done until the waist disappears. Hemodynamic measurements are repeated.

Inoue balloon flotation technique[18]

A simple algorithm for negotiating the tricuspid valve is:

Step 1. Simply float the Inoue balloon into the right ventricle like the Swan–Ganz catheter (Figure 20.2).
Step 2. If step 1 fails, use the J stylet with clockwise rotation.[19]
Step 3. If step 2 fails, use the J stylet and utilize the Swan–Ganz property of the Inoue balloon to enter the right ventricle.
Step 4. If step 3 fails, use the over the wire technique or a special loop in the right atrium for distorted right atrial anatomy (Figure 20.3).

Transjugular approach[20]

The right internal jugular vein is cannulated percutaneously and a 14 Fr Mullins sheath is advanced into the right atrium. The left arm non-invasive blood pressure is monitored throughout the procedure. A tip hole balloon flotation catheter is advanced through the tricuspid and pulmonary valves into the right or left pulmonary artery, and then, through the central hole, a 0.035 inch 260 cm long decron coated exchange guidewire is positioned deep into the lower lobe pulmonary artery. That tip hole balloon catheter is then withdrawn. A double lumen catheter is then advanced over this wire into the right ventricle. Simultaneous right atrial and right ventricular pressures are recorded and then the double lumen catheter is withdrawn. The tricuspid valve is dilated using a cylindrical balloon (NuMed) or an Inoue balloon positioned across the tricuspid valve over the wire.

Complications

Because of the proximity of the atrial–ventricular conduction system to the tricuspid annulus, balloon dilatation of the tricuspid valve may be associated with atrio-ventricular delay due to barotrauma. Transient heart block has been reported.[12]

Antibiotic prophylaxis

The patient must receive antibiotic prophylaxis prior to the procedure and two doses at 8 hour intervals.

Follow-up

Patients should be re-evaluated every 3 months for the first year and at 6 month intervals thereafter. A detailed clinical and echocardiographic (2D, continuous wave Doppler and color flow imaging) assessment is done at each visit. Restenosis is defined as >50% loss of increase in the valve area achieved after valvuloplasty or a valve area of < 1.5 cm², or both.[21]

Therapeutic results

Following tricuspid balloon valvuloplasty (TBV), satisfactory immediate hemodynamic results have been consistently reported in various case reports[12,13,17] and small series.[16,22] Most of the cases of TBV apart from bioprosthesis were performed concomitantly with mitral, aortic, or pulmonary balloon dilatation. The procedure has been technically successful with a significant increase in tricuspid valve area, a fall in transtricuspid gradient, and a decrease in right atrial pressures along with improvement in clinical symptoms. However, no criteria for optimal valvuloplasty have been defined; they may be considered to be the same as for the mitral valve, i.e., a valve area of ≥ 1.5 cm² and/or an increase in the valve area of at least 25% with < 3 + degree of regurgitation.[23] Sharma et al[16] combined balloon mitral valvuloplasty with dilatation of the tricuspid valve in 10 patients using the Mansfield double balloon technique in 6 and the Inoue single balloon in 4 patients. Hemodynamic parameters revealed an increase in the tricuspid valve area from 1.11 ± 0.41 cm² to 2.52 ± 0.69 cm² ($p < 0.0005$), a fall in the mean valve gradient from 11.80 ± 4.70 to 4.14 ± 3.40 mmHg, along with an increase in the cardiac index from 2.47 ± 0.38 to 3.46 ± 0.42 liters per minute per square meter ($p < 0.005$). The ratio of the effective balloon to annulus diameter measured on right ventricular angiography was 90 to 110% in nine patients in whom the degree of tricuspid regurgitation remained unchanged.[24] Significant tricuspid regurgitation occurred in one patient, which was attributed to larger balloon size (25 + 18 mm) where the annulus measurement was not quantified. No patient was subjected to tricuspid valve repair or replacement. Bahl et al[17] also obtained optimum results with a balloon to annulus diameter (28 mm) ratio of efficiency 100%, with a decline in the mean diastolic gradient from 10 to 2 mmHg and an increase in tricuspid valve area (TVA) from 0.85 to > 3 cm² without any increase in trivial tricuspid regurgitation.[17]

Multi-valvular heart disease is not well tolerated during pregnancy and TBV has been successfully performed in symptomatic patients along with mitral and aortic valve dilatation.[25] The specific impact of isolated TS on pregnancy is not known. Gamra et al[26] found recurrent miscarriages in a patient with TS, and that patient had a normal pregnancy after successful dilatations.[26] The mechanism by which TS could be the cause of miscarriages has been ascribed to low cardiac output, resulting in an impairment of uterine blood flow. In addition, elevated venous pressure may have some adverse effects on venous drainage of the uterus/placenta and thus reduce both placental and fetal viability.

Although a potential drawback of the procedure is restenosis, no such problem has been reported. Ribeiro et al reported four cases of TBV and none of them had restenosis at up to 3 years of follow-up.[22] Similarly, Sharma et al[16] showed continous relief of stenosis after 3–24 months in four patients. Nevertheless, larger series and longer follow-up are needed.

Discussion

The fundamental approach to the management of severe TS has been surgical after intensive medical therapy, mainly salt and water restriction plus diuretics to diminish the impact of hepatic congestion. Since it is almost always associated with mitral valve disease, the decision on the tricuspid valve therapeutic modality is usually made on the operating table at the time of mitral commissurotomy or mitral valve replacement, when the mean diastolic gradient exceeds 5 mmHg and the tricuspid valve area is approximately 2 cm² or less. During the procedure of open valvotomy, the stenotic tricuspid valve is converted into a functionally bicuspid one, which may result in substantial improvement.[27] The commissures between the anterior and septal leaflets are opened. It is not advisable to open the commissure between the anterior and posterior leaflets for fear of producing severe regurgitation. For this very reason it was felt that simple finger fracture may not result in significant hemodynamic improvement but may merely substitute severe regurgitation for stenosis. The feasibility of TBV has been demonstrated with reasonable safety and efficacy, although the procedure involves mechanical dilatation without visualization.[16,17,22]

The technical aspects of tricuspid valvuloplasty present certain issues:

1. *Balloon sizing.* This may be a problem; however, careful measurement of the tricuspid annulus diameter by 2D echo is very helpful in determining the size of balloon to be used. Although not well defined for the tricuspid valve, effective balloon diameter, which is 80% of the total balloon diameter used, should be 90–110% of the annulus diameter for optimum dilatation.[16,17]

2. *Balloon selection.* The valve is usually dilated to a greater extent than the mitral valve, with some studies preferring the use of two balloons (cylindrical, bifoil, and trefoil), of total cross-sectional area 7 to 10 cm², than a single Inoue balloon of 25 to 28 mm to achieve adequate dilatation.[28] However, large balloons may lead to significant tricuspid regurgitation,[16] the clinical importance of which is determined to a large extent by the severity of coexisting mitral stenosis and

the adequacy of concurrently performed balloon mitral valvuloplasty. Sometimes a small single cylindrical balloon is used in the presence of grade 3 (significant) tricuspid regurgitation.[20]

3. *Balloon positioning.* This is a common problem during the TBV and is judged by

   (i) indentation of the stenosed tricuspid valve in the middle of both balloons[16]

   (ii) injection of contrast medium into the right atrium

   (iii) withdrawal of the side catheter from the right ventricle with pressure recordings to locate the tricuspid valve.[29]

But with the Inoue balloon, this problem is easily overcome by virtue of its unique design. The different compliance of distal, mid, and proximal portions of the balloon makes it ideal for fitting snugly across the tricuspid orifice while pulling back from the right ventricular cavity after distal inflation.

4. *Guidewire positioning.* The guidewire can be placed in the right ventricular apex, but positioning in the left lower lobe of the pulmonary artery provides a more stable position and also avoids the risk of perforation and arrhythmias.[26]

5. *Distorted anatomy.* The Inoue balloon is preferred in a grossly enlarged right atrium which makes the placement of the tubular balloon across the tricuspid valve difficult.

6. *Transjugular approach.* A balloon flotation catheter easily crosses the stenotic valve and tends to go to the right pulmonary artery, where a stable position coaxial with the tricuspid valve orifice can be obtained. If femoral wires are positioned into the right ventricular apex, they are coaxial with the tricuspid orifice but do not give adequate support.

The jugular approach can potentially simplify tricuspid valve crossing with the Inoue balloon without the use of wire and also allow coaxial orientation with the orifice. This approach is mainly used in the presence of inferior vena cava obstruction. It is not routinely used as there are the limitations of transjugular interatrial septal puncture, more radiation, and limited working space.

In patients with combined mitral and tricuspid stenosis, the mitral valve is usually dilated first. This is especially relevant to patients with pre-existing tricuspid regurgitation, as dilating the mitral valve first provides the opportunity to confirm a satisfactory split of the mitral valve and a fall in pulmonary artery pressure before dilating the tricuspid valve. Because of the high right atrial pressures, a close watch should be kept for hypoxemia developing due to right to left shunt across the interatrial septum.[16] In such an event, the tricuspid valve has to be dilated as quickly as possible. If attempted before the mitral valve, to prevent right

to left shunt and clinical compromise, there is a possibility of worsening the pulmonary congestion due to the increase in blood flow, given the extremely high left atrial pressure and transmitral gradient. If there is associated aortic or pulmonary valve stenosis, dilatation of these valves is attempted before tricuspid stenotic valve. When two stenotic lesions exist in tandem, the manifestations of the more proximal of the two tend to mask those produced by the distal lesion. This is particularly true if the proximal lesion is more severe than the distal one.

Conventional options for management of medically refractory patients with valvular disease during pregnancy have been therapeutic abortion or valve surgery.[30] A single valve replacement is associated with a maternal mortality of 3%, which is normally slightly higher relative to non-pregnant values, and a fetal mortality as high as 33%.[31] Mitral stenosis is the most frequently encountered disorder complicating pregnancy. It usually results in acute pulmonary edema, which parallels increased maternal age and parity. The presence of tricuspid stenosis adds to the hemodynamic complexity. During labor, hypotension from vagotonia, blood loss, or anesthesia may result in circulatory collapse, placing the mother and fetus at risk. In developing countries, where the majority of patients with rheumatic valvular lesions are young, not only is balloon valvuloplasty being performed for mitral stenosis as the procedure of choice during pregnancy, even dilatation of coexisting aortic/tricuspid stenosis has resulted in satisfactory results.[23,25]

Conclusion

Balloon vavuloplasty of the tricuspid valve can provide satisfactory clinical and hemodynamic benefits which are also sustained at intermediate term follow-up. This procedure offers an alternative safe and efficacious therapeutic modality avoiding multiple valve surgery, not only for elderly and sick patients with comorbid conditions of chronic obstructive pulmonary disease, renal failure, etc., but also for young patients, in developing countries especially those with rheumatic heart disease and other stenotic valvular lesions. However, the complication of tricuspid regurgitation may necessitate valve replacement[32] or lead to refractory heart failure.[33]

Although rheumatic valvular disease is less frequent in the USA and Western Europe because of the decline in acute rheumatic fever in the past three decades, it is still prevalent in the underdeveloped countries of the world. By virtue of its cost effectiveness, the non-surgical procedure of relieving valvular stenosis has proven to be a great advance in medical care, not only in places where surgical facilities are not readily available, as it has the advantages of avoiding the risks of thoracotomy, cardiopulmonary bypass, and problems related to valve replacement.

References

1. Braunwald E. Valvular heart disease. In Braunwald E, ed. Heart Disease, 4th edition. Philadelphia, PA: WB Saunders Co, 1992: 1053.
2. Kitchin A, Turner R. Diagnosis and treatment of tricuspid stenosis. Br Heart J 1964; 26: 354–79.
3. Mahapatra RK, Agarwal JB, Wasir HS. Rheumatic tricuspid stenosis. Ind Heart J 1978; 30: 138–43.
4. Hollman A. The anatomical appearance in rheumatic tricuspid valve disease. Br Heart J 1957; 19: 211–16.
5. Carbello BA. Advances in the hemodynamic assessment of stenotic cardiac valves. J Am Coll Cardiol 1987; 10: 912–19.
6. Joyner CR, Hey EB, Johnson J, Reid JM. Reflected ultrasound in the diagnosis of tricuspid stenosis. Am J Cardiol 1967; 19: 66–73.
7. Shimala R, Takshita A, Nakamura M et al. Diagnosis of tricuspid stenosis by M-mode and two dimensional echocardiography. Am J Cardiol 1984; 53: 164–8.
8. Fawzy ME, Dunn MB, Amri MA, Andaya W. Doppler echocardiography in the evaluation of tricuspid stenosis. Eur Heart J 1989; 10: 1985–90.
9. Kan JS, White RI, Mitchell SE, Gardner TJ. Percutaneous balloon valvuloplasty: a new method for treating congenital pulmonary valve stenosis. N Engl J Med 1982; 307: 540–2.
10. Cribier A, Savin T, Berland J et al. Percutaneous transluminal balloon valvuloplasty of adult aortic stenosis. Report of 92 cases. J Am Coll Cardiol 1987; 9: 381–6.
11. Inoue K, Owaki T, Nakamura T et al. Clinical application of transvenous mitral commissurotomy by a new balloon catheter. J Thorac Cardiovasc Surg 1984; 87: 394–402.
12. Khalilullah M, Tyagi S, Yadav BS et al. Double balloon valvuloplasty of tricuspid stenosis. Am Heart J 1987; 114: 1232–3.
13. Goldenberg IF, Pederson W, Olson J et al. Percutaneous double balloon valvuloplasty for severe tricuspid stenosis. Am Heart J 1989; 118: 417–19.
14. Trace HD, Bailey CP, Wendhos MH. Tricuspid valve commissurotomy with a one year followup. Am Heart J 1954; 47: 613–17.
15. Guyer DE, Gillam LD, Foale RA et al. Comparison of the echocardiographic and haemodynamic diagnosis of rheumatic mitral stenosis. J Am Coll Cardiol 1984; 3: 1135–44.
16. Sharma S, Loya YS, Desai DM, Pinto RJ. Percutaneous double valve balloon valvotomy for multivalve stenosis: immediate results and intermediate term followup. Am Heart J 1997; 133: 64–70.
17. Bahl VK, Chandra S, Sharma S. Combined dilatation of rheumatic mitral and tricuspid stenosis with Inoue balloon catheter. J Interven Cardiol 1993; 42: 178–81.
18. Bhargava B, Mathur A, Chandra S, Bahl VK. Tricuspid balloon valvuloplasty – a simple algorithm. Cathet Cardiovasc Diagn 1997; 40: 334.
19. Patel TM, Dani SI, Shah SC, Patel TK. Tricuspid balloon valvuloplasty – a more simplified approach using Inoue balloon. Cathet Cardiovasc Diagn 1996; 37: 86–8.
20. Joseph G, Rajendran G, Rajpal K. Transjugular approach to concurrent mitral-aortic and mitral-tricuspid balloon valvuloplasty. Cathet Cardiovasc Interven 2000; 49: 335–41.
21. Abascal VM, Wilkins GT, Oshea JP et al. Prediction of successful outcome in 130 patients undergoing percutaneous balloon mitral valvotomy. Circulation 1990; 82: 448–56.
22. Ribeiro PA, Al Zaibag M, Idris MT. Percutaneous double balloon tricuspid valvotomy for severe tricuspid stenosis – 3year follow-up study. Eur Heart J 1990; 11: 1109–12.
23. Arora R, Kalra GS, Singh S et al. Percutaneous transvenous mitral commissurotomy – immediate and longterm followup results. Cathet Cardiovasc Interven 2002; 55: 450–6.
24. Helmcke F, Nanda NC, Hsiung MC et al. Colour Doppler assessment of mitral regurgitation with orthogonal planes. Circulation 1987; 75: 175–83.
25. Savas V, Grines CL, O'Neill WW. Percutaneous tricuspid valve balloon valvuloplasty in a pregnant woman. Cathet Cardiovasc Diagn 1991; 24: 288–94.
26. Gamra H, Betbout F, Ayari M et al. Recurrent miscarriages as an indication for percutaneous tricuspid valvuloplasty during pregnancy. Cathet Cardiovasc Diagn 1997; 40: 283–6.
27. Peterffly A, Jonasson R, Henze A. Haemodynamic changes after tricuspid valve surgery. Scand J Thorac Cardiovasc Surg 1981; 15: 161.
28. Konugres GS, Lau FYK, Ruiz CE. Successive percutaneous double balloon mitral, aortic & tricuspid valvotomy in rheumatic trivalvular stenosis. Am Heart J 1991; 119: 663–6.
29. Shrivastava S, Radhakrishnan S, Dev V. Concurrent balloon dilatation of tricuspid and calcific mitral valve in a patient of rheumatic heart disease. J Interven Cardiol 1988; 20: 133–7.
30. Chen CR, Lo ZX, Huang ZD, Cheng TO. Concurrent percutaneous balloon valvuloplasty for combined tricuspid and pulmonic stenosis. Cathet Cardiovasc Diagn 1988; 15: 55–60.
31. Vosloo S, Reichart B. The feasibility of closed mitral valvotomy in pregnancy. J Thorac Cardiovasc Surg 1987; 93: 675–9.
32. Bourdillon PDV, Hookman LD, Morris SN, Waller BF. Percutaneous balloon valvuloplasty for tricuspid stenosis, hemodynamic and pathological findings. Am Heart J 1989; 117: 492–5.
33. Shaw TRD. The Inoue balloon for dilatation of the tricuspid valve; a modified over the wire approach. Br Heart J 1992; 67: 263–5.

21

Pulmonary atresia

Jospesh V De Giovanni

Anatomy

Pulmonary atresia can be an isolated defect with an intact ventricular septum, maybe associated with a ventricular septal defect, or it can be part of a more complex congenital heart defect. The latter is usually palliated surgically, but the first two may be amenable to intervention for palliation or as definitive treatment.[1–5]

Pulmonary atresia with a ventricular septal defect may be palliated by intervention if there are native pulmonary arteries which are confluent and linked to a well developed main pulmonary artery and if the infundibulum is also well developed. In general, however, the atresia in this situation is muscular with a long distance between the right ventricle and pulmonary artery and hence surgical palliation is more commonplace.

In pulmonary atresia with intact ventricular septum, which forms 1–3% of critically ill infants with congenital heart disease, however, intervention has become the treatment of choice depending on the anatomy of the right ventricle, size of the tricuspid valve, and the presence/number of ventriculo-coronary communications.[6–8] Although the prognosis has improved for this condition, this does not apply to the subgroup with severe tricuspid regurgitation due to Ebstein's anomaly of a dysplastic tricuspid valve.[9] The rest of this chapter will concentrate on interventional procedures for pulmonary atresia with intact ventricular septum.

Pathophysiology

Pulmonary atresia with intact ventricular septum is usually associated with confluent native pulmonary arteries and patients are cyanosed and duct dependent. The cyanosis is contributed to by the reduced pulmonary blood flow as well as right to left shunting at atrial level. Treatment can be palliative or definitive, depending on the size and morphology of the right ventricle.[10] The treatment objective is to establish a secure pulmonary blood flow in order to improve oxygen saturation and to stop dependence on a patent arterial duct. In addition, relief of the right ventricular outflow obstruction provides an opportunity for right ventricular growth and development depending on the morphologic status prior to intervention; in other words, a small, non-tripartite right ventricle with a small tricuspid valve will not grow to an anatomic or functionally normal right ventricle, even if the pulmonary valve is fully opened. The variation in anatomy implies that some cases can proceed to biventricular repair whereas some can only hope for a Fontan type procedure as the definitive treatment.[11] There is a group in between where a one and a half cavopulmonary connection is possible.[12–14]

In pulmonary atresia with intact ventricular septum the infundibulum is usually well developed and the pulmonary valve is replaced by a 'membrane' and thus this is referred to as a membranous atresia. The membrane is sometimes perforated with a pinhole and reasonably well formed cusps. Although this is functionally the same as pulmonary atresia, it is referred to as critical pulmonary stenosis and is often associated with a better anatomy of the right ventricle. The main pulmonary artery is usually well developed and the pulmonary artery branches are often confluent but small and supplied by a patent arterial duct. The distance between the right ventricle and pulmonary artery is usually very short.

Diagnosis and management

The diagnosis can be made antenatally on echocardiography because of the right ventricular and tricuspid valve size as well as the absence of antegrade flow through the pulmonary valve on color Doppler. There may be associated hydrops. Postnatally, the patients are cyanosed and duct dependent. If the atrial communication is restrictive, this can result in hepatomegaly and a low cardiac output state. The initial management consists of intravenous prostaglandin therapy (PGE1 infusion, 5–20 nanograms/kg per minute) followed by a detailed evaluation and strategy plan which can consist solely of intervention, surgery, or a combination of both.

Intervention either by catheter or surgery is indicated in the early neonatal period unless the baby is very small (<2 kg) in which case extended treatment with prostaglandins to allow for further growth is acceptable.

Catheter interventional options objectives include:

1. relieving the right ventricular outflow tract obstruction by intervention or surgery
2. enlarging the atrial communication when indicated
3. stenting the arterial duct
4. stents to the right ventricular outflow tract when the obstruction is muscular
5. avulsion of the tricuspid valve/obliteration of the right ventricular cavity when dictated by the coronary artery anatomy (nowadays not considered as an option).

Surgical options include:

1. relief of the right ventricular outflow tract obstruction by closed or open valvotomy
2. the insertion of a systemic to pulmonary artery shunt (e.g., modified Blalock–Taussig or central shunt) or a combination of both 1 and 2
3. surgery may also include transannular patch enlargement, right ventricular overhaul, and a septectomy if the right ventricle is considered non-viable
4. closure of the tricuspid valve orifice.

History

Surgical relief of the right ventricular outflow tract in pulmonary atresia with intact ventricular septum[15,16] has gradually been replaced by interventional methods. The initial transitional step between surgery and intervention, an early form of hybrid procedure, consisted of introducing a valvuloplasty balloon under direct vision during surgery, placed across the atretic pulmonary valve, followed by inflation under vision.[17] Catheter procedures designed to cross the atretic pulmonary valve have developed since, including the use of a stiff end of a coronary guidewire,[18–20] laser therapy delivered through a fiber optic cable,[21,22] or radiofrequency perforation.[23–26]

Initial assessment is done by echocardiography and the systemic venous anatomy must be identified as this can determine the approach or suitability for intervention. Absence of the inferior vena cava with azygos replacement, for instance, will dictate that the approach should be through the umbilical or internal jugular vein; some operators have described the retrograde approach from the aorta through the arterial duct in order to perforate the membranous atresia. The diagnosis of pulmonary atresia with intact ventricular septum is made on cross sectional and color flow Doppler assessment, although it is not always possible to distinguish between pulmonary atresia and critical pulmonary stenosis without selective angiography.[27]

The following echocardiographic observations are essential:

1. Tricuspid valve size: ideally 10 mm or larger; if below 8 mm there is a higher chance of requiring repeated procedures, greater probability of a Fontan-type procedure, and higher mortality. A Z score of -0.58 or higher implies a better outlook.
2. Tricuspid regurgitant jet, including velocity.
3. Right ventricular size including the inlet, trabecular, and outlet portions. A right ventricular volume of 30 ml/m^2 very often results in a single procedure and/or a biventricular circulation.
4. Infundibulum and its diameter. A pulmonary valve of 7 mm or more is favorable.
5. Distance between the infundibulum and main pulmonary artery, and identifying whether the pulmonary artery branches are confluent.
6. Patent arterial duct with respect to size, shape, origin, and course.
7. Atrial communication, size, and restriction.
8. Evidence of ventriculo-coronary communications/fistulae.

If an interventional approach is considered as the first or best option, the surgical team needs to be involved as part of the decision-making process as well as for support should surgical intervention be required.

Informed consent should encompass the options available as well as the risks, which include perforation, infection, thrombo-embolic events (including stroke), tamponade, need for emergency surgery, failure of the procedure, and death.

Technique

Cardiac catheterization should be done with biplane fluoroscopy and an ultrasound machine available in the catheterization laboratory. A pericardiocentesis kit must be available. A minimum of 2 units of blood should be cross-matched in advance. The procedure is best carried out under general anesthesia with endotracheal intubation. Inhalation anesthesia using nitrous oxide and servofluorane together with fentanyl is a common combination.

The usual catheterization approach is through the femoral vein percutaneously. The umbilical approach is possible, but less favorable as it is difficult to achieve optimal orientation of the catheter tip within the infundibulum from this approach. The jugular vein approach is very rarely used when the traditional approach is technically not feasible. The retrograde approach[28,29] is less attractive, partly because the duct may go into spasm, but the course is less favorable and this approach is only resorted to in exceptional circumstances.

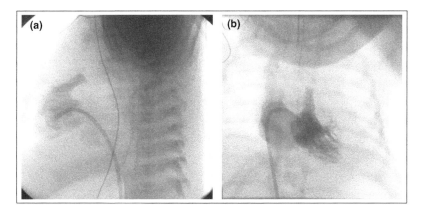

Figure 21.1
Right ventriculogram in membranous pulmonary atresia with intact septum showing tripartite right ventricle with obstruction at pulmonary valve level and no coronary sinusoids/fistulae.(a): 90° left anterior oblique, LAO; (b): antero-posterior, AP; (b) shows tricuspid regurgitation.

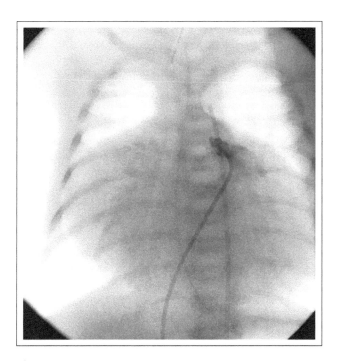

Figure 21.2
Hand angiogram below the atretic pulmonary valve in association with Ebstein's anomaly of the tricuspid valve. Note the gross cardiomegaly.

Hemodynamic information is obtained including atrial and ventricular pressures. The right ventricular pressure is usually suprasystemic and the right atrium pressure is higher than the left.

Angiography is essential prior to intervention and biplane images add to the detail and, hence, the safety of the intervention. The antero-posterior and lateral projections are standard. If the catheter procedure is carried out entirely from a venous approach, the atrial communication is crossed to reach the left ventricle for a left ventriculogram. It is also worth considering an aortogram, mainly to see the arterial duct and its detail, to look at the pulmonary arteries with respect to size and confluence, and to identify the proximal end of the main pulmonary artery and its orientation and relationship to the infundibulum. Using a Terumo wire (Terumo Corporation, Tokyo, Japan) to reach the aorta from the left ventricle is a smooth procedure. A multipurpose or Gensini 5 Fr catheter is commonly used for angiography. A right ventriculogram is essential to determine whether the ventricle has the expected three components, namely an inlet, outlet, and a trabecular portion (Figure 21.1). The overall size of the right ventricle is also helpful, although this does not always predict the outcome in as much as the size can become considerably smaller once the ventricle is depressurized. The same applies to right ventricular function, which cannot be assessed accurately until the obstruction is relieved. In addition to the right ventricular anatomy, the right ventriculogram will demonstrate the tricuspid regurgitation as well as any ventriculo-coronary communications, some of which may contraindicate relief of the pulmonary atresia. Unless the tricuspid valve is intrinsically abnormal, the degree of tricuspid regurgitation does not determine whether the pulmonary atresia should be relieved (Figure 21.2).

If angiography confirms membranous pulmonary atresia suitable for intervention, the catheter is changed to a Judkins right coronary catheter with a 3.5 or 4 cm curve, or a cobra catheter (Cordis Corporation, Florida, USA), depending on which one provides the best orientation perpendicular to the atretic membrane. Once the catheter is in the infundibulum, a hand angiogram is essential in two planes to determine whether there is a pinhole through the membrane or if this is totally atretic (Figure 21.3). My

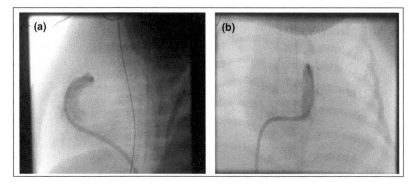

Figure 21.3
Hand angiogram through Judkins right coronary guide catheter, just beneath the atretic pulmonary valve. This helps to distinguish between critical stenosis and atresia and with fine-tuning of the catheter tip position prior to perforation.
(a): 90° LAO; (b): AP.

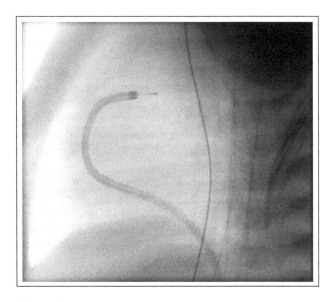

Figure 21.4
Baylis radiofrequency wire perforating the pulmonary valve and delivered through Judkins right coronary guide catheter. Projection in 90° LAO.

personal preference is to use a Judkins right guide catheter 5 Fr (Brite tip, Cordis) as this provides stability, reaches the target point, has a soft visible tip, and a large lumen. Precise positioning of the delivery catheter involves fine-tuning of the tip position. From the right ventricular cavity, clockwise rotation of the catheter places the tip in the infundibulum and, once this is below the atretic membrane, gentle forward pushing of the catheter with a mild anti-clockwise rotation will optimize the tip position against the membrane and direct it towards the main pulmonary artery. The main pulmonary artery position may have to be confirmed by an aortogram or by placement of a coronary wire from the aorta through the arterial duct. Some

operators have used cross-sectional echocardiography to optimize the catheter tip position prior to perforation.

The procedure is covered with heparin, usually 50 units/kg, and repeated if the procedure is prolonged. Antibiotic cover with cefuroxime or a combination of amoxicillin/flucloxacillin is used in our practice. Operator and patient preparation with respect to sterility should be of the highest level and the same as for open heart surgery.

Once the guide catheter is in an optimal and secure position, perforation of the membrane is carried out. Several techniques have been used although, nowadays, radiofrequency is the commonest modality used because it is the most successful and most easily available:[30,31]

1. *Mechanical perforation.* Using the stiff end of a 0.014 inch coronary guidewire through the guide catheter, the membrane is perforated to enter the main pulmonary artery. The stiff end sometimes moves the tip of the guide catheter or retracts the catheter as the wire hits the membrane. If this technique is successful, however, an over the wire 3 mm coronary balloon is rail-roaded across the atretic segment and inflated. This can be followed by a larger valvuloplasty balloon, the size being determined by the size of the main pulmonary artery. Generally, the balloon size to pulmonary artery diameter is a ratio of between 1 and 1.3. This technique of wire perforation is rarely performed as it provides little control and there are better alternatives.

2. *Laser beam.* The membranous atresia can be perforated using a fiber optic 0.018–0.021 inch trimedyne wire (Trimedyne Inc, California, USA) linked to an excimer or NdYag laser generator. The cable is not as radio-opaque as a wire and the laser beam can extend beyond the membrane, resulting in perforation of the main pulmonary artery. In addition, not all units are equipped with expensive and bulky laser generators and

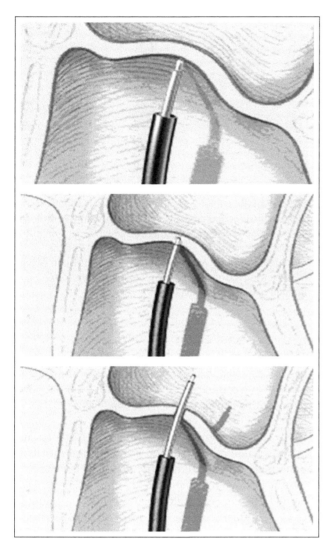

Figure 21.5
Animation showing delivery catheter and Baylis radiofrequency wire below the atretic pulmonary valve (top), perforating the membrane (middle), and through into the main pulmonary artery (bottom).

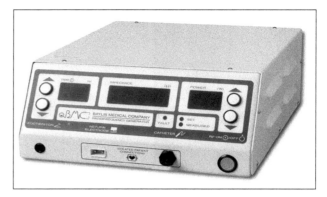

Figure 21.6
Baylis Medical Corporation radiofrequency generator. It has windows showing time, impedance, and power, with up and down arrows for adjustment. The lower front central panel shows the socket for the indifferent electrode (left) and the module socket for the RF wire (right).

this method is rarely used nowadays. When used, strict protocols apply to protect the staff from retinal eye damage, and special protective glasses must be worn by all the staff in the catheterization theater.

3. *Radiofrequency perforation (RF).* This is the commonest modality used today because of its efficacy, simplicity of use, availability, and customized equipment designed for this purpose (Figure 21.4). There are two types of radiofrequency systems both using 500 kHz frequency:

(i) Ablation: this is based on the radiofrequency system used for ablation for arrhythmia substrates and is delivered through the same generator, such as the Hat 200 (Osypka). Originally a 5 Fr ablation catheter was used, but this can produce a large hole;[32,33] should the catheter perforate the infundibulum or main pulmonary artery, tamponade usually results. For this method, a high power of 30–50 watts, a lower voltage of 30–50 volts, and a long duration of application of up to 60–120 seconds are used and an impedance of between 90 and 130 ohms is reached. A customized 2 Fr radiofrequency perforation wire with a 2 mm tip was designed specifically for pulmonary atresia perforation (Cereblate, Osypka) and this requires a short application of energy (usually 5 seconds), but this has been superseded by the Baylis wire.

(ii) Perforation with the Baylis radiofrequency co-axial system (Baylis Medical Company). This system has been specifically designed for tissue perforation and uses a high voltage (150–280 volts), lower power (5–10 watts), reaches a high impedance (up to 7000 ohms), and has a short duration of application of between 1 and 5 seconds. The system has a specifically designed wire as well as a customized radiofrequency generator which can produce an output of 16 watts (Figures 21.5 and 21.6). If the impedance goes outside the range, the generator will cut out. The radiofrequency wire for this system is a 0.024 inch wire with a length of 260 cm. The metal tip is 2 mm and the rest of the wire is covered with Teflon. The distal end can be shaped for better orientation if this cannot be achieved solely by the guide catheter. The Baylis system also comes with a fine catheter which can go over the wire once the latter has crossed the atretic segment, thus creating a co-axial system. This design allows for the radiofrequency wire to be removed and replaced by a guidewire for graded balloon dilatation of the atretic segment.

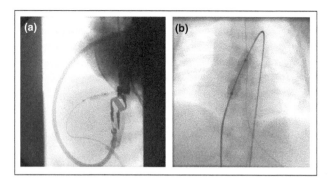

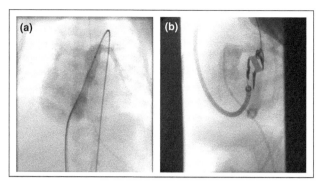

Figure 21.7

(a) Inflation of the coronary balloon across the atretic pulmonary valve with a waist at the level of the valve (90° left anterior oblique, LAO). (b) Pulmonary valvuloplasty with an 8 mm Cristal balloon in the antero-posterior (AP) projection and with a waist prior to full inflation; note the different guidewire size in the two images and that in (b) the wire crosses the duct into the descending aorta.

Figure 21.8

Right ventriculogram post-valvuloplasty. (a) Right ventriculogram post-valvuloplasty in the AP projection and through a multi-track catheter; the guidewire crosses the arterial duct into the descending aorta. (b) Angiogram in the right ventricular outflow tract showing the opened atretic pulmonary valve. Note infundibular narrowing in (a).

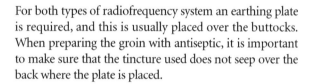

For both types of radiofrequency system an earthing plate is required, and this is usually placed over the buttocks. When preparing the groin with antiseptic, it is important to make sure that the tincture used does not seep over the back where the plate is placed.

The RF wire, which is easily radio-opaque, is pushed through the tip of the guide catheter once this has been placed optimally under the atretic membrane. Test angiography using biplane fluoroscopic imaging can be carried out through the side arm of a Tuohy–Borst Y connector in order to achieve the best position and orientation prior to perforation. Repeated small hand injections and fine-tuning of the catheter tip are absolutely essential prior to perforation. Once this has been achieved the guide catheter must be kept stable by the operator and the RF generator is activated either by a foot pedal or by a button on the generator. The output is set between 3 and 5 watts initially, although this can be increased to 10 watts. Perforation is usually achieved within less than 5 seconds. As the generator is activated, the radiofrequency wire is pushed forward until the membrane is crossed, when radiofrequency administration should be stopped. The lateral fluoroscopic projection is preferred during this part of the procedure. The tip of the radiofrequency wire is soft and can be pushed forward either into one of the pulmonary artery branches or through the duct into the aorta. If the course of the wire is not in keeping with the position of the main pulmonary artery, its branches, or descending aorta, or if it courses the cardiac silhouette, it is likely that the pericardial space has been entered and the wire should be withdrawn. The hole created by this wire is usually very small and less likely to create tamponade, but this must be monitored by transthoracic echocardiography. Once the radiofrequency wire is

well away from the pulmonary valve, the fine catheter can be sleeved over the radiofrequency wire and the latter replaced by a coronary 0.014 inch wire for an initial valvuloplasty with a 3 mm coronary balloon (Figure 21.7a). This balloon can then be replaced by a catheter which can take a larger diameter guidewire for further dilatation using a larger balloon. The balloon size is determined by the pulmonary artery diameter, but is usually between 6 and 10 mm in diameter and 2 cm in length (Figure 21.7b). Several valvuloplasty balloons are available, including the Opta by Cordis, Cristal by Balt, and Tyshak by NuMed.

Once the waist on the balloon is abolished, the balloon is deflated and removed. A multi-track catheter can be used to measure the gradient as well as perform a right ventriculogram in order to assess the result and decide whether further dilatation is required (Figure 21.8). Moreover, it is important to look for extravasation within the pericardium. Finally, there is often a residual gradient which is usually dynamic and due to infundibular hypertrophy.

If it proves difficult to cross the atretic segment with a balloon, stabilizing the wire helps. This can be achieved by pushing the coronary guidewire into the descending aorta through the arterial duct towards the femoral artery. Once this is achieved, external compression over the femoral artery stabilizes the wire, allowing the balloon to be pushed forward across the membrane. An alternative is to create an arterio-venous loop by catheterizing the aorta through the femoral artery or the umbilical artery.[34] With this technique, it is important to avoid tension on the wire as this may cut through tissue when it goes round corners, especially the aortic end of the arterial duct. At the end of the procedure it is essential to carry out an echocardiogram to exclude a pericardial effusion and to document the velocity across the right ventricular outflow tract.

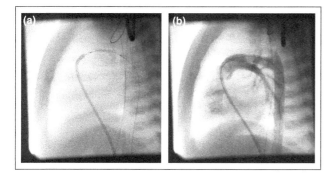

Figure 21.9
(a) Deployment of a stent in a patent arterial duct in a patient who had successful opening of the atretic pulmonary valve but remained dependent on prostaglandin. (b) Angiogram demonstrating full deployment of the stent within the arterial duct. Both images in 90° LAO.

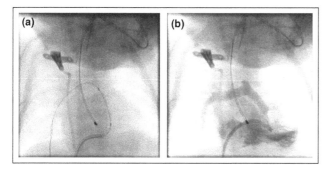

Figure 21.10
(a) Stent placement in the right ventricular outflow tract in muscular atresia with ventricular septal defect. (b) Right ventricular angiogram post-stent showing wide open subpulmonary area but with residual muscular obstruction within the right ventricular body.

Aftercare and follow-up

The post-operative care consists of regular clinical observation, assessment of the entry sites, and pulse rate, blood pressure, respiration, and saturations. If the patient is clinically unwell, blood gases, acid–base status, and lactate must be measured.

Prostaglandin therapy is usually continued and weaned appropriately if the saturations are maintained so long as there is a satisfactory opening of the right ventricular outflow tract as seen by echo/Doppler. Most patients remain somewhat desaturated even after a successful result due to poor right ventricular compliance and persistent right to left shunting at atrial level. Generally, saturations above 80% in air are acceptable and merit a trial withdrawal of prostaglandin. Sometimes, however, prostaglandin may have to be continued for 2–3 weeks before it can be

weaned or withdrawn. If prostaglandin therapy cannot be withdrawn because of right ventricular size or poor compliance, the options include stenting of the arterial duct[2,35,36] or a surgically modified Blalock–Taussig shunt (Figure 21.9). If right ventricular outflow tract obstruction persists and if this is mainly infundibular, beta-blockers such as propranolol can be prescribed, usually to a maximum dose of 6 mg/kg per day, given in three divided doses. If beta-blockers are required they are often prescribed for several months.

When the atresia is muscular or if there is a major subpulmonary component to the right ventricular outflow tract obstruction, one option is to implant a stent in the outflow tract, especially if the arterial duct is closed or if the atresia is associated with a ventricular septal defect[37] (Figure 21.10).

When there is a right ventricular dependent coronary circulation, the right ventricle should not be decompressed as this will lead to myocardial ischemia. Ventriculocoronary communication as well as stenosis or interruption of coronary arteries must be assessed by detailed angiography prior to any intervention.

If the patient requires duct stenting or a systemic to pulmonary artery shunt, heart failure therapy must be prescribed as a high pulmonary blood flow can result in circulatory collapse. This may not happen immediately, but usually occurs once the pulmonary vascular resistance drops.

Follow-up assessment is targeted at clinical progress, development and growth of the right ventricle,[38–40] measurement of the estimated right ventricular pressure on Doppler, the degree of tricuspid regurgitation, right ventricular outflow tract velocity, ductal patency, orientation of the interatrial septum, and the size of the atrial communication, as well as saturation by pulse oximetry.

Further pulmonary valvuloplasty may be required in some patients. If desaturation persists despite adequate growth of the right ventricle and with no material gradient across the right ventricular outflow tract, the atrial communication may be closed after a test occlusion with a balloon.[41] This is unlikely to be required before the age of 2 years and most devices can be used, although the Amplatzer (AGA Medical Corporation) or Helex (WL Gore) septal occluders are more commonly used. If the arterial duct is stented and if its patency is no longer required, this may have to be closed by transcatheter means using a coil or a plug, but this is unlikely to be required within the first year.

When membranous pulmonary atresia is diagnosed antenatally, relief of the outflow obstruction may encourage growth and development of the right ventricle, although this depends on the anatomy and gestational age. Intrauterine fetal pulmonary valvuloplasty has been performed only in a few cases.[42]

Antibiotic prophylaxis for surgery or potentially septic situations is essential for life.

Prognosis

Over the past three decades, major advances in surgical and interventional procedures have evolved and developed, with a resulting improvement in the outcome for patients with pulmonary atresia with intact ventricular septum. There remains, however, an appreciable mortality and morbidity associated with this condition and with treatment procedures. Between 30 and 40% will finish with a biventricular repair through either intervention, surgery, or a combination of both. The mortality over the first 5 years is still around 20%. The rest will benefit from a Fontan type procedure.

REFERENCES

1. Cheatham JP. The transcatheter management of the neonate and infant with pulmonary atresia and intact ventricular septum. J Interven Cardiol 1998; 11: 1–24.
2. Alwi M, Kandavello G, Choo KK et al. Risk factors for augmentation of the flow of blood to the lungs in pulmonary atresia with intact ventricular septum after radiofrequency valvotomy. Cardiol Young 2005; 15(2): 141–7.
3. Mi YP, Chau AK, Chiu CS et al. Evolution of the management approach for pulmonary atresia with intact ventricular septum. Heart 2005; 91(5): 657–63.
4. Yoshimura N, Yamaguchi M, Ohashi H, et al. Pulmonary atresia with intact ventricular septum: strategy based on right ventricular morphology. J Thorac Cardiovasc Surg 2003; 126(5): 1417–26.
5. Sano S, Ishino K, Kawada M et al. Staged bi-ventricular repair for pulmonary atresia or stenosis with intact ventricular septum. Ann Thorac Surg 2000; 70(5): 1501–6.
6. Godart F, Fall AL, Francart C et al. Pulmonary atresia with intact interventricular septum. Arch Mal Coeur Vaiss 2005; 98(5): 466–70.
7. Satou GM, Perry SB, Gauvreau K, Geva T. Echocardiographic predictors of coronary artery pathology in pulmonary atresia with intact ventricular septum. Am J Cardiol 2000; 85(11): 1319–24.
8. Coles JG, Freedom RM, Lightfoot NE et al. Long term results in neonates with pulmonary atresia and intact ventricular septum. Ann Thorac Surg 1989; 47(2): 213-17.
9. Stellin G, Santini F, Thiene G et al. Pulmonary atresia, intact ventricular septum, and Ebstein's anomaly of the tricuspid valve. Anatomic and surgical considerations. J Thorac Cardiovasc Surg 1993; 106(2): 255–61.
10. Fedderly RT, Lloyd TR, Mendelsohn AM, Beekman RH. Determinants of successful balloon valvotomy in infants with critical pulmonary stenosis or membranous pulmonary atresia with intact ventricular septum. J Am Coll Cardiol 1995; 25(2): 460–5.
11. Mair DD, Julsrud PR, Puga FJ, Danielson GK. The Fontan procedure for pulmonary atresia with intact ventricular septum; operative and late results. J Am Coll Cardiol 1997; 29: 1359–64.
12. de Leval M, Bull C, Stark J et al. Pulmonary atresia and intact ventricular septum; surgical management based on a revised classification. Circulation 1982; 66: 272–80.
13. Miyaji K, Shimada M, Sekiguchi A et al. Pulmonary atresia with intact ventricular septum: long term results of 'one and a half ventricular repair'. Ann Thorac Surg 1995; 60(6): 1762–4.
14. Numata S, Uemura H, Yagihara T et al. Long term functional results of the one and one half ventricular repair for the spectrum of patients with pulmonary atresia/stenosis with intact ventricular septum. Eur J Cardiothorac Surg 2003; 24(4): 516–20.
15. Cobanoglu A, Metzdorff MT, Pinson CW et al. Valvotomy for pulmonary atresia with intact ventricular septum. A disciplined approach to achieve a functioning right ventricle. J Thorac Cardiovasc Surg 1985; 89(4): 482–90.
16. Moulton AL, Bowman FO Jr, Edie RN et al. Pulmonary atresia with intact ventricular septum. Sixteen year experience. J Thorac Cardiovasc Surg 1979; 78(4): 527–36.
17. Hamilton JR, Fonseka SF, Wilson N, Dickinson DF, Walker DR. Operative balloon dilatation for pulmonary atresia with intact ventricular septum. Br Heart J 1987; 58(4): 374–7.
18. Piechaud JF, Ladeia AM, DaCruz E et al. Perforation-dilatation of pulmonary atresia with intact ventricular septum in neonates and infants. Arch Mal Coeur Vaiss 1993; 86(5): 581–6.
19. Gournay V, Piechaud JF, Delogu A et al. Balloon valvotomy for critical stenosis or atresia of pulmonary valve in newborns. J Am Coll Cardiol 1995; 26(7): 1725–31.
20. Siblini G, Rao PS, Singh GK et al. Transcatheter management of neonates with pulmonary atresia and intact ventricular septum. Cathet Cardiovasc Diagn 1997; 42(4): 403–4.
21. Qureshi SA, Rosenthal E, Tynan M et al. Transcatheter laser-assisted balloon pulmonary valve dilation in pulmonic valve atresia. Am J Cardiol 1991; 67: 428–31.
22. Gibbs JL, Blackburn ME, Uzun O et al. Laser valvotomy with balloon valvuloplasty for pulmonary atresia with intact ventricular septum: five years experience. Heart 1997; 77(3): 225–8.
23. Rosenthal E, Qureshi SA, Chan KC et al. Radiofrequency-assisted balloon dilatation in patients with pulmonary valve atresia and an intact ventricular septum. Br Heart J 1993; 69: 347–51.
24. Reddington AM, Cullen S, Rigby M. Laser or radiofrequency pulmonary valvotomy in neonates with pulmonary atresia and intact ventricular septum: description of a new method avoiding arterial catheterisation. Cardiol Young 1992; 2: 387–90.
25. Alwi M, Geetha K, Bilkis AA et al. Pulmonary atresia with intact ventricular septum percutaneous radiofrequency-assisted valvotomy and balloon dilatation versus surgical valvotomy and Blalock–Tausig shunt. J Am Coll Cardiol 2000; 35(2): 468–76.
26. Justo RN, Nykanen DG, Williams WG et al. Transcatheter perforation of the right ventricular outflow tract as initial therapy for pulmonary valve atresia and intact ventricular septum in the newborn. Cathet Cardiovasc Diagn 1997; 40(4): 414–15.
27. Walsh KP, Abdulhamed JM, Tometzki JP. Importance of right ventricular outflow tract angiography in distinguishing critical pulmonary stenosis from pulmonary atresia. Heart 1997; 77(5): 456–60.
28. Hijazi ZM, Patel H, Cao QL, Warner K. Transcatheter retrograde radiofrequency perforation of the pulmonic valve in pulmonary atresia with intact ventricular septum, using a 2 French Catheter. Cathet Cardiovasc Diagn 1998; 45(2): 151–4.
29. Coe JY, Chen RP, Dyck J, Byrne P. Transaortic balloon valvuloplasty of the pulmonary valve. Am J Cardiol 1996; 78(1): 124–6.
30. Wang JK, Wu MH, Chang CI et al. Outcomes of transcatheter valvotomy in patients with pulmonary atresia and intact ventricular septum. Am J Cardiol 1999; 84(9): 1055–60.
31. Gibbs JL. Interventional catheterisation. Opening up 1: the ventricular outflow tracts and great arteries. Heart 2000; 83(1): 111–15.
32. Akagi T, Hashino K, Maeno Y et al. Balloon dilatation of the pulmonary valve in a patient with pulmonary atresia and intact ventricular septum using a commercially available radiofrequency catheter. Pediatr Cardiol 1997; 18(1): 61–3.
33. Wright SB, Radtke WA, Gillette PC. Percutaneous radiofrequency valvotomy using standard 5 French electrode catheter for pulmonary atresia in neonates. Am J Cardiol 1996; 77(15): 1370–2.
34. Webber HS. Initial and late results after catheter intervention for neonatal critical pulmonary valve stenosis and atresia with intact ventricular septum: a technique in continual evolution. Cathet Cardiovasc Interven 2002; 56(3): 394–9.

35. Schneider M, Shranz D, Michel-Behnke I, Oelert H. Transcatheter radiofrequency perforation and stent implantation for palliation of pulmonary atresia in a 3060 gm infant. Cathet Cardiovasc Diagn 1995; 34(1): 46–7.

36. Bokenkamp R, Kaulitz R, Paul T, Hausdof G. Stepwise interventional approach in a neonate with pulmonary valve atresia and intact ventricular septum. Eur J Pediatr 1998; 157(11): 885–9.

37. Hausdorf G, Schulze-Neick I, Lange PE. Radiofrequency-assisted 'reconstruction' of the right ventricular outflow tract in muscular pulmonary atresia with ventricular septal defect. Br Heart J 1993; 69(4): 343–6.

38. Ovaert C, Qureshi SA, Rosenthal E et al. Growth of the right ventricle after successful transcatheter pulmonary valvotomy in neonates and infants with pulmonary atresia and intact ventricular septum. J Thorac Cardiovasc Surg 1998; 115(5): 1055–62.

39. Humpl T, Soderberg B, McCrindle BW et al. Percutaneous balloon valvotomy in pulmonary atresia with intact ventricular septum: impact on patient care. Circulation 2003; 108(7); 826–32.

40. Agnoletti G, Piechaud JF, Bonhoeffer P et al. Perforation of the atretic pulmonary valve. Long term follow-Up. J Am Coll Cardiol 2003; 41(8): 1399–1403.

41. Atiq M, Lai L, Lee KJ, Benson LN. Transcatheter closure of atrial septal defects in children with hypoplastic right ventricle. Cathet Cardiovasc Interven 2005; 64(1): 112–16.

42. Tulzer G, Arzt W, Franklin RC et al. Fetal pulmonary valvuloplasty for critical pulmonary stenosis or atresia with intact septum. Lancet 2002; 360(9345): 1567–8.

22

Transcatheter valve replacement of the aortic valve

Alain Cribier, Helene Eltchaninoff, and Vasilis Babaliaros

History of the procedure

Steps toward the development of transcatheter valve replacement began as early as 1965. Inspired by the success of the Hufnagel ball valve, Hywel Davies investigated the possibility of reproducing this surgical treatment by a percutaneous approach.[1] He was able to mount a parachute valve onto a catheter tip and temporarily treat the untoward effects of aortic regurgitation. Like Davies, other groups[2,3] with similar devices tried to duplicate the surgical approach percutaneously, but were never able to apply the techniques to humans due to limitations discovered during animal experimentation. In 1985, balloon aortic valvuloplasty (BAV) emerged as a treatment for non-surgical patients with degenerative aortic stenosis.[4] Though BAV could effectively palliate the symptoms of congestive heart failure and diminish the rate of rehospitalization in this group, the duration of benefits remained unpredictable and rarely lasted more than 1 year because of valve restenosis.[5–11]

With the advent of stent technology, a new era for percutaneous treatment of valvular disease flourished. In 1992, Andersen and his colleagues reported the first trial in which a bioprosthetic valve attached to a wire-based stent could be mounted on a balloon valvuloplasty catheter, and successfully deployed into a porcine aorta.[12] Despite encouraging results, technical limitations again precluded human application. Eight years later, Bonhoeffer and colleagues reported the successful percutaneous implantation of a bovine jugular valve attached to a platinum–iridium stent platform in children and young adults.[13,14] In April 2002, the first percutaneous valve was implanted in an elderly male with inoperable aortic stenosis.[15] Since this landmark case, percutaneous heart valve (PHV) implantation has been attempted in a series of 40 profoundly ill patients with aortic stenosis on a compassionate basis at our institution. The results of the earliest cases are already partially reported and are very encouraging.[16,17]

Indications for treatment and baseline evaluation

Currently, PHV implantation for the treatment of aortic stenosis is available only by a study protocol. Eligibility for entry into the study requires the presence of severe aortic valve stenosis ($\leq 0.7 \, cm^2$) and associated symptoms (dyspnea class IV by NYHA classification) that are expected to benefit from isolated valve replacement. Patients must be refused for standard aortic valve replacement by two cardiac surgeons and classified as high operative risk by a Parsonnet's score ≥ 30.[18,19] Patients are excluded if they have any of the following: intracardiac thrombus, unprotected stenosis of the left main coronary artery not amenable to percutaneous intervention, myocardial infarction within 7 days, prosthetic heart valves, active infection, active bleeding, coagulopathy, or significant vascular disease that precludes access. Patients who cannot be fully dilated with a 23 mm aortic valvuloplasty balloon (notable waist) and patients with a native aortic valve annulus size > 25 mm or < 19 mm are also excluded. Within the week preceding PHV implantation, echocardiography, heart catheterization, and BAV should be done as part of the baseline assessment. Echocardiography and heart catheterization can identify associated cardiac and extracardiac disease which can complicate the procedure (associated valvular, coronary, or peripheral vascular disease). Supra-aortic angiography can define the relation of the native valve to the coronary orifices and anatomic details of the valve calcification. The amount and distribution of valve calcification, the size of the aortic valve annulus, and the relative size of the BAV balloon at maximal inflation are three pieces of data that we use to decide whether the 23 mm PHV is appropriately sized for a particular patient. As an example, a patient with a small annulus size (< 20 mm) and a heavily calcified valve that can be fully expanded with a 23 mm balloon would be an excellent candidate. These anatomic data, together with details of the clinical status, are crucial for the therapeutic decision.

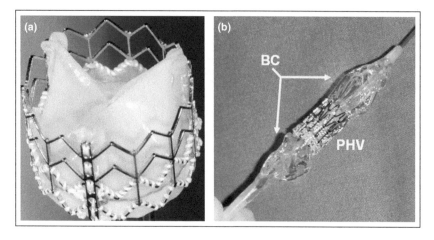

Figure 22.1
(a) Top view of the percutaneous heart valve (PHV) in the closed position. The pericardial leaflets are securely sutured onto the stent frame. (b) PHV is crimped over a balloon catheter (BC); in the collapsed position, the PHV is compatible with a 24 Fr introducer.

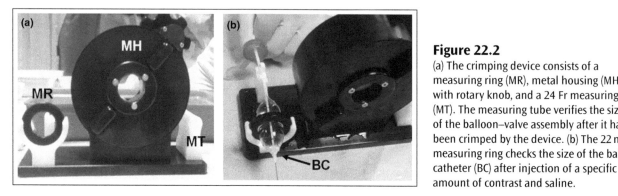

Figure 22.2
(a) The crimping device consists of a measuring ring (MR), metal housing (MH) with rotary knob, and a 24 Fr measuring tube (MT). The measuring tube verifies the size of the balloon–valve assembly after it has been crimped by the device. (b) The 22 mm measuring ring checks the size of the balloon catheter (BC) after injection of a specific amount of contrast and saline.

Device description

The PHV is a trileaflet bioprosthetic valve made of equine pericardium that is securely sutured to a stainless steel, balloon expandable stent (Figure 22.1a). The stent is 23 mm at its maximum diameter and 14 mm in length; the crimped diameter is less than 8 mm (Figure 22.1b). The valve is preserved in low concentrations of glutaraldehyde in the open position.

The crimping tool is a compression device that symmetrically collapses the PHV over the delivery balloon catheter. The crimper comprises a metal housing and a compression mechanism which is manually closed by the means of a rotary knob located on the housing (Figure 22.2a). The crimper is equipped with a 24 Fr tube to verify the size of the balloon/PHV assembly has been suitably crimped to fit a 24 Fr introducer (Cook, Bjaeverskov, Denmark). The crimper also has a 22 mm measuring ring which verifies the delivery balloon diameter at full inflation (Figure 22.2b).

The delivery balloon catheter is a commercially available 22 mm × 3 cm Z-MED II (NuMED, Inc, Hopkinton, New York, USA) percutaneous transluminal balloon catheter. The catheter length is 120 cm, which is necessary in larger patients with significant vessel tortuosities. The balloon catheter is purged of air before mounting the stent. A 20 ml

syringe is used to determine the exact amount of solution (1:9 contrast/saline) necessary to obtain a 22 mm expanded diameter (typically 17 ml after purging).

Percutaneous aortic valve replacement procedure

Vascular access, right heart catheterization, and supra-aortic angiography

The procedure is performed under local anesthesia and mild sedation such as that used during a routine interventional procedure. Aspirin (160 mg) and a loading dose of clopidogrel (300 mg) are administered 24 hours before intervention, and antibiotics (first generation cephalosporin, intravenous administration) are given just before the procedure and continued for 48 hours afterwards (oral administration).

Vascular access begins with a 6 Fr introducer in the right common femoral artery (mainly for pressure monitoring) and an 8 Fr introducer in the left common femoral artery and both femoral veins. Though two arterial access sites are preferable and allow for more alternatives during the procedure, one site for arterial access will suffice. If arterial access in the femoral vessels is not possible, the right brachial artery can be used. We prefer vascular cut down of the brachial artery in this situation for better control of hemostasis, particularly when using larger introducers. Depending on the size of the patient, we rarely use a sheath greater than 10 Fr in the upper extremity.

Right heart catheterization is performed with a Swan–Ganz catheter; cardiac output is measured later when the aortic valve has been crossed and the transvalvular gradient has been measured. Oxygen saturations from the pulmonary artery, aorta, superior and inferior vena cava should be taken with the patient off supplemental oxygen if possible. These saturations will be compared to those measured at the end of the procedure to evaluate for significant intracardiac shunting.

A 6 Fr pigtail is advanced from the left femoral artery to the level of the aortic valve. A supra-aortic angiogram is performed to detail the anatomy of the valve and the relation of the coronary arteries. Typically, the antero-posterior (AP) view is selected so that the plane of the aortic valve is perpendicular to the screen. In some cases, caudal angulation is needed as the aortic valve is pointed posteriorly. A still frame on an adjoining screen will be used as a road map at the time of PHV implantation.

Rapid pacing, crossing the stenotic valve, and valvuloplasty

The technique of rapid pacing, crossing the stenotic valve, and valvuloplasty is covered in detail in the chapter on BAV (Chapter 16). Briefly, a 6 Fr pacing lead (Soloist, Medtronic, Inc, Minneapolis, MN) is advanced into the right ventricle from the left femoral vein and connected to an external pulse generator capable of pacing at rates > 200 beats/min (Medtronic, Inc, Model 5348). A test of rapid stimulation should be performed to find the rate (typically 200–220 beats/min) at which rapid stimulation causes a predictable and sudden drop in blood pressure to 30–40 mmHg. This rate is required to stabilize the balloon during inflation across the aortic valve, allowing effective valve pre-dilatation and precise PHV delivery. Rapid pacing should always be tested before balloon valvuloplasty or PHV implantation; a demand rate of 80 beats/min should be set to prevent episodes of significant bradycardia.

The native valve is crossed with the help of an Amplatz or Sones (B type) catheter and a straight guidewire. Heparin 5000 IU is given intravenously before crossing the valve. In our experience, this method is safe for the patient even if transseptal catheterization is performed later. Retrograde dilatation of the native valve with a 23 mm balloon is done over a stiff guidewire (0.035 inch, 270 cm, Amplatz, Extra Stiff, Cook). Before use, the flexible end of this wire must be reshaped into an exaggerated pigtail curve to decrease the

risk of left ventricular trauma or arrhythmia. Pre-dilatation of the native valve is mandatory before proceeding to valve implantation. Special attention to the size of the balloon within the aortic valve and the presence of a waist during inflation is invaluable for determining suitability of the patient for a PHV. If the patient cannot be dilated retrogradely, antegrade dilatation is possible (see the antegrade technique), though this increases the risk of atrial septal damage and should be done with caution. After pre-dilatation, PHV implantation can proceed by either the antegrade transseptal or the retrograde approach.

Antegrade transseptal approach for PHV implantation

The antegrade transseptal approach has been the primary mode of valve delivery. Though more technically demanding, the advantages of this approach have been facilitated implantation of the device in heavily diseased valves, and the lower risk of inserting a 24 Fr sheath in the femoral vein rather than the femoral artery.

Transseptal catheterization

Transseptal catheterization is performed using a standard technique. A 6 Fr pigtail catheter is advanced to the level of the aortic valve from the left femoral artery, and an 8 Fr Mullins sheath and dilator are advanced to the level of the superior vena cava from the right common femoral vein. The Brockenbrough needle is advanced until the tip is 3–4 cm from the distal end of the Mullins dilator; the entire assembly is pulled back into the right atrium in the AP projection until the dilator is below the level of the pigtail catheter (Figure 22.3a). We prefer to puncture the septum in the left lateral view, at the distal third of a virtual line connecting the aortic valve (the distal tip of the pigtail catheter) to the posterior border of the heart (Figure 22.3b). In our experience, a lower puncture facilitates the rest of the valve procedure (establishing and maintaining the guidewire loop, passage of the PHV through the septum). Appropriate puncture is confirmed by pressure measurement through the crossing needle and fluoroscopic visualization. Once the position is verified, the dilator and sheath are advanced over the needle into the left atrium. Subsequently, the needle and dilator are removed and the Mullins sheath is flushed.

Guidewire placement

Through the Mullins sheath, a 7 Fr Swan–Ganz catheter (Edwards Lifesciences, Irvine, CA, 0.035 inch guidewire compatible) is advanced into the left atrium, across the mitral valve, and into the left ventricle. Normally, the tip of

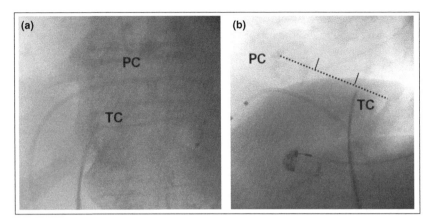

Figure 22.3
(a) Mullins sheath and dilator with Brockenbrough needle (TC, transseptal catheterization assembly) is pulled below the level of a pigtail catheter (PC) in the antero-posterior projection. (b) Atrial septum is punctured in the lateral view at the distal third of an imaginary line from the aortic valve to the lateral border of the heart. TC, transseptal catheterization assembly; PC, pigtail catheter.

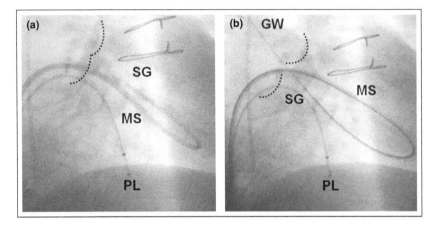

Figure 22.4
(a) Swan–Ganz catheter (SG) is advanced through the Mullins sheath (MS) into the left ventricle, and the tip faces the aortic valve (dotted lines). PL, pacer lead. (b) A guidewire (GW) is used to guide the Swan–Ganz catheter across the aortic valve (dotted lines).

the Swan–Ganz catheter will turn upwards and exit the left ventricle without difficulty (Figure 22.4a). If this does not occur by simply pushing the catheter, the Mullins sheath can be advanced into the left ventricle and another effort can be made. If the distal tip faces the left ventricular outflow tract but does not advance, a 0.032 inch Terumo wire (Terumo Corp, Tokyo, Japan) is used to cross the aortic valve antegradely (Figure 22.4b), and the Swan–Ganz catheter is advanced over the wire with the balloon deflated. Once in the ascending aorta, the balloon is re-inflated, and the catheter is advanced in the descending aorta.

A long guidewire (0.035 inch, 260 cm) is used to exchange the Swan–Ganz catheter for a 6 Fr pigtail catheter (Figure 22.5). The pigtail catheter is very important as it serves as a conduit through which wire exchanges and manipulations can be done without damaging the mitral valve leaflets. The final wire exchange is for a 0.035 inch 360 cm stiff guidewire (Amplatz, Extra Stiff, Cook), which is advanced through the pigtail catheter to the level of the abdominal aorta. The guidewire is snared (Figure 22.6) (Microvena, Amplatz Goose Neck, GN 2500, White Bear Lake, MN) through an 8 Fr sheath in the left common femoral artery and externalized under fluoroscopic visualization in order to maintain the guidewire loop in the left

ventricle. This maneuver requires the second operator to push the guidewire forward through the right femoral vein while the first operator pulls the wire from the left femoral artery. If this maneuver is not done carefully, the guidewire loop will be straightened, causing traction on the anterior mitral leaflet, severe mitral regurgitation, and eventually, hemodynamic collapse. The externalized parts of the wire should be equivalent on both sides (approximately 100 cm).

Dilatation of the interatrial septum

Over the stiff guidewire, a 10 Fr sheath is introduced into the right femoral vein, and a 10 mm balloon septostomy catheter (Owens balloon, Boston-Scientific Scimed, Inc, Maple Grove, MN) is advanced into the interatrial septum. A 30:70 contrast/saline solution in a 10 ml syringe is used to inflate the balloon (Figure 22.7); at least two balloon inflations are performed and held for 30 seconds to adequately dilate this area. Dilatation of the septum is a critical step to allow unrestricted passage of the PHV; it should be thoroughly done and subsequently checked with the partially inflated septostomy balloon traversing the septum without resistance. In some cases, septal dilatation is done before establishment of the guidewire loop; a larger septal orifice

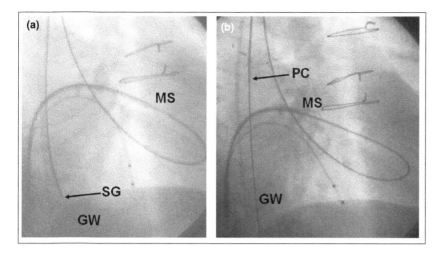

Figure 22.5

(a) A long guidewire is advanced through the Swan–Ganz catheter (SG) into the descending aorta. MS, Mullins sheath. (b) A pigtail catheter (PC) is advanced over the long guidewire (GW) in the descending aorta to serve as a conduit for further wire exchanges.

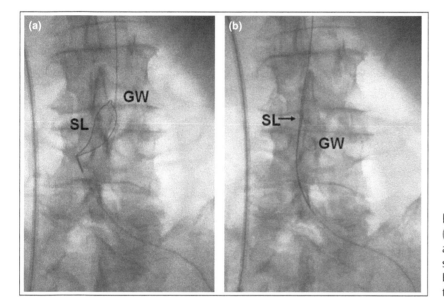

Figure 22.6

(a) The guidewire (GW) in the descending aorta is approached with the lasso (SL) of the snaring system. (b) The guidewire is caught by the lasso and will be externalized through the left femoral artery.

allows unrestricted motion of the Mullins sheath, facilitating Swan–Ganz manipulation in the left ventricle prior to guidewire placement as described above.

PHV implantation

The 10 Fr sheath in the right femoral vein is exchanged for a 24 Fr introducer (Cook). This exchange requires supplemental local anesthesia and an initial pass with the dilator. From the left femoral artery, a 7 Fr Sones (B type) catheter is advanced over the stiff guidewire until its distal tip is positioned in the middle of the left ventricle (Figure 22.8a). The PHV/balloon assembly is then introduced from the 24 Fr sheath, over the guidewire, and across the interatrial septum. The PHV should advance easily through the left atrium, across the mitral valve, and into the left ventricle until its distal tip faces the native aortic valve. Movement of

the PHV involves traction on the guidewire which can change the configuration of the guidewire loop. In this situation, the Sones catheter is invaluable for maintaining the guidewire loop in the left ventricle; valve implantation during hemodynamic collapse is an unfavorable situation.

As the PHV approaches the native valve, the Sones catheter is withdrawn so the tip is 2 cm above the calcifications (Figure 22.8b). Careful positioning of the PHV/balloon assembly across the native diseased valve requires tracking the guidewire from the right femoral vein or applying pressure to the Sones from the left femoral artery. Using the reference image obtained during supra-aortic angiography and fluoroscopy, the horizontal equator of the PHV stent should be transected by the leaflet calcifications (Figure 22.9a). A final test of rapid pacing is performed before deployment; in some cases rapid pacing causes forward movement of the PHV, which can be adjusted for with final positioning.

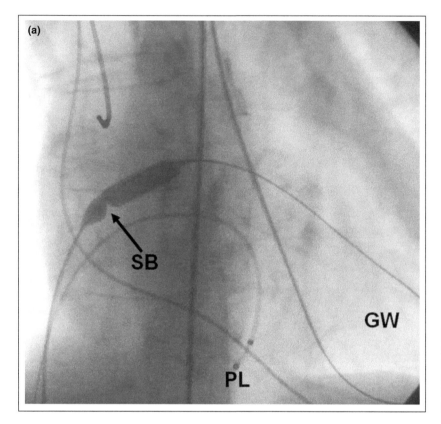

Figure 22.7
Atrial septum is dilated with a septostomy balloon (SB) to allow unobstructed passage of the percutaneous heart valve to the left side of the heart. PL, pacer lead; GW, guidewire loop.

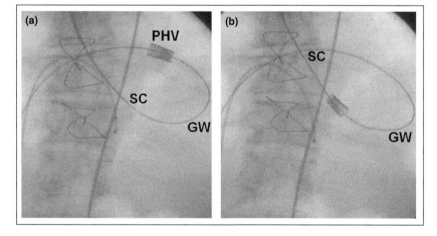

Figure 22.8
(a) During movement of the percutaneous heart valve (PHV), the Sones catheter (SC) is positioned in the left ventricle to maintain the guidewire loop (GW). (b) As the PHV approaches the aortic valve, the Sones catheter is pulled back into the aorta.

If the test of rapid pacing and positioning of the PHV is satisfactory, the delivery balloon is quickly inflated with the commencement of pacer induced hypotension. The entire amount of pre-measured contrast/medium solution in the 20 ml syringe is used to expand the PHV (Figure 22.9b). After full inflation, the balloon is deflated and withdrawn from the valve orifice; rapid pacing is interrupted when the balloon is completely deflated. The total duration of rapid pacing and balloon inflation is less than 10 seconds. The balloon catheter is then exchanged for a 6 Fr pigtail catheter. With the tip of the pigtail and Sones catheter in contact, the guidewire is rapidly withdrawn. Changes in catheters and guidewire removal should be done quickly, because only after their

removal will the PHV function and hemodynamics return to normal. The pigtail in the left ventricle is used to measure transvalvular gradients. Normally, the transvalvular gradient measured invasively is less than 5 mmHg (Figure 22.10).

Retrograde approach for PHV implantation

The retrograde approach has an attractive advantage of being a faster and simpler procedure. The two major limitations, however, are cannulating the femoral artery with a 24 Fr sheath and crossing the aortic valve with the PHV. This approach, therefore, should be limited to patients with

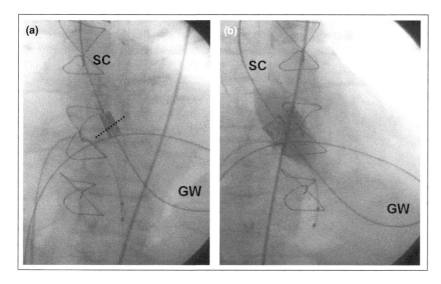

Figure 22.9
(a) The percutaneous heart valve (PHV) is positioned so the valve calcifications (dotted line) transect the middle of the stent frame. SC, Sones catheter; GW, guidewire loop.
(b) The PHV is deployed by the antegrade approach.

femoral and iliac vessels that are adequate in size (inner diameter >7 mm), without significant tortuosity or disease, and to patients with mild valvular calcification. Other than pre-closure of the femoral puncture site, the retrograde technique is exactly the same as the antegrade up until the transseptal catheterization. Pre-closure of the femoral puncture site is performed at the beginning of the procedure using two 10 Fr Prostar XL devices (Abbott Vascular Devices, Redwood City, CA).[20] Below, the retrograde approach is described after pre-dilatation of the aortic valve.

Percutaneous insertion of the 24 Fr sheath and PHV implantation

The balloon–catheter is withdrawn while leaving the stiff guidewire in the left ventricle. The 12 Fr sheath is removed while hemostasis is obtained with manual compression. Additional local anesthesia is administered, and the femoro-iliac axis is carefully pre-dilated using three polyethylene dilators (18, 20, and 22 Fr). Pre-dilatation should be performed under fluoroscopic visualization. After successful dilatation, the 24 Fr sheath can be introduced into the femoro-iliac arteries.

The PHV/balloon assembly is prepared as previously described. Through the 24 Fr sheath, this device is advanced over the guidewire, and pushed across the aortic valve. Using the calcification of the leaflets and the reference image obtained during thoracic aortography as markers, the PHV is accurately positioned in the native valve and deployed during rapid pacing as described in the antegrade approach (Figure 22.11). The balloon catheter is subsequently removed and the guidewire position should be maintained in the left ventricle. If the patient has unfavorable hemodynamics, the guidewire should be removed to allow the PHV to function normally.

Final measurements and follow-up

Following implantation of the valve, right and left heart catheterization is performed to re-assess baseline parameters. The transvalvular gradient and cardiac outputs are measured to calculate the new aortic valve area. If a guidewire or catheter is not in the left ventricle after valve implantation, use of transthoracic echocardiography (TTE) is satisfactory and re-crossing the PHV is not necessary. The valve area is typically 1.7 cm²; invasive measurements may be flawed by the lack of transvalvular gradient. Final blood samples are collected for measurement of oxygen saturation and assessment of interatrial shunting. If the patient does not have renal insufficiency or has not been exposed to a significant amount of dye, a left ventriculogram and supra-aortic angiogram can be done to assess the results of the procedure (Figure 22.12), though this information can be obtained by echocardiography. All catheters are subsequently removed, leaving vascular access sites for closure. In cases where the retrograde approach has been used, the femoral artery entry site is closed using the pre-delivered Prostar XL sutures, or a surgical repair in case of failure. A pneumatic compression device or hand pressure is applied to venous entry sites.

The patients are closely monitored during follow-up. Clinical evaluation and echocardiographic examination are performed immediately post-procedure, at day 1, day 7, 1 month, and every 3 months thereafter (TTE and transesophageal echocardiography (TEE) at day 1, TTE thereafter). Post-procedural treatment includes 75 mg of clopidogrel daily for 1 month and 160 mg of daily aspirin indefinitely. Subcutaneous low molecular weight heparin is administered during the hospitalization stay, and oral antibiotics are continued for 48 hours. Oral anticoagulants are given only in patients with chronic atrial fibrillation, starting 2 days before discharge.

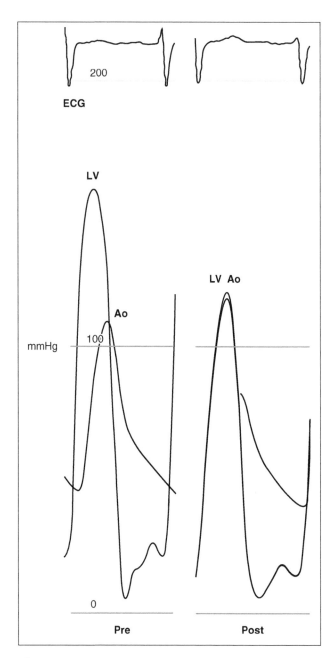

Figure 22.10
Significant improvement in transvalvular pressure gradient post-valve implantation. LV, left ventricular pressure; Ao, aortic pressure; ECG, electrocardiographic tracing.

Complications of PHV implantation

Renal failure requiring hemodialysis post-procedure, stroke, and tamponade

Renal failure requiring hemodialysis post-procedure is the result of excessive contrast administration, pre-procedural

renal dysfunction, intraprocedural hypotension, and embolic phenomena to the kidney. Careful assessment of pre-procedure serum creatinine, maintenance of intraprocedural hemodynamics, and limited contrast administration are paramount to prevent this complication. Once it has occurred, supportive therapy and careful control of volume status should foster recovery. Dialysis, which can retard the recovery of acute renal failure, should be reserved for appropriate clinical situations.

The complication of stroke has been previously discussed in the chapter on BAV (Chapter 16) and does not differ for PHV implantation. Pericardial tamponade has occurred in one patient after placement of the right ventricular pacing lead, and in one patient after heroic transseptal catheterization. Use of echocardiography to guide transseptal puncture in patients with distorted anatomy and to diagnose tamponade in patients with hypotension is very useful.

Mitral valve and atrial septal injury

Damage to the mitral valve and the atrial septum is seen exclusively with the antegrade method for PHV implantation. In one case outside of our series, the anterior leaflet of the mitral valve was transected during guidewire placement. All guidewire maneuvers, such as removal or externalization to the arterial system, should be done through a pigtail catheter to prevent this complication. In another case, also outside of our series, the atrial septum was damaged after antegrade BAV prior to PHV deployment. In this situation, the edges of the deflated dilatation balloon caused significant damage during removal; since this case, we have performed all our aortic valvuloplasties by the retrograde approach if possible. Persistent atrial septal defect after antegrade PHV implantation is not seen in our series.

Moderate to severe paravalvular insufficiency and valve migration

The risk of paravalvular leak is increased in patients with heavy valve calcifications that can prevent apposition of the PHV. A notable waist in the 23 mm pre-dilatation balloon during inflation should preclude these patients from valve implantation. Currently, new techniques are being developed to remedy this problem once it has occurred. In cases of aortic annulus/PHV size mismatch, implantation of a larger size stent valve (26 mm in place of the original 23 mm) will prevent paravalvular leak.

Valve migration can occur if the PHV is undersized or placed too high. Patients with a large aortic annulus (>23 mm) and mild valvular calcification are at risk for this complication. Once it has occurred, the valve can be moved distally into the descending aorta and deployed without clinical sequelae.

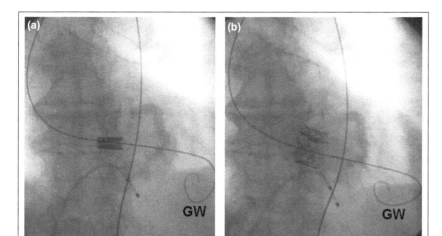

Figure 22.11
(a) Retrograde positioning of the percutaneous heart valve prior to deployment. GW, guidewire tip with exaggerated curve. (b) Retrograde deployment of the percutaneous heart valve.

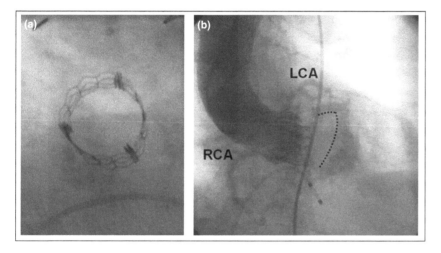

Figure 22.12
(a) Cranial view of the stent frame from the right anterior oblique projection shows complete and symmetric expansion. (b) Supra-aortic angiogram reveals minimal aortic regurgitation and subcoronary position of the percutaneous heart valve. LCA, left coronary artery; RCA, right coronary artery; dotted line, mitral annulus calcification.

Transient hemodynamic collapse and death

Intraprocedural transient hemodynamic collapse can lead to cardiac arrest and subsequent death, if not managed quickly. This complication can occur in patients with depressed left ventricular function, cardiogenic shock, or even small hypercontractile ventricles if antegrade implantation is attempted. In this situation, the Sones catheter can maintain the shape of the guidewire loop to prevent traction on the anterior mitral leaflet by the guidewire. If this maneuver does not work, the guidewire should be withdrawn into the left atrium, and the patient should be allowed to recover to a normal systemic pressure before trying again. Proceeding to valve implantation during a state of shock can be catastrophic.

Conclusion

Implantation of a percutaneous bioprosthesis in the position of the aortic valve is a novel method to treat inoperable patients with aortic stenosis. Current advances in the technique and hardware include (1) the use of a steerable catheter to facilitate retrograde implantation, (2) a lower profile delivery system, and (3) a 26 mm PHV which should further simplify the procedure and reduce the risk of complications. Though surgical valve replacement remains the standard of care for most patients, percutaneous valve implantation will become a realistic way for the interventional cardiologist to treat a select group with aortic stenosis.

References

1. Davies H. Catheter mounted valve for temporary relief of aortic insufficiency. Lancet 1965; 1: 250.
2. Moulopoulos SD, Anthopoulos L, Stamatelopoulos S, Stefadouros M. Catheter-mounted aortic valves. Ann Thorac Surg 1971; 11(5): 423–30.
3. Phillips SJ, Ciborski M, Freed PS et al. A temporary catheter-tip aortic valve: hemodynamic effects on experimental acute aortic insufficiency. Ann Thorac Surg 1976; 21(2): 134–7.
4. Cribier A, Savin T, Saoudi N et al. Percutaneous transluminal valvuloplasty of acquired aortic stenosis in elderly patients: an alternative to valve replacement? Lancet 1986; 1(8472): 63–7.

5. National Heart, Lung and Blood Institute participants group. Percutaneous balloon aortic valvuloplasty. Acute and 30-day follow-up results in 674 patients from the NHLBI Balloon Valvuloplasty Registry. Circulation 1991; 84(6): 2383–97.

6. Cribier A, Letac B. Two years' experience of percutaneous balloon valvuloplasty in aortic stenosis. Herz 1988; 13(2): 110–18.

7. Cribier A, Letac B. Percutaneous balloon aortic valvuloplasty in adults with calcific aortic stenosis. Curr Opin Cardiol 1991; 6(2): 212–18.

8. Letac B, Cribier A, Eltchaninoff H et al. Evaluation of restenosis after balloon dilatation in adult aortic stenosis by repeat catheterization. Am Heart J 1991; 122(1 Pt 1): 55–60.

9. Lieberman EB, Bashore TM, Hermiller JB et al. Balloon aortic valvuloplasty in adults: failure of procedure to improve long-term survival. J Am Coll Cardiol 1995; 26(6): 1522–8.

10. Otto CM, Mickel MC, Kennedy JW et al. Three-year outcome after balloon aortic valvuloplasty. Insights into prognosis of valvular aortic stenosis. Circulation 1994; 89(2): 642–50.

11. Safian RD, Berman AD, Diver DJ et al. Balloon aortic valvuloplasty in 170 consecutive patients. N Engl J Med 1988; 319(3): 125–30.

12. Andersen HR, Knudsen LL, Hasenkam JM. Transluminal implantation of artificial heart valves. Description of a new expandable aortic valve and initial results with implantation by catheter technique in closed chest pigs. Eur Heart J 1992; 13(5): 704–8.

13. Bonhoeffer P, Boudjemline Y, Saliba Z et al. Transcatheter implantation of a bovine valve in pulmonary position: a lamb study. Circulation 2000; 102(7): 813–16.

14. Bonhoeffer P, Boudjemline Y, Saliba Z et al. Percutaneous replacement of pulmonary valve in a right-ventricle to pulmonary-artery prosthetic conduit with valve dysfunction. Lancet 2000; 356(9239): 1403–5.

15. Cribier A, Eltchaninoff H, Bash A et al. Percutaneous transcatheter implantation of an aortic valve prosthesis for calcific aortic stenosis: first human case description. Circulation 2002; 106(24): 3006–8.

16. Bauer F, Eltchaninoff H, Tron C et al. Acute improvement in global and regional left ventricular systolic function after percutaneous heart valve implantation in patients with symptomatic aortic stenosis. Circulation 2004; 110(11): 1473–6.

17. Cribier A, Eltchaninoff H, Tron C et al. Early experience with percutaneous transcatheter implantation of heart valve prosthesis for the treatment of end-stage inoperable patients with calcific aortic stenosis. J Am Coll Cardiol 2004; 43(4): 698–703.

18. Parsonnet V, Dean D, Bernstein AD. A method of uniform stratification of risk for evaluating the results of surgery in acquired adult heart disease. Circulation 1989; 79(6 Pt 2): I3–12.

19. Gabrielle F, Roques F, Michel P et al. Is the Parsonnet's score a good predictive score of mortality in adult cardiac surgery: assessment by a French multicentre study. Eur J Cardiothorac Surg 1997; 11(3): 406–14.

20. Solomon LW, Fusman B, Jolly N et al. Percutaneous suture closure for management of large French size arterial puncture in aortic valvuloplasty. J Invas Cardiol 2001; 13(8): 592–6.

23

Transcatheter valve replacement of the pulmonary valve

Sachin Khambadkone and Philipp Bonhoeffer

Anatomy/pathophysiology

Pulmonary valve replacement (PVR) is required for residual right ventricular outflow tract (RVOT) lesions usually seen after repair of:

- pulmonary atresia, ventricular septal defect
- tetralogy of Fallot
- absent pulmonary valve syndrome
- common arterial trunk (truncus arteriosus)
- rastelli type repair of transposition, ventricular septal defect with pulmonary stenosis (TGA, VSD, PS) or pulmonary atresia
- homograft in the subpulmonary outflow, e.g. after Ross operation.

Stenosis results from:

- small conduit
- residual narrowing due to angulation, kinking, or twisting of the conduit
- intimal proliferation
- degenerative calcification.

Regurgitation may be due to:

- resection of the valve leaflets during surgery in the native RVOT
- degeneration of the valvular mechanism (for, e.g., homograft degeneration).

Calcified outflow tracts may lead to concomitant severe stenosis. Regurgitation may be caused by a transannular patch and usually leads to aneurysmal dilatation of the RVOT (most common with an autologous pericardial patch).

Indications for pulmonary valve replacement

These are not very clearly defined. Consensus indications are:[1]

- Symptomatic patients with severe pulmonary regurgitation (PR) with right ventricle (RV) dysfunction and/or dilatation.
- Patients with symptomatic arrhythmias and severe PR with RV dysfunction/dilatation needing intervention.
- Severe pulmonary regurgitation and evidence of RV dysfunction (on echo/magnetic resonance imaging (MRI)/ radionuclide angiography) and objective evidence of decreased exercise tolerance in asymptomatic patients.
- Patients with moderate or severe PR and additional lesions (residual ventricular septal defect, branch pulmonary artery stenosis, tricuspid regurgitation (TR)) needing intervention, with or without symptoms.

History

Transcatheter replacement of the pulmonary valve was first described by Philipp Bonhoeffer et al in 2000.[2] The first eight cases in Paris were reported to have no regurgitation and relief of stenosis.[3] Up to now 91 patients have received 99 valves, with a second implantation in eight patients, with no procedural or late mortality.[4]

Pre-catheter assessment

- History incuding New York Heart Association (NYHA) functional class assessment.

- Electrocardiogram (ECG), look for RV hypertrophy, QRS duration.
- Holter monitoring for asymptomatic ventricular or supraventricular arrhythmias.
- Echocardiography
  assess RV and right atrial (RA) dilatation
  look for associated lesions, e.g. severe TR or residual VSD
  TR jet interrogation by continuous wave (CW) Doppler to assess RV pressure on 4 chamber and RV inflow view on parasternal long axis planes, RVOT velocity

  a. pulse wave, PW Doppler
  b. CW Doppler – may indicate level of RVOTO

  (remember the limitation of the modified Bernouilli equation for multi-level obstruction).

- Magnetic resonance imaging (MRI)

  1. Retrospective-gated steady state free precession (SSFP) cine MR images of the heart are acquired in the vertical long axis, four-chamber view, and short axis, covering the entirety of both ventricles (9–12 slices).
  2. Pulmonary artery flow data are acquired using a flow sensitive gradient echo sequence (TR 9 ms, TE 5 ms, flip angle 15°, slice thickness 5–7 mm, matrix $128-192 \times 256$) during free breathing. Image planes are located at the mid-point of the main pulmonary artery/conduit pre-procedure, and just above the stent following percutaneous pulmonary valve implantation (PPVI), to avoid any stent artifacts after the procedure.
  3. End-diastolic and end-systolic volumes are calculated using Simpson's rule for each ventricle and from these volumes, stroke volume and ejection fraction are calculated. Where pulmonary regurgitation is present, an effective right ventricle (RV) stroke volume (SV) is calculated to reflect the net forward blood flow into the pulmonary arteries:

$$\text{effective RV SV} = \text{RV SV} - \text{pulmonary regurgitation volume}$$

Tips for case selection

- Low velocity TR jet ($V_{max} < 3$ m/s on CW Doppler) indicates absence of significant stenosis despite an RVOT Doppler velocity indicating stenosis.
- Assess calcification of the RVOT.
- Assess the dynamic nature of the RVOT in patients with aneurysmal RVOT.
- Chest X-ray to assess calcification of the RVOT.
- MRI three-dimensional (3D) reconstruction and black blood images help in selecting the site of implantation.

Procedure

Anesthesia

- General.

Access

- Femoral vein and femoral artery.
- Has been performed through internal jugular vein (IJV).

Sheaths

- Start with an 8 French (Fr) venous sheath
- Arterial sheath 5 Fr
  for systemic pressure monitoring, to assess hemodynamics for aortography, coronary angiography, or any other concomitant interventions on the arterial side.

Steps

1. Right heart catheterization for hemodynamics with Judkins right coronary catheter, JR 3.5 or any other catheter with a curved tip. Cross the tricuspid valve with a balloon-tipped catheter or with a convex curve of a catheter with a right atrial loop to prevent getting caught in chordae tendinae. Use a hydrophilic coated guidewire (e.g. Terumo. 0.035 inch) to get a good distal position in the right or left pulmonary artery and follow it with a good distal position of the catheter. Exchange the catheter with a stiff exchange wire (e.g Cook. 0.035 inch Ultra-stiff 260 cm). Put a curve on the wire to match the curve of the RVOT and branch PA. Use a multi-track angiographic catheter (NuMed Inc.) over the stiff wire to obtain the hemodynamics and assess the gradients on pullback.

2. Tips

   - The stiff end of the Terumo wire may be used to provide support for the multi-track catheter to facilitate crossing a tight or tortuous RVOT. A proximal loop in the RA may also facilitate this, provided the distal shaft of the multi-track has its axis parallel to the guidewire axis.
   - The stiff wire should be kept free from the inner surface of the right heart and within the lumen of the vessel (for example, branch pulmonary artery in this case) while the multi-track catheter is advanced, by gentle traction.
   - The wire should be held within the lumen of the vessel before contrast injection, using a power injector to prevent dissection of the vessel wall and an intra-mural contrast injection.

Pressures: RA, RV (including end diastolic pressure (EDP)), pulmonary artery, femoral artery, aorta, left ventricle.
Gradients: RVOT pullback.

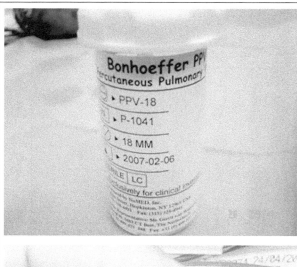

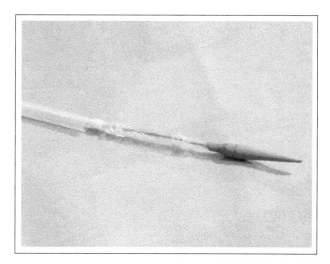

Figure 23.2
Delivery system with BIB balloon and outer sheath.

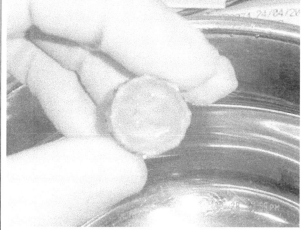

Figure 23.1
Bonhoeffer PPV.

3. Angiography is performed in the RVOT, also branch PA anatomy is assessed to rule out any distal obstruction if MRI or computerized tomography has not been done to assess bifurcation and PA anatomy.
   Projections:
   RVOT:
   anteroposterior/lateral
   lateral with caudal tilt (10–20°)
   RAO to open up the length of the stenosis
   for PA bifurcation:
   four chamber projection for PA bifurcation (LAO/cranial 60/40).

4. If suitable for PPVI, open the valve to rinse off the glutaraldehyde preservative, followed by three 5 minute washes in normal saline. Avoid handling or manipulating the valve leaflets. Do not remove the label (Figure 23.1).

5. During the wash, remove the multi-track and the introducer sheath, dilate the femoral vein with a 14 Fr and 22 Fr dilator to provide easy entry of the delivery system through the skin.

6. Prepare the delivery system by flushing the guidewire lumen and side arm of the outer shaft of the delivery system (Figure 23.2).

7. Prepare the inner (color indigo) and outer (color orange) balloons after de-airing with one-third strength contrast diluted with saline. A 10 ml luer-lock syringe is used to inflate the inner balloon and a 20 ml one for the outer balloon.

8. The valve is then crimped down in a 2 ml syringe, by a symmetric squeezing and elongating (milking) action, until it loosely fits in the body of the syringe.

9. Ensure the correct orientation of the valve while crimping and subsequently loading it on to the balloon in balloon (BIB):

   (i) by checking the label which indicates the 'distal' end of the valve
   (ii) by matching the sutures in the valve stent with the delivery system.

   Tips: The blue suture matches the blue 'carrot' shaped dilator of the delivery system, which is the distal end of the BIB balloon, and the white suture matches the white of the proximal end of the BIB balloon catheter. This should be checked and signed off by lab personnel not scrubbed for the procedure (nurse, radiographer, anesthetist) and recorded.

10. Load the valve onto the BIB balloon of the delivery system, which is uncovered by withdrawing the outer sheath (Figure 23.3).

11. Crimp the valve over the BIB balloon, with the same symmetric, elongating, squeezing and rolling action with thumb and fingers of both hands pulling away from the center to the proximal and distal ends of the valve stent.

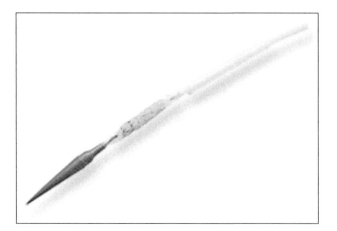

Figure 23.3
Appropriate loading of the PPV on the BIB balloon of the delivery system.

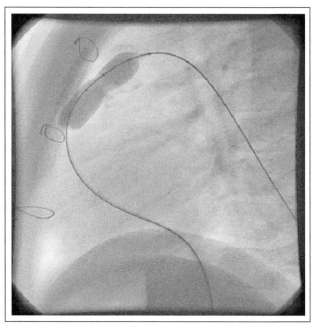

Figure 23.4
Pre-dilatation of a calcified conduit.

12. Maintain the position of the stent on the center of the BIB.
13. Bring the outer sheath over the stent–valve assembly; ensure that all the proximal struts of the stent are covered by the outer sheath as it covers the stent from its proximal end and do not move it from the center of the balloon as it reaches to cover the distal end.
14. Flush the side arm of the outer shaft as it covers the BIB–valve–stent assembly and engages the proximal end of the dilator tip (carrot).
15. The delivery system is now loaded with the assembly.
16. The 22 Fr dilator is removed and a small incision can be made on the skin with a blade.
17. The delivery system is advanced over the stiff guidewire and tracked to reach the RVOT in projections which are deemed most suitable for implantation.
18. Manipulation of the delivery system over the stiff wire requires manipulation of both, to advance the system into tortuous and stenosed RVOTs. The standard rules of guidewire/balloon catheter/sheath manipulation apply. For example, to facilitate advancement of the delivery system, pull on the guidewire without losing the position of the distal end, pull the guidewire away from the wall of the RVOT, and try to keep the guidewire in the center of the lumen with the optimum tension.

    Tips: partial uncovering of the valve–stent assembly may help in advancing the delivery system. Avoid complete uncovering of the valve before reaching the site of implantation.
19. Pre-dilatation may be required for severely stenosed and calcified conduits to facilitate advancement of the delivery system. The preferred balloon size is usually at least 2 mm less than the large balloon of the delivery system used to implant the valve. Beware

of dissection and rupture of conduit during pre-dilatation (Figure 23.4). Signs are:

- hypotension, which remains sustained after deflation of the balloon and may require intravenous fluids
- opacification of the hemithorax on fluoroscopy
- hemodynamic compromise
- angiographic diagnosis – on an RVOT angiogram after pre-dilatation.

20. Use the following rules for the site of the valve implantation:

    - away from the bifurcation
    - the stent does not lie in the muscular RVOT
    - the length of the stenosis in the conduit is covered by the stent without the first two rules.

    Tip: Sternal wires, clips on shunts, an endotracheal tube, or a pigtail in the aortic root could be used to mark the implantation site.
21. Once the site of implantation is reached, uncover the valve. This is done by bringing back the outer shaft of the delivery system over the shaft of the balloon catheter up to the black double ring marker on it. The distal end of the outer sheath is not radio-opaque and uncovering would be seen only as a change in the alignment of the valve–stent assembly. Always pull back on the shaft of the outer sheath and not on the side arm.

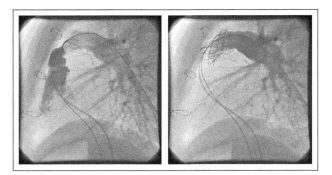

Figure 23.5
Before and after percutaneous pulmonary valve implantation.

22. Angiography can be performed from the side arm of the outer sheath to reassess the position.
23. Once a good position is achieved, the balloons are inflated in sequence. The inner balloon is inflated and the position confirmed, check angiography can be repeated if required.
24. With the inner balloon inflated, the second operator inflates the outer balloon to its full dimension to implant the valve stent assembly.
25. Both balloons are deflated simultaneously.
26. The delivery system is removed while the guidewire is held in the center of the valve with appropriate tension.
27. Careful manipulation of the delivery system during its withdrawal through the implanted valve is important to prevent dislodgement.
28. The multi-track catheter is advanced over the wire for hemodynamics (RA, RV, PA pressure, RVOT gradient).
29. If acceptable, angiography is performed above the valve to assess valvar and paravalvar regurgitation.
30. If a residual gradient is present, a high pressure balloon (e.g. Mullins balloon) of the same size as the outer diameter of the BIB is advanced over the guidewire and inflated with an indeflator to 10 atm.
31. Hemodynamics and angiography are repeated (Figure 23.5).
32. If acceptable, any catheter or guidewire across the valve is removed under screening.
33. Hemostasis and local anesthesia to the groin.

Choice of delivery system

- Systems currently available are 18 mm, 20 mm, 22 mm, and 24 mm (indicates the size of the outer balloon of the BIB).
- Choose the size equal to the size of the homograft. If the homograft is < 18 mm, choose 18 mm, if the homograft

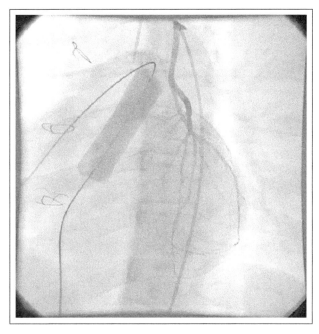

Figure 23.6
Simultaneous balloon inflation in the RVOT with coronary angiography in an unusual coronary anatomy – a case of anomalous left coronary artery from pulmonary artery (ALCAPA) repair.

is dilated, choose the system larger than the largest measured diameter on MRI.

Unusual anatomy

1. Remember the juxtaposition of the atrial appendages (left juxtaposition of right appendage) in transposition can make entry into the RV difficult.
2. The coronary anatomy should be delineated before the procedure from previous catheter, MRI, or operative notes. The relation to the RVOT and the impact of stent implantation on the coronary arteries should be considered (Figure 23.6).
3. If the coronary anatomy is unusual or unknown, inject the coronary arteries selectively with balloon inflation in the RVOT. Look for ST segment changes and hemodynamic compromise during balloon inflation.
4. Extra-anatomic conduits (Rastelli procedure for TGA, VSD, PS, or pulmonary atresia with conduits) usually require difficult manipulation to achieve a good position (Figure 23.7).
5. Retrosternal conduits with calcifications may not allow expansion of the stent to its full diameter and may leave residual stenosis (Figure 23.8).
6. In RVOTs which are of the appropriate size but have a very elastic/dynamic nature, a sizing balloon (PTS, AGA Medical) may be helpful to assess the dimensions of the RVOT.

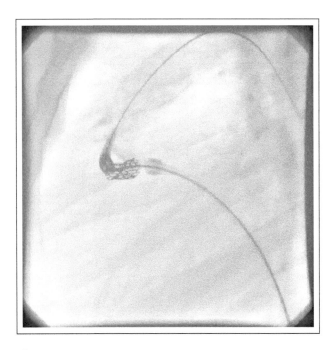

Figure 23.7
Difficult course of the delivery system in an extra-anatomic
conduit in the right ventricle.

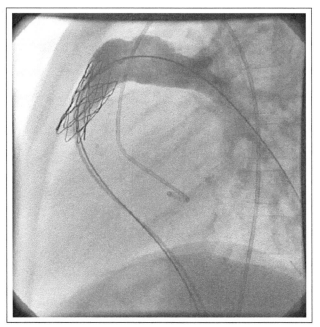

Figure 23.8
Residual stenosis in a retrosternal conduit.

Post-procedure

1. Routine observations as indicated after an interventional catheterization.
2. Echocardiography:

    (i)   look for pericardial effusion
    (ii)   look for worsening of TR
    (iii) assess hemodynamics, TR velocity, RVOT velocity, PR
    (iv)   position of the valve.

3. Chest X-ray PA and lateral on the following day.
4. Aspirin, if not contraindicated, for 3 to 6 months.
5. May need pain control overnight and, very occasionally, opiates.
6. Febrile episodes may be seen which are not dissimilar to those seen after surgical homograft placements with elevated inflammatory markers, but negative blood cultures, needing anti-inflammatory medications.

Follow-up

1. Clinical follow-up.
2. Echocardiography to assess hemodynamics and the RVOT gradient, and to grade PR.

3. Chest X-rays to rule out stent fractures if there are clinical concerns, or routinely, particularly in patients with important residual stenosis and compression of the stent with the cardiac cycle.
4. Antibiotic prophylaxis against infective endocarditis.

References

1. Davlouros PA, Karatza AA, Gatzoulis MA, Shore DF. Timing and type of surgery for severe pulmonary regurgitation after repair of tetralogy of Fallot. Int J Cardiol 2004; 97(Suppl 1): 91–101.
2. Bonhoeffer P, Boudjemline Y, Saliba Z et al. Percutaneous replacement of pulmonary valve in a right-ventricle to pulmonary-artery prosthetic conduit with valve dysfunction. Lancet 2000; 356(9239): 1403–5.
3. Bonhoeffer P, Boudjemline Y, Qureshi SA et al. Percutaneous insertion of the pulmonary valve. J Am Coll Cardiol 2002; 39(10): 1664–9.
4. Khambadkone S, Coats L, Taylor A et al. Percutaneous pulmonary valve implantation in humans: results in 59 consecutive patients. Circulation 2005; 112(8): 1189–97.

24

Transcatheter valve repair for mitral insufficiency – direct repair

Peter C Block

The Evalve cardiovascular valve repair system consists of a steerable (one plane) guide catheter and a clip delivery system (CDS) which includes a steerable sleeve (two planes), a clip delivery catheter, and a clip (MitraClip™ Evalve, Inc., Menlo Park, CA) (Figures 24.1 and 24.2). The clip is placed on the free edges of the central anterior and posterior mitral leaflet scallops which results in permanent approximation similar to the suture-based, surgical edge-to-edge repair technique.[1,2] The CDS has at its tip a detachable clip (Figure 24.2) used to grasp the mitral leaflets from the ventricular side. Once the leaflets are grasped the 'gripper' is lowered onto the atrial side of the leaflets and the clip is partially closed, securing the leaflets. Reduction of mitral regurgitation (MR), the establishment of a double orifice, and adequate leaflet insertion within the clip are then evaluated. If these criteria are met, the clip is closed further to reduce MR. Once MR is adequately reduced and there is good insertion of the mitral leaflets into the clip, the clip can be released. If the results of the grasp are not adequate, the 'gripper' can be raised, the clip re-opened and other attempts at grasping can be performed after repositioning of the CDS, if needed.

For the interventional cardiologist, imaging of the heart and great vessels has had its basis in fluoroscopy and cineangiography. A percutaneous direct repair of mitral valve regurgitation requires a departure in thinking in that transesophageal (TEE) and sometimes additional transthoracic echocardiography (TTE) are the most helpful and primary imaging modalities. Interestingly, multiple imaging views may be more of a hindrance than a help. Before the case, the operator and the echocardiographer should determine a minimum number of echocardiographic views as the 'working' views. The operator should be knowledgeable in understanding the TEE views needed and should be the person determining which view is the best for the next interventional step. It is critical that the operator and the echocardiographer have a common 'vocabulary' to identify a limited number of TEE views, so that clear communications can be maintained throughout the procedure. Fluoroscopy is helpful in only limited portions of the procedure: initial transseptal catheter positioning for transseptal puncture, initial CDS steering to move the clip towards the plane of the mitral valve, opening of the clip and raising of the 'gripper' prior to grasping, release of the clip, and removal of the guide catheter and CDS once the clip is released. TEE guidance is used for three-dimensional positioning of the CDS within the left atrium in relation to the planes of the mitral valve, alignment of the clip arms perpendicular to the line of co-aptation, passage of the clip through the mitral valve into the left ventricle, actual grasping and evaluation of the result of the grasp, and the evaluation of the amount of residual MR before and after clip release.

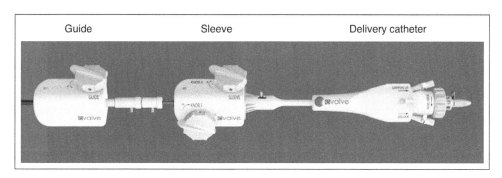

Figure 24.1
System handles and positioning controls.

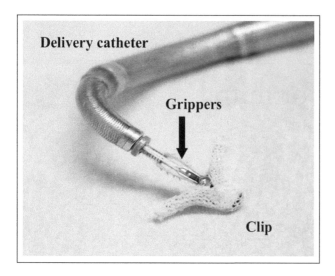

Figure 24.2
Evalve MitraClip and delivery catheter.

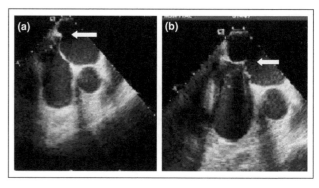

Figure 24.3
Short axis transesophageal view at the base. (a) Transseptal puncture target site in the fossa, positioned anterior to the line of co-aptation of the mitral valve. (b) Short axis transesophageal view at the base showing the transseptal puncture target site in the fossa, positioned well relative to the line of co-aptation of the mitral valve. Note tenting of the fossa ovalis in both pictures that determines the location of the puncture.

Transseptal puncture

Because of the need to approach the mitral valve at appropriate angles in all three planes of the valve so as to assure successful and adequate grasping of the mitral leaflets, it is critical that the transseptal puncture be placed relatively posterior and relatively 'high' or cephalad in the fossa ovalis. The 'high' puncture allows an adequate working space/distance above the mitral leaflets for catheter manipulations, clip opening, and clip retraction during the grasp. If the transseptal puncture is placed 'low' in the fossa, the guide catheter tip may lie just above and too close (<2.5–3.0 cm) to the mitral annular plane. Subsequent orientation of the CDS to position the clip appropriately and grasp the leaflets may not be possible if there is inadequate space in the left atrium above the annular plane. The transseptal puncture should also be optimally positioned from an anterior-posterior perspective, to enable tip positioning near the line of co-aptation. Two key echo views are used to optimize the location of the puncture. To first evaluate the position of the puncture site a short axis TEE view of the base of the heart is used. 'Tenting' of the atrial septum can be seen as the transseptal catheter is pushed against it. The catheter tip should be close to the center of the fossa ovalis in this view so as to place the guide catheter in the same plane as the line of mitral valve co-aptation. Then, in the long axis four-chamber view, the catheter tip should be moved to as 'high' a position as possible, however still within the fossa ovalis. Actual puncture should only be done if such tenting is clearly seen in both views (Figures 24.3 and 24.4).

Once an adequate transseptal puncture is achieved using standard transseptal puncture devices, a 0.038 inch transfer wire is placed in the left atrium and the guide catheter and dilator are introduced over it. Placement of the tip of the transfer wire is important. Entrance into a pulmonary

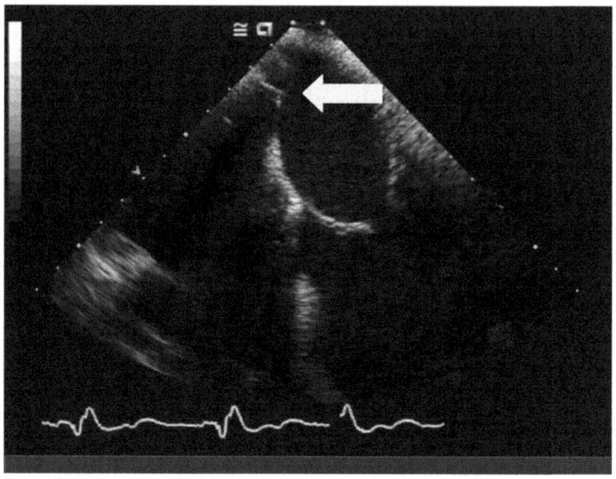

Figure 24.4
Long axis four-chamber transesophageal echo view. The arrow indicates 'tenting' of the atrial septum by a transseptal catheter in a 'high' position, giving more working room than a position 'lower' in the septum and closer to the mitral valve plane.

vein may not be possible and a transmitral valve position with the tip of the wire in the left ventricle may produce unwanted ventricular ectopy. Pre-forming a large (3–5 cm diameter) loop in the tip of the transfer wire usually allows it to remain looped in the left atrium against the wall. Inadvertent atrial or atrial appendage damage is also avoided by using this technique. The guide catheter is then brought up to the atrial septum and the puncture hole dilated to accommodate the 22 Fr guide catheter by gentle pressure and forward movement of the dilator tip, which has echocardiographically visible coils embedded. Once the dilator tip is half to three-quarters across the atrial septum, a 30 second wait is often useful to allow the atrial septum to stretch. Advancement of the guide catheter tip across the atrial septum is then easier. It is critical not to place the guide catheter too far into the left atrium, but rather to achieve a position of the tip about 1–2 cm across the atrial septum, away from any left atrial tissue. This can be easily seen under TEE guidance as the tip of the guide catheter has a 'ribbed' appearance.

It must then be determined if the distal tip of the guide catheter is positioned primarily perpendicular or planar to the mitral valve plane. Using the short and long axis views by TEE the guide catheter is slowly rotated. This determines if such rotation produces a 'sweep' parallel to or perpendicular to (toward and away from) the mitral valve plane. Ideally, the initial transseptal puncture site positions the guide catheter so that clockwise rotation moves its tip posterior and cephalad, so as to achieve even more height above the mitral valve line of co-aptation if needed. If the guide catheter tip is not in a favorable position, tip deflection can be added. The anatomic effect of the tip deflection in relation to the plane of the mitral valve and line of co-aptation is monitored by TEE during these maneuvers.

Positioning of the CDS over the mitral valve

Once the guide catheter tip is in position about 1–2 cm across the atrial septum it is critical to carefully de-air the guide catheter to be certain that no air is introduced when the CDS is advanced. As the CDS exits the guide catheter tip, careful TEE monitoring is necessary to ensure that the tip of the clip remains away from the atrial wall. In general, the best views for evaluation of clip positioning and mitral leaflet grasping are the mid-esophageal two-chamber long axis ('intercommissural'), the mid-esophageal five chamber long axis left ventricular outflow tract ('LVOT view'), and the transgastric short axis ('transgastric short axis'). If the transgastric short axis view is not easily obtained, a surface 'transthoracic short axis' view frequently substitutes well and may be superior for clip alignment perpendicular to the mitral valve line of coaptation (Figures 24.5–24.7).

Once the clip and the CDS are safely outside the guide catheter tip, the first adjustments in position are to direct the clip medially toward the apex. Small adjustments (in mm) in steering can be used incrementally to align the clip and delivery catheter parallel with the long axis of the heart and perpendicular to the mitral valve opening. To image this maneuver, the 'intercommissural' view is most helpful. Incremental steering changes of the CDS allow movement of the clip tip to a position just over the middle scallop of the anterior (A2) and posterior (P2) leaflets of the mitral valve. Though this view shows the clip position relative to the medial and lateral scallops of the valve (Figure 24.5), its

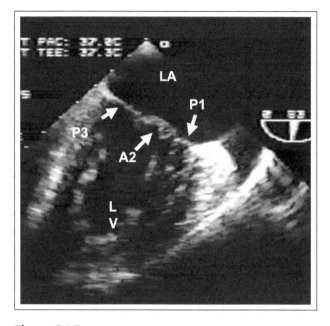

Figure 24.5
Mid-esophageal two-chamber long axis ('intercommissural') transesophageal echocardiographic view. This view allows initial medial–lateral positioning of the clip over the central scallop of the mitral leaflets (A2 and P2 (see text)) so that it is is axially aligned without significant medial or lateral deviation. P1, 'lateral' posterior scallop; P3, 'medial' posterior scallop, LV, left ventricle; LA, left atrium.

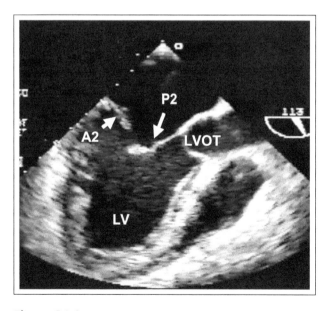

Figure 24.6
Mid-esophageal five-chamber long axis transesophageal echocardiographic view ('LVOT view'). This view allows anterior-posterior positioning of the clip so that it is axially aligned without significant anterior or posterior deviation. P2, central scallop of posterior mitral leaflet; A2, central scallop of anterior leaflet; LVOT, left ventricular outflow tract; LV, left ventricle.

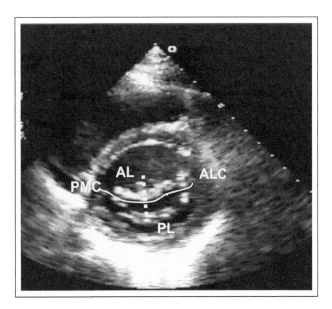

Figure 24.7
'Transthoracic (surface) short axis' echocardiograhic view of the mitral valve at the line of co-aptation. This view allows positioning of the open clip arms perpendicular to and central within the mitral line of coaptation. Solid line, line of coaptation; dashed line, perpendicular position of the clip arms before grasping; AL, anterior mitral leaflet; PL, posterior mitral leaflet; PMC, postero-medial ('medial') commissure; ALC, antero-lateral ('lateral') commissure.

anterior-posterior orientation is not apparent in this view. The LVOT view (Figure 24.6) is then assessed and further fine steering movements in the antero-posterior direction are made to move the clip to the appropriate position. One must check these two views at least twice to be certain that movement in one plane has not changed the other planar position, and appropriate fine adjustments can be made to correct any unwanted deviation.

The delivery catheter is then advanced to assess the 'trajectory' of the clip. Once in position in both planes, color flow is evaluated. If orientation of the CDS is correct, the clip can be seen in the LVOT view and intercommissural view to 'split' the mitral regurgitation jet. The guide catheter and the CDS as a unit can also be advanced or pulled back slightly, thereby moving the clip medially or laterally to help position the clip over the origin of the regurgitant jet. The clip is then opened to 180° and the 'gripper' raised under fluoroscopy. The 'transgastric short axis' or 'transthoracic short axis' (whichever is best) view is then used to rotate the clip so the orientation of the clip arms is perpendicular to the line of mitral valve co-aptation (Figure 24.7). This is a critical maneuver since significant deviation from a perpendicular orientation may result in an inadequate grasp of mitral leaflet tissue. To remove any hysteresis from the system the delivery catheter is advanced and retracted

several times above the valve (taking care not to traverse the mitral valve), leaving the open clip just above the line of co-aptation of the mitral valve. Once proper alignment is achieved the clip is advanced through the mitral valve into the left ventricle, so that the arms are well under the free edges of the mitral leaflets. Free motion of the leaflet edges is important to note and restriction of the leaflets by the clip arms means it is not far enough below the free edges to achieve a successful grasp. This is best done in the LVOT view and a final check of the perpendicular orientation in the LVOT and short axis views is done with the clip in the ventricle, to be sure there has been no deviation of clip orientation relative to the mitral leaflets. If deviation is significant, the clip should be further opened to the inverted position and withdrawn into the left atrium, where adjustments in position can be made and another passage through the valve can be performed. Adjusting clip position while it is in the left ventricle should be limited. Significant anterior-posterior or medio-lateral movement of the clip may ensnare the mitral chordae and result in inability to easily retract the CDS or produce a higher likelihood of an inadequate grasp of the leaflets.

Leaflet grasping and clip closure

The leaflets are grasped by retracting the delivery catheter as the mitral leaflets are closing in systole. If the patient is in normal sinus rhythm this maneuver can be timed with the onset of systole as expected. If atrial fibrillation is present this maneuver may not be as easy and more than one attempt to capture both leaflets is frequently needed. Retraction should be done in a smooth manner, yet quickly enough to capture the edges of the mitral leaflets as they close. The distance of CDS movement varies with each patient, but rarely is more than 2–3 cm. If the leaflets are successfully immobilized by the open clip (as seen in the LVOT view) the gripper is quickly lowered and the clip is closed to about 35–45°. A successful grasp captures the mitral leaflets and produces a double orifice mitral valve with reduction in mitral regurgitation. Two key questions are then answered by TEE evaluation. First: is there adequate 'capture' of both mitral leaflets within the clip? The LVOT view is critical in evaluating this most important question. Although the clip may appear to be in a good position, careful views of the amount of insertion of the leaflets into the anterior and posterior arms of the clip must be obtained and assessed. If there is significant motion of the mitral leaflet just as it enters the clip the resulting 'grasp' may not be adequate for a long term result. Release of the clip and repeat grasping is mandatory. If the leaflets are 'stable' and immobile at the clip entry point an adequate grasp has been achieved. The presence of a stable double orifice is best seen in the 'short axis' views. Second: is MR adequately reduced? Multiple TEE views with color and pulsed wave Doppler should be used to evaluate the reduction in MR. The short axis, LVOT, intercommissural, pulmonary vein and, if needed, transthoracic views may all help in this determination. Note that the clip has not been completely closed before this first evaluation, but despite this a significant reduction in mitral regurgitation should be evident. If so, while viewing the best TEE view of the remaining MR jet the clip is incrementally closed further – hopefully reducing MR adequately.

Since the gripper can be raised and the clip re-opened, nothing is cast in stone at this point. If the amount of residual MR is too large, the clip is simply re-opened and another grasp is attempted with the clip in a different position. Alternatively, a second clip may be placed. There is one further important evaluation to assure the completeness of repair. At the end of the MR assessment, prior to deciding to deploy the clip, the patient's systolic blood pressure should be raised to the normal awake pressure for the patient and the extent of residual MR measured. MR is affected by both pre-load and afterload – hence a final check under 'real life' conditions helps to anticipate post-clip hemodynamics.

If the desired endpoint has been achieved the clip is released under fluoroscopic guidance. Despite having a successful result at this juncture it is important to remember that the tip at the distal end of the delivery catheter where the clip was attached must be carefully retracted back into the guide catheter without damage to the left atrium. Careful, reverse steering with slow retraction of the CDS (now without its clip) back into the guide catheter is done using TEE guidance. Fluoroscopy does not help in evaluating the distance of the tip of the release 'pin' from the left atrial wall(s); hence TEE guidance is needed. Once the CDS is retracted, the guide catheter is withdrawn into the right atrium and the procedure is completed.

References

1. Alfieri O, Maisano F, De Bonis M et al. The double-orifice technique in mitral valve repair: a simple solution for complex problems. J Thorac Cardiovasc Surg 2001; 122: 674–81.
2. Maisano F, Caldarola A, Blasio A et al. Midterm results of edge-to-edge mitral valve repair without annuloplasty. J Thorac Cardiovasc Surg 2003; 126(6): 1987–97.

25

Transcatheter valve repair for mitral insufficiency – annuloplasty

Motoya Hayase and Martin B Leon

New therapy for functional mitral regurgitation

Heart failure is a major public health problem; nearly 5 million patients are under active treatment in the United States alone.[1] The most significant etiology of congestive heart failure (CHF) is coronary artery disease leading to myocardial infarction, initiating left ventricular dilatation, which stretches the mitral valve annulus and chordae, eventually causing mitral regurgitation (MR). This class of MR is generally called functional MR or ischemic MR (IMR).[2–4]

It is estimated that 15% of the approximately 20 million CHF patients worldwide suffer from clinically significant MR (>2+ grade).[5–11] The compound effect of MR in CHF patients is a serious problem with an extremely detrimental impact on survival.[12–14] In the past 5 years there has been a growing recognition of the clinical significance of IMR and the potential benefits of appropriately timed correction.[15–17] The current standard of care for heart failure patients with MR is open surgical valve repair via placement of an annuloplasty ring, or mitral apparatus reconstruction, or mitral valve replacement.[5,18] Surgical mitral annuloplasty is designed to reduce the anterior and posterior annulus diameter and improve the co-aptation of the mitral valve leaflets, and therefore reduce MR.[5,18,19] Mitral annuloplasty is generally effective in producing a durable reduction in mitral regurgitation. However, mortality rates associated with mitral valve surgery limit its application, particularly in the already compromised CHF patients who suffer differentially higher surgical morbidity and mortality.[5,6,12,16,20,21] Over the past 5 years, a high procedure morbidity and mortality has propelled the development of various novel approaches, including both surgical and percutaneous means. This section will focus on the present status of a proposed alternative method, the percutaneous transvenous mitral annuloplasty

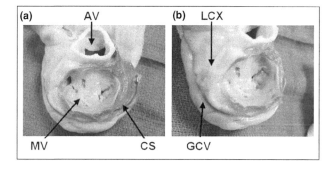

Figure 25.1
CS and mitral annulus in swine. (a) The CS and GCV travel in the atrioventricular groove in close proximity to the posterior mitral annulus. (b) The LCX crosses over the GCV. MV, mitral valve; AV, aortic valve; LCX, left circumflex coronary artery; CS, coronary sinus; GCV, great cardiac vein.

(PTMA) via a coronary sinus (CS) approach. These efforts are still in the pre-clinical stage.

Coronary sinus and mitral annulus

Figure 25.1 shows a gross anatomic short-axis view of the mitral valve apparatus in swine. The CS and great cardiac vein (GCV) form a gentle curve in the arterio-ventricular groove, and are separated from the posterior mitral annulus by a thin band of atrial muscle and connective tissue. The CS and GCV generally follow the course of the posterior mitral annulus from its ostium in the right atrium to the origin of the anterior interventricular vein (AIV), from commissure to commissure of the mitral valve. These anatomic characteristics, coupled with the ease of percutaneous access to the CS, led to the hypothesis that mitral annuloplasty could be successfully performed percutaneously by a PTMA device in the CS.[22–24]

Concept of percutaneous transvenous mitral annuloplasty

The general concept of PTMA is to place a device percutaneously in the CS–GCV venous continuity that remodels the surrounding cardiac anatomy to effect a favorable change in the mitral geometry. The device would be placed in a catheterization lab setting with the patient sedated and MR observed continuously, as contrasted with the classic open chest surgical setting with the patient on cardiopulmonary bypass. The geometric correction induced by a surgical annuloplasty is generally well understood. The objective of an annuloplasty is to reduce the anterior-posterior dimension of the mitral annulus by approximately 10 mm without inducing other unfavorable geometric changes.[25] In addition, it is well understood that in expert hands surgical annuloplasty includes various fine geometric corrections to best optimize treatment effect for a given patient's specific anatomic presentation.[18,26] The anterior-posterior correction is required to compensate for the adverse changes imposed on the valve by the characteristic left ventricular dilatation associated with CHF.[18,19] Any percutaneous means of correction must impose a similar, durably effective correction. The various proposed concepts of percutaneous mitral annuloplasty have thus included various means of adjusting the magnitude and character of the treatment effect in response to the observed effects on the severity of mitral regurgitation.

Over the past 3 years, several acute and chronic experimental studies of various approaches to PTMA have been reported in the literature and presented in conference settings. The literature has demonstrated acute, short and long term safety and efficacy of PTMA devices in experimental MR models induced with coronary ligations, rapid ventricular pacing in large animals, and chronic models of infarction and CHF.[27–31] These PTMA concepts have included various design concepts: stent-like implant anchors and interspersed tensioners, C-shape implant devices, straight or curved shape implant devices, wire-based implant devices, heat energy approaches, and transventricular suture-based annuloplasty.[32] Various other percutaneous methods are under development that target regurgitation originating due to leaflet prolapse, but are generally not expected to be effective in the isolated setting of IMR. These devices, however, may ultimately have a role in combination with the PTMA devices discussed here.[33]

Patient pre-screening

For successful PTMA, patient pre-screening will be crucial. Non-invasive imaging technology such as three-dimensional (3D) echocardiography, multi-slice computed tomography, and magnetic resonance imaging can provide tremendous insight into the unique spatial and transverse anatomic relationships between the CS and mitral annulus.[34–37] The objectives and methods of pre-screening can be expected to continuously evolve as percutaneous treatment methods emerge, and the understanding of the ideal characteristics of candidates for medical, percutaneous, and surgical techniques is refined. Each of the imaging modalities is experiencing exciting and significant evolution that will continue to challenge clinical decision strategies for this patient cohort.

It is well understood that there is considerable variation in both the coronary venous system and also in the underlying valvular architecture and ventricular dimensions leading to the presentation of IMR in a CHF patient. The critical factors associated with the venous anatomy that we have to evaluate before the PTMA procedure include:

1. abnormal anatomy, such as angulation, narrowing, or hypoplasia of the CS or GCV[38]
2. the length between the ostium of the CS and the distal GCV
3. the location of cross-over between the GCV and left circumflex coronary artery (LCX)
4. the size of the CS and GCV
5. the relative position or transverse relation between CS and mitral annulus, and
6. mitral annulus calcification.

Of course, favorable and unfavorable anatomic variants will be device and technique specific. As our clinical experience with the various percutaneous and surgical alternatives evolves, specific anatomic inclusions and exclusions will be defined.

Figure 25.2 (see also color plate section) represents the 3D overlay of venous and arterial pathways from multi-slice CT data from 10 human subjects with ischemic MR and chronic heart failure. Multi-slice CT data clearly show the length from the ostium of the CS to the ostium of the AIV, the location of the cross-over between the GCV and LCX, and the relative position or transverse relation between the CS and mitral annulus.

The relative position between the CS and the mitral annulus is very important for a successful PTMA implant. Von Ludinghausen et al[39] examined 240 human hearts (Figure 25.3). The widely postulated location of the coronary sinus in the left posterior coronary sulcus was found in only 12% of the case studies. In most specimens, the coronary sinus was in a displaced position towards the posterior wall of the left atrium. The displacement or elevation was

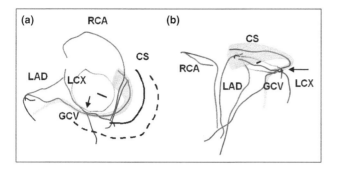

Figure 25.2
Multi-slice CT 3D model data. Overlay of anatomy from multi-slice CT data from 10 human subjects with ischemic mitral regurgitation with chronic heart failure. Panel (a) is a short axis view and panel (b) shows the long axis. Red lines show the coronary arteries; the blue line is the coronary vein, and the yellow line indicates the mitral annulus. The long arc (broken line) is the length between the ostium of the CS and distal GCV. The short arc (solid line) is the distance between the CS ostium and the cross-over between the GCV and LCX. The short line in the mitral annulus is a 1 cm calibration. An arrow indicates the crossover between the GCV and LCX. LAD, left anterior descending coronary artery; LCX, left circumflex coronary artery; RCA, right coronary artery; CS, coronary sinus; GCV, great cardiac vein; (Reproduced courtesy of Dr. Richard White and Dr. Randy Setser of the Cleveland Clinic Foundation. (See also color plate section.)

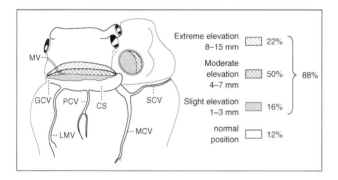

Figure 25.3
Relative position between the CS and mitral annulus. The displacement or elevation of the CS towards the posterior wall of the left atrium was slight (1–3 mm) in 16% of the cases, moderate (4–7 mm) in 50%, and extreme (8–15 mm) in 22%. CS, coronary sinus; GCV, great cardiac vein; LMV, left marginal vein; MV, Marshall's vein, oblique vein of the left atrium; MCV, middle cardiac vein; PCV, posterior cardiac vein, posterior vein of the left ventricle; SCV, small cardiac vein.[40]

slight (1–3 mm) in 16% of the cases, moderate (4–7 mm) in 50%, and extreme (8–15 mm) in 22%.[23,39,40] If the CS and GCV are extremely displaced from the mitral annulus towards the posterior wall of the left atrium, efficacy in reducing the IMR will be diminished. The size of the CS and

GCV must also be evaluated to prevent major complications related to the PTMA procedure. If the CS is too small,[22,37,38] the patient should be excluded because the device can occlude the CS and GCV, which would cause venous stasis and a possible hemorrhagic infarction.[41]

Transthoracic echocardiography will remain the fundamental, non-invasive imaging technology employed for the screening of CHF-IMR patients. Early pre-clinical experience suggests that good candidates for the PTMA procedure will present with a generally central jet of MR. The tenting angle of the leaflets also must not be excessive. Finally, the origins of the MR must be appropriate. The ideal patient will have ischemic and functional mitral regurgitation with generally symmetric mitral annulus dilatation and will usually have a normal appearing mitral apparatus; the regurgitation is caused by changes in left ventricular and mitral annular geometry that prevent normal leaflet co-aptation. MR due to mitral valve prolapse will be addressed by other surgical or percutaneous means. As clinical experience evolves with PTMA devices, other inclusion and exclusion criteria are expected to emerge. Most particularly, the overall cardiac functional status of the patient will be a key element in appropriate patient selection for PTMA, surgical annuloplasty, or medical management. PTMA will most likely be best indicated for a cohort of patients that are at moderately high risk for surgery, but whose overall cardiac functional status suggests they might favorably benefit from a reduction in MR. Surgical annuloplasty will likely continue to be the preferred option for patients undergoing concomitant surgical revascularization. If we stratify patients through careful pre-screening, we can best optimize the introduction of these new treatment options to the evolving clinical armamentarium. Of course rigorous registry and randomized trials in varying cohorts and methods will be required to guide the evolution of these technologies.[42]

Access and procedures

Electrophysiologists routinely practice CS intervention, most commonly for the placement of biventricular pacing leads in branch veins terminating in the CS or the GCV. There is extensive literature and experience documenting the critical aspects of safe percutaneous technique within these delicate venous structures.[43–47] Meisel et al reported successful cannulation of the CS in 96% of 129 patients.[24] Electrophysiologists have achieved high procedure safety rates; however, interventional cardiologists are not familiar with CS access and coronary venous intervention and should be cautious as to the differences between conventional arterial access and venous access. Looking ahead to PTMA procedures, the most important aspect of CS access is inserting these potentially relatively larger devices, compared to the current pacemaker leads, without complication. Also, once in place, these devices are not only somewhat larger than state-of-the-art pacing leads, but the various proposed PTMA actions will place treatment loads into the surfaces of these venous structures. The potential acute and chronic adverse interactions must be carefully understood for these proposed methods to be successful. It is quite certain that special attention must be given to prevent tamponade caused by perforation or dissection during engagement of CS sheath, wire manipulation, or contrast injection within the target venous anatomy.

To minimize the risk of thrombus formation during PTMA procedures, heparin must be administered intravenously at the beginning of the procedure following standard percutaneous guidelines.

Access procedures for PTMA follow fairly standard methods. Following local anesthesia, 5 Fr sheaths are placed in the femoral artery and vein, and an 8 or 9 Fr coronary sinus sheath is placed in a jugular or subclavian vein using the standard Seldinger technique.

Via the femoral artery, the left coronary artery is cannulated with a 5 Fr diagnostic catheter under fluoroscopic guidance, and baseline coronary angiography with venous follow-through is performed with left anterior oblique (LAO) angle and right anterior oblique (RAO) angle (Figure 25.4). As appropriate, a 5 Fr standard angiographic pigtail catheter is also advanced retrograde into the LV using a 0.035 inch guidewire. Left ventriculography (LVG) and hemodynamic measurements are then performed. Via the femoral vein, a 5 Fr Swan–Ganz catheter is advanced into the pulmonary artery to measure the pulmonary wedge pressure. Via the jugular or subclavian vein the CS is selectively cannulated with an 8 or 9 Fr standard coronary sinus access sheath appropriate for the vessel used for access, either subclavian left or right, or jugular vein (e.g. SafeSheath, Pressure Products, San Pedro, CA).

There are two techniques for engaging the coronary sinus guiding sheath into the CS. The first one is to engage it based on the venous follow-through roadmap by coronary angiography with an LAO view. The second method is to use the pressure wave of the right ventricle (RV) and right atrium (RA). Following sheath advancement into the RA, the sheath and a wire are inserted into the RV, and then retracted slowly into the RA. Once in the RA, torque counterclockwise towards the posterior wall; the CS is located just infero-posterior to the tricuspid valve. The wire is advanced and the SafeSheath is engaged into the CS. The wire will then be replaced with a 0.025 inch hydrophilic angled Glidewire (Terumo Corporation, Tokyo, Japan). The Glidewire is advanced from the CS to the distal AIV. Over the Glidewire, a PTMA device can be delivered to the ostium of the CS and the GCV.

The preferential wire choice is a hydrophilic coated wire over a coil wire. Coil wires tend to induce higher friction along the delicate vein wall and can easily create hemorrhage in the coronary vein.

The safest way to manipulate the wire within the coronary vein is to make a tight curve at the distal tip before insertion. Once it is advanced in the coronary vein, make a

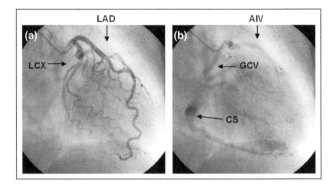

Figure 25.4
Left coronary angiography (a) and venous follow-through (b) with a 30° right anterior oblique view in a human. LAD, left anterior descending coronary artery; LCX, left circumflex coronary artery; CS, coronary sinus; GCV, great cardiac vein; AIV, anterior ventricular vein.

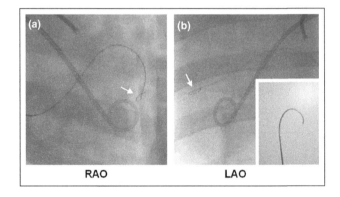

Figure 25.5
A pigtail catheter is placed in the left ventricle. A Glidewire is placed in the distal anterior ventricular vein (AIV) with RAO (a) and LAO (b). The right lower corner represents the tip of the Glidewire with a tight J curve. The white arrow shows a loop in the wire tip within the AIV. The loop of the Glidewire is important to prevent a perforation in the coronary vein. RAO, right anterior oblique angle; LAO, left anterior oblique angle.

loop in the wire tip within the vein by prolapsing the distal wire tip with a torquing and advancing motion. The wire can then be advanced more safely and atraumatically into the distal AIV (Figure 25.5).

Baseline data collection

Baseline hemodynamic measurements and electrocardiography are performed before the PTMA device deployment. A venous road map, as well as information on the relationship between the LCX and GCV, is obtained with simultaneous coronary angiography and venography or angiography with a venous follow-through phase. It is estimated that in 81%

of patients, the GCV crosses over the LCX in the atrioventricular groove[37] (Figure 25.1a). Coronary angiography and venography are necessary to avoid possible LCX occlusion from compression with the PTMA device deployment in the CS. Venography via CS with a Safesheath or a wedge balloon can also provide precise anatomic information on the length and curvature of the CS and GCV. The size of the PTMA device is selected based on the distance between the CS and the origin of the AIV. When the venography is performed, it is safe to keep the wire in place through the Safesheath or wedge balloon and monitor the pressure wave from the distal end of the catheter to prevent a wedge injection. The presence and severity of MR are evaluated with transthoracic echocardiography (TTE) as a standard pre-operative assessment. Echocardiography is performed using the modes of two-dimensional (2D) imaging and real-time 3D color Doppler imaging to evaluate the following factors:

1. LV volumes and ejection fraction
2. 2D image of the mitral valve, and
3. color Doppler imaging of the MR jet.

While transesophageal echo (TEE) is also a possibility, for the proposed patient cohort the advantage of avoiding general anesthesia is considerable and thus transthoracic echocardiography will likely be preferred, except in cases where the thoracic echo window is truly inadequate and the patient can be appropriately interrogated via TEE. For TTE, a real-time 3D system is the preferred choice. Intracardiac echocardiography and real-time 3D TEE is also likely to emerge as important tools as these procedures are established. A further consideration is the need for regular echo follow-up during the early clinical development of these various methods. It may be appropriate to exclude patients who do not present a suitable transthoracic imaging window.

Devices

Over the past 4 years, the author has contributed to development of one particular embodiment of a percutaneous mitral annuloplasty device (Viacor, Wilmington, MA).[27,30] Based upon extensive animal and initial human experience with this technique, and some limited exposure to various alternative approaches under development, the general techniques relevant to PTMA will be described.

Device description

Figure 25.6 (see also color plate section) represents the fundamental concept of the Viacor PTMA device. The device and method are based upon the progressive insertion of initially straight percutaneous mitral annuloplasty devices into the venous continuity, which then bend in response to

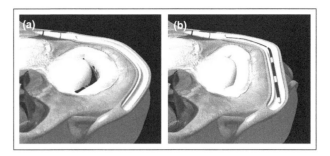

Figure 25.6
Straight shape percutaneous mitral annuloplasty device. (a) Catheter placed in the CS. (b) Reshaping of the mitral annulus via the coronary sinus utilizing a 'rigid bar'. The device pushes forward the posterior annulus, thereby increasing leaflet co-aptation. (Reproduced courtesy of Viacor Inc., Wilmington, MA, USA.) (See also color plate section.)

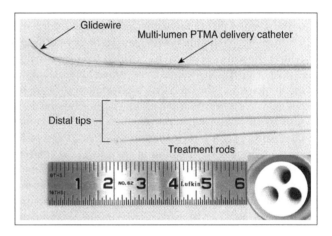

Figure 25.7
PTMA device (Viacor, Wilmington, MA). Distal portion of guidewire and multi-lumen delivery catheter with tips of three different treatment rods. The right lower corner demonstrates a magnified cross-section of the multi-lumen delivery catheter. By varying the number of devices, up to three, and the stiffness of each device, the total stiffness can be magnified, increasing the force delivered to the posterior mitral annulus. (Reproduced courtesy of Viacor Inc., Wilmington, MA, USA.)

placement and push forward the posterior annulus, thereby increasing leaflet coaptation.

Figure 25.7 shows the PTMA device. There are two components: a delivery catheter and treatment devices. The delivery catheter is designed to be advanced over the wire into the CS, GCV, and AIV. The catheter is compatible with a standard 0.025 inch diameter Glidewire (Terumo Corporation, Tokyo, Japan). The distal tip of the delivery catheter is a soft, atraumatic, molded silicone material. The main shaft of the catheter is a 7 Fr, multi-lumen PTFE (Teflon R) extrusion. The distal end of the PTFE extrusion and the proximal end

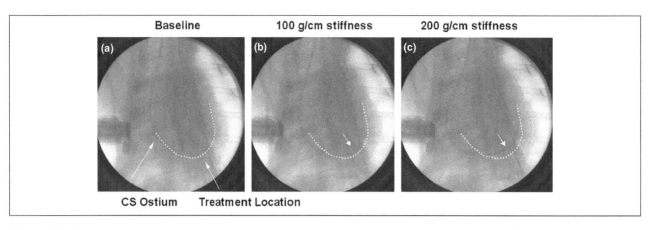

Figure 25.8
PTMA devices and fluoroscopic images. (a) Baseline catheter position without treatment rods in the CS and GCV; (b) stiffness of 100 g/cm was delivered; (c) 200 g/cm delivered. The 200 g/cm stiffness shifted the catheter position 6 mm towards the anterior direction compared to the baseline catheter position. CS, coronary sinus; GCV, great cardiac vein. (Reproduced courtesy of Viacor Inc., Wilmington, MA, USA.)

of the silicone tip are fitted internally with custom Nitinol (a binary nickel–titanium alloy) stiffeners that stabilize the catheter once it is advanced fully within the target anatomy. The PTFE extrusion includes three parallel lumens that travel the full length of the catheter. The treatment rods are solid Nitinol wires that are custom ground to establish the desired stiffness properties. When placed within the delivery catheter, these will apply pressure to the mitral annulus to decrease the anterior-posterior dimension of the valve. The treatment rods are supplied in two stiffnesses, nominally 100 g/cm and 200 g/cm, and nine configurations ranging from a treatment length of 75 mm to 125 mm. The treatment rods are fitted with a proximal handle that limits the maximum distal travel of the device within the delivery catheter. By selectively increasing the number, length, and stiffness of the treatment rods, the mitral annulus can be incrementally reshaped.

PTMA diagnostic procedure

Device sizing

Before treatment, a measurement device is inserted into the PTMA delivery catheter. The measuring device is similar to conventional measuring guidewires in that it is fitted with standard radio-opaque markers at 1 cm increments along its length, thus facilitating routine measurement of functional lengths between relevant anatomic landmarks: the length between the CS ostium and the ostium of AIV, and the distance between the CS ostium and the LCX junction. Based on these measurements, the initial size of the treatment rod will be carefully selected because it will be most critical to the success of the procedure, both by assuring appropriate device stability and efficacy, and also to prevent possible LCX occlusion. In summary, the initial treatment rod is intended to span as much as possible of the arc of the

CS–GCV, while delivering the optimal treatment effect to the mitral annulus. Experience has shown that the annulus is typically centered slightly proximal along the CS–GCV arc.

At this point data collection should be performed. Transthoracic echocardiography, hemodynamic measurement, and fluoroscopic images are obtained while the measurement device is in the PTMA delivery catheter.

Device implantation

Fluoroscopy

The treatment rods are introduced into the CS through the lumens of the delivery catheter under fluoroscopic guidance. After adjustment of each treatment rod, fluoroscopy is used to visualize the radio-opaque delivery catheter and treatment rods and to evaluate CS shape and posterior annulus movement as compared to the baseline position. Figure 25.8 represents the effect of rod stiffness within the delivery catheter. Figure 25.8a shows the baseline catheter position without rods in the CS and GCV. Figure 25.8b shows 100 g/cm stiffness, with treatment rods delivered, and Figure 25.8c shows 200 g/cm delivered; 200 g/cm stiffness shifted the catheter position 6 mm in the anterior direction.

Transthoracic echocardiography

After the adjustment of each treatment rod, 2D and real-time 3D echocardiographic images are obtained. Two-dimensional echocardiography in the parasternal long-axis view demonstrates the device position and AP change (Figure 25.9). To obtain 2D and real-time 3D echo images, a phased array 3.5 to 5 MHz probe and a matrix array hand-held transducer (×4 transducer) are used respectively, with a Sonos 7500 ultrasound system (Philips, WA). All 3D echo

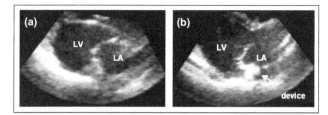

Figure 25.9
Representative example of the baseline and device implant on two-dimensional echocardiography in the short-axis view. The PTMA device significantly reduced area and AP diameter in the mitral annulus (b) compared to baseline (a) in chronic IMR. LV, left ventricle; LA, left atrium.[30] (Reproduced courtesy of Viacor Inc., Wilmington, MA, USA.)

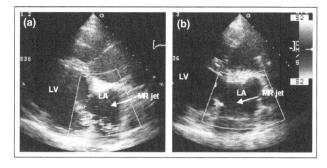

Figure 25.10
The PTMA device significantly reduced the MR jet area (b), compared to baseline (a) in chronic IMR. LV, left ventricle; LA, left atrium.[30] (Reproduced courtesy of Viacor Inc., Wilmington, MA, USA.) (see also color plate section.)

images are stored digitally on compact disk and all 2D echo images are stored digitally on magneto-optical disks for off-line analysis. The MR grade is evaluated by the jet area using the color Doppler technique with 2D echocardiography in the parasternal long-axis view, with the integrated evaluation program in the ultrasound system (Figure 25.10, see also color plate section).[30]

We use 3D computer software (TomTec, Co) to evaluate LV wall motion and dimensions, left atrial dimensions, and geometry of the mitral apparatus. For evaluating geometry of the mitral apparatus, the diameter of the mitral annulus in two directions (AP, anterior-posterior, and CC, commissure-commissure) and the mitral annular area at systole and diastole must be assessed.[27,30] Figure 25.11 shows the 2D images of the mitral annulus at baseline and with the device in place.

There is a significant reduction in AP diameter from 2.5 mm to 1.9 mm and in mitral annular area from 8.7 mm² to 6.4 mm² in this animal. There is no difference in CC from 4.1 mm to 3.9 mm.

The most important use of the echo is the real-time 3D echo to view the orthogonal images of the MR. When the central MR jet is treated with a PTMA device, the device often creates split jets, causing the grade of MR to be underestimated. Adequate and balanced correction must be applied to reduce the total presentation of MR.

Angiography and venous follow-through

Coronary angiography as well as electrocardiography will warn of pinching of the coronary artery by the device. Venous follow-through can show the contrast flow in the venous system from the AIV, through the GCV to the CS, and into the right atrium. Venous stasis in the CS would cause a hemorrhagic infarction. If venous stasis is seen in the CS, the device should be safely removed. Direct retrograde

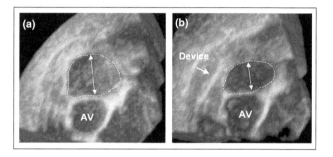

Figure 25.11
Representative example of the baseline and device implant on two-dimensional echocardiography in the short-axis view. The PTMA device significantly reduced AP diameter (white arrow) and mitral annular area (white broken line circle) (b), compared to baseline (a) in chronic IMR. There is a significant reduction in AP diameter from 2.5 mm to 1.9 mm and mitral annular area from 8.7 mm² to 6.4 mm² in this animal. AV, Aortic valve. (Reproduced courtesy of Viacor Inc., Wilmington, MA, USA.)

coronary venography is not recommended after device placement to avoid dissection/disruption of the CS. The contrast injection and pressurization of the venous system might cause hemorrhage or perforation.

Whenever a stable position of the treatment rods is obtained at the treatment site, hemodynamic measurements, electrocardiography, fluoroscopic assessment, echocardiography, and coronary angiography are performed.

When the maximum reduction of MR is achieved, the treatment rods with the delivery catheter are left in place for 30–60 minutes. As the device itself is slowly adjusting in the heart, a 30–60 minute observation is needed. When the PTMA device has been stable at the treatment site for 60 minutes, hemodynamic measurements, electrocardiography, fluoroscopic assessment, echocardiography, and coronary angiography are performed again.

Endpoint for diagnostic PTMA

There is as yet no single clinical definition of a successful diagnostic PTMA procedure. Many patient characteristics must be considered. In general, the objective of the procedure is to reduce the MR grade to less than 1+, or alternatively, to achieve at least a 2 grade reduction from baseline.

The reduction of the ratio of the MR jet area to the left atrial area by ≥50% and the reduction of the AP diameter compared to the baseline were used as indicators to evaluate the endpoint in the pre-clinical experiments. In the clinical studies, quantitative grading of MR and measurement of the orifice of the mitral regurgitation remain good indicators.[15] In an ovine study, Liddicoat et al demonstrated a 6 mm reduction in septal-lateral diameter, which is similar to that observed with open surgical annuloplasty.[18,27,48]

If the reduction of the MR jet and AP diameter is satisfactory, careful PTMA device placement should be performed and the following factors should be evaluated:

1. coronary angiography showing good LCX flow and no ischemia
2. good venous follow-through, no venous stasis
3. no symptoms or signs of discomfort
4. no arrhythmia and no ST change, and
5. no tamponade.

During the diagnostic procedure, the MR reduction is evaluated. If there is no significant MR reduction, or there are acute complications, such as ECG evidence of ischemia, difficulty in device manipulation, or elevated heart rate, the procedure should be stopped and the patient should be excluded from PTMA treatment.

Temporary and permanent implantation

Since the PTMA device will be adjusted gradually, close observation of the patient should be maintained when either the temporary or the permanent devices are placed. Symptoms, transthoracic echocardiography, and chest X-ray should be checked post-procedure, and 2 hours after implant, the next day, and one week later. Tamponade, device perforation, and device migration have to be monitored for carefully via echocardiography and fluoroscopy. In the specific case of the Viacor device, the principal concept of PTMA implantation and the transition from temporary to permanent implant are the same as for a pacemaker implant. The PTMA implant device is placed in an equivalent fashion to the diagnostic catheter. The PTMA treatment devices are then placed, ideally directly following the devices predicted by the diagnostic procedure. The PTMA

implant device is fitted with an integral proximal hub that facilitates placement of the devices and closure of the system to biofluids. The hub is then implanted in a subclavian pocket in a fashion identical to a pacemaker.

The most crucial requirement for any PTMA implant is that it remains retrievable during the temporary implant in case removal becomes necessary. Experience with this disease state has indicated that there is some risk of unexpected interactions between the device and cardiac function. In the event of unexpected adverse functional evolution, the device must be removed and the patient stabilized.

Permanent human implantation of PTMA devices is anticipated in 2006 using multiple devices. Given the complex device interactions with the cardiac anatomy, rigorous follow-up will be required to assure patient safety as experience is gained with these new devices. After permanent PTMA device implantation, symptoms, transthoracic echocardiography, and chest X-ray will be checked every week until the device and patient status are stable. Ongoing follow-up up to 5 years will be indicated, given both clinical and regulatory imperatives. During late follow-up, one intriguing potential advantage of a percutaneous system is the opportunity to address late changes in clinical status. When the MR reduction improves heart function and size, the device might become too large for the heart and have to be adjusted for long term placement. Alternatively, progressive adverse remodeling may result in a recurrence of significant MR. Ideally, treatment effect could feasibly be increased or decreased with the PTMA device or system to compensate for these late cardiac changes.

Additional techniques for PTMA

Concept and device description

In recent years, exploration of the PTMA concept has resulted in multiple additional development programs, each with unique features. These methods include: C-shaped adjustable implants, stent-like 'cinching' devices, wire anchor cinching implants, heat energy contraction methods, and transventricular suture-based annuloplasty. Each method is being evolved by combined industry and clinical teams.

Mitralife/ev3 C-Cure device (sold to Edwards LifeSciences) (Figure 25.12a)

This method proposed a C-shaped percutaneous mitral annuloplasty device that was fixed at the CS ostium and reduced the arc of the mitral annulus. This device was employed in a first series of temporary human evaluations

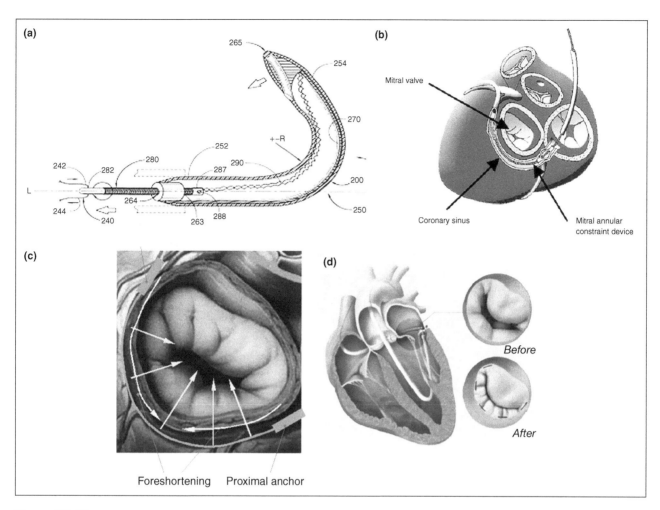

Figure 25.12

New techniques for percutaneous mitral transvenous annuloplasty. This method proposed a C-shaped percutaneous mitral annuloplasty device that was fixed at the CS ostium and reduced the arc of the mitral annulus. (a) Schematic drawing of the prototype annuloplasty system (C-Cure, ev3, Plymouth, MN). (b) This system is a wire-based percutaneous mitral annuloplasty device. Distal and proximal anchors are collapsed before insertion and the device is delivered to the CS via a guide catheter. A distal anchor is deployed in the distal CS or GCV and locked in place. Tension is then applied via the delivery system until satisfactory acute efficacy with stable coronary perfusion is documented. The proximal anchor is then deployed and locked in the proximal CS and then the delivery system is uncoupled and removed. This device is proceeding towards initial human implants. (Reproduced courtesy of Cardiac Dimensions, Kirkland, WA, USA.) (c) This device is a stent-based percutaneous mitral annuloplasty device. The device consists of three elements: two anchor stents to be deployed into the CS and GCV respectively, and a middle stent or constricting device for shortening to make the posterior leaflet attach to the anterior leaflet. Among the embodiments proposed is a delayed constriction device disposed between the two anchoring stents. By this method, the stents would endothelialize for several weeks before treatment effect would be induced via the constricting device (Edwards Lifescience, Irvine, CA). (Reproduced courtesy of Edwards LifeScience, Irvine, CA, USA.) (d) Transventricular suture-based annuloplasty. This procedure entails, first, positioning one magnet-tipped guidance catheter in the CS adjacent to the posterior side of the mitral valve and an opposite pole magnet-tipped catheter retrograde into the left ventricle. Magnetic attraction guides the catheter in the left ventricle into position under the mitral valve annulus. There, catheters deliver a series of implants into the annulus. The implants are tensioned together to cinch down the annulus then they are locked into place, reducing the circumference of the dilated valve and eliminating mitral regurgitation. The catheter in the CS, since used for guidance only, is removed, leaving nothing behind in that critical vessel. CS, coronary sinus; GCV, great cardiac vein. (Reproduced courtesy of Mitralign, Salem, NH, USA.) (see also color plate section.)

in 2002 (Condata, Caracas, Venezuela). Figure 25.12a shows a schematic drawing of the prototype annuloplasty system (C-Cure, ev3, Plymouth, MN). The underlying technology of the Mitralife device has been acquired by Edwards LifeSciences.

Cardiac Dimensions (Figure 25.12b)

This system is a wire-based percutaneous mitral annuloplasty device. Distal and proximal anchors are collapsed before insertion and the device is delivered to the CS via a guide catheter. A distal anchor is deployed in the distal CS or GCV and locked in place. Tension is then applied via the delivery system until satisfactory acute efficacy with stable coronary perfusion is documented. The proximal anchor is then deployed and locked in the proximal CS and then the delivery system is uncoupled and removed. This device is proceeding towards initial human implants[28,29] (Cardiac Dimensions, Kirkland, WA).

Edwards (JoMed) (Figure 25.12c)

This device is a stent-based percutanous mitral annuloplasty device. The device consists of three elements: two anchor stents to be deployed into the CS and GCV respectively, and a middle stent or constricting device for shortening to make the posterior leaflet attach to the anterior leaflet. Among the embodiments proposed is a delayed constriction device disposed between the two anchoring stents. By this method, the stents would endothelialize for several weeks before treatment effect would be induced via the constricting device. This device was recently deployed in the first permanent human implant (Edwards Lifescience, Irvine, CA).

Mitralign transventricular suture-based annuloplasty (Figure 25.12d)

The catheter in the CS is only used for guidance. The procedure entails, first, positioning one magnet-tipped guidance catheter in the CS adjacent to the posterior side of the mitral valve and an opposite pole magnet-tipped catheter retrograde into the left ventricle. Magnetic attraction guides the catheter in the left ventricle into position under the mitral valve annulus. There, catheters deliver a series of implants into the annulus. The implants are tensioned together to cinch down the annulus then locked into place, reducing the circumference of the dilated valve and eliminating mitral regurgitation. The catheter in the CS is removed, leaving nothing behind in that critical vessel.

QuantumCor

This device is a heat energy annuloplasty device. The principle of this device is to shrink annular collagen by the heat generated with a CS probe, improving mitral competence without implanted materials (QuantumCor, Irvine, CA).

Possible complications

Possible adverse events associated with PTMA device delivery include the following: cardiac/CS dissection and perforation, cardiac tamponade, CS venous thrombosis, death, device migration and pocket erosion, endocarditis, induced atrial or ventricular arrhythmia, infection, local tissue reaction, intimal growth and possible occlusion in the vein, and myocardial irritability.

The PTMA procedure is similar to the implantation of a pacemaker in the CS for a biventricular-pacing device. Recent electrophysiologic literature provides useful information, especially related to complications associated with CS access.[43,45] There are five major concerns for complications by the PTMA procedure.

1. *Perforation and tamponade from wire or device.* Since patients with ischemic MR take aspirin and plavix (Clopidogrel bisulfate) (ev3 Inc., Plymouth, MN, USA), they tend to have more problems with bleeding and oozing compared to patients not on medication. They should be carefully followed up with chest X-rays and echo. CS dissection may be caused by vigorous advancement of the guiding catheter,[43,44] or by injection of the contrast medium through a catheter with the tip pressed against the vessel wall. Kuhlkamp[45] reported that the incidence of CS dissection was 4.0%. If perforation from the device has occurred, surgical treatment should be considered. As the device seals the perforation, it should not be removed in the catheterization laboratory without a surgical preparation for sealing the perforation.

2. *Coronary occlusion.* Intermittent coronary angiography, as well as electrocardiography, will warn of pinching of the coronary artery, which leads to myocardial ischemic injury, acute myocardial infarction, and unstable angina or coronary spasm.[29] A significant additional concern is the possibility for late migration of the PTMA device or progressive remodeling of the anatomy in the vicinity of the device, resulting in the initiation of arterial impingement and myocardial ischemia. Careful, progressive experience with anatomic variations, device implantation techniques, and clinical evaluation will be required to establish optimally safe and effective methods.

3. *Coronary sinus thrombosis.* If the device size is not matched to the CS and obstructs the blood flow, CS venous stasis is likely and would lead to a hemorrhagic infarction. CS thrombosis occurs in up to 35% of patients with CS transvenous pacemaker lead placement.[49–51] Generally, venous stasis will be well tolerated if the magnitude is sufficiently small to be compensated for via collateral flow, or if the stasis evolves slowly in response to device implantation. Appropriate anticoagulation regimes will have to be established, with careful attention paid to the various clinical considerations.

4. *Device migration.* If device migration occurs, the device has to be retrieved, either percutaneously or surgically. Of the devices proposed, several offer the option of acute or diagnostic evaluation of device stability prior to permanent implantation. The directly implanted PTMA devices will not likely be removable except via surgery, and thus must be deployed with confidence as to the late course.[45,52]

5. *Infection.* The risk of infection with the Viacor-style PTMA device is similar in clinical risk and consequence to a pacemaker implantation. If infection has occurred, the device has to be removed completely and the patient treated with antibiotic medications. The directly implanted devices are unlikely to become infected, as their deployment is similar to conventional coronary stent deployment.[45]

Limitations

The recent literature has demonstrated acute, short and long term safety, and efficacy of a PTMA device in an experimental MR model induced with coronary ligations or rapid ventricular pacing in large animals.[27–31] However, there is no animal model that perfectly resembles structural valve disease that occurs in humans. Although the safety and feasibility of PTMA can be evaluated in the experimental studies, the treatment efficacy for human MR with CHF cannot be assessed in any animal model.[28,30] This concept and the efficacy have to be carefully proven in human patients. Additionally, each proposed device employs differing operating characteristics. Clinically important advantages and disadvantages to each will likely be exposed during early human cases and appropriate associated selection criteria established.

Conclusions

Careful patient selection, device positioning, and sequential angiography during device placement are necessary in clinical settings. With a preliminary decision based on a non-invasive imaging technique such as CT, echo, or MRI, patients have to be selected and then an accurate diagnostic procedure with an appropriate size of the PTMA device has to be performed using echo, hemodynamic measurements, and fluoroscopy. Moreover, close observation should be maintained of the temporary and permanent implants.

The most crucial requirement is that the PTMA device has to be safe and retrievable during the diagnostic procedure and temporary placement, and be adjustable for the permanent implant. Percutaneous mitral transvenous annuloplasty in the cath lab is an exciting new technique, in an area of large clinical need.

Although the concept is very simple, the device implantation for long term treatment has to be further evaluated in terms of safety and possible complications.

Acknowledgements

We acknowledge the expert preparation of the manuscript by Jonathan M Rourke and Jennifer Cara McGregor.

References

1. Hunt SA, Baker DW, Chin MH et al. ACC/AHA guidelines for the evaluation and management of chronic heart failure in the adult: executive summary. A report of the American College of Cardiology/American Heart Association Task Force on Practice Guidelines (Committee to revise the 1995 Guidelines for the Evaluation and Management of Heart Failure). J Am Coll Cardiol 2001; 38: 2101–13.

2. Gheorghiade M, Bonow RO. Chronic heart failure in the United States: a manifestation of coronary artery disease. Circulation 1998; 97: 282–9.

3. Otsuji Y, Handschumacher MD, Schwammenthal E et al. Insights from three-dimensional echocardiography into the mechanism of functional mitral regurgitation: direct in vivo demonstration of altered leaflet tethering geometry. Circulation 1997; 96: 1999–2008.

4. Yu HY, Su MY, Liao TY et al. Functional mitral regurgitation in chronic ischemic coronary artery disease: analysis of geometric alterations of mitral apparatus with magnetic resonance imaging. J Thorac Cardiovasc Surg 2004; 128: 543–51.

5. Gillinov AM, Wierup PN, Blackstone EH et al. Is repair preferable to replacement for ischemic mitral regurgitation? J Thorac Cardiovasc Surg 2001; 122: 1125–41.

6. Grossi EA, Goldberg JD, LaPietra A et al. Ischemic mitral valve reconstruction and replacement: comparison of long-term survival and complications. J Thorac Cardiovasc Surg 2001; 122: 1107–24.

7. Akins CW, Hilgenberg AD, Buckley MJ et al. Mitral valve reconstruction versus replacement for degenerative or ischemic mitral regurgitation. Ann Thorac Surg 1994; 58: 668–75; discussion 675–6.

8. Cooper HA, Gersh BJ. Treatment of chronic mitral regurgitation. Am Heart J 1998; 135: 925–36.

9. Seidl K, Rameken M, Vater M, Senges J. Cardiac resynchronization therapy in patients with chronic heart failure: pathophysiology and current experience. Am J Cardiovasc Drugs 2002; 2: 219–26.

10. Kannel WB, Belanger AJ. Epidemiology of heart failure. Am Heart J 1991; 121: 951–7.

11. Eriksson H. Heart failure: a growing public health problem. J Intern Med 1995; 237: 135–41.

12. Grigioni F, Enriquez-Sarano M, Zehr KJ et al. Ischemic mitral regurgitation: long-term outcome and prognostic implications with quantitative Doppler assessment. Circulation 2001; 103: 1759–64.

13. Trichon BH, Felker GM, Shaw LK et al. Relation of frequency and severity of mitral regurgitation to survival among patients with left ventricular systolic dysfunction and heart failure. Am J Cardiol 2003; 91: 538–43.

14. Robbins JD, Maniar PB, Cotts W et al. Prevalence and severity of mitral regurgitation in chronic systolic heart failure. Am J Cardiol 2003; 91: 360–2.

15. Enriquez-Sarano M, Avierinos JF, Messika-Zeitoun D et al. Quantitative determinants of the outcome of asymptomatic mitral regurgitation. N Engl J Med 2005; 352: 875–83.

16. Calafiore AM, Gallina S, Di Mauro M et al. Mitral valve procedure in dilated cardiomyopathy: repair or replacement? Ann Thorac Surg 2001; 71: 1146–52; discussion 1152–3.

17. Bax JJ, Braun J, Somer ST et al. Restrictive annuloplasty and coronary revascularization in ischemic mitral regurgitation results in reverse left ventricular remodeling. Circulation 2004; 110: II103–8.

18. Miller DC. Ischemic mitral regurgitation redux – to repair or to replace? J Thorac Cardiovasc Surg 2001; 122: 1059–62.

19. Bolling SF, Pagani FD, Deeb GM, Bach DS. Intermediate-term outcome of mitral reconstruction in cardiomyopathy. J Thorac Cardiovasc Surg 1998; 115: 381–6; discussion 387–8.

20. Wu AH, Aaronson KD, Bolling SF et al. Impact of mitral valve annuloplasty on mortality risk in patients with mitral regurgitation and left ventricular systolic dysfunction. J Am Coll Cardiol 2005; 45: 381–7.

21. Enriquez-Sarano M, Schaff HV, Orszulak TA et al. Congestive heart failure after surgical correction of mitral regurgitation. A long-term study. Circulation 1995; 92: 2496–503.
22. von Ludinghausen M. Clinical anatomy of cardiac veins v. cardiacae. Surg Radiol Anat 1987; 9: 159–68.
23. Mohl W. Coronary Sinus Interventions in Cardiac Surgery, 2nd edition. Georgetown: Eurekah.com/Landes Bioscience, 2000: 18–34.
24. Meisel E, Pfeiffer D, Engelmann L et al. Investigation of coronary venous anatomy by retrograde venography in patients with malignant ventricular tachycardia. Circulation 2001; 104: 442–7.
25. Timek TA, Dagum P, Lai DT et al. Pathogenesis of mitral regurgitation in tachycardia-induced cardiomyopathy. Circulation 2001; 104: I47–53.
26. Boltwood CM, Tei C, Wong M, Shah PM. Quantitative echocardiography of the mitral complex in dilated cardiomyopathy: the mechanism of functional mitral regurgitation. Circulation 1983; 68: 498–508.
27. Liddicoat JR, Mac Neill BD, Gillinov AM et al. Percutaneous mitral valve repair: a feasibility study in an ovine model of acute ischemic mitral regurgitation. Cathet Cardiovasc Interven 2003; 60: 410–16.
28. Kaye DM, Byrne M, Alferness C, Power J. Feasibility and short-term efficacy of percutaneous mitral annular reduction for the therapy of heart failure-induced mitral regurgitation. Circulation 2003; 108: 1795–7.
29. Maniu CV, Patel JB, Reuter DG et al. Acute and chronic reduction of functional mitral regurgitation in experimental heart failure by percutaneous mitral annuloplasty. J Am Coll Cardiol 2004; 44: 1652–61.
30. Daimon M, Shiota T, Gillinov AM et al. Percutaneous mitral valve repair for chronic ischemic mitral regurgitation. A real-time three-dimensional echocardiographic study in an ovine model. Circulation 2005; 111: 2183–89.
31. Byrne MJ, Kaye DM, Mathis M et al. Percutaneous mitral annular reduction provides continued benefit in an ovine model of dilated cardiomyopathy. Circulation 2004; 110: 3088–92.
32. Yacoub MH, Cohn LH. Novel approaches to cardiac valve repair: from structure to function: Part II. Circulation 2004; 109: 1064–72.
33. Fann JI, St Goar FG, Komtebedde J et al. Beating heart catheter-based edge-to-edge mitral valve procedure in a porcine model: efficacy and healing response. Circulation 2004; 110: 988–93.
34. Gerber TC, Sheedy PF, Bell MR et al. Evaluation of the coronary venous system using electron beam computed tomography. Int J Cardiovasc Imag 2001; 17: 65–75.
35. Ortale JR, Gabriel EA, Iost C, Marquez CQ. The anatomy of the coronary sinus and its tributaries. Surg Radiol Anat 2001; 23: 15–21.
36. Pejkovic B, Bogdanovic D. The great cardiac vein. Surg Radiol Anat 1992; 14: 23–8.
37. Schaffler GJ, Groell R, Peichel KH, Rienmuller R. Imaging the coronary venous drainage system using electron-beam CT. Surg Radiol Anat 2000; 22: 35–9.
38. Schumacher B, Tebbenjohanns J, Pfeiffer D et al. Prospective study of retrograde coronary venography in patients with posteroseptal and left-sided accessory atrioventricular pathways. Am Heart J 1995; 130: 1031–9.
39. von Ludinghausen M, Schott C. Microanatomy of the human coronary sinus and its major tributaries. In: Meerbaum ES, ed. Retroperfusion, Coronary Venous Retroperfusion. Darmstadt: Steinkopff, 1990: 93–122.
40. Mohl W. Coronary sinus interventions: from concept to clinics. J Cardiol Surg 1987; 2: 467–93.
41. Oesterle SN, Reifart N, Hayase M et al. Catheter-based coronary bypass: a development update. Cathet Cardiovasc Interven 2003; 58: 212–8.
42. Vassiliades TA, Jr., Block PC, Cohn LH et al. The clinical development of percutaneous heart valve technology: a position statement of the Society of Thoracic Surgeons (STS), the American Association for Thoracic Surgery (AATS), and the Society for Cardiovascular Angiography and Interventions (SCAI). Endorsed by the American College of Cardiology Foundation (ACCF) and the American Heart Association (AHA). J Am Coll Cardiol 2005; 45: 1554–60.
43. Langenberg CJ, Pietersen HG, Geskes G et al. Coronary sinus catheter placement: assessment of placement criteria and cardiac complications. Chest 2003; 124: 1259–65.
44. Stellbrink C, Breithardt OA, Hanrath P. Technical considerations in implanting left ventricular pacing leads for cardiac resynchronisation therapy. Eur Heart J 2004; 6: D43–46.
45. Kuhlkamp V. Initial experience with an implantable cardioverter-defibrillator incorporating cardiac resynchronization therapy. J Am Coll Cardiol 2002; 39: 790–7.
46. Trigano JA, Paganelli F, Ricard P et al. [Heart perforation following transvenous implantation of a cardiac pacemaker.] Presse Med 1999; 28: 836–40.
47. Von Sohsten R, Kopistansky C, Cohen M, Kussmaul WG 3rd. Cardiac tamponade in the 'new device' era: evaluation of 6999 consecutive percutaneous coronary interventions. Am Heart J 2000; 140: 279–83.
48. Timek TA, Dagum P, Lai DT et al. Will a partial posterior annuloplasty ring prevent acute ischemic mitral regurgitation? Circulation 2002; 106: 133–39.
49. O'Cochlain B, Delurgio D, Leon A. Biventricular pacing using two pacemakers and the triggered VVT mode. Pacing Clin Electrophysiol 2001; 24: 1284–5.
50. Mitrovic V, Thormann J, Schlepper M, Neuss H. Thrombotic complications with pacemakers. Int J Cardiol 1983; 2: 363–74.
51. Antonelli D, Turgeman Y, Kaveh Z et al. Short-term thrombosis after transvenous permanent pacemaker insertion. Pacing Clin Electrophysiol 1989; 12: 280–2.
52. Purerfellner H, Nesser HJ, Winter S et al. Transvenous left ventricular lead implantation with the EASYTRAK lead system: the European experience. Am J Cardiol 2000; 86: K157–64.

26

Percutaneous closure of paravalvular leaks

Jean-François Piéchaud

A paravalvular leak may be the result of valve rupture of early or late occurrence, or endocarditis, with possible low-intensity heart murmurs, that sometimes has gone unnoticed. These leaks, when large, may cause hemodynamic changes and hemolysis, especially when they result in a high-velocity flow jet. Implantation of a device for paravalvular leak closure was initially attempted by Jim Lock.[1]

Leaks can be relatively small, almost circular, or larger, located around the whole circumference of the valve or crescent-shaped. They can also form a tunnel between the two chambers, especially in the presence of endocarditis like a sterilized abscess.

Accurate diagnosis of the number, size, and location of the leaks can be achieved through transthoracic echocardiography (TTE) and transesophageal echocardiography (TEE), which absolutely must be performed during the closure procedure. Angiography has a minor role, except for assessing the final result. The best angiographic view depends on the leak location and should be in the annulus projection. Small jets can be more accurately visualized than large defects. Magnetic resonance imaging (MRI) and CT scan examinations are not very useful.

Patient selection

Many of the patients eligible for such a procedure have had multiple valve replacements, and are at high risk for surgery. Optimal selection is usually performed in view of the transeosophageal echographic aspect. In the presence of large defects around the annulus, the chances of success are so small that such cases should be rejected. The shape of the leak plays a minor role if it is not too large.

Prostheses

There are no specifically dedicated devices available for treatment of this pathology. The following prostheses have already been used and some are commercially available:

- Rashkind PDA occluder (Bard Inc., Murray Hill, NJ, USA)
- Cardioseal/Starflex (NMT Medical, Boston, MA, USA), small-size
- Controlled-delivery rigid coils, especially PDA Jackson coil (Cook Medical Inc., Bloomington, IN, USA) for small leaks
- Amplatzer PDA device of various sizes, positioning of the disk in the ventricle (AGA Medical, Golden Valley, MN, USA)
- Small-size ASD device or VSD muscular (AGA)
- Amplatzer plug for tunnel-shaped leaks (AGA).

Use of heparin

Optimal anticoagulation must be achieved even in patients already treated. The activated cephaline time (ACT) level must be regularly monitored. An ACT of 300 seconds is recommended.

Aortic position

Vascular approach

Femoral artery: a relatively large (7 Fr) sheath may be inserted into the artery used for device implantation. Another catheter placed through the contralateral artery may be useful for angiographic assessment.

Delivery system

The length of the delivery system is a major issue which requires extreme caution. It should be measured before the procedure (approximately 1 m for devices implanted in adults). There are very few sheaths of this size. Long ones are available from the DAIG catalog (St Jude Medical Inc., Saint Paul, MN, USA). The delivery system must be longer than the sheath. When the Amplatzer device is used, two delivery cables should be securely screwed together in order to obtain a longer one.

Procedure

A prior coronary angiogram is performed in order to visualize the position of the coronary arteries and their location in relation to the prosthetic aortic valve. Crossing of the leak is achieved with a right Judkins shape coronary diagnostic catheter combined with an angulated 0.035 inch Terumo wire (Terumo Medical Corp, Somerset, NJ, USA) followed by insertion of a 0.035 inch exchange wire (normal or rigid, as required).

Sizing

A balloon catheter may be used in order to measure the size of the leak and to determine the exact number of leaks. One can use a 7 Fr capillary wedge pressure catheter, with one-third contrast medium, two-thirds saline. A 10 ml luer-lock syringe is filled with a maximum of 2 ml for easy balloon deflation by means of a strong aspiration (by applying negative pressure). The balloon catheter is then advanced on the wire, inflated in the left ventricle, and withdrawn up to the prosthetic valve. The completeness of the closure and the potential presence of additional leaks are then assessed by TTE or TEE.

Device selection

In the aortic position, the defect is often circular and usually small. The best device currently available seems to be the Amplatzer PDA Occluder which is 2 mm larger than the hole, as for a PDA closure. Its distal disk remains in the left ventricle while the proximal part is positioned inside the defect. An Amplatzer muscular VSD device with its two disks could be useful for bigger leaks.

Placement of the device

A long sheath in proportion to the size of the device used is advanced on the wire. The device is pushed forward inside the sheath. The part of the device to be positioned in the ventricle is opened and then pulled against the valvular ring. Device position and efficacy are then assessed by means of TTE, TEE, or angiogram, then the proximal part of the device is opened. Free movement of the mechanical valve leaflets and coronary arteries must be ensured. Amplatzer devices and coils can be easily removed, withdrawn, or re-implanted, which is not the case with umbrellas.

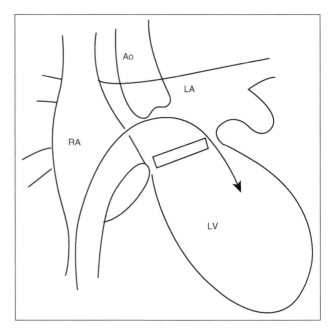

Figure 26.1
The leak can be crossed antegrade after transseptal puncture. RA, right atrium; LA, left atrium; LV, left ventricle; Ao, aorta.

Mitral position
Vascular approaches

They may vary according to the closure technique used. Femoral vein and possibly jugular vein approaches are used when the closure is performed from the left atrium (LA) to the left ventricle (LV). An arterial approach may be used for crossing the leak or for positioning the device from the LV.[2] Some teams have suggested the transventricular approach by direct puncture of the heart. This may require a surgical closure of the left ventricular entry at the end of the procedure.

Procedure
Crossing of the leak

From the left atrium: In some instances, the leak may be crossed directly from the LA to the LV after transseptal puncture (Figure 26.1). This is generally performed with a right Judkins catheter and a Terumo wire. The operator must check by means of multiple views whether the catheter is correctly positioned around the circumference of the valve and not in the valve. A large introducer sheath (10 Fr or 12 Fr Mullins, Cook) must be positioned immediately across the interatrial septum in order to avoid further sheath exchanges. However, due to the often powerful flow jet induced by the leak, or to the position of the leak next to the interatrial septum, the probabilities of crossing the leak successfully from the LA are low.

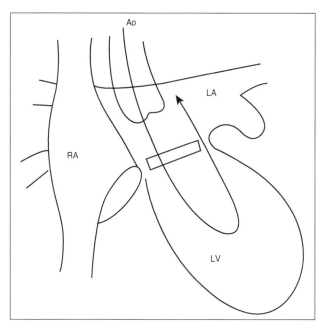

Figure 26.2
The leak can be crossed retrograde by the arterial approach. RA, right atrium; LA, left atrium; LV, left ventricle; Ao, aorta.

From the left ventricle: Crossing of the leak may also be attempted from the LV via the retrograde arterial approach (Figure 26.2). Though the presence of a mechanical valve in the aortic position may complicate this strategy, it should be attempted for a few minutes. From the LV using either a right Judkins catheter engaged towards the LA direction or a left Judkins one, with the help of an angled 0.035 inch Terumo wire, manipulated with a torquer, the leak can be crossed and the catheter pushed through. Then a usual 0.035 inch exchange wire replaces the Terumo one. If the leak is crossed successfully, the operator must catch the wire in the atrium after a transseptal puncture using a snare (Amplatzer Gooseneck Snare, ev3, Plymouth, MN, USA) in order to create a circuit (Figure 26.3a). This circuit will allow the subsequent crossing of the leak from the LA to the LV. If the leak is located on the side of the valve opposite the interatrial septum, the operator must use a femoral venous approach so that the delivery system may form a perfect curve. Thus the captured wire is pulled out through the femoral vein access (Figure 26.3b). Conversely, if the leak is located next to the interatrial septum, the operator should preferably use the jugular venous approach. In such a case, a more complex circuit must be formed. The wire is caught

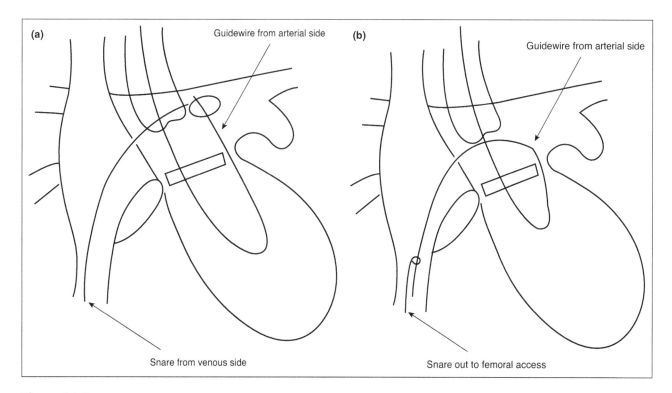

Figure 26.3
Creation of a circuit to implant the device from the inferior vena cava (IVC). (a) Guidewire snared in the left atrium from the IVC; (b) guidewire pulled down in the IVC.

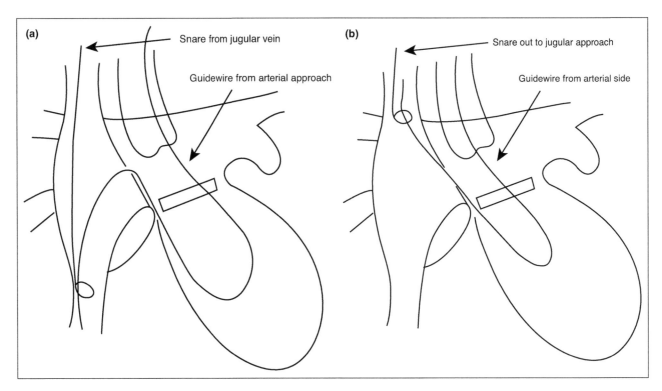

Figure 26.4
Creation of a circuit to implant the device from the superior vena cava (SVC). (a) Guidewire snared in the IVC from the SVC; (b) guidewire pulled up in the SVC.

(captured) as above and pulled down in the IVC. The wire is then left free in the inferior vena cava (IVC) and captured again, but through the jugular vein access (Figure 26.4a). It is pulled out up to the neck and the circuit is then obtained (Figure 26.4b). The wire must be retrieved from the aortic valve as soon as possible.

The leak can also be crossed by direct puncture of the LV. Very few cases have been reported, to my knowledge. However, since the patient has been operated on several times, the risk of bleeding around the access during the procedure seems low. Nevertheless, in the reported cases, surgical closure was performed at the end of the procedure.

Sizing

The size of the leak may be assessed by TEE. The leak may be very large and/or comprise several orifices separated by stitches. There may be multiple leaks. Sizing under TEE guidance is useful. A capillary wedge pressure catheter or low pressure sizing balloon catheter (AGA Medical or NuMed Inc., Hopkinton, NY, USA) can be used.

Device selection

In the case of very small leaks, a simple Gianturco or Jackson coil can be used (Cook, Inc.).[3] Usually one of the Amplatzer range devices is adequate: an Amplatzer PDA

device for small defects, with the distal disk in the LV,[4] and an Amplatzer VSD or ASD device for bigger holes. They remain in place because of their two disks, and they assume an oval rather than a circular position around the defect.

Implantation of the device

In most instances, the device is positioned from the LA. In order to achieve a smooth curve, the delivery guiding catheter should be advanced on the wire, from the femoral vein if the leak is far from the interatrial septum, or from the jugular vein if it is close to it. Implantation of the device can also be performed from the left ventricle via the retrograde arterial approach or via the transventricular approach. The delivery system is then advanced on the wire. The device is deployed in the left ventricle and potential interference with the valve leaflets is carefully monitored. Several devices may be positioned side by side or in multiple leaks.

Potential problems

- Residual leaks or leaks not visualized previously may appear at the end. Several procedures may be necessary, especially in the presence of defects which are close to one another, when further manipulation might dislodge the devices already in place.

- Successful closure of a large leak around the circumference of the valve is unlikely.
- An Amplatzer device of excessive diameter may enlarge the size of the defect. The operator should start with a smaller device.
- Embolization remains a potential adverse event. Devices for retrieval must be available in the cath lab, such as large, long Mullins sheaths (Cook), large diameter Amplatzer gooseneck snares (EV3), and biopsy forceps. A complication may occur if the prosthesis is embolized inside the ventricle, in between two mechanical valves.
- Usually the sheath types used are those recommended by the manufacturer. It may be necessary to use other types of long sheaths. For example, with a Mullins sheath made by Cook, the device could be loaded into a short introducer in the hemostatic valve.

References

1. Hourihan M, Perry SB, Mandell VS et al. Transcatheter umbrella closure of valvular and paravalvular leaks. J Am Coll Cardiol 1992; 20(6): 1371–7.
2. Piéchaud JF. Percutaneous closure of mitral paravalvular leak. J Interven Cardiol 2003; 20(2): 153–5.
3. Pate G, Webb J, Thompson C et al. Percutaneous closure of a complex prosthetic mitral paravalvular leak using transesophageal echocardiographic guidance. Can J Cardiol 2004; 20(4): 452–5.
4. Webb J, Pate JE, Munt BI. Percutaneous closure of an aortic prosthetic paravalvular leak with an Amplatzer duct occluder. Cathet Cardiovasc Interven 2005; 65(1): 69–72.

27

Catheter closure of perforated sinus of Valsalva

Ramesh Arora

Introduction

Perforated sinus of Valsalva (PSOV) aneurysm, a well recognized entity, is usually congenital, occurs in adolescence to early childhood, and very rarely such communication has been observed following infective endocarditis or aortic valve replacement.[1,2] It has been described in medical literature since 1840 and may occur as an isolated defect or with other congenital cardiac anomalies. The incidence varies from 0.14 to 3.5% of all congenital anomalies.[3,4] It is five times more prevalent in Asian countries than the Western population, and three times more common in males.[5]

The unperforated aneurysm of sinus of Valsalva is usually asymptomatic; however, when it perforates into one of the cardiac chambers, the hemodynamic effects are profound and nearly 80% of the patients are symptomatic.[6] Symptoms are variable, either acute heart failure or sudden death, but it may have insidious onset like any left to right shunt/regurgitant lesion, depending upon the site of perforation. If left untreated the predicted life expectancy is 1 to 3.9 years.[7,8]

The conventional treatment of these aneurysms has been surgical repair with patch closure at both ends under cardiopulmonary bypass.[9] Although the mortality is low (<2%), the potential morbidity from cardiopulmonary bypass and thoracotomy including the scar are the underlying hazards. Even though the long term results of a successful operation are usually good, recurrence or the presence of a residual shunt may necessitate a second operation which carries a higher risk.[10] To avoid repeat sternotomy, percutaneous closure of a congenital perforated aneurysm was described by Cullen et al in 1994, using a Rashkind umbrella device (RUD) in a patient with a recurrence after prior surgical repair.[11] However, even before that, an acquired aorta to right ventricular fistula following aortic valve replacement was attempted by Hourihan et al in 1992.[2] That successful attempt to close the high-risk surgical candidates opened the possibility for transcatheter device closure of PSOV.[12]

Materials and methods

Diagnostic criteria

A perforated aneurysm of sinus of Valsalva can be diagnosed precisely by careful non-invasive evaluation with cross-sectional and color Doppler echocardiography (Figure 27.1, see color plate section). The criteria for diagnosis are:[13]

- root of the aneurysm above the aortic annulus
- saccular shaped aneurysm
- normal size of aorta above the aneurysm
- continuous systolic–diastolic turbulence detected by the pulsed wave Doppler just distal to the area of perforation at high velocities
- color flow mapping with mosaic turbulence across the perforated aneurysm in real time.

Patient selection

Patients are selected on the basis of transthoracic/transesophageal echocardiography with perforated aneurysm of sinus of Valsalva into the right atrium and right ventricle with:

- left to right shunt > 1.5:1
- right ventricle volume overload (RVID) > 1.5 cm/m^2
- margin of the defect at least 5 mm from the right coronary ostia
- past history of infective endocarditis.

Exclusion criteria

- Patients with PSOV into the pulmonary artery and left ventricle.
- Presence of associated defects – ventricular septal defect and aortic regurgitation.

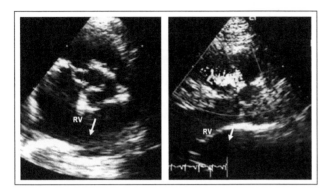

Figure 27.1
Two-dimensional echo and color flow mapping showing PSOV from right coronary sinus into right ventricle (RV). (see also color plate section.)

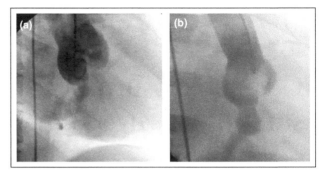

Figure 27.2
Aortic root angiogram showing an aneurysm of non-coronary cusp. (a) Perforation into the right atrium; (b) perforation into the right ventricle.

- Aneurysmal opening within < 5 mm of coronary ostia.
- Right to left shunting with systemic saturation < 94%.
- Patients with pulmonary vascular resistance (PVR) > 7 wood's units.
- Significant right ventricle/left ventricle dysfunction with left ventricular ejection fraction (LVEF) < 30%.

Procedure

The procedure is attempted under local/dissociated anesthesia with fluoroscopic and transthoracic/transesophageal echocardiographic guidance. Percutaneous access to the femoral vein and artery is obtained by the Seldinger technique and hemostatic sheaths are inserted. Unfractionated heparin 80–100 units/kg and antibiotic prophylaxis are given intravenously. Routine right and left heart cardiac catheterization is performed to obtain pressure data and to assess the magnitude of the left to right shunt. Selective coronary angiography is done for assessment of coronary anatomy, specially for ostia of the right coronary artery when the aneurysm of PSOV arises from the right coronary sinus. An aortic root cineangiogram is performed in at least two orthogonal views to delineate the opening of the PSOV, its fistulous connection to the cardiac chambers, and its dimensions (Figure 27.2). Then a 6 Fr right coronary or multi-purpose coronary catheter (Cordis, Miami, FL) is advanced from the right femoral artery until the mouth of the sinus of Valsalva aneurysm and the defect is crossed with a 0.035 inch exchange length (260 cm) Terumo wire (Terumo Medical Corp., Somerset, NJ, USA) (Figure 27.3). The right coronary/multi-purpose catheter is then advanced over it. The Terumo wire is then removed and exchanged with a J-tipped decron coated 260 cm long guidewire. Using a 10 mm goose neck snare (Microvena, White Bear Lake, MN), advanced through the 7 Fr right femoral venous sheath, the wire is snared from the pulmonary artery/superior vena cava and exteriorized out

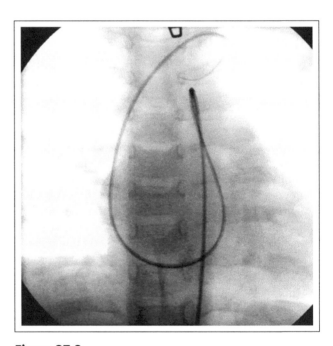

Figure 27.3
The defect crossed and the wire lying in the superior vena cava.

through the femoral vein, establishing an arteriovenous guidewire circuit (Figure 27.4).

Sizing of the defect

The procedure involves the occlusion technique. An end-hole balloon-tipped catheter with a central lumen diameter of 0.038 inch (6 Fr or 7 Fr wedge pressure Swan–Ganz catheter) is passed antegradely from the femoral vein across the defect over the wire. The balloon is inflated with dilute contrast medium to a size bigger than the defect. The inflated balloon is pulled slowly back to the opening in the ascending aorta. While the operator applies gentle traction on the balloon catheter, the assistant deflates the balloon

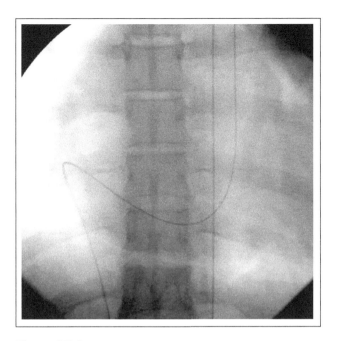

Figure 27.4
Arteriovenous circuit established by snaring the wire out to the femoral vein.

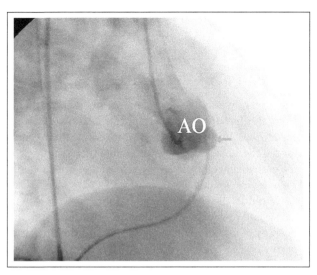

Figure 27.5
Swan–Ganz catheter at the aortic opening (AO) showing occlusion of the defect.

slowly till it fits snugly into the defect and occludes it. To avoid rupture of the edges, do not let the balloon pop out of the defect. To judge the occlusion of the defect, a cine-angiogram is performed with the pigtail catheter positioned at the aortic root (Figure 27.5) and by concomitant color Doppler echocardiography. This pigtail catheter is passed from the femoral artery hemostatic sheath after pulling the guidewire from the venous side, trying to keep the arterial end of the guidewire as low as possible in the iliac arteries; or a smaller size of pigtail catheter is passed from the femoral artery hemostatic sheath from the side of the guidewire in position. The deflated balloon is then withdrawn, keeping in the syringe the measured amount of contrast. The smallest diameter of the inflated balloon can be measured on fluoroscopic frame of digital imaging system with online quantitative analysis and also by inflating the exteriorized balloon on the measuring plate to obtain the size of the defect. Sizing with a static balloon technique (Numed, Hopkinton, NY) should be avoided to prevent stretching of the defect as there is weakness of the aortic wall and rupture of the fistulous tract (Figure 27.6).

Selection of the device

- Amplatzer Duct Occluder (ADO): the selected size of ADO should be 1–2 mm greater than the measured defect size.
- Gianturco Grifka occlusion vascular device (GGOVD): this is another alternative from the venous route. If the

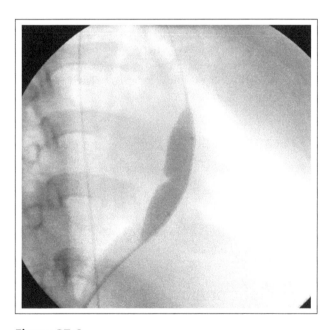

Figure 27.6
Balloon sizing with a static balloon.

fistulous tract is long, very careful selection of the device needs to be done from the available sizes 3, 5, 7 and 9 mm. The sack diameter should be more than 1.5 mm of the measured defect and the length of the fistulous tract 1.5 to 2 times the sack diameter. However, the mechanism of its use is awkward and not precise.
- Coils: the use of 0.052 inch Gianturco coils is very attractive, being less expensive. It is possible to deploy it especially in the fistulous tract, as has been successfully

done in one case by Rao et al,[14] with a coil size twice the narrowest exit in the fistulous tract.

Placement of the device

Subsequently, after the hemostatic sheath has been removed from the femoral vein, the appropriate size of Mullins sheath, 7 Fr to 11 Fr (one size more than the one required for the chosen device), is advanced into the ascending aorta; the exchange wire need not be removed to obtain stability. The device loaded on to the delivery system is then advanced to the tip of the Mullins sheath. With the distal device end opened, the entire assembly is withdrawn to the opening of the defect on the aortic side. Aortography is then performed to confirm the position and occlusion status. Simultaneously, transthoracic echocardiography/transesoephageal echocardiography (TTE/TEE) is done for aortic incompetence or any residual shunt. The guidewire is then withdrawn and, with a steady traction on the delivery rod, the whole device is opened by carefully withdrawing the Mullins sheath. The proper position of the device is confirmed and, if all findings are satisfactory, the device is released (Figure 27.7). Selective coronary angiography is performed again to rule out any encroachment of the device. At times, a right coronary sinus aneurysm may rupture in more than one chamber, e.g. right atrium and right ventricle; the devices should be appropriately deployed at the exit openings.[15]

Precautions

While closing PSOV into the right ventricular outflow tract, avoid protrusion of the device across the pulmonary valve and subpulmonic obstruction (Figure 27.8). Technically, one must try to achieve complete occlusion to prevent hemolysis and the risk of infective endocarditis from residual shunting (Figure 27.9).

Antibiotic prophylaxis

The patient must receive antibiotic prophylaxis prior to the procedure and two doses at 8 hours apart. Continue with antiplatelet agents – clopidogrel plus aspirin for 6 months and infective endocarditis prophylaxis for 6 months, if required.

Pulmonary artery hypertension

In patients with severe pulmonary artery hypertension, balloon occlusion as for large patent ductus arteriosus should be done. A decline in pulmonary artery pressure to half of the systemic pressure is predictive of a favorable outcome after closure.[16]

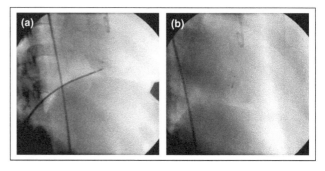

Figure 27.7
Device deployed (a) before release, (b) after release.

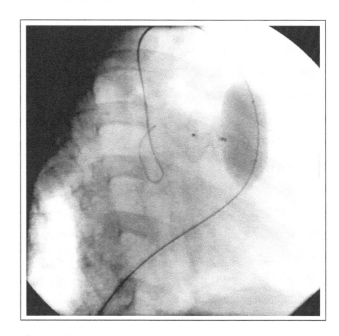

Figure 27.8
Balloon dilatation after right ventricular outflow tract gradient.

Results

The literature is scanty and there are few case reports, with one small series.[2,11,12,15] The first case was of acquired aorta to right ventricle para-aortic fistula following aortic valve replacement.[2] The closure was attempted with a 17 mm RUD for an angiographically determined fistulous diameter of 6 mm. There was residual shunt followed by hemolysis, which disappeared after embolization of the device during the next 12 hours. After retrieval of two embolized 17 mm devices, the third 23 mm RUD was successfully deployed. In fact, the 17 mm RUD was of inadequate size for a 6 mm fistulous tract, as has been shown by significant residual shunts following closure of patent ductus arteriosus more than 5 mm in diameter.[17] The disappearance of hemolyis following device embolization highlighted the appropriate selection of a device of a larger than usual size for defects across the high pressure gradients. The patient was clinically

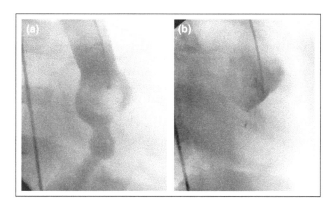

Figure 27.9
PSOV into right ventricular outflow tract (a) before occlusion, (b) after occlusion with an Amplatzer Duct Occluder.

in NYHA class 1 after 32 months. Encouraged by this, Cullen et al[11] attempted catheter closure after recurrence of perforated sinus of Valsalva 10 years following surgical repair with excellent result.

The introduction of the Amplatzer duct/septal occluders and the high occlusion rate of patent ductus arteriosus prompted attempts to correct this defect.[12,15] Fedson et al[16] reported successful deployment of two ADO devices at the site of non-coronary sinus aneurysm rupture into the right atrium and right ventricle. An attempt to place a Flipper coil (Cook, Canada and Stouffville, Ontario) retrogradely from the aneurysm into the second rupture site failed and resulted in distal coil embolization into the trabeculations of the right ventricle. In the author's experience of eight male patients, symptomatic class III–IV, age range 14–35 years, with a defect size of 6–13 mm, the procedure was technically successful in all but one patient, with perforation into the right ventricular outflow tract.[12] After device placement, that patient had a peak systolic gradient of 40 mmHg just below the pulmonary valve. Dilatation with an Inoue balloon shifted the device towards the aorta and the gradient decreased to 10 mmHg. Then the patient developed hemolysis after 24 hours and residual shunt was detected. Even after a repeat procedure with a second device in position, intermittent hemolysis persisted and surgical repair was contemplated. Echocardiographic follow-up of seven patients for 18–96 months revealed no device embolization, residual shunt, infective endocarditis, or aortic regurgitation. Six patients were in NYHA class I, however one who had congestive heart/multi-organ failure showed initial improvement but died after 6 months of progressive congestive heart failure.

Discussion

With the improvement in cardiac imaging and availability of various catheter materials, including occlusion devices,

non-surgical closure of various intracardiac defects is becoming a primary alternative to open surgical repair.[18,19] However, PSOV is a rare congenital defect; the natural history is not well defined but, if left untreated, the prognosis is poor.[7,8] Pathologically, there is thinning of the aortic media, an incomplete fusion of the bulbar septum and truncal ridges with malfusion of the aortic media, and annulus fibrosis resulting in aneurysmal formation.[3,20] Although sinus of Valsalva aneurysm may involve all three sinuses, it arises more frequently from the right coronary sinus (80–85%) than from the non-coronary sinus (5–15%).[5] Perforation most often occurs into either the right atrium or right ventricle, but may also occur into the left ventricle, pulmonary artery, superior vena cava, and mediastinum. The acquired aneurysms which may result from endocarditis or degenerative and inflammatory diseases, e.g. Marfan's syndrome and Behçet's disease, tend to involve more than one of the sinuses of Valsalva and at times the aortic root. Ventricular septal defect (VSD) and aortic regurgitation are common associated defects. When an aneurysm ruptures into the right ventricular outflow tract a coexistent subarterial VSD is likely, but if the VSD is small and the diameter of the aneurysm wall increases, it may contact the opposite margin of the VSD, which then closes by adhesion.[21]

It has been shown that conventional surgical repair of PSOV carries low morbidity and mortality, since it was first attempted under cardiopulmonary bypass by Lillehei and colleagues,[22–24] but development of postoperative infective endocarditis and septicemia may be fatal.[23] Not only as a means to avoid second open heart surgery after recurrence of left to right shunt and following development of acquired fistula, transcatheter closure has a number of potential advantages over surgical repair. The need for both sternotomy and cardiopulmonary bypass can be avoided, which is especially important in cases where there is hemodynamic instability as a result of acute perforation.

The procedure is attempted like VSD, by retrograde crossing of the defect from the arterial side and snaring the wire from the femoral vein, establishing an arteriovenous monorail system.[19] All devices are usually delivered from the antegrade venous route to avoid arterial damage with large sheaths and also having an arterial catheter for contrast injection to delineate the proper position of the device prior to release. Although Cullen et al[11] and Rao et al[14] have used the arterial route for device deployment, technically the antegrade venous approach not only provides a more stable position,[25] but also avoids puncture of the second femoral artery on the other side and the introduction of a large sheath into the artery.

The devices used so far have been the RUD (no longer in use for technical reasons), Amplatzer Duct/Septal Occluder, and Gianturco coils.[12,14] The GGOVD can find application in long fistulous tracts, but Starflex/Sideris buttoned devices do not appear suitable for this particular anatomy.

Although no devices have been specially designed for these defects, the Amplatzer Duct Occluder has the distinct advantage of being user friendly and easy to retrieve and reposition, and it has more complete occlusion rates, as evident from closure of other defects.[17,18]

Conclusion

Transcatheter closure of PSOV has the definite advantage of obviating open heart surgery under cardiopulmonary bypass and its inherent risk problems. In addition, high surgical risk candidates who are hemodynamically unstable and, if left untreated, have a poor prognosis now have an alternative therapeutic approach. Although the number of case reports so far is small, the procedure appears safe and efficacious. Long-term results need to be established.

References

1. Goldberg N, Krasnon N. Sinus of valsalva aneurysm. Clin Cardiol 1990; 13: 631–6.
2. Hourihan M, Perry SB, Mandell VS et al. Transcatheter umbrella closure of valvular and para-valvular leaks. J Am Coll Cardiol 1992; 6: 131–7.
3. Tanabe T, Yokota A, Sugie S. Surgical treatment of aneurysms of the sinus of valsalva. Ann Thorac Surg 1979; 27: 133–6.
4. Taguchy K, Sasaki N, Mastura Y, Uemura R. Surgical treatment of aneurysms of sinus of valsalva: a report of 45 consecutive patients including 8 with total replacement of the aortic valve. Am J Cardiol 1969; 23: 180–91.
5. Chen TO. About sinus of valsalva aneurysm. J Thorac Cardiovasc Surg 2000; 41: 647.
6. Kirklin JW, Barratt-Boyes BG. Congenital aneurysm of sinus of Valsalva; In: Kirklin JW, Barratt-Boyes BG eds. Cardiac Surgery, Vol I, 2nd edition. New York: John Wiley and Sons, 1993: 825.
7. Sawyer JL, Adam JE, Scott HW Jr. Surgical treatment for aneurysms of the aortic sinuses with aortic atrial fistula. Surgery 1957; 41: 46–8.
8. Sakakabara S, Konno S. Congenital aneurysm of the sinus of valsalva anatomy and classification. Am Heart J 1962; 63: 405–24.
9. Vural KM. Approach to sinus of valsalva aneurysm – a review of 53 cases. Eur J Cardio Thorac Surg 2001; 20: 71–6.
10. Chao Dong, Qing-Yu Wu, Yue Tang. Ruptured sinus of valsalva aneurysm – a Beijing experience. Ann Thorac Surg 2002; 74: 1621–4.
11. Cullen S, Somerville J, Redington A. Transcatheter closure of ruptured aneurysm of sinus of valsalva. Br Heart J 1994; 71: 479–80.
12. Arora R, Trehan V, Rangashetty UMC et al. Transcatheter closure of ruptured sinus of valsalva. J Interven Cardiol 2004; 17: 53–8.
13. Ssahasakul Y, Panchavinnin P, Chaithiraphan S, Sakiyalak P. Echocardiographic diagnosis of a ruptured aneurysm of the sinus of valsalva: operation without catheterization in seven patients. Br Heart J 1990; 64: 195–98.
14. Rao PS, Bromberg BI, Jureidini SB, Fiore AC. Transcatheter sinus of valsalva aneurysm – innovative use of available technology. Cathet Cardiovasc Interven 2003; 58: 130–4.
15. Francis E, Anil SR, Sivakumar K, Kumar RK. Trial balloon occlusion for large patent ductus arteriosus with elevated pulmonary vascular resistance. Ind Heart J 2002; 54: 499, abstract 57.
16. Fedson S, Jolly N, Lang RM, Hizazi JM. Percutaneous closure of a ruptured sinus of valsalva aneurysm using the Amplatzer duct occluder. Cathet Cardiovasc Interven 2003; 58: 406–11.
17. Arora R, Kalra GS, Nigam M et al. Transcatheter occlusion of patent ductus arteriosus by RUD – followup results. Am Heart J 1994; 178: 539–41.
18. Arora R, Singh S, Kalra GS. Patent ductus arteriosus: catheter closure in the adult patient. J Interven Cardiol 2001; 14: 255–9.
19. Arora R, Trehan V, Kumar A et al. Transcatheter closure of congenital ventricular septal defect: experience with various devices. J Interven Cardiol 2003; 16: 83–91.
20. Edwards JE, Burchell HB. The pathological anatomy of deficiencies between aortic root and the heart including aortic sinus aneurysms. Thorax 1957; 12: 125–39.
21. Choudhary SK, Bhan A, Sharma R et al. Sinus of valsalva aneurysm; 20 years experience. J Card Surg 1997; 12: 300–8.
22. Lillehei CW, Stanlet P, Varco L. Surgical treatment of ruptured aneurysm of the sinus of valsalva. Ann Surg 1957; 146: 459–71.
23. Hamid IA, Jothi M, Rajan S et al. Transaortic repair of ruptured aneurysm of sinus of valsalva – 15 year experience. J Thorac Cardiovasc Surg 1994; 107: 1464–8.
24. Wink Kuk AU, Shiu-wah Chill, Chekeung et al. Repair of ruptured sinus of valsalva aneurysm – determinants of long term survival. Ann Thorac Surg 1998; 66: 1604–10.
25. Hizazi JM. Ruptured sinus of valsalva aneurysm: management options. Cathet Cardiovasc Interven 2003; 58: 135–6.

Section VII

Septal defects

28

Closure of secundum atrial septal defect using the Amplatzer Septal Occluder

Yun-Ching Fu, Qi-Ling Cao, and Ziyad M Hijazi

Introduction

Most secundum type of atrial septal defects (ASD) are amenable for transcatheter closure. The Amplatzer Septal Occluder (ASO) is a unique device that combines the advantage of being a double-disk device with a self-centering mechanism.[1] It is the first and only device to ever receive full approval in 2001 for clinical use from the United States Food and Drug Administration (FDA). Since its initial human use in 1995,[2] it is now the most popular and effective device to close the ASD worldwide.

The device

The ASO device (AGA Medical Corp, Golden Valley, Minnesota, USA) is a self-expandable double-disk device made of a nitinol (55% nickel; 45% titanium) wire mesh (Figure 28.1).[1–3] The ASO device is constructed from a 0.004–0.0075 inch nitinol wire mesh that is tightly woven into two flat disks. There is a 3–4 mm connecting waist between the two disks, corresponding to the thickness of the atrial septum. Nitinol has superelastic properties with shape memory. This allows the device to be stretched into an almost linear configuration and placed inside a small sheath for delivery and then reform to its original configuration within the heart when not constrained by the sheath. The device size is determined by the diameter of its waist and is constructed in various sizes ranging from 4 to 40 mm (1 mm increments up to 20 mm; 2 mm increments up to the largest device currently available at 40 mm). The two flat disks extend radially beyond the central waist to provide secure anchorage. Patients with secundum ASD usually have left-to-right (L–R) shunt. Therefore, the left atrium (LA) disk is larger than the right atrium (RA) disk. For devices 4–10 mm in size, the LA disk is 12 mm and the RA disk is 8 mm larger than the waist. However, for devices

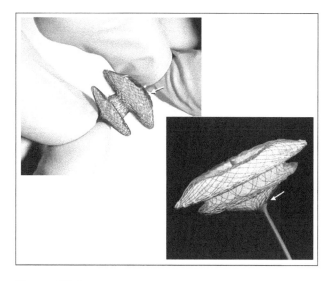

Figure 28.1
Top left, the Amplatzer Septal Occluder (ASO) consists of three components: a left atrial disk (arrow), a connecting waist, and a right atrial disk. Polyester fabric fills these three components. Bottom, the device is attached to the cable which is inside the delivery sheath (arrow).

larger than 11 mm and up to 34 mm in size, the LA disk is 14 mm and the RA disk is 10 mm larger than the connecting waist. For devices larger than 34 mm, the LA disk is 16 mm larger than the waist and the RA disk is 10 mm larger than the waist. Both disks are angled slightly towards each other to ensure firm contact of the disks to the atrial septum. There are a total of three Dacron polyester patches sewn securely with polyester thread into each disk and the connecting waist to increase the thrombogenicity of the device. A stainless steel sleeve with a female thread is laser welded to the RA disk. This sleeve is used to screw the delivery cable to the device. For device deployment, we recommend using a

6 Fr delivery system for devices < 10 mm in diameter, a 7 Fr delivery system for devices 10–15 mm in diameter, an 8 Fr sheath for devices 16–20 mm in diameter, a 9 Fr sheath for devices 22–28 mm in diameter, a 10 Fr sheath for devices 30–34 mm, a 12 Fr sheath for the 36 and 38 mm devices and a 14 Fr sheath for the 40 mm device.

Amplatzer delivery system

The delivery system is supplied sterilized and separate from the device. It contains all the equipment needed to facilitate device deployment. It consists of:

- A delivery sheath of specified French size and length and appropriate dilator.
- A loading device, used to collapse the device and introduce it into the delivery sheath.
- A delivery cable (internal diameter (ID) = 0.081 inch), the device is screwed onto its distal end and it allows for loading, placement, and retrieval of the device.
- A plastic pin-vice; this facilitates unscrewing of the delivery cable from the device during device deployment.
- A Touhy–Borst adapter with a side arm for the sheath, to act as a one-way stop-bleed valve.

All delivery sheaths have a 45° angled tip. The 6 Fr sheath has a length of 60 cm, the 7 Fr is available in lengths of 60 and 80 cm, and the 8, 9, 10, and 12 Fr sheaths are all 80 cm in length.

Optional but recommended equipment
Amplatzer sizing balloon

Double-lumen balloon catheter with a 7 Fr shaft size: the balloon is made from nylon and is very compliant, making it ideal for sizing secundum ASD by flow occlusion and preventing overstretching of the defect. The balloon catheter is angled at 45° and there are radio-opaque markers proximal to the balloon for calibration at 2, 5, and 10 mm. The balloon catheters are available in two sizes, 24 mm (maximum volume 30 ml, used to size defects ≤ 22 mm) and 34 mm (maximum volume 90 ml, used to size defects ≤ 40 mm).

NuMED sizing balloon

An alternative to the above balloon is the NuMED sizing balloon (NuMED Inc, Hopkinton, NY), available in sizes 20 mm × 3 cm, 25 mm × 3 cm, 30 mm × 3–5 cm, 40 mm × 3–5 cm. There are radio-opaque markers for calibration inside the balloon at 10–15 mm intervals. The shaft size is 8 Fr.

Amplatzer super stiff exchange guide wire 0.035 inch

This is used to advance the delivery sheath and dilator into the left upper pulmonary vein.

Patient selection

The indication for ASD closure using the ASO is the secundum type ASD demonstrated by echocardiography with

1. symptomatic or hemodynamically significant shunt (Qp/Qs > 1.5 or evidence of right ventricular enlargement for body surface area); we usually do not depend on the Qp/Qs ratio to determine the importance of the shunt, but rather on the size of the right ventricle, or
2. patients with a small atrial defect and a history of paradoxical embolization resulting in either a stroke, transient ischemic attack, or peripheral embolism.

Contraindications for the use of the ASO include

1. patients with an associated anomalous pulmonary venous drainage
2. patients with sinus venosus defects
3. patients with primum ASD
4. a deficient rim (< 5 mm) from the ASD to the superior or inferior vena cava, right upper or lower pulmonary vein, coronary sinus, mitral or tricuspid valve (a deficient anterior rim toward the aorta is not a contraindication for the ASO)
5. associated other cardiac anomalies requiring surgical repair
6. pulmonary vascular resistance of greater than 8 Woods units
7. sepsis, or
8. contraindication to antiplatelet therapy.

Pre-catheterization evaluation

Echocardiographic assessment of the type, size, and number of ASDs is of paramount importance for planning the device closure.[4] Transesophageal echocardiography (TEE) can provide superior anatomic detail of the defect and the surrounding structures. Figure 28.2 details the TEE views that need to be obtained in order to assess suitability for device closure. Transthoracic echocardiography (TTE) is usually sufficient for children with good imaging windows. It is essential to assess whether there is associated anomalous pulmonary venous drainage and to assess the

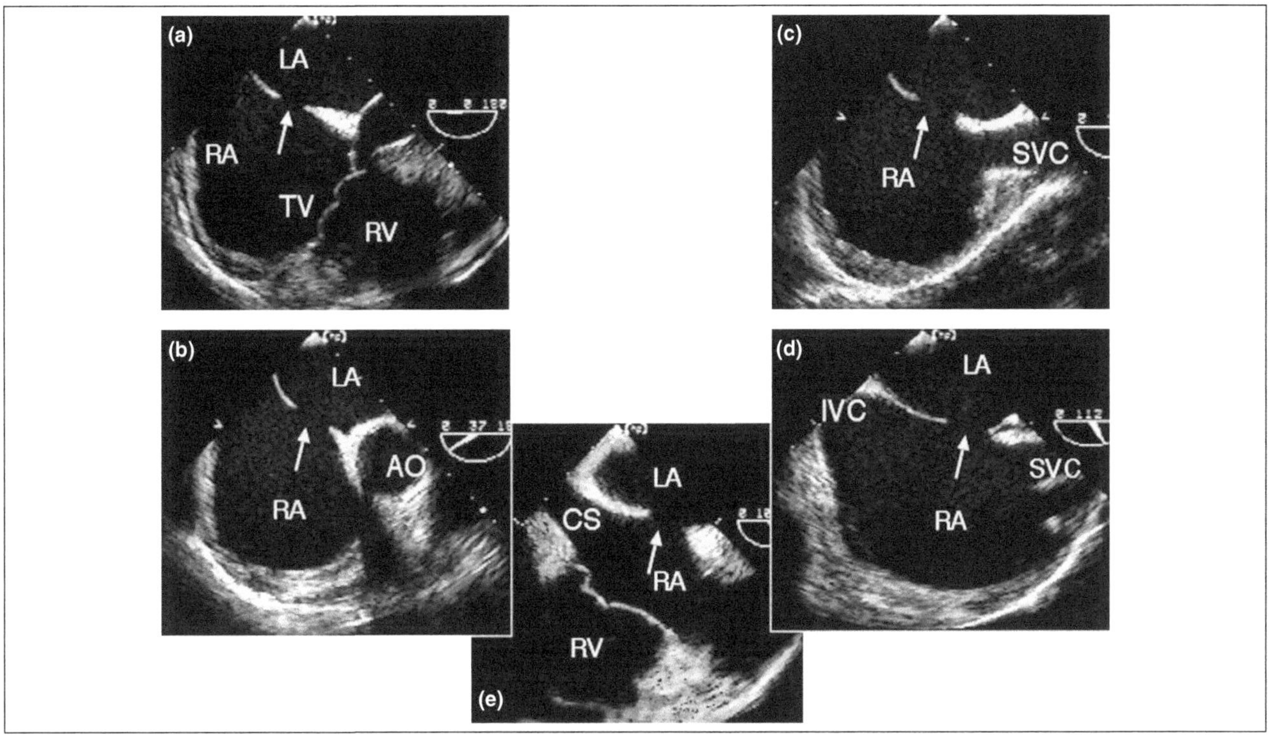

Figure 28.2

Transesophageal echocardiographic images in a patient with secundum atrial septal defect demonstrating the essential views for selection of patients to undergo device closure using the Amplatzer Septal Occluder. (a) Four-chamber view (0° omniplane) showing the defect (arrow), the inferior anterior rim, and the inferior-posterior rim. (b) Classic short axis view at about 35° demonstrating the defect (arrow), the anterior rim, and the posterior rim. (c) Bicaval view at about 120° demonstrating the superior rim and the inferior rim and the defect (arrow). (d) Same view as above with slight rightward rotation to open up the inferior vena cava. This view again demonstrates the defect (arrow), the entire inferior rim, and the superior rim. (e) Bicaval view with slight posterior rotation of the probe to open up the coronary sinus. The defect is shown here as well (arrow). LA, left atrium; RA, right atrium; RV, right ventricle, TV, tricuspid valve; SVC, superior vena cava; IVC, inferior vena cava; CS, coronary sinus.

adequacy of all rims. If the septum has more than one hole, the bigger hole is usually located in the supero-anterior septum, while the smaller hole is located in the infero-posterior septum. Three-dimensional echocardiography may provide a better defect morphology and structural relationships. Nevertheless, the accuracy of its reconstructed images is heavily dependent on the technical expertise of the echocardiographer. Forty-eight hours prior to the procedure, patients are asked to take aspirin 3–5 mg/kg per day.

Transcatheter closure of secundum ASD: step by step technique

Materials and equipment

- Single or biplane cardiac catheterization laboratory. We prefer to work with the single plane fluoroscopy system;

this allows more room for the echo machine and for anesthesia if needed.
- TEE or intracardiac echocardiography (ICE). We prefer the ICE technology using the AcuNAV catheter (Acuson, a Siemens Company).
- Full range of device sizes, delivery and exchange (rescue) systems.
- Sizing balloon catheters.
- A multi-purpose catheter to engage the defect and the left upper pulmonary vein.
- Supra stiff exchange length wire; we prefer the 0.035 inch Amplatzer supra stiff exchange length guidewire with a 1 cm floppy tip, but any extra-stiff J-tipped wire may be used.

Personnel

- Interventional cardiologist appropriately proctored to perform device closure.
- Cardiologist, non-invasive, to facilitate TEE or ICE.

- Anesthesiologist, if the procedure is performed under TEE guidance.
- Nurse certified to administer unconscious sedation if performed under ICE guidance.
- Catheterization laboratory technicians.

Procedure

The right femoral vein is accessed using a 7–8 Fr short sheath. An arterial monitoring line can be inserted in the right femoral artery, especially if the patient's condition is marginal or if the procedure is performed under TEE and general endotracheal anesthesia. If the femoral venous route is not available, we advocate the transhepatic approach. The subclavian or internal jugular venous approach makes it very difficult to maneuver the device deployment, especially with large defects. We administer heparin to achieve an activated clotting time (ACT) > 200 seconds at the time of device deployment. Antibiotic coverage for the procedure is recommended. We usually use cefazolin 1 g intravenously, the first dose at the time of procedure and two subsequent doses 6–8 hours apart.

Routine right heart catheterization should be performed in all cases to ensure the presence of normal pulmonary vascular resistance. The left to right shunt can also be calculated. Echocardiographic assessment of the secundum ASD should be performed simultaneously, either by TEE or ICE (Figure 28.2). A comprehensive study should be performed, looking at all aspects of the ASD anatomy (location, size, presence of additional defects, and adequacy of the various rims). Figures 28.3 and 28.4 (see also color plate section) are examples of two cases of secundum ASD that underwent closure of the defect under TEE guidance. One patient (Figure 28.3) had balloon sizing of the defect and the other patient (Figure 28.4) did not.

The important rims to look for are:

- Superior/superior vena cava (SVC) rim: this is best achieved using the bicaval view.
- Superior-posterior/right upper pulmonary vein rim.
- Anterior-superior/aortic rim: this is the least important rim. Often, many patients lack this rim. This is best seen in the short axis view.
- Inferior/inferior vena cava (IVC) and coronary sinus rim: this is an important rim to have. Best seen in the bicaval view.
- Posterior rim: this can be seen best in the short axis view at the aortic valve level.

How to cross the ASD

Use a multi-purpose catheter; the MP A2 catheter has the ideal angle. Place the catheter at the IVC/RA junction. The IVC angle should guide the catheter to the ASD; keep

a clockwise torque on the catheter while advancing it towards the septum (posterior). If unsuccessful, place the catheter in the SVC and slowly pull the catheter into the RA and keep a clockwise posterior torque to orient the catheter along the atrial septum until it crosses the defect. TEE/ICE can be very useful to guide the catheter across difficult defects.

Right upper pulmonary vein angiogram

It can be useful to perform an angiogram in the right upper pulmonary vein (Figure 28.5a) in the hepatoclavicular projection (35° LAO/35° cranial). This delineates the anatomy, shape, and length of the septum. This may become handy when the device is deployed but not released; the operator can position the I/I in the same view of the angiogram and compare the position of the device with that obtained during the deployment (Figure 28.5f).

Defect sizing

Position the MP A2 catheter in the left upper pulmonary vein. Prepare the appropriate sizing balloon according to the manufacturer's guidelines. We prefer to use the 34 mm balloon since it is longer and, during balloon inflation, it sits nicely over the defect. Pass an extra stiff floppy/J-tipped 0.035 inch exchange length guidewire (Amplatzer super stiff wire). This gives the best support within the atrium for the balloon, especially in large defects. Remove the MP A2 catheter and the femoral sheath. We advance the sizing balloon catheter over the wire directly without a venous sheath. Most sizing balloons require an 8 or 9 Fr sheath. The balloon catheter is advanced over the wire and placed across the defect under both fluoroscopic and echocardiographic guidance. The balloon is then inflated with diluted contrast until the left to right shunt ceases as observed by color flow Doppler TEE/ICE (flow occlusion). The best echo view for measurement is to observe the balloon in its long axis (Figure 28.3h). In this view the indentation made by the ASD margins can be visualized and precise measurements made.

Fluoroscopic measurement

Angulate the X-ray tube so the beam is perpendicular to the balloon. This can be difficult but the various calibration markers can help. Ensure that the markers are separated and discrete. Measure the balloon diameter at the site of the indentation as per the diagnostic function of the laboratory (Figure 28.5b). If a discrepancy exists between the echocardiographic and the fluoroscopic measurements we have found that the echocardiographic measurement is usually more accurate.

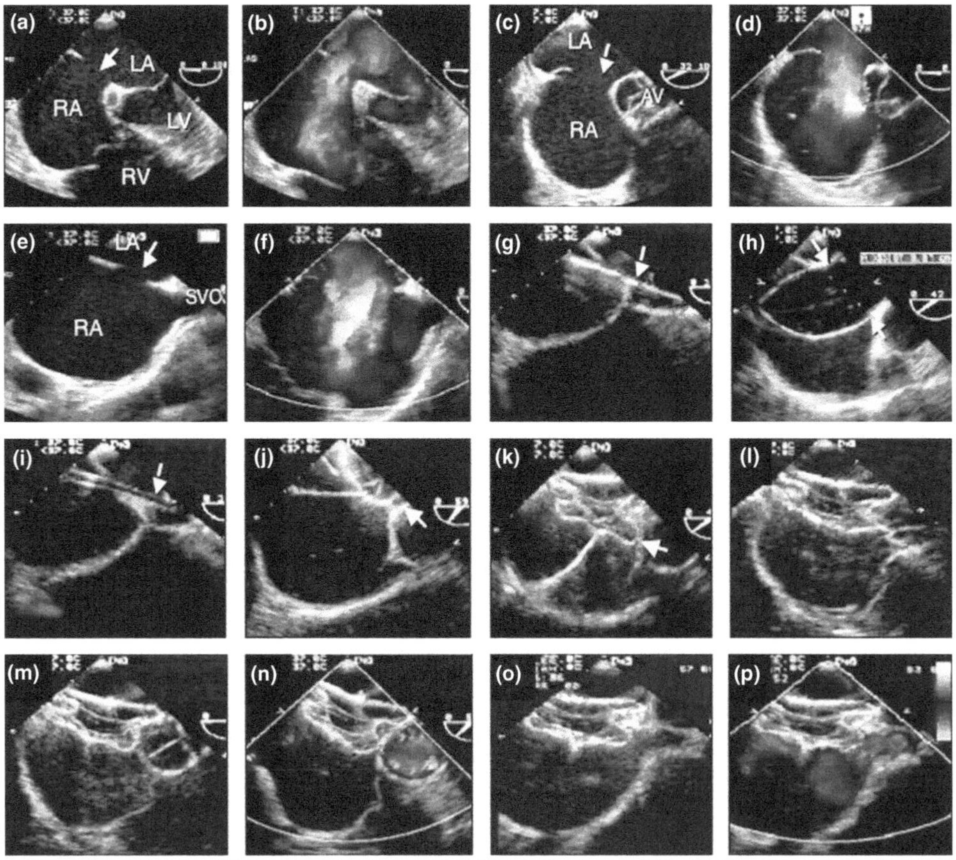

Figure 28.3

Transesophageal echocardiographic images in a 53-year-old patient with a secundum atrial septal defect measuring 30 mm demonstrating the various steps of closure. (a) and (b) Four-chamber view (0° omniplane) showing the defect (arrow), the inferior/anterior rim is deficient, the inferior/posterior rim is adequate, and the left-to-right shunt. (c) and (d) Short axis view at about 15° demonstrating the defect (arrow), the anterior rim, the posterior rim, and the left-to-right shunt. (e) and (f) Bicaval view at about 120° demonstrating the superior rim, the inferior rim, and the defect (arrow). (g) and (h) Wire passage and balloon sizing indicating the stretched diameter (arrows). (i) Passage of the delivery sheath (arrow) through the defect. (j) Deployment of the left disk (arrow) of a 38 mm Amplatzer device in the left atrium. (k) Deployment of the right disk (arrow) in the right atrium in short axis view. (l) Bicaval view after the device has been released. (m) and (n) Short axis views without and with color Doppler after the device has been released indicating good device position and no residual shunt. (o) and (p) Bicaval views without and with color Doppler after the device has been released indicating good device position and no residual shunt. LA, left atrium; RA, right atrium; LV, left ventricle; RV, right ventricle; SVC, superior vena cava. (see also color plate section.)

Once the size is determined, deflate the balloon and pull it back into the RA/IVC junction, leaving the wire in the left upper pulmonary vein. This is a good time to recheck the ACT and give the first dose of antibiotics.

Device selection

If the defect has adequate rims (>5 mm), we usually select a device 0–2 mm larger than the balloon stretched diameter. However, if the superior/anterior rim is deficient (5–7 mm), we select a device 4 mm larger than the balloon stretched diameter. Lately, we have been closing ASDs without balloon sizing. Our choice for the device size depends on the echocardiographic measurements of the defect (ICE). In adults, we choose a device about 4–6 mm larger than the two-dimensional (2D) size by color Doppler; in children, we choose a device no more than 2 mm larger than the 2D size by color Doppler. Once the device size is selected, open the appropriate size delivery system. Flush the sheath and dilator. The proper size delivery sheath is advanced over the guidewire to the left upper pulmonary vein (Figures 28.3g and 28.4g). Both dilator and wire are removed, keeping the tip of the sheath inside the left upper pulmonary vein.

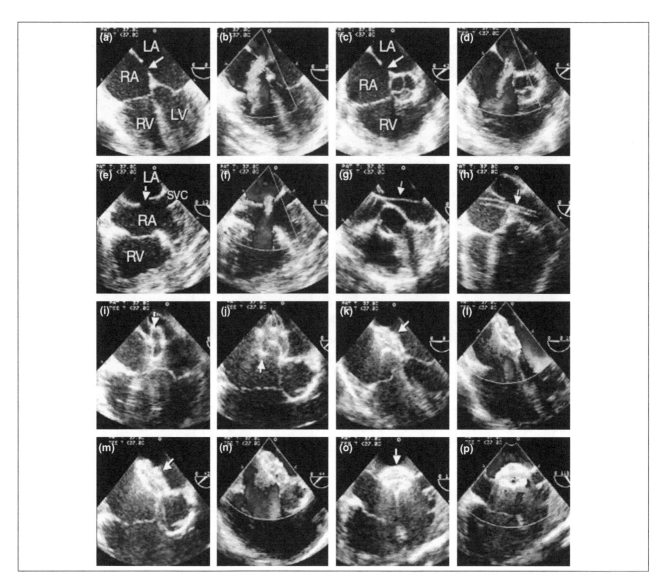

Figure 28.4

Transesophageal echocardiographic images in a 1.2-year-old patient with a secundum atrial septal defect measuring 7 mm demonstrating the various steps of closure. (a) and (b) Four-chamber view (0° omniplane) showing the defect (arrow), both inferior-anterior and inferior-posterior rims are adequate, and the left-to-right shunt. (c) and (d) Short axis view at about 15° demonstrating the defect (arrow), the anterior rim (deficient), the posterior rim (adequate), and the left-to-right shunt. (e) and (f) Bicaval view at about 120° demonstrating the superior rim (adequate), the inferior rim (adequate), and the defect (arrow). (g) and (h) Wire and delivery sheath passage (arrows). (i) Four-chamber view demonstrating deployment of the left disk (arrow) of an 8 mm Amplatzer device in the left atrium. (j) Short axis view demonstrating deployment of the right disk (arrow) in the right atrium. (k) and (l) Four-chamber view without and with color Doppler after the device has been released demonstrating good device position (arrow) and no residual shunt. No mitral or tricuspid valve regurgitations. (m) and (n) Short axis view without and with color Doppler demonstrating good device position and no residual shunt. (o) and (p) Bicaval view without and with color Doppler demonstrating good device position and no residual shunt. LA, left atrium; RA, right atrium; LV, left ventricle; RV, right ventricle; SVC, superior vena cava. (see also color plate section.)

Extreme care must be exercised not to allow passage of air inside the delivery sheath. An alternative technique to minimize air embolism is passage of the sheath with the dilator over the wire until the inferior vena cava, then the dilator is removed and the sheath is advanced over the wire into the left atrium while continuously flushing the side arm of the sheath. The device is then screwed to the tip of the delivery cable, immersed in normal saline or blood, and drawn into the loader underwater seal to expel air bubbles out of the system. A Y-connector is applied to the proximal end of the loader to allow flushing with saline. The loader containing the device is attached to the proximal hub of the

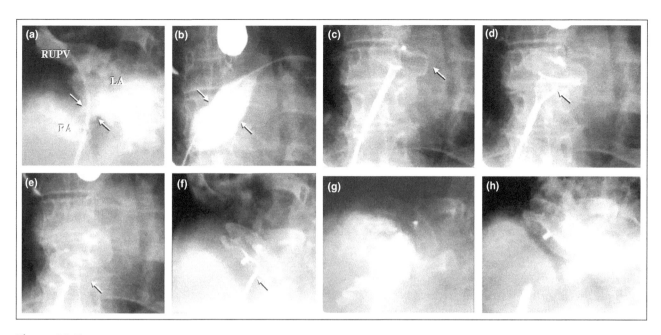

Figure 28.5

Cine fluoroscopic images demonstrating the steps of closure. (a) Angiography in the right upper pulmonary vein in the hepatoclavicular projection demonstrating a secundum type ASD (arrows). (b) Cine image demonstrating the sizing balloon with a waist (arrows) indicating the stretched diameter or stop-flow diameter. (c) The left atrial disk (arrow) has been deployed in the left atrium. (d) Deployment of the connecting waist (arrow) partly in the left atrium and partly in the defect. (e) Deployment of the right atrial disk (arrow) in the right atrium. (f) The device has been released from the delivery cable (arrow). (g) Angiogram in the right atrium demonstrating good device position (the RA disk opacifies, indicating it is all in the RA, and the LA disk does not opacify). (h) Pulmonary levophase of the previous angiogram showing that the LA disk opacifies, indicating it is in the LA, and the RA disk does not opacify, indicating it is in the right atrium. LA, left atrium; RA, right atrium; RUPV, right upper pulmonary vein.

delivery sheath. The cable with the ASO device is advanced to the distal tip of the sheath, taking care not to rotate the cable while advancing it in the long sheath to prevent premature unscrewing of the device. Both cable and delivery sheath are pulled back as one unit to the middle of the left atrium. The position of the sheath can be verified using cine fluoroscopy or TEE/ICE.

The LA disk is deployed first under fluoroscopic (Figure 28.5c) and/or echocardiographic guidance (Figures 28.3j and Figure 28.4i). Caution should be taken not to interfere with the left atrial appendage. Part of the connecting waist should be deployed in the left atrium, very close (a few mm) to the atrial septum (the mechanism of ASD closure using the ASO is stenting of the defect) (Figure 28.5d). While applying constant pulling of the entire assembly and withdrawing the delivery sheath off the cable, the connecting waist and the right atrial disk are deployed in the ASD itself and in the RA, respectively (Figures 28.5e, 28.3k, and 28.4j). Proper device position can be verified using different techniques:

1. Fluoroscopy in the same projection as that of the angiogram. Good device position is evident by the presence of two disks that are parallel to each other and separated from each other by the atrial septum

(Figure 28.5f). In the same view the operator can perform the 'Minnesota wiggle' (the cable is pushed gently forward and pulled backward). A stable device position manifests by the lack of movement of the device in either direction.

2. TEE/ICE: the echocardiographer should make sure that one disk is in each chamber. The long axis view should be sufficient to evaluate the superior and inferior part of the septum and the short axis view for the anterior and posterior part of the disk (Figures 28.3(m)–(p) and 28.4(k)–(p)).

3. The last method to verify device position can be achieved by angiography. This is done with the camera in the same projection as the first angiogram to profile the septum and device using either the side arm of the delivery sheath or via a separate angiographic catheter inserted in the sheath used for ICE, or via a separate puncture site. Good device position manifests by opacification of the right atrial disk alone when the contrast is in the right atrium and opacification of the left atrial disk alone on pulmonary levophase (Figure 28.5(g), (h)).

If device position is not certain or questionable after all these maneuvers, the device can be recaptured entirely or partly and repositioned following similar steps. Once device position is verified, the device is released by counter clockwise rotation of the delivery cable using a pin vice. There is often a notable change in the angle of the device as it is released from the slight tension of the delivery cable and it self-centers within the ASD and aligns with the interatrial septum. To assess the result of closure, repeat TEE/ICE with color Doppler and angiography in the four-chamber projection in the RA with pulmonary levophase are performed (Figure 28.5(g),(h)). Patients receive a dose of an appropriate antibiotic (commonly cephazolin at 1 g) during the catheterization procedure and two further doses at 8-hour intervals. Patients are also asked to take endocarditis prophylaxis when necessary for 6 months after the procedure, as well as aspirin 81–325 mg orally once daily for 6 months. Full activity including competitive sports is usually allowed after 4 weeks of implantation. Magnetic resonance imaging (if required) can be done any time after implantation.

Once the procedure is complete, recheck the ACT and, if appropriate, remove the sheath and achieve hemostasis. If the ACT is above 250 seconds, we have been reversing the effect of heparin by using protamine sulfate.

Post-procedure monitoring

Patients are recovered overnight in a telemetry ward. Some patients may experience an increase in atrial ectopic beats. Rarely, some patients may have sustained atrial tachycardias. Resume aspirin therapy 81–325 mg per day after the procedure and continue it for 6 months. The following day an ECG, a CXR (PA and lateral), and a TTE with color Doppler should be performed to assess device position and the presence of residual shunt. Recheck ECG, CXR, and a TTE/TEE at 6 months post-procedure to assess everything. If device position is good with no residual shunt, follow-up can be annual for the first 2 years, then every 3–5 years. We suggest long term follow-up so that long term device performance can be assessed and any new information communicated to the patient. The patient is asked not to engage in contact sports for one month after the procedure.

Post-procedure medications

Aspirin as described above. Infective endocarditis prophylaxis for 6 months should be given when needed. After 6 months, if there is no residual shunt, prophylaxis and aspirin can be discontinued.

Results

The initial human use of ASO in 30 patients showed a complete closure rate of 80% at 24-hour follow-up.[2] At that time, the result was very encouraging compared to all other contemporary devices. With the improvement of device and

deployment technique, the result became more and more promising. The ASO was approved by the US FDA in December 2001. The data presented to the FDA for the approval revealed that the procedure's success rate was 97.6% (413/423). The complete closure rate at 1-day, 6-month and 12-month follow-up was 96.7% (404/418), 97.2% (376/387), and 98.5% (326/331). Major adverse events occurred in only 7 (1.6%) out of 442 patients, including device embolization in 4, cardiac arrhythmia requiring major treatment in 2, and delivery system failure in 1. Minor adverse events occurred in 27 (6.1%) out of 442 of patients, including cardiac arrhythmia with minor treatment in 15 (3.4%), thrombus formation in 3 (0.7%), headache in 2, allergic reaction in 2, delivery system failure in 2, device embolization with percutaneous removal in 1, extremity tingling in 1, and urinary tract disturbance in 1.

Complications/problems encountered during ASD closure

1. *Device embolization/migration*: this complication is rare (about 1%) and usually occurs in patients with a large ASD and deficient rims. Most of these embolizations do not cause acute hemodynamic collapse. The device can be snared and retrieved percutaneously; however, a larger sheath (+2 Fr) than the one used for delivery may be needed. The presence of a cardiovascular surgeon in house is essential for device closure of ASD.

2. *Arrhythmia*: the study with an ambulatory electro-cardiographic monitoring showed that supraventricular ectopy was noted in 26 (63%) out of 41 patients immediately after device closure, including 9 patients (23%) with non-sustained supraventricular tachycardia.[5] Changes in atrioventricular (AV) conduction occurred in 3 patients (7%). Complete AV block is a potential risk but rare (<1%). Suda et al[6] reported that 10 out of 162 (6.2%) patients presented with new-onset (n = 9) or aggravation of pre-existing (n = 1) AV block. Three of them occurred during the procedure, 7 patients were first noted 1 to 7 days later. All AV blocks (first degree in 4, second degree in 4, and third degree in 2) resolved or improved spontaneously, with no recurrence at mid-term follow-up.

3. *Cardiac erosion or perforation*: Amin et al[7] reported that the ASO may cause cardiac erosion in 0.1% of patients, which all occurred at the dome of the atria, near the aortic root. The risks for erosions may be seen in patients with deficient aortic rim and/or superior rim, or with the use of an oversized ASO. Divekar et al[8] reported the similar findings that ASO-associated cardiac perforations uniquely involve the antero-superior atrial walls and adjacent aorta. Most (66.6%) of the cardiac perforations occurred after the patients' discharge. One cardiac perforation occurred 3 years after device closure. The above findings imply that high risk patients

need closer follow-up. Our protocol to diagnose erosions includes performing an echocardiogram the following day. If there is a new pericardial effusion or an increasing one, we repeat the echocardiogram after 12 hours and re-assess. If the effusion is stable, then we discharge the patient and bring them back after 3 days for a repeat echocardiogram.

4. *Cobra-head formation*: the left disk maintains a high profile when deployed, mimicking a cobra head. This can occur if the left disk is opened in the pulmonary vein or left atrial appendage, or if the left atrium is too small to accommodate the device size. It can also occur if the device is defective or if the device has been loaded with unusual strain on it. If this occurs check the site of deployment; if appropriate recapture the device, remove it and inspect it, and if the 'cobra head' forms outside the body use a different device. If the disk forms normally try deploying the device again. Do not release a device that has a cobra head appearance to the left disk.

5. *Recapture of the device*: to afford the smallest sheath size for device delivery, its wall thickness is small with a resultant decrease in sheath strength. To recapture a device prior to its release, the operator should hold the sheath at the groin with his/her left hand and with his/her right hand pull the delivery cable forcefully inside the sheath. If the sheath is damaged/kinked (accordion effect) use the exchange (rescue) system to change the damaged sheath. First, extend the length of the cable by screwing the tip of the rescue cable to the proximal end of the cable attached to the device. Then remove the sheath or, if the sheath is 9 or 12 Fr, introduce the dilator of the rescue system over the cable inside that sheath until it reaches a few cm near the tip of the sheath. This dilator will significantly strengthen the sheath, allowing the operator to pull back the cable with the dilator as one unit inside the sheath. Then the operator can decide what to do next (change the entire sheath system or the device).

6. *Release of the device with a prominent Eustachian valve*: to avoid the possibility of cable entrapment during release, advance the sheath to the hub of the right disk. Then release the cable and immediately draw back inside the sheath before the position of the sheath is changed.

General remarks

1. *ASO versus surgical closure of ASD*: a multi-center, non-randomized concurrent study was performed in 442 patients with ASO closure and 154 patients with surgical closure from March 1998 to March 2000, which showed that the early, primary, and secondary efficacy success rates were not statistically different between the two groups.[9] However, the complication rate was lower and the length of hospital stay was shorter for device closure than for surgical closure. Kim et al[10] reported that ASO closure not only had equal effectiveness but also cost less compared to surgical closure (11 541 versus 21 780 US dollars).

2. *Echocardiographic guidance*: TEE has been successfully used for guiding transcatheter closure of ASD.[11–14] However, TEE requires general anesthesia. ICE using an AcuNav catheter (Acuson Corporation, Siemens Medical, Iselin, NJ) can eliminate the need for general anesthesia and has been proved to be effective to guide device closure of ASD with less fluoroscopy and a shorter procedure time compared to TEE.[15–19] Please refer to Chapter 4 by Koenig et al.

3. *Multiple ASDs*: multiple ASD closure is more challenging than a single ASD. If the septum has more than one hole, the bigger hole is usually located in the supero-anterior septum, while the smaller hole is located in the infero-posterior septum. Because the LA disk is 12–16 mm larger than the waist and the stenting of the larger defect may squeeze the smaller defect, the two close defects may be closed with one device.[20] For two defects with a wide separation (>7 mm), two devices are required to achieve successful closure. Rarely, three devices are needed to close three defects. Cao et al[21] reported 22 patients with more than one ASD who were successfully closed with more than one device. The smaller device is usually deployed first, but not released until the larger device is positioned across the defect. If stability of both devices is confirmed, the devices are released sequentially, starting with the smaller device. Chun et al[22] described a case of multiple atrial septal defects that were 'consolidated' into a single defect using blade atrial septostomy for successful closure with a single ASO;[22] we do not advocate this technique.

4. *Large ASD*: to date, an ASO is the only device suitable for a large ASD up to 40 mm in diameter. However, a large defect, especially associated with deficient rims, is still challenging. In such circumstances, oftentimes, when deploying the LA disk, the disk becomes perpendicular to the atrial septum, resulting in prolapse into the right atrium. There are several techniques that can be used to overcome such difficulties in aligning the LA disk to be parallel to the atrial septum that will result in a successful procedure.[23]

   (i) *Hausdorf sheath (Cook, Bloomington, IN)*: a specially designed long sheath with two curves at its end.[24] The two posterior curves help align the left disk parallel to the septum. This sheath is available in sizes 10–12 Fr. Under fluoroscopic and echocardiographic guidance, if the initial deployment of the left disk is not ideal, counterclockwise rotation of the sheath will orientate the tip posterior and further deployment of the left disk will be parallel to the septum.

   (ii) *Right upper pulmonary vein technique*: this technique is only recommended in larger patients. The delivery sheath is carefully positioned in the right upper pulmonary vein, the device is advanced to the tip of the sheath then the left disk is partially deployed in the right upper pulmonary vein.[25–27] The sheath is quickly retracted to deploy the remainder of the left disk; this will result in the disk jumping from that location to be parallel to the atrial septum. Quick and successive deployment of the connecting waist and the right disk is carried out before the sheath may change its position or prior to the left disk prolapsing through the defect to the RA.

(iii) *Left upper pulmonary vein technique:* this technique can be used in children as well as in adults. The delivery sheath is carefully positioned in the left upper pulmonary vein. The device is advanced to the tip of the sheath and the left disk is then deployed inside the vein. Deployment of the waist and right disk is continued to create an 'American football' appearance within the vein.[26] As the sheath reaches the RA, the left disk disengages from the pulmonary vein and the disk jumps to be parallel to the atrial septum. Continuous retraction of the sheath over the cable with pulling of the entire assembly towards the RA will result in parallel alignment of the left disk to the septum.

(iv) *Dilator assisted technique:* after deployment of the left disk, a long dilator (usually of the delivery sheath being used) is advanced into the LA by an assistant to hold the superior anterior part of the left disk to prevent it from prolapsing into the RA, while the operator continues to deploy the waist and right disk in their respective locations.[24] Once the right disk is deployed in the RA, the assistant withdraws the dilator back to the RA.

(v) *Balloon assisted technique:* Dalvi et al[28] reported a new balloon-assisted technique to facilitate device closure of large ASDs and to prevent prolapse of the left disk into the RA. In essence it is similar in concept to the dilator technique. During device deployment, they used a balloon catheter to support the left disk of the ASO, preventing its prolapse into the RA.

(vi) *Right coronary Judkins guide catheter technique:* this technique is used only if the device size is less than 16 mm. An 8 Fr delivery sheath is positioned in the LA. The device is then pre-loaded inside the 8 Fr Judkins coronary guide catheter (inner lumen 0.098 inch). The entire assembly (device/cable/guide catheter) is then advanced inside the delivery sheath until the catheter reaches the tip of the sheath. The sheath is brought back to the inferior vena cava, keeping the coronary catheter in the LA. Due to the curve of the catheter, once the left disk is deployed in the LA, counterclockwise rotation of the guide will result in alignment of the left disk to be parallel to the septum. Deployment of the waist and right disk in their respective locations is continued. We found this technique to be of use in small children.

References

1. Hamdan MA, Cao QL, Hijazi ZM. Amplatzer septal occluder. In: Rao PS, Kern MJ, eds. Catheter Based Devices for the Treatment of Non-coronary Cardiovascular Disease in Adults and Children. Philadelphia, PA Williams and Wilkins, 2003: 51–9.

2. Masura J, Gavora P, Formanek A, Hijazi ZM. Transcatheter closure of secundum atrial septal defects using the new self-centering Amplatzer septal occluder: initial human experience. Cathet Cardiovasc Diagn 1997; 42: 388–93.

3. Omeish A, Hijazi ZM. Transcatheter closure of atrial septal defects in children & adults using the Amplatzer Septal Occluder. J Interven Cardiol 2001; 14: 37–44.

4. Harper RW, Mottram PM, McGaw DJ. Closure of secundum atrial septal defects with the Amplatzer septal occluder device: techniques and problems. Cathet Cardiovasc Interven 2002; 57: 508–24.

5. Hill SL, Berul CI, Patel HT et al. Early ECG abnormalities associated with transcatheter closure of atrial septal defects using the Amplatzer septal occluder. J Interven Cardiol Electrophysiol 2000; 4: 469–74.

6. Suda K, Raboisson MJ, Piette E et al. Reversible atrioventricular block associated with closure of atrial septal defects using the Amplatzer device. J Am Coll Cardiol 2004; 43: 1677–82.

7. Amin Z, Hijazi ZM, Bass JL et al. Erosion of Amplatzer septal occluder device after closure of secundum atrial septal defects: review of registry of complications and recommendations to minimize future risk. Cathet Cardiovasc Interven 2004; 63: 496–502.

8. Divekar A, Gaamangwe T, Shaikh N et al. Cardiac perforation after device closure of atrial septal defects with the Amplatzer septal occluder. J Am Coll Cardiol 2005; 45: 1213–8.

9. Du ZD, Hijazi ZM, Kleinman CS et al. Larntz K. Amplatzer Investigators. Comparison between transcatheter and surgical closure of secundum atrial septal defect in children and adults: results of a multicenter nonrandomized trial. J Am Coll Cardiol 2002; 39: 1836–44.

10. Kim JJ, Hijazi ZM. Clinical outcomes and costs of Amplatzer transcatheter closure as compared with surgical closure of ostium secundum atrial septal defects. Med Sci Monit 2002; 8: CR787–91.

11. Hijazi ZM, Cao Q, Patel HT et al. Transesophageal echocardiographic results of catheter closure of atrial septal defect in children and adults using the Amplatzer device. Am J Cardiol 2000; 85: 1387–90.

12. Mazic U, Gavora P, Masura J. The role of transesophageal echocardiography in transcatheter closure of secundum atrial septal defects by the Amplatzer septal occluder. Am Heart J 2001; 142: 482–8.

13. Figueroa MI, Balaguru D, McClure C et al. Experience with use of multiplane transesophageal echocardiography to guide closure of atrial septal defects using the Amplatzer device. Pediatr Cardiol 2002; 23: 430–6.

14. Latiff HA, Samion H, Kandhavel G et al. The value of transesophageal echocardiography in transcatheter closure of atrial septal defects in the oval fossa using the Amplatzer septal occluder. Cardiol Young 2001; 11: 201–4.

15. Hijazi Z, Wang Z, Cao Q et al. Transcatheter closure of atrial septal defects and patent foramen ovale under intracardiac echocardiographic guidance: feasibility and comparison with transesophageal echocardiography. Cathet Cardiovasc Interven 2001; 52: 194–9.

16. Koenig P, Cao QL, Heitschmidt M et al. Role of intracardiac echocardiographic guidance in transcatheter closure of atrial septal defects and patent foramen ovale using the Amplatzer device. J Interven Cardiol 2003; 16: 51–62.

17. Koenig PR, Abdulla RI, Cao QL, Hijazi ZM. Use of intracardiac echocardiography to guide catheter closure of atrial communications. Echocardiography 2003; 20(8): 781–7.

18. Alboliras ET, Hijazi ZM. Comparison of costs of intracardiac echocardiography and transesophageal echocardiography in

monitoring percutaneous device closure of atrial septal defect in children and adults. Am J Cardiol 2004; 94: 690–2.

19. Bartel T, Konorza T, Arjumand J et al. Intracardiac echocardiography is superior to conventional monitoring for guiding device closure of interatrial communications. Circulation 2003; 107: 795–7.

20. Roman KS, Jones A, Keeton BR, Salmon AP. Different techniques for closure of multiple interatrial communications with the Amplatzer septal occluder. J Interven Cardiol 2002; 15: 393–7.

21. Cao Q, Radtke W, Berger F et al. Transcatheter closure of multiple atrial septal defects. Initial results and value of two- and three-dimensional transoesophageal echocardiography. Eur Heart J 2000; 21: 941–7.

22. Chun TU, Gruenstein DH, Cripe LH, Beekman RH 3rd. Blade consolidation of multiple atrial septal defects: a novel approach to transcatheter closure. Pediatr Cardiol 2004; 25: 671–4.

23. Fu YC, Cao Q, Hijazi ZM. Device closure of large ASDs: technical considerations. Ital Heart J (in press).

24. Wahab HA, Bairam AR, Cao QL, Hijazi ZM. Novel technique to prevent prolapse of the Amplatzer septal occluder through large atrial septal defect. Cathet Cardiovasc Interven 2003; 60: 543–5.

25. Berger F, Ewert P, Abdul-Khaliq H et al. Percutaneous closure of large atrial septal defects with the Amplatzer Septal Occluder: technical overkill or recommendable alternative treatment? J Interven Cardiol 2001; 14: 63–7.

26. Varma C, Benson LN, Silversides C et al. Outcomes and alternative techniques for device closure of the large secundum atrial septal defect. Cathet Cardiovasc Interven 2004; 61: 131–9.

27. Kannan BR, Francis E, Sivakumar K et al. Transcatheter closure of very large (> or = 25 mm) atrial septal defects using the Amplatzer septal occluder. Cathet Cardiovasc Interven 2003; 59: 522–7.

28. Dalvi BV, Pinto RJ, Gupta A. New technique for device closure of large atrial septal defects. Cathet Cardiovasc Interven 2005; 64: 102–7.

29

Atrial septal defect closure with Starflex device

Mario Carminati, Massimo Chessa, Gianfranco Butera,
Luciane Piazza, and Diana Negura

Devices

The original Clamshell double umbrella device,[1-3] designed for transcatheter closure of atrial septal defects (ASDs), was subsequently modified and the CardioSEAL (CS) became available.[4,5] This device consists of two square-shaped umbrellas connected in the center. The wire skeleton is made of Mp35n, a non-ferromagnetic alloy with a woven Dacron fabric cover. Each arm has three spring coils, which allow variable positions of each arm, rendering the device highly flexible.

The StarFlex (SF)[6-8] (Figure 29.1) is the latest generation of the device. It differs from the CS by the addition of a unique self-centering mechanism, fabricated from a single nitinol microcoil spring. The microspring is attached to alternating sides of the umbrella arm tips and provides a self-adjusting positioning mechanism which assists to centrally locate the implant within the defect. This increases the apposition of the implant arms to the septal wall, while maintaining the low septal profile and high conformability. The low profile of the device and smooth transition between the frame and fabric surface are designed to conform to individual patient anatomy. The inherent porosity achieved by selecting a knitted design should enhance the integration of tissue ingrowth into the fabric, thus promoting uniform and smooth endothelialization. The SF device is available in different sizes: 23, 28, 33, and 40 mm (the measure indicates the diagonal diameter); more recently two additional devices with six arms (38 and 43 mm in size) became available.

Technique of implantation

Device implantation is performed under fluoroscopic and echocardiographic control, either by using transesophageal or intracardiac echo transducers.[9] Echocardiographic interrogation allows the exact position and diameter of the defect,

as well as the characteristics of the rims and the length of the entire septum itself.[10,11] Angiography is generally unnecessary; an injection into the right upper pulmonary vein in the left anterior oblique view with cranial angulation may give some additional information in selected cases. After the basal hemodynamic data set has been obtained, heparin (100 U/kg) and antibiotic prophylaxis are administered. Measurement of the 'stretched' diameter of the defect is then obtained;[12] an endhole catheter (usually a multi-purpose) is advanced into the left upper pulmonary vein and a superstiff guidewire is recommended to advance the sizing balloon to stabilize it during inflation. Although balloon sizing is not performed routinely in some centers, we think that it still plays an important role in device size selection. An approximate 2:1 ratio between the device and the stretched defect size is recommended. A 10 Fr Mullins sheath is introduced into the left upper pulmonary vein. A larger Mullins sheath should not be used, as the proximal arms of the device can get twisted within a larger sheath during repositioning maneuvers and can interlock within the sheath. The device is advanced into the sheath until the distal umbrella is deployed in the left atrial cavity. The most important distal arm during deployment of the device is usually the right upper arm of the distal umbrella, which is pointing to 11o'clock in the frontal plane; the entire system is pulled towards the atrial septum, until the most anterior arm is barely touching the atrial septum (a short axis view on transesophageal echocardiography (TEE) is the most useful to verify the position); the long sheath is withdrawn, keeping the delivery wire stable, to allow the proximal umbrella to spring open on the right side of the septum (Figure 29.2, see also color plate section). An excessive pull of the system towards the septum may cause the most anterior arm to prolapse through the defect; in this case, provided the proximal umbrella is still folded within the sheath, the device should be re-advanced into the left atrium and the sheath rotated clockwise and pulled back to the septum again. Sometimes it is helpful to pull the distal arms back into the Mullins

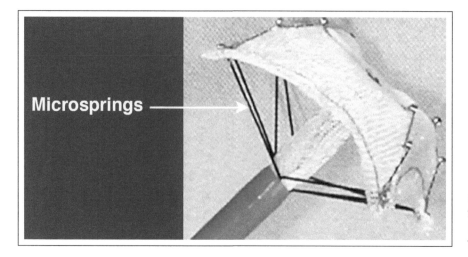

Figure 29.1
Starflex device: the proximal umbrella is folded into the sheath, for best visualization of nitinol microsprings.

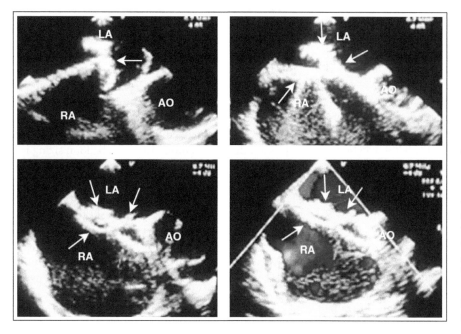

Figure 29.2
Transesophageal monitoring of device implantation. Top right: the distal umbrella is deployed in the left atrium. Top left: both umbrellas are deployed, with the device still attached to the delivery cable. Bottom right: the device was released; note the flat appearance of both umbrellas, as a 'sandwich' on the atrial septum. Bottom left: no evidence of residual shunt at color flow interrogation. (See also color plate section.)

sheath, rotate the sheath clockwise, and advance it into the right upper pulmonary vein. Within the right upper pulmonary vein, the distal arms of the device are partially opened and the device is gently pulled back, again under echocardiographic guidance (longitudinal plane), which is of paramount importance. Prolapse of one arm through the defect is likely to cause a residual leak (Figures 29.3 to 29.6; see also color plate section for Figures 29.3 and 29.4) and, more importantly, instability that may lead to device embolization. To prevent the problem it must be taken into account that when the self-centering mechanism is activated and the nitinol microsprings are exposed, they apply some tension on the distal umbrella, so that the arms of the distal umbrella

are curved towards the septum. Thus, the effective diameter of the device is reduced. To enlarge the distal umbrella by straightening the arms, the sheath should be re-advanced. When the arms are in contact with the septum the sheath is pulled back again to expose the microsprings again.

Multi-fenestrated defects may be successfully closed by using a device large enough to cover the fenestrated septum. In the presence of multiple defects which are widely spaced, implantation of multiple devices is necessary and compatible with a successful procedure[13–15] (Figure 29.7 and 29.8, see color plate section).

Some potential technical problems that can occur should be addressed and they are listed below.

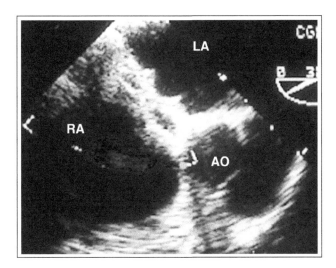

Figure 29.3
TEE short axis view of a well positioned device, with no residual shunt. (See also color plate section.)

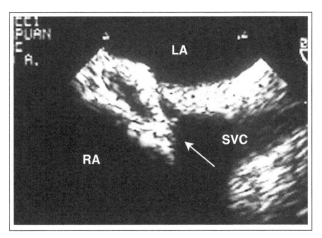

Figure 29.5
TEE long axis view of a malpositioned device, partially prolapsing through the atrial septum.

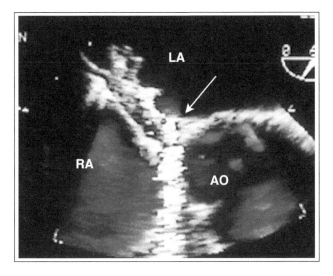

Figure 29.4
TEE short axis view in another case with deficient anterior rim and small residual shunt as assessed by the color flow jet. (See also color plate section.)

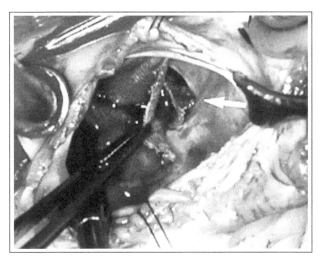

Figure 29.6
Intraoperative view of the same case as shown in Figure 29.5, demonstrating the prolapsing device. This patient was electively sent to surgery for a substantially residual shunt and the possible risk of device embolization.

The *proximal umbrella is not opening*. This can be due to:

- A large Eustachian valve/Chiari network. By use of a pigtail catheter the proximal arms can be liberated.
- Too large a sheath and twisting and interlocking of the proximal arms. By re-advancing the Mullins sheath into the partially opened proximal umbrella, this can be opened.
- Inadequate loading with distortion of the proximal arms. Thus it is critical that loading is performed gently without applying force.
- The sheath pulled back too far, with only the most distal spring coils of the arms that remain within the sheath,

and therefore the Dacron is no longer covered by the sheath and it can unfold, so that force is needed to pull the proximal arms back into the sheath, resulting in distortion of these arms. If this occurs, retrieval of the device is an adequate solution.

The device is not releasing. This occurs rarely and the solution is simple. Rotate the wire of the delivery catheter in one direction until the device releases.

Device malposition/embolization. To retrieve a device it is necessary to snare it with a goose neck or a basket snare and fold it back into a larger sheath, a 14 Fr is recommended,

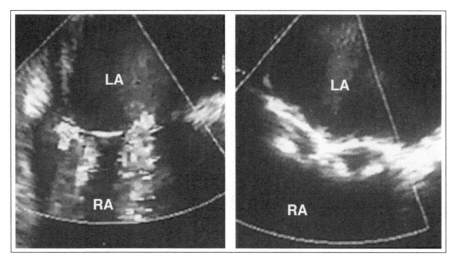

Figure 29.7

TEE image of a case of multi-fenestrated atrial septum (right part of the figure), as clearly demonstrated by multiple color flow jets. A single large device (left part of the figure) is covering all the fenestrations, with no residual shunt. (See also color plate section.)

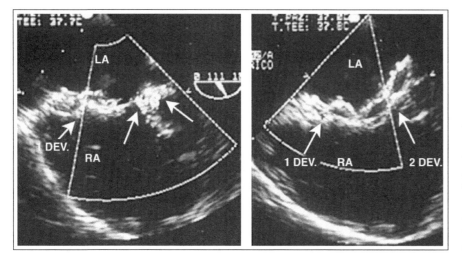

Figure 29.8

TEE of a case of double defects. One defect was closed with a device, but there was evidence of a large additional hole, as shown by the color flow (right part of the figure). A second device was successfully implanted, closing the second hole (left part of the figure). (See also color plate section.)

making it possible to retrieve the device percutaneously (Figure 29.9). It is possible to avoid surgery in most instances.[9]

Discharge and follow-up

Patients are usually discharged after 24 hours, with an anti-aggregation (ASA 300 mg/daily) therapy for the following 6 months. A double anti-aggregation or anticoagulation therapy is not absolutely necessary.

An echocardiographic evaluation at 1–6 and 12 months after the procedure is mandatory: to evaluate residual shunting, the presence of a thrombus on the right or left 'patch', and AV valve problems due to the device. Some small residual leaks may spontaneously disappear with time.[13]

The problem of arm fractures, very common with the original Clamshell and also observed with the CS, became less frequent with the SF; however, arm fractures can also occur with SF devices (Figure 29.10).[10] Fortunately it is very unlikely that arm fractures will cause clinical consequences; paradoxically, from the clinical point of view, it is preferable to have arm fractures instead of cardiac perforation due to a device too stiff to accommodate itself into the cardiac chambers. Arm fractures, as well as other complications like significant residual leaks or device malposition/embolization, usually occur with large devices (particularly the 40 mm SF).

In conclusion, the SF device can give satisfactory results, comparable to the Amplatzer that is the most commonly used device in the majority of centers, in small to moderate size defects. The SF device is not recommended for closing defects larger than 20 mm in diameter.[17]

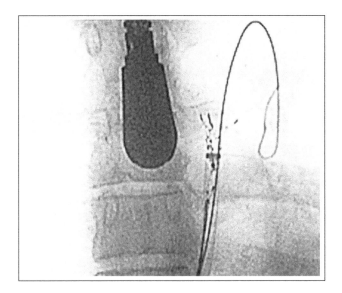

Figure 29.9
A device embolized to the pulmonary artery was snared and retrieved into a 14 Fr long sheath. (See also color plate section.)

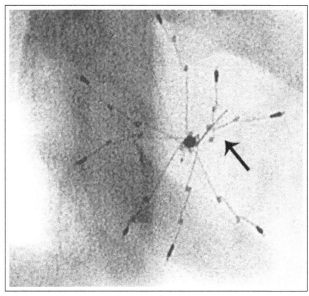

Figure 29.10
Fluoroscopic picture of a device with an arm fracture (indicated by arrow).

References

1. Rome JJ, Keane JF, Perry SB et al. Double-umbrella closure of atrial septal defects: initial clinical application. Circulation 1990; 82: 751–8.
2. Lock JE, Rome JJ, Davis R et al. Transcatheter closure of atrial septal defects : experimental studies. Circulation 1989; 79: 1091–9.
3. Bridges ND, Newburger JW, Mayer JR. Transcatheter closure of the secundum ASD in the pediatric patients: the first year's experience. Am J Cardiol 1990; 66: 522.
4. Kaulitz R, Paul T, Hausdorf G et al. Extending the limits of transcatheter closure of atrial septal defects with double umbrella device (CardioSEAL). Heart 1998; 80: 54–9.
5. Carminati M, Hausdorf G, Tynan M et al. Initial clinical experience of transcatheter closure of secundum atrial septal defect with a septal occlusion system: a multicenter European study (abstract). Eur Heart J 1997; 18(Suppl): 136.
6. Hausdorf G, Kaulitz R, Paul T et al. Transcatheter closure of atrial septal defects with a new flexible, self-centering device: initial experience with the Starflex occluder. Am J Cardiol 1999; 84: 1113–16.
7. Carminati M, Giusti S, Hausdorf G et al. European multicentric experience using the CardioSEAL and Starflex double umbrella devices to close interatrial communication holes within the oval fossa. Cardiol Young 2000; 10: 492–9.
8. Carminati M, Chessa M, Butera G et al. Transcatheter closure of atrial septal defects with the STARflex device: early results and follow-up. J Interven Cardiol 2001; 14: 319–24.
9. Hellenbrand W, Fahey JT, McGowan FX et al. Transesophageal echocardiography guidance of transcatheter closure of atrial septal defect. Am J Cardiol 1990; 66: 207–13.
10. Chan KC, Godman MJ. Morphological variations of fossa ovalis atrial septal defects (secundum): feasibility for transcutaneous closure with the clam-shell device. Br Heart J 1993; 69: 52–5.
11. Ferreira SM, Ho SY, Anderson RH. Morphological study of defects of the atrial septum within the oval fossa: implications for transcatheter closure of left-to-right shunt. Br Heart J 1992; 67: 316–20.
12. Rao PS, Langhough R, Beekman RH et al. Echocardiographic estimation of balloon stretched diameter of secundum atrial septal defect for transcatheter occlusion. Am Heart J 1992; 124: 172–5.
13. Chessa M, Carminati M, Butera G et al. Early and late complications associated with transcatheter occlusion of secundum atrial septal defect. J Am Coll Cardiol 2002; 39: 1061–5.
14. Chessa M, Butera GF, Giamberti A et al. Transcatheter closure of residual atrial septal defects after surgical closure. J Interven Cardiol 2002; 15: 187–9.
15. Cao QL, Radtke W, Berger F et al. Transcatheter closure of multiple atrial septal defects: initial results and value of two and three-dimensional transesophageal echocardiography. Eur Heart J 2000; 21: 941–7.
16. Boutin C, Musewe NN, Smallhorn JF et al. Echocardiographic follow-up of atrial septal defect after catheter closure by double umbrella device. Circulation 1993; 88: 621–7.
17. Butera GF, Carminati M, Chessa M et al. CardioSEAL/Starflex versus Amplatzer devices for percutaneous closure of small to moderate (up to 18 mm) atrial septal defects. Am Heart J 2004; 148: 507–10.

30

Atrial septal defect closure using the Helex device

Neil Wilson

Closure of secundum atrial septal defects (ASDs) is indicated when there are typical clinical signs supported by diagnostic evidence of a significant left to right shunt. Such evidence includes an ECG pattern of rSR splintering in the right sided chest leads, enlargement of the right atrium seen on chest X-ray, and echocardiographic evidence of right atrial and right ventricular volume loading. Dilation of the right ventricle beyond two standard deviations from the mean is also usually associated with abnormal septal motion seen as dyskinesia, sometimes descibed as 'paradoxical septal motion'. ASD closure is advocated to avoid the long term effects of right heart dilation. These include effort intolerance, atrial tachydysrhythmias, particularly atrial fibrillation, and right heart failure secondary to pulmonary hypertension progressing to pulmonary vascular disease. A very small number of patients with an ASD present with a paradoxic embolic event such as stroke, transient ischemic attack, or systemic arterial embolism. Whilst interventional closure of secundum ASDs with devices is commonplace, surgical closure is still required for very large defects.

The Helex device is a non-self-centering double disk device consisting of a 0.012 inch nitinol wire frame on which is bonded a curtain of hydrophilic ePTFE (Goretex, WL Gore & Associates, Flagstaff, AZ, USA). The hydrophilic ePTFE greatly enhances the echogenicity of the device. The nitinol is wound as two opposing spirals such that when the device is constituted it configures in two planar parallel disks which sit either side of the atrial septum (Figure 30.1).

The Helex device is supplied in an integral delivery catheter, necessitating only a short 10 or 12 Fr gauge venous introducer sheath. A sheath protected by a hemostatic valve is preferred. The device is available in five sizes of 15, 20, 25, 30, and 35 mm diameter. It has gained popularity on account of the proven compatibility of Goretex in the cardiovascular system, having been used for some 30 years initially as vascular graft tubes and subsequently as patch material to close intracardiac defects. The 0.014 inch nitinol

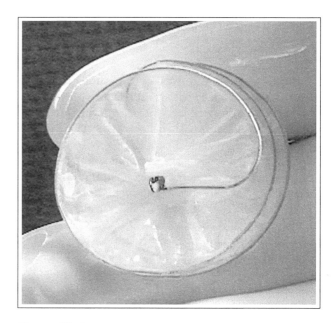

Figure 30.1
Right atrial aspect of the Helex device. When the device is wet prior to implantation the ePTFE assumes an almost transparent appearance.

imparts flexibility and this furthers the 'tissue friendly' feel to the device which is appealing when implanting in growing hearts. Its low profile and the low thrombogenicity of Goretex with rapid endothelialization further its attraction as an intracardiac prosthesis (Figure 30.2).

Following *in-vitro* and *in-vivo* feasibility and biocompatibility studies,[1] the first human implants of the Helex device were performed in 1999.[2] Subtle modifications have been introduced since then to enhance the practicality of implantation, including the use of hydrophilic ePTFE, adjustment of the winding pattern of the disks, and most recently changes in the delivery system.

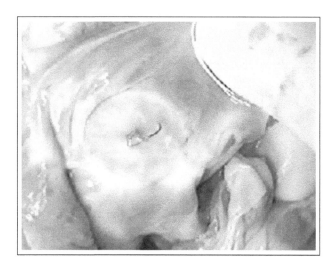

Figure 30.2
Right atrial aspect of the Helex device showing full
endothelialization 3 months post-implantation.

Patient selection, as with any device, is important. With a
recommended device to defect ratio in the region of 1.8–2
the largest defect closeable with a Helex device is 18–19 mm
in diameter, as measured on balloon sizing. There is a pro-
viso, however, in that children with large ASDs have a relatively small left atrium and experience has shown that
the 30 and 35 mm devices do not sit effectively on the left
atrial side of the septum in children weighing less than
25 kg. Pre-catheter imaging is usually transthoracic and/or
transesophageal echocardiography (TOE). Some operators
choose not to balloon size, particularly for patent foramen
ovale and smaller defects. When dealing with smaller ASDs
of less than 15 mm diameter it is my personal practice to
choose a device:defect ratio of 2:1 on the basis of imaging
alone, providing there are well developed margins to the
septum. In the face of a deficient anterior-superior rim,
adjacent to the aorta, oversizing is recommended. The
device can be used for all types of ASDs within the recommended sizing criteria. This includes fenestrated, aneurysmal, and multiple defects.[3,4] The device is also widely used
in the closure of patent foramen ovale (see above),[5–7] and
for closing fenestrations of the Fontan type circulation.[8]

Implantation procedure

General endotracheal anesthesia is employed in all children
and most adults. Access is percutaneously, preferentially to
the right femoral vein using a 10 Fr sheath. In children it is
usual to start with a smaller sheath and then upsize. Arterial
access is not essential unless systemic blood pressure monitoring is preferred by the operator or the anesthetist, or a saturation run for Fick estimation of shunt size is desired.
Heparin 100 U/kg is administered intravenously, as for other

devices. Activated clotting time (ACT) may be checked
should the procedure be prolonged over 1 hour, in which case
further heparin is given to maintain the ACT in the region of
220–250 U/kg. Most institutions give a single dose of broad
spectrum antibiotic intravenously, some continue for 24
hours or more. Endocarditis on the device is exceptionally
rare. It is usual to check intracardiac pressures, particularly
pulmonary artery pressure prior to closure. Elevation of pulmonary artery pressure is not unusual in older patients with
larger defects. A full discussion on the merits and limitations
of ASD closure in the presence of pulmonary artery hypertension is beyond the scope of this chapter, but general guidelines are that caution should be exercised with pulmonary
artery pressure beyond half the systemic level. Whilst the
catheter operator is recording pressures, the transesophageal
operator should be performing a full study to confirm
anatomy with particular reference to left ventricular size and
function and pulmonary venous anatomy. The atrial septum is examined critically for number and size of defects,
assessing the presence of the atrial septal rim and where it
may be deficient. It is not so unusual that, despite good
quality transthoracic echocardiography prior to the catheter
procedure, multiple defects are identified on TOE. Alternatively, some adult centers have developed a routine whereby,
under sedation and local anesthesia, initial catheter aspects
of the procedure including balloon sizing and sheath placement are performed and a device size chosen. Just prior to
implantation of the device the transesophageal probe is
introduced, minimizing the length of discomfort for the
patient.

The introduction of intracardiac echocardiography
(ICE)[9] has also avoided the need for general anesthesia in
adults, and the emergence of an 8 Fr intracardiac echo
probe will make some impact along these lines in older children who may be able to undergo interventional ASD with
sedation and local anesthesia.

At cardiac catheter the atrial septum is crossed using an
appropriate sized diagnostic endhole catheter such as a
multi-purpose. The catheter is directed under fluoroscopic
control superiorly and posteriorly towards the left shoulder
into the left atrium. With a little clockwise torque and
advancement it is usually very easy to enter the left upper
pulmonary vein. Here a heavy duty exchange length
guidewire such as the Amplatz Superstiff is positioned in
the pulmonary vein and the diagnostic catheter removed.
A PTA (NMT Medical) or Amplatz (AGA, Golden Valley,
MN, USA) balloon sizing catheter is advanced over the
guidewire until it is judged to be astride the atrial septum.
The sizing catheters are made with very compliant balloon
material and are filled with dilute contrast until a satisfactory waist is seen on fluoroscopy (Figure 30.3). Fluoroscopy
is usually performed with the image intensifier in the left
anterior oblique position at 30–45°. It is usual for the TOE
operator also to measure the diameter of the inflated balloon and to check for residual flow at that or any other

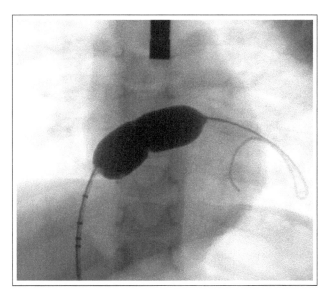

Figure 30.3
Balloon sizing maneuver. The indentation in the central portion of the balloon identifies the constraints of the atrial septum and thus sizes the ASD.

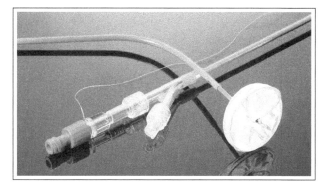

Figure 30.4
Helex device presented attached to the integral green delivery catheter. The control catheter is seen attached to the red cap. The safety suture is seen locked into position by the red safety cap. The mandrel is controlled by the short side arm, which can be locked into position using the Luer lock. (See also color plate section.)

occult defect which may have been revealed by the sizing maneuver. It is not always possible to achieve a clean 'section' of the balloon sizing catheter on TOE. If the fluoroscopy image is likewise distorted, the image intensifier should be rotated until a satisfactory profile is obtained.

Once the defect has been sized the appropriate sized device is chosen according to the ratio of 1.8–2:1. The Helex device is supplied in an integral delivery catheter (Figure 30.4) such that a long femoral vein to the left atrial sheath is unnecessary. The device is loaded into the flushed green delivery catheter in the small 'water bath' provided in the packaging by pulling the gray control cathetar, and is flushed further with saline until all air has been expelled.

Once loaded, the delivery catheter is advanced from the groin into the right atrium and across the ASD to the left atrium. Using a series of 'push, pinch, and pull' maneuvers the left atrial disk is constituted under fluoroscopic control and is pulled to the atrial septum. Subsequently the right atrial disk is configured by keeping the green delivery catheter immobile and advancing the gray pusher catheter. The position and configuration of the device are assessed using TOE. At this stage it is possible to make small adjustments in device position if necessary by gentle manipulation of the green catheter. Should the device configuration be undesirable, the device can be withdrawn into the delivery catheter using the same method as for the initial loading. Assuming satisfactory device position, at which stage it is usual to see a small amount of flow through the device on TOE, the device is locked by first removing the red safety cap and exerting a firm pull on the mandrel. The delivery catheter assembly is then removed by withdrawing gently, allowing the safety suture to pass through the right atrial

eyelet and out of the patient. If for any reason the device had misplaced during the locking procedure then it may still be removed by replacing the red cap and pulling the device, via the suture, into the green delivery catheter and out of the venous sheath in the groin. Figure 30.5 outlines the stages in device configuration as seen using fluoroscopic control. Figure 30.6 shows the appearance of the device on transesophageal echo after full deployment and release.

When the ASD is sited superior-inferior close to the aorta and where there is a deficient rim, by necessity the left and right aspects of the device have to sit astride the aorta. In this instance there is a certain amount of 'splaying' of the device, evident under fluoroscopy. This must not be interpreted as abnormal configuration. TOE will demonstrate the disks astride the aorta and effective closure. An understanding of the anatomy of such defects bears this out. Figure 30.7 demonstrates a device astride the aorta producing effective closure.

When the procedure is performed under local anesthetic with sedation, most patients can be discharged home the same day. With general anesthesia the patient may be retained overnight. Current practice is an antiplatelet dose of aspirin given once daily for 6 months. Some adult operators add clopidogrel for 2 months after the procedure. A transthoracic echocardiogram and ECG is prudent prior to discharge.

As described above, intracardiac echocardiography (ICE) can be used as an alternative to TOE, giving excellent imaging quality and avoiding general anesthesia. Figure 30.8 outlines the closure procedure using ICE.

Complications

Serious complications following Helex closure of an ASD are rare. Cardiac perforation and tamponade have not yet

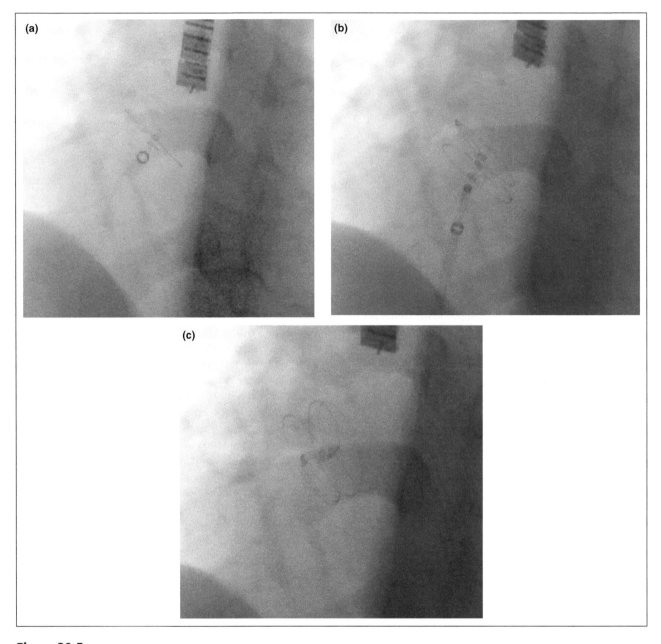

Figure 30.5
(a) Left atrial disk at septum; (b) both disks applied either side of the septum prior to locking; (c) post-device locking and removal of delivery catheter.

been reported. Embolization occurs, but almost always the device can be retrieved using a snare device and a long 10 Fr sheath. Wire fractures have been seen in a small percentage of patients and are usually of no consequence as the wire is held secure by the fabric of the device and its comprehensive endothelialization, as in Figure 30.2. Figure 30.9 demonstrates a device which has embolized to the pulmonary artery, from whence it was retrieved using a goose neck snare.

Conclusion

The Helex device has gained popularity as a consequence of its reputation as a biocompatible implant with a low profile and tissue friendly flexibility, which is particularly attractive in children and in patients such as those with patent foramen ovale where avoidance of thrombotic events is clearly the aim.[10] Implantation technique is enhanced by attention to detail, particularly using TEE,[11] and recent modification

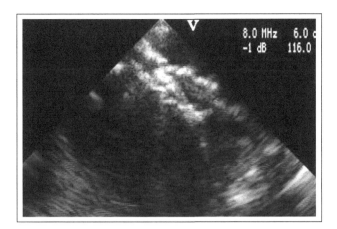

Figure 30.6
TOE image of the device in place at the end of the procedure.

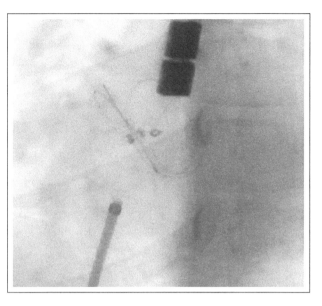

Figure 30.7
Left and right atrial disks appear splayed as they sit astride the aorta in this anterior-superior situated ASD.

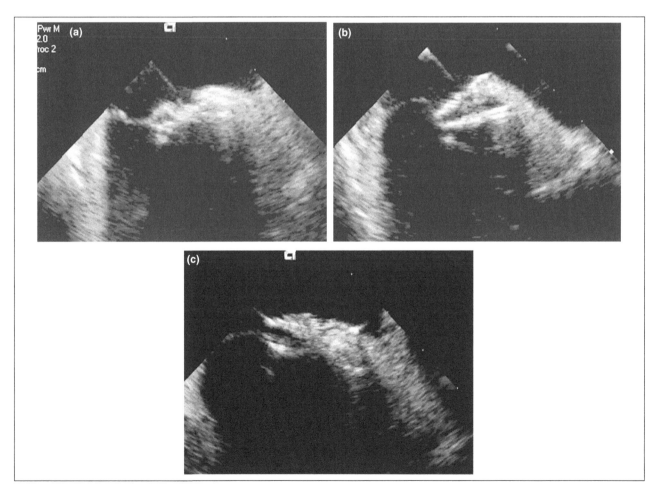

Figure 30.8
ICE images of ASD closure: (a) left atrial disk opposed to septum; (b) both disks deployed prior to locking and Release; (c) device apppearance post-release.

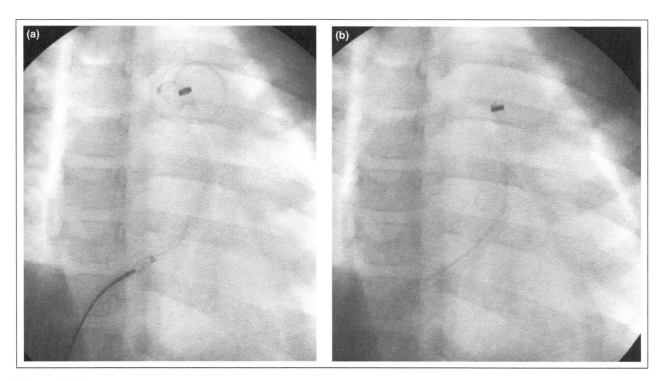

Figure 30.9
(a) Helex device which has embolized to the main pulmonary artery and has been snared with a goose neck snare and partially withdrawn into the long sheath; (b) device fully recovered into the long sheath.

of the delivery system has simplified the loading and implant procedure. Operators wishing to gain experience with the Helex device, as with any new technology, are advised to seek proctoring in technique. Most new operators are aware of a 'learning curve',[12,13] and it is the cardiologist's responsibility to minimize this by whatever means. The availability of 'live case' demonstrations in interventional meetings continues to educate in a manner which is particularly appealing and helpful to a subspeciality where dexterity, technique, and experience are paramount.

References

1. Zahn EM, Wilson N, Cutright W, Latson LA. Development and testing of the Helex septal occluder, a new expanded polytetrafluoroethylene atrial septal defect occlusion system. Circulation 2001; 104: 711–16.

2. Latson LA, Zahn EM, Wilson N. Helex septal occluder for closure of atrial septal defects. Curr Interven Cardiol Rep 2000; 3: 268–73.

3. Pedra CA, Pedra SR, Esteves CA et al. Transcatheter closure of secundum atrial septal defects with complex anatomy. J Invasive Cardiol 2004; 16(3): 117–22.

4. Dobrolet NC, Iskowitz S, Lopez L et al. Sequential implantation of two Helex septal occluder devices in a patient with complex atrial septal anatomy. Cathet Cardiovasc Interven 2001; 2: 242–6.

5. Krumsdorf U, Keppeler P, Horvath K et al. Catheter closure of atrial septal defects and patent foramen ovale in patients with an atrial septal aneurysm using different devices. J Interven Cardiol 2001; 1: 49–55.

6. Sievert H, Horvath K, Zadan E et al. Patent foramen ovale closure in patients with transient ischemia attack/stroke. J Interven Cardiol 2001; 2: 261–6.

7. Onorato E, Melzi G, Casilli F et al. Patent foramen ovale with paradoxical embolism: mid-term results of catheter closure in 256 patients. J Interven Cardiol 2003; 1: 43–50.

8. Peuster M, Beerbaum P. A novel implantation technique for closure of an atypical fenestration connecting the right atrial appendage to an extracardiac conduit by use of a 15 mm Helex device in a patient with a total cavopulmonary connection. Z Kardiol 2004; 10: 818–23.

9. Koenig PR, Abdulla RI, Cao QL, Hijazi ZM. Use of ICE to guide catheter closure of atrial communications. Echocardiography 2003; 20: 781–7.

10. Lopez L, Ventura R, Welch EM et al. Echocardiographic considerations during deployment of the Helex septal occluder for closure of atrial septal defects. Cardiol Young 2003; 3: 290–8.

11. Krumsdorf U, Ostermayer S, Billinger K et al. Incidence and clinical course of thrombus formation on atrial septal defect and patent foramen ovale closure devices in 1000 consecutive patients. J Am Coll Cardiol 2004; 2: 302–9.

12. Vincent RN, Raviele AA, Diehl HJ. Single center experience with the Helex septal occluder for closure of atrial septal defects in children. J Interven Cardiol 2003; 1: 79–82.

13. Pedra CA, Pedra SF, Esteves CA et al. Initial experience in Brazil with the Helex septal occluder for percutaneous occlusion of atrial septal defects. Arq Bras Cardiol 2003; 5: 435–52.

31

Patent foramen ovale – Amplatzer PFO occluders

Bernhard Meier

Introduction

The Amplatzer patent foramen ovale (PFO) occluder (AGA Medical Corporation, Golden Valley, Minnesota, USA) is a derivative of the Amplatzer atrial septal defect occluder. It consists of two flat self-expandable retention disks interconnected by a short, thin, and flexible waist. The disks are formed by 0.005 inch nitinol wire and filled with polyester fabric (Dacron). The currently available sizes are depicted in Figure 31.1.

The first Amplatzer PFO occluder was implanted on 10 September 1997 (by the author in the presence of Kurt Amplatz). It has since supplanted all other techniques to close PFOs at our center and gained the largest acceptance of all PFO devices worldwide.

Technique of Amplatzer PFO occluder implantation

The main steps are summarized in Table 31.1. Some centers prefer to use echocardiographic guidance or size the PFO with a balloon. The most recent roughly 800 PFO closures

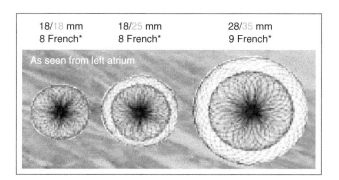

Figure 31.1
Amplatzer PFO occluders. The disk diameters are indicated in mm (black: left-sided disk, gray: right-sided disk). *Minimally required sheath size (1 French = 0.3 mm).

at our center have been done without these measures. In none of the few problems encountered was it deemed that peri-procedural echocardiography or balloon sizing would be of help. Stripping the technique of the procedure to the bare essential has allowed costs to be curbed and cut down procedure time to less than 30 minutes, with only a few minutes of fluoroscopy use.

Echocardiographic properties relevant for PFO closure

The PFO can be found during catheterization with very few exceptions in case the PFO has unequivocally been demonstrated in a transesophageal echocardiogram at the pre-intervention work-up. Figure 31.2 (see also color plate section) depicts the rare instance with a demonstrable color

Table 31.1 *Technique with Amplatzer PFO occluder*
• Pre-intervention work-up, preferably with TEE
• ≤ 1 night at hospital
• Local anesthesia
• No echocardiographic guidance
• Access: right femoral vein
• 0.035 inch ordinary or exchange wire (preferably with U-tip)
• Multi-purpose catheter to cannulate PFO unless wire passed spontaneously
• No balloon gauging
• 8 Fr sheath for 18 and 25 mm occluder, 9 Fr for 35 mm occluder
• Right atrial dye injections (by hand, LAO cranial)
• Antibiotics (0–3 doses)
• Acetylsalicylic acid 100 mg (5 months) and clopidogrel 75 mg (1 month)
• Prophylaxis against endocarditis (for 3–6 months)

Fr, French; LAO, left anterior oblique; PFO, patent foramen ovale; TEE, transesophageal echocardiography.

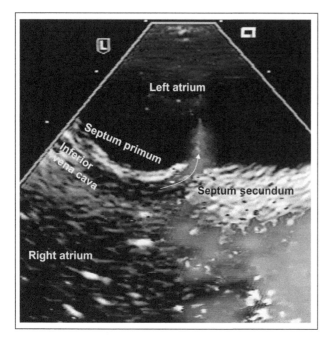

Figure 31.2
Transesophageal echocardiogram performed for suspicion of paradoxical stroke through a PFO immediately after a prolonged Valsalva maneuver. A flame of red color indicates a temporary right to left shunt through the PFO (curved arrow). (See also color plate section.)

Doppler right to left shunt. Figures 31.3 to 31.5 show the typical and proper diagnosis of a PFO with transesophageal echocardiography pointing out some of the salient features. False negative diagnosis by transesophageal echocardiogram may occur in the case of the wrong echocardiographic plane being assessed, insufficient contrast medium (aerated saline, Hemaccel, Echovist, Levovist, etc.) concentration, absent or insufficient Valsalva maneuver, or poor coordination between the Valsalva maneuver and contrast medium

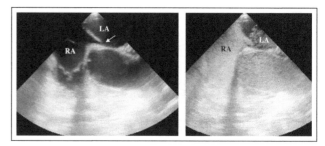

Figure 31.3
Transesophageal echocardiogram performed for demonstration of a PFO. Left: high suspicion of a PFO (arrow). Right: the PFO is ultimately proved by a bubble transit after a Valsalva maneuver. LA, left atrium; RA, right atrium.

injection. The Valsalva maneuver should be maintained for at least 20 seconds. This results in reduced filling of the entire heart. At the time of the release of the Valsalva maneuver, the venous blood pooled in the lower body rushes back to the right atrium. This results in the right atrium being well filled while the left atrium remains temporarily underfilled. The physiologic situation will be re-established a few seconds later, when the blood wave has circulated through the lungs. Hence, the bubbles typically pass the PFO only for a few heart beats. This makes it even more important to be ready in the optimal echocardiographic plane to catch and document the bubble passage. This plane is typically found somewhere with a 60–90° rotation of the multi-planar probe.

Although the maximum PFO gaps can often be measured (Figure 31.5), they are of little value for PFO closure with the Amplatzer technique. First, the PFO may be a slit of more than 20 mm length and the gap between the lips forming the valve-like PFO is smaller towards the edges of the slit. Second, when inserting a device to close a PFO the septum

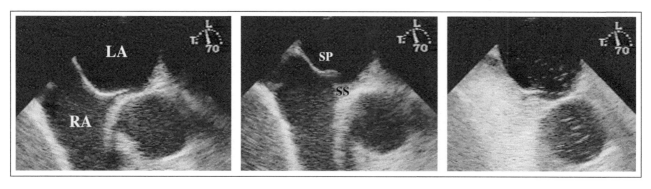

Figure 31.4
Transesophageal echocardiogram performed for demonstration of a PFO. Left: during the Valsalva maneuver the septum primum is usually deviated towards the right atrium (RA). The picture indicates that a possible PFO will be of the tunnel type. Center: after releasing the Valsalva maneuver, the mobile septum primum (SP) moves away from the triangular wedge-like septum secundum (SS). This is highly suggestive of a PFO. Right: the arrival of contrast bubbles immediately after the release of the Valsalva maneuver and their passage through the PFO tunnel into the left atrium (LA) unequivocally document the PFO and redemonstrate its tunnel shape.

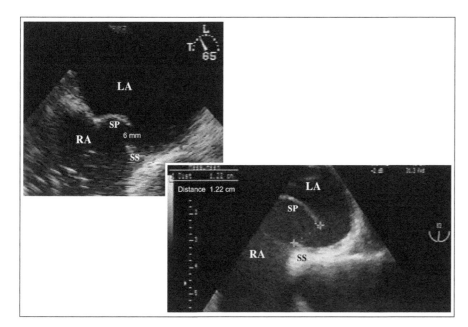

Figure 31.5
Attempts to echocardiographically size the maximum gap of PFOs after a proper Valsalva maneuver. The 6 mm or 1.22 cm distances indicated between the edges of the septum primum (SP) and the septum secundum (SS) are not relevant for the technique or choice of device with Amplatzer PFO occluders. LA, left atrium; RA, right atrium.

primum will be pulled towards the septum secundum by the left atrial device before deploying the right atrial device. This can be compared to sticking a folded umbrella through a door ajar. Opening it on the other side of the door, and trying to pull the umbrella back through the door, the door will be pulled shut. It is irrelevant how far it can maximally be opened.

The presence and extent of a hypermobile septum primum (atrial septal aneurysm) (Figure 31.6), a Chiari network (Figure 31.7), or a Eustachian valve (Figures 31.8 and 31.9) can be nicely demonstrated by transesophageal echocardiography. Again they are not important for the Amplatzer technique notwithstanding a few exceptions discussed below.

Occasionally it is possible to diagnose a PFO quite reliably with transthoracic echocardiography. However, while the diagnosis of a floppy septum primum (atrial septal aneurysm) is quite easy transthoracically, PFOs are more difficult to document (Figure 31.10). This is one of the reasons why atrial septal aneurysms were considered risk factors per se for stroke before transesophageal echocardiography was available. The PFO was simply overlooked.

Implantation procedure

Different protocols exist for percutaneous Amplatzer PFO closures. The one used at our center (Table 31.1) has stood the test of time in hundreds of implantations. It allows accomplishment of the procedure in less than 30 minutes, with the patient returning to full physical activities as early as a few hours later.

The right femoral vein is punctured and a regular 0.035 inch U-tipped guidewire is advanced through the needle up to the right atrium. In about every third case it will pass the PFO without further ado as the PFO is situated directly opposite the exit of the inferior vena cava into the right atrium. In the remainder of the cases a multi-purpose catheter is advanced directly through the skin without an introducer. With the catheter tip below the hepatic vein and pointing medially, the guidewire is advanced towards the atrial septum. This will cross the PFO in another third of the patients. Should that fail even after straightening the U-tip of the guidewire, the PFO is looked for usually in a frontal projection by sliding along the interatrial septum with the tip of the multi-purpose catheter pointing from 8 to 2 o'clock and torquing it in both directions as soon as the tip gets caught in the region of the fossa ovalis. Only rarely a straight Terumo guidewire or even a steerable coronary guidewire is required to negotiate the PFO. Particularities in crossing the PFO are discussed later. As soon as the PFO is crossed or earlier, 5000 units of heparin are given. The guidewire in the left atrium, preferably in a left pulmonary vein, provides for advancing the deployment sheath into the left atrium. To make place for it, the multi-purpose catheter (if one had been used) is withdrawn into the inferior vena cava but not yet removed from the groin to prevent venous oozing while the Amplatzer PFO occluder is prepared.

An 8 or 9 Fr Amplatzer introducer set is opened (9 Fr set if a 35 mm PFO occluder (or a larger ASD occluder) is going to be used). A 35 mm PFO occluder may become necessary, if the selected 25 mm occluder, i.e., its 18 mm left-sided disk, is pulled through the PFO without having exerted exaggerated traction during an attempt to place it at the septum (Figure 31.11). A 35 mm Amplatzer PFO occluder may be used without first attempting a 25 mm model in the presence of a huge atrial septal aneurysm for fear of embolization (Figure 31.6), an extremely long tunnel

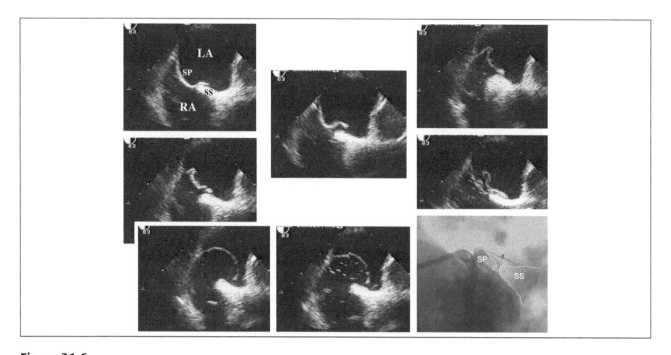

Figure 31.6

Atrial septal aneurysm, an expression for a redundant septum primum (SP), in different positions. While the position at the bottom left strongly suggests a PFO, the proof needs the visualization of bubbles passing through the gap (bottom center). The insert at the bottom right shows a right atrial dye injection during fluoroscopy, in this case after positioning a 35 mm Amplatzer PFO occluder in the projection used for the echocardiographic pictures. While the device sits tight on the tongue-like septum secundum (SS) the curtain-like SP is still ondulating between the caudal disk halves (dotted lines). LA, left atrium; RA, right atrium.

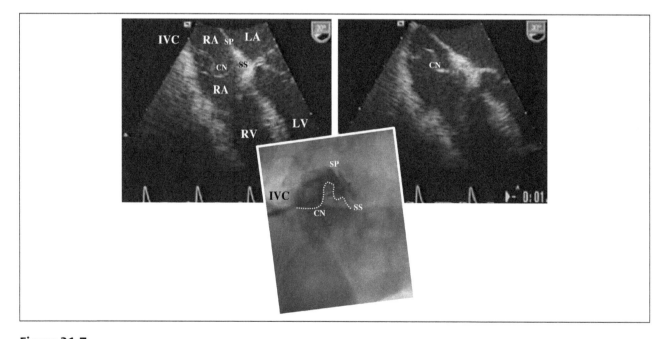

Figure 31.7

Transesophageal echocardiogram showing a Chiari network (CN). It is seen spanning the right atrium (RA) from the inferior vena cava (IVC) to the septum secundum (SS). It must not be confounded with a mobile septum primum (SP), i.e., an atrial septal aneurysm. In this patient the SP is clearly distinguishable from the CN and non-mobile. The lower insert shows a right atrial dye injection during fluoroscopy in the same patient after implantion of a 25 mm Amplatzer PFO occluder in the PFO using the same projection. Again it is important not to mix up the CN with the SP which would lead to the misdiagnosis of erroneous placement of the caudal part of the device in the left atrium. LA, left atrium; LV, left ventricle; RV, right ventricle.

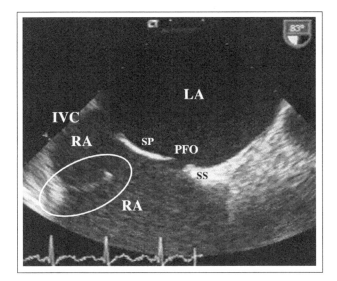

Figure 31.8
Transesophageal echocardiogram showing a Eustachian valve (circle) protruding from the lateral orifice of the inferior vena cava (IVC) towards the PFO or, in this case, rather a small ASD because the septum primum (SP) falls short of reaching the septum secundum (SS). In contrast to the Chiari network, the Eustachian valve only partially traverses the right atrium (RA).

for fear of running out of material on the right disk of a 25 mm device before reaching the right atrium at the end of the tunnel (Figures 31.12 and 31.13), or (exquisitely rarely) in a case with a particularly thick septum secundum or a large aortic root protruding close to the fossa ovalis for fear for aortic erosion by the device disks (Figure 31.14).

The pusher cable is screwed into the central female screw of the right atrial disk of the Amplatzer PFO occluder. To make sure that it will unscrew properly at the time of release, the screw is not completely tightened down (the first millimeter of unscrewing is the most difficult one, in analogy to automobile wheel nuts). The device is then pulled backwards into the short loader sheath in a water bowl. It is pushed out and retracted once or twice to get rid of air bubbles. The tip is left peeping out the few millimeters to avoid an air space between the loader tip and the tip of the device.

Once the device is ready, the multi-purpose catheter is pulled out of the femoral vein. In case a short 0.035 mm guidewire is being employed, a liquid filled syringe is hooked up to the end of the multi-purpose catheter at the time the wire disappears at its hub while the tip of the catheter has not yet left the patient. With a powerful hand injection the wire is kept across the interatrial septum while withdrawing the multi-purpose catheter further until the

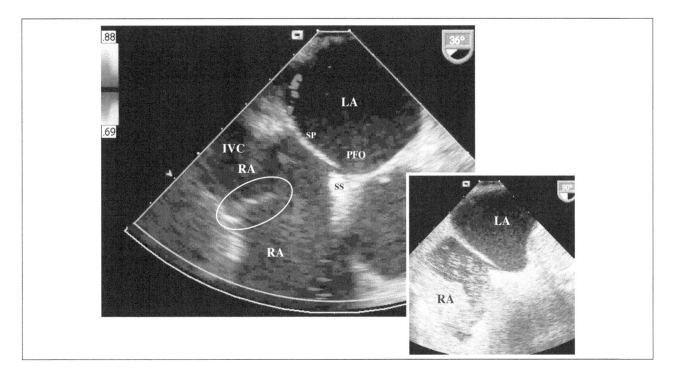

Figure 31.9
Transesophageal echocardiogram showing a Eustachian valve (circle), similar to the one in Figure 31.8, in the presence of a PFO. There is a spontaneous left to right shunt through the PFO (red Doppler flow signal). The flow from the inferior vena cava (IVC) through the right atrium (RA) following the Eustachian valve is shown by blue color Doppler flow signals. The insert in the right bottom corner shows the situation during a bubble test with the Eustachian valve (outlined by a dotted line) separating the almost bubble-free inflow from the IVC from the bubble-laden blood coming from the superior vena cava (lower part of the right atrium). Some of the bubbles still manage to cross the PFO. It is understandable that, in the presence of a Eustachian valve, a bubble studied through the arm may be falsely negative and fail to diagnose a PFO. LA, left atrium; SP, septum primum; SS, septum secundum. (See also color plate section.)

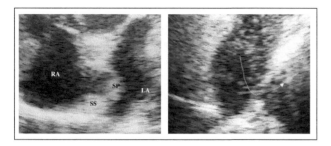

Figure 31.10
Transthoracic echocardiogram in an apical four-chamber view showing an atrial septal aneurysm (left) and a train of bubbles crossing the septum after a Valsalva maneuver (dotted arrow, right). LA, left atrium; RA, right atrium; SP, septum primum; SS, septum secundum.

tip is born. This maneuver is not necessary with a long wire. However, a long wire is more cumbersome throughout the remainder of the procedure. The bleeding ensuing after removal of the multi-purpose catheter is scrutinized for absence of arterial blood. Arterial bleeding would indicate that the puncture has been carried out involving an artery while getting into the vein. In that case a new puncture should be done before introducing the large Fr sheath to avoid an arteriovenous fistula.

The introducer sheath is then advanced over the guidewire. When entering the groin the end of the guidewire is moved in a short to and fro fashion to avoid kinking of the wire at the tip of the sheath transgressing the groin tissue and the wall of the vein. Once the tip of the sheath is within the vein, progress is easy and the wire wiggling maneuver

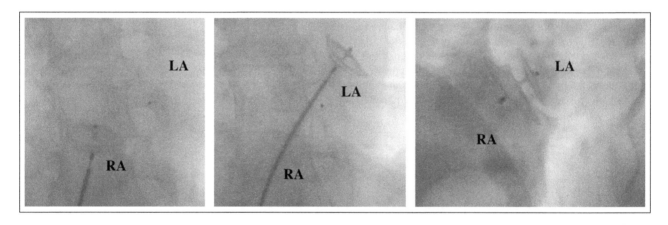

Figure 31.11
Hypermobile septum primum (atrial septal aneurysm) preventing anchorage of a 25 mm Amplatzer PFO occluder which is dislocated into the right atrium (RA, left panel) and the left atrium (LA, center panel) at three consecutive deployment attempts. Substituting a 35 mm Amplatzer occluder solves the problem (right panel). The incorrect positions of the device are recognized by two criteria: parallel position of the disks with no space in between them (well shown in the center panel) and free movability of the device away from the region of the interatrial septum.

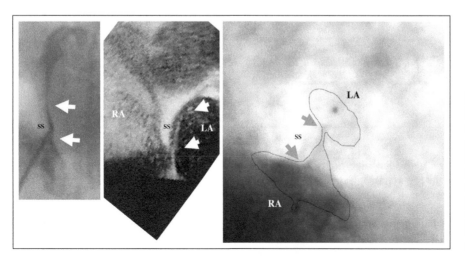

Figure 31.12
Particularly long PFO tunnel (ends marked by arrows, left and center panel) requiring a 35 mm device (right panel). The angiographic (left and right panel) and the echocardiographic (center panel) pictures are aligned in a similar projection for easier understanding. LA, left atrium; RA, right atrium; SS, septum secundum.

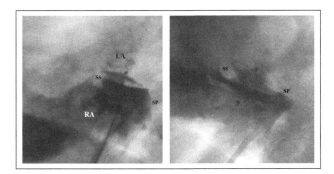

Figure 31.13
Incorrect position of a 25 mm Amplatzer PFO occluder (left panel). The septum secundum (SS) cannot be properly engaged because the septum primum (SP) yields easily, allowing the device to shift away from the SS. This is overcome by a 35 mm Amplatzer PFO occluder (right panel) in spite of continued significant indentation of the SP by the delivery catheter. LA, left atrium; RA, right atrium.

can be stopped. Some operators prefer a stiff guidewire. Yet, the straight path for PFO closure does not impose it.

The tip of the obdurator of the sheath is stopped proximal to the end of the wire in the left atrium and the introducer sheath itself is advanced while keeping the obdurator put. Once it has reached a position in the middle of the left atrium, the obdurator and the guidewire are withdrawn, keeping the hub of the sheath below heart level. The hub of the sheath is closed with a finger as soon as the obdurator and the wire have been removed completely. The sheath is

then flushed with a syringe of saline just like any end hole catheter. Flushing is not necessary if backflow is abundant and the device is ready for insertion.

It has been recommended to leave the introducer in the right atrium when removing the obdurator and advance it only into the left atrium after it has been flushed. This may reduce the risk of air embolism into the left atrium. On the other hand, the diameter mismatch between the small guidewire and the large bore introducer to be advanced over it through the PFO occasionally precludes the advancement, the rim getting caught at the edge of the septum secundum. Since air embolism has virtually been eliminated by using the introducer without the side arm for the initial part of the procedure outlined above, this precaution appears no longer warranted.

Keeping the sheath hub below heart level, usually lateral to the right thigh, the short loading sheath with the device peaking out a few millimeters is hooked up to the sheath placed in the left atrium, making sure that there is backflow from the sheath at that moment.

The device is then advanced without fluoroscopy until the plastic coated part of the pusher cable has entered the sheath. From this moment on fluoroscopy should be used.

A left oblique cranial projection is ideal to position the device. In this projection first the left disk is pushed out of the sheath and the sheath and pusher cable are pulled back as a unit under fluoroscopic control. As soon as the left disk reaches the PFO, it will pull the valve closed and change its position to one parallel to the interatrial septum (Figure 31.15). Maintaining tension on the pusher cable, the sheath is then further withdrawn until the right-sided disk is born.

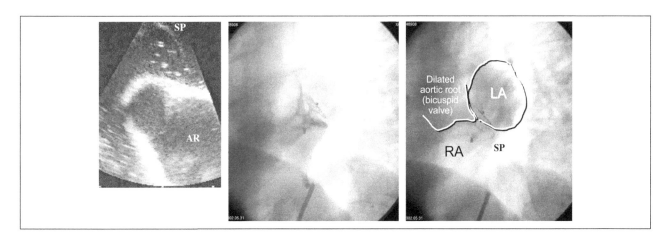

Figure 31.14
Implantation of a 35 mm Amplatzer PFO occluder (rather than a 25 mm) in a patient with a dilated aortic root because of a bicuspid valve. It was deemed that a larger device would embrace the aortic root rather than indenting it with its sharp rim, thereby decreasing the risk of erosion. The transesophageal echocardiographic picture on the left shows the dilated aortic root (AR), the mobile septum primum (SP), and bubbles passing through the PFO. The angiographic picture in a left anterior oblique projection is shown with and without labels (center and right panels). LA, left atrium; RA, right atrium.

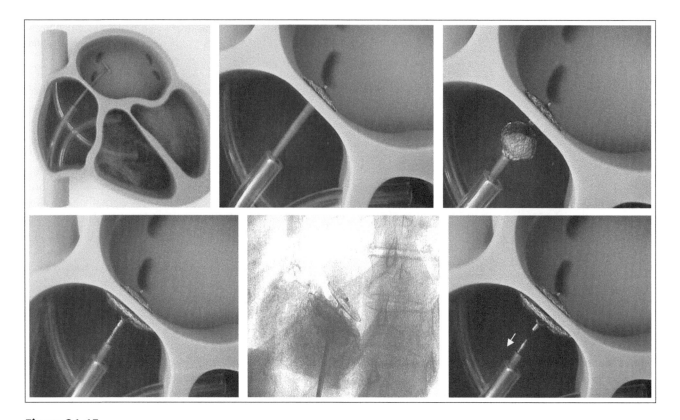

Figure 31.15

Steps for implantation of a 25 mm Amplatzer PFO occluder from top left to bottom right. After an 8 Fr introducer has been placed centrally in the left atrium, the left-sided disk (diameter 18 mm) is deployed (top left) and the introducer and device are pulled back as a unit until stopped by the septum (top center). While keeping traction on the pusher cable, the right-sided disk is produced (top right). Relaxing the introducer and the pusher cable allows the right-sided disk to accommodate to the septum (bottom left). Before releasing the device a hand injection of 10 ml of contrast medium through the introducer in a projection delineating the device as two parallel disks (usually left anterior oblique with cranial tilt) is used to ascertain the correct position of the device (bottom center). Finally, the device is released by unscrewing it from the pusher cable (arrow, bottom right).

Relaxing both the sheath and the cable, the right-sided disk will accommodate itself to the right face of the interatrial septum. The fluoroscopy angle is adjusted to see the two disks perpendicularly, i.e. as two lines. These should be forming a V-shape open to the top left (Figures 31.14 and 31.15). This proves that the septum secundum is sandwiched between the disks. Before setting the device free by unscrewing it counterclockwise, a hand injection of contrast medium into the right atrium is performed (Figure 31.15). For this purpose the side arm adapter of the sheath (part of the delivery set) is inserted on the pusher cable and connected to the sheath. The sheath is then flushed. First arterial blood remaining in the sheath from the left atrium will be aspirated, followed by dark blood from the right atrium. The dye injection will ascertain the correct position of the device (Figure 31.15), which then can be released. For documentation an additional hand injection through the sheath will be done after readjusting the X-ray plane to see the device again in a perpendicular fashion in case it has shifted at release (Figure 31.16).

The sheath is then removed and light manual pressure is maintained on the femoral vein. This can be carried out by the patient himself. After keeping the groin still for about 1 hour, the patient can usually get up without risk of bleeding and will be immediately able to perform any type of physical activity he desires. He is allowed to drive unless significant tranquilizers have been administered.

During the intervention an intravenous antibiotic is administered which can be repeated a few hours later if the patient is still at the hospital. Acetylsalicylic acid (100 mg per day) and clopidogrel (75 mg per day) are prescribed, starting the day of intervention, for 5 and 1 months, respectively. The patient is instructed to observe the usual prophylaxis against endocarditis at least for a couple of months. All medications can usually be stopped once a (preferably transesophageal) echocardiogram proves a tight seat of the device without any sign of thrombosis at least 4 months after the intervention and preferably a few weeks after stopping antiplatelet therapy.

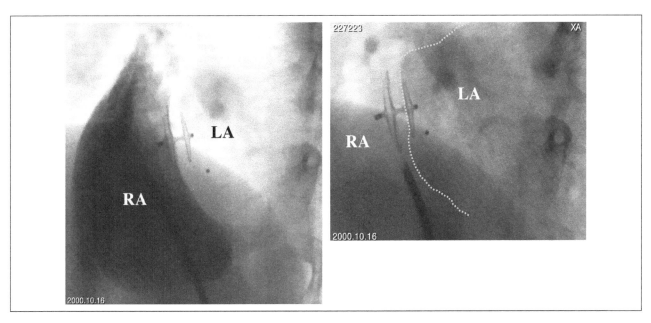

Figure 31.16
Angiographic documentation of Amplatzer PFO occlusion by hand injections of contrast medium through the introducer in a left anterior oblique projection with cranial angulation. The right atrium (RA) is clearly delineated (left panel). After the dye has passed through the lungs, the left atrial border is also visible (right panel, dotted line) albeit more faintly. LA, left atrium.

Important points to check before releasing the device

Proof of correct position before release from the pusher cable is of paramount importance. While some centers deem transesophageal or intracardiac echocardiography necessary, we have defined a number of angiographic features that appear equally reliable and are easier to obtain.[1] The most important one is the so-called Pacman sign. It is explained in Figures 31.17–31.24. The angiographic examples convincingly demonstrate that the quality of the transesophageal echocardiographic demonstration of correct position (Figure 31.24) can be paralleled by angiography.

Follow-up examinations after Amplatzer PFO occlusion

It is recommended to perform a transesophageal echocardiography at 4–6 months' distance from the implantation. A good position of a thrombus-free device will be found in over 95% of cases (Figure 31.25).

Although the rapidity of endocardial coverage of the device is not known, animal studies and examination of devices removed at different time periods after implantation proved that coating with fibrinogen occurs within the first hours and endocardialization is complete at the latest at 4 months (Figure 31.26).

Thrombotic problems with the Amplatzer occluders are exquisitely rare. This constitutes one of the significant advantages of this device over competitors.[2] In our personal experience with almost 1000 Amplatzer shunt occluders and routine 6-month follow-up transesophageal echocardiography, a single case with a drop-like thrombus attached to the left-sided nipple of an Amplatzer PFO occluder occurred (Figure 31.27). The patient was orally anticoagulated for a year but the finding persisted. It has been followed conservatively for over 6 years with no clinical events.

Erosion of the superior atrial wall (left or right) into the pericardium or into the aorta has been described with most devices, including the Amplatzer PFO occluder.[3] Debate is ongoing whether the risk of such a complication is dependent on the size of the device. It is obvious that a device not reaching the aorta will be less prone to erosion as the main mechanism is rubbing against the aorta. On the other hand, such a small device will have a higher risk for incomplete closure of the PFO, although it may not always be necessary to cover the entire width of the mouth of the PFO (closing one half of a valve should prevent the other half from opening). A large device might embrace the aorta rather than poking it with its sharp edge and therefore, again, have less propensity for erosion. Again, the complete occlusion rate may be jeopardized because of the failure to snugly hug the interatrial septum. The advantages or disadvantages of small or large devices are explained in Figure 31.28. The compromise is to use the 25 mm medium-sized Amplatzer PFO occluder for the routine case. It is fairly reliable in

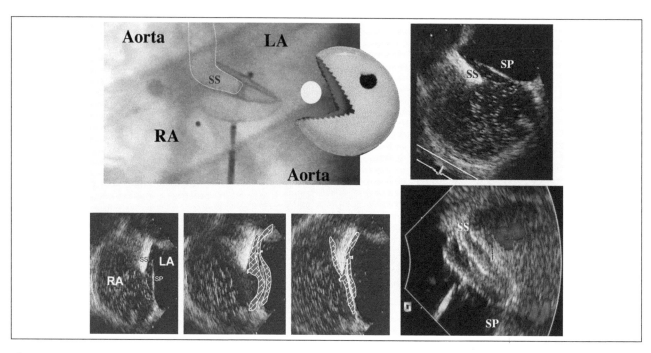

Figure 31.17
Pacman sign for correct placement of PFO occluder. The top left panel shows a 25 mm Amplatzer PFO occluder placed correctly. Even without dye injection the V-shape of the two disks can be appreciated. Separation of left side of the disks is caused by the muscular septum secundum (dotted outline), while the paper-thin septum primum to the right does not separate the two disks ostensibly. The right panels show the transesophageal echocardiographic picture in an analogous projection without (top) and with (bottom) the device. The bottom left panels show the echocardiographic situation in the projection used angiographically with an incorrectly (center) and correctly (right) placed superimposed Amplatzer PFO occluder. LA, left atrium; RA, right atrium; SP, septum primum; SS, septum secundum. (See also color plate section.)

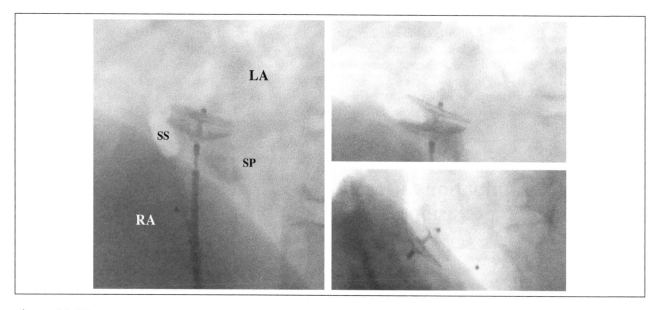

Figure 31.18
Enhanced visibility of the Pacman sign with hand injection of contrast medium into the right atrium (RA). The uvula-like septum secundum (SS) is clearly delineated by the contrast medium. On the left it is not between the two disks of this 18 mm Amplatzer PFO occluder. The right disk had to be withdrawn into the introducer and again released with more tension to obtain the correct position (right) before (top) and after (bottom) release. LA, left atrium; SP, septum primum.

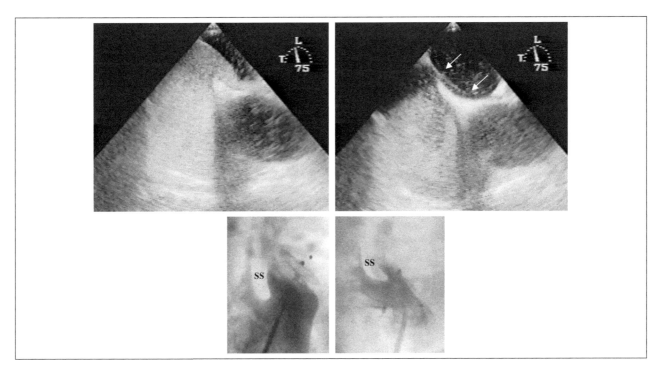

Figure 31.19
Tunnel-shaped PFO demanding particular attention to the Pacman sign. Top panels: transesophageal echocardiography with bubble test. The right panel exhibits the length of the tunnel (arrows). A first attempt with a 25 mm Amplatzer PFO occluder resulted in a negative Pacman sign (bottom left). This could be corrected by withdrawal and redeployment of the right disk (bottom right).

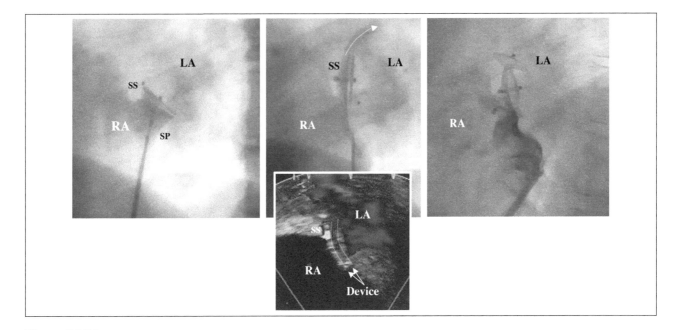

Figure 31.20
Amplatzer 18 mm PFO occluder erroneously released without a reliable Pacman sign. Left panel: the right atrial disk of the device is barely indenting (rather than embracing) the septum secundum (SS). After release from the pusher cable, the right atrial disk slips into the PFO tunnel, resulting in a significant residual shunt (center panel, arrow). The device should have been replaced for a 25 mm PFO occluder to safely embrace the septum secundum before release. The residual shunt was still present at the 6-month follow-up transesophageal echocardiogram (bottom insert). At that time it was remedied with the implantation of a second Amplatzer PFO occluder (right panel). LA, left atrium; RA, right atrium; SP, septum primum. (See also color plate section.)

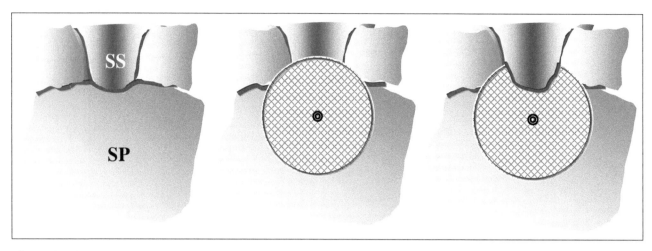

Figure 31.21

Artist's rendering of the Pacman sign situations as seen from the right atrium in Figures 31.17–31.20. The tongue-like septum secundum (SS) encompasses only a small segment of the upper septum (left). The correct position of the Amplatzer occluder is depicted in the center and the incorrect position in the right panel. Although there is little risk of complete embolization of the device, the incorrect position harbors a high propensity of a residual shunt (Figure 31.20).

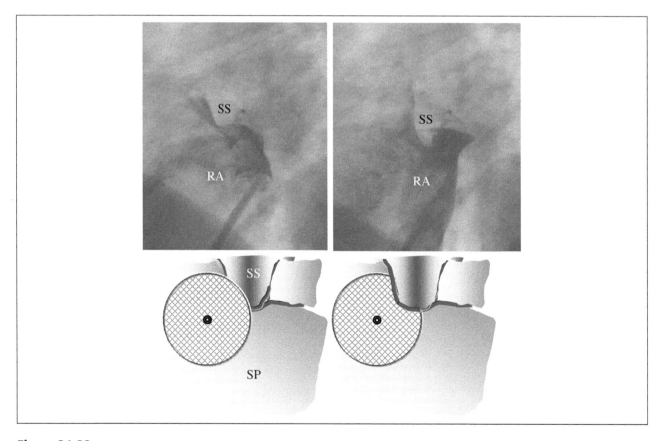

Figure 31.22

Situation with a partially prolapsing Amplatzer PFO occluder at the septum secundum (SS). An eccentric placement of the device is visible by a contrast medium injection into the right atrium (RA, top panels). At first, a correct sandwich position of the septum secundum between the two disks appears. However, during washout of the dye, a lateral prolapse of the SS beyond the right atrial disk becomes apparent. The situation is schematically explained (bottom panel) with the potential risk of partial prolapse of the right atrial disk into the left atrium, like the case in Figure 31.20 (bottom right). SP, septum primum.

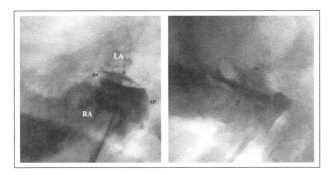

Figure 31.23
Rare occasion where a 25 mm Amplatzer PFO occluder is too small to produce a positive Pacman sign (left, septum secundum (SS) cannot be straddled between the disks). This is remedied by substituting a 35 mm Amplatzer PFO occluder (right). LA, left atrium; RA, right atrium; SP, septum primum.

establishing a positive Pacman sign during implantation, has a low risk of eroding the aorta (albeit not zero), and a high potential for complete or sufficient coverage of

the PFO mouth (about 90% complete permanent closure of the PFO).

To explain incomplete closure, several mechanisms have been considered, with an insufficiently large device placed eccentrically being the most common one (Figures 31.21, 31.22, 31.28, and 31.29). Remedy requires implantation of a second device (Figure 31.29).

Use of the Amplatzer atrial septal defect occluder for PFO closure

In some patients the septum primum does not reach the septum secundum, thereby creating an atrial septal defect of the secundum type. If the gap is just a few mm by transesophageal echocardiography, we generally use a PFO device just the same. Gaps 10 mm or larger may be better treated with balloon sizing and an appropriate atrial septal defect device. Before the Amplatzer PFO occluder became

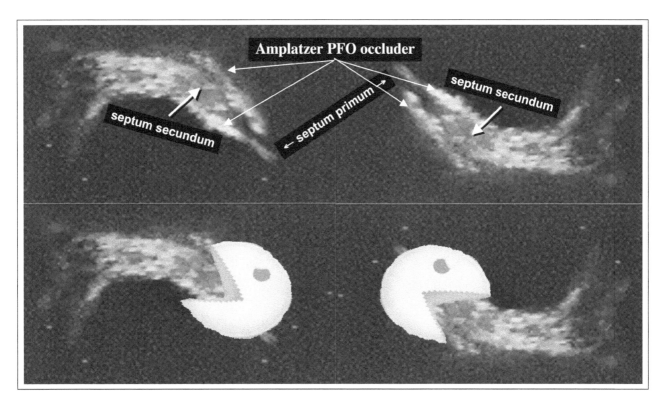

Figure 31.24
Left: demonstration of a positive Pacman sign by transesophageal echocardiography in the projection usually seen during fluoroscopy. The bottom panel explains where the name 'Pacman sign' derives from. Right: the same situation seen in the projection typical for transesophageal echocardiography.

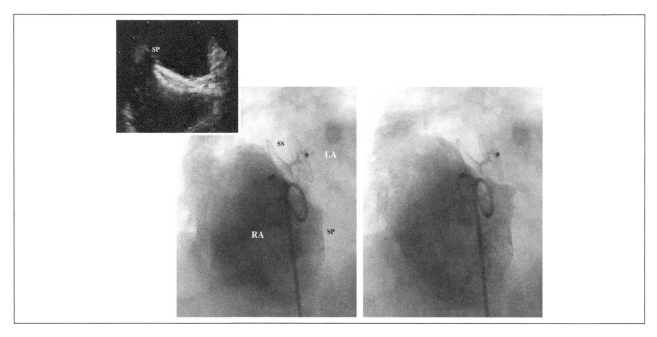

Figure 31.25
Transesophageal echocardiography (left top) and right atrial angiography (right bottom) examination at 6-month follow-up after successful and complete PFO closure with a 25 mm Amplatzer PFO occluder. The left angiographic picture was taken during and the right after a prolonged Valsalva maneuver. While the septum secundum (SS) remains immobile, the thin and flaccid septum primum (SP, atrial septal aneurysm) is pushed towards the right atrium (RA) during and freely prolapses into the left atrium (LA) after the Valsalva maneuver.

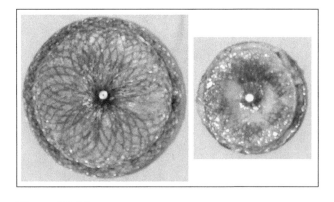

Figure 31.26
Endothelialization depicted on the example of two Amplatzer atrial septal defect occluders (same material as PFO occluders) removed at different time points (seen from the right atrial view). The left is a 34 mm device removed 5 hours after implantation. It already shows homogeneous coverage with fibrin. The right is a 24 mm device removed at 4 months. It shows complete coverage with a glistening new endocardium.

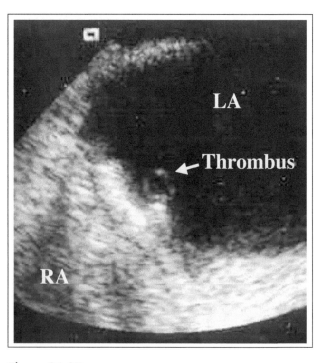

Figure 31.27
Drop-like mobile but organized thrombus attached to the left-sided nipple of an Amplatzer 25 mm PFO occluder at a 6-month follow-up transesophageal echocardiogram. The right atrium (RA) is filled with bubbles and proving the tightness of the occlusion as no bubbles transit into the left atrium (LA).

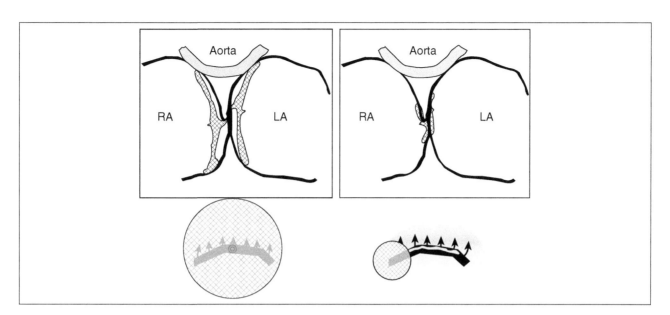

Figure 31.28
Didactic depiction of advantages and disadvantages of large and small PFO occluder devices. Left: the large device will fairly reliably cover the entire PFO mouth (bottom). However, it will not be hugging the septum in a snug fashion and it has the potential of eroding the atrial wall while rubbing against the aorta. Right: a small device will conform perfectly to the septum and will be devoid of the risk of eroding a free atrial wall. However, it may only cover part of the PFO mouth (bottom), particularly when placed eccentrically, which cannot be avoided by fluoroscopy or by transesophageal echocardiography during implantation. LA, left atrium; RA, right atrium.

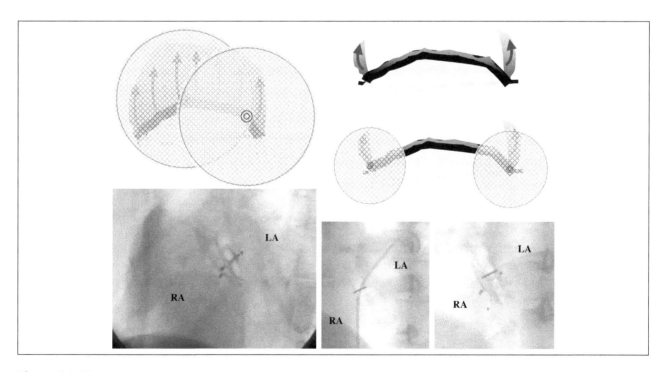

Figure 31.29
Examples for an incomplete closure of a PFO. Left top: eccentrically placed first 25 mm Amplatzer PFO occluder too small to cover the entire width of the PFO. The PFO can be completely closed by implantation of a second occluder. Right top: most of the PFO is fused except for the two edges of the mouth. This is best treated by two small devices being implanted separately (right center). The left bottom panel shows the aspect of two 25 mm Amplatzer PFO occluders side by side with the contour of the right atrium (RA) delineated by contrast medium. The right bottom panels show the implantation of a 25 mm Amplatzer PFO occluder to remedy a leaky PFO Star occluder implanted several months earlier (left: catheter across the septum through the PFO Star occluder; right: Amplatzer PFO occluder straddling the PFO Star occluder). The left atrium (LA) is faintly outlined by contrast medium.

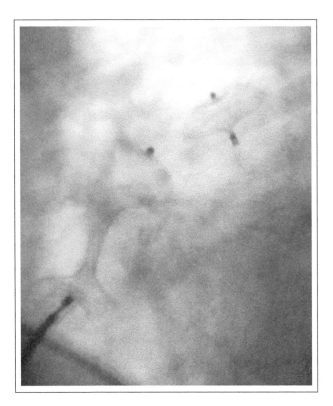

Figure 31.30
Poor choice of device. A 15 mm Amplatzer atrial septal defect occluder was used to close a funnel-shaped PFO. While it occluded the PFO the left atrial disk remained distorted. A 10 mm Amplatzer atrial septal defect occluder had been previously placed in the left atrial appendage to avoid anticoagulation in this 70-year-old patient with atrial fibrillation and a history of coumadin necrosis. The 15 mm Amplatzer atrial septal defect occluder device had been found too large for the left atrial appendage and was afterwards employed for the PFO closure for availability.

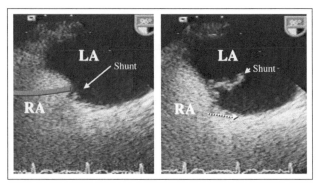

Figure 31.31
Impossibility of cannulating a PFO suspected from a clearly demonstrated bubble crossing on transesophageal echocardiography. The left panel shows a bubble about to cross close to the junction of the septum secundum with the septum primum, which is aneurysmatic (left side). The right panel shows more bubbles appearing in the left atrium, but this time their point of transit is less clear. It proved impossible to cannulate the suspected hole because the catheter (superimposed in the left panel) wound up in the aneurysmatic pouch when looking for the hole and the actual foramen ovale canal (dotted arrow) proved tight. LA, left atrium; RA, right atrium.

available, Amplatzer atrial septal defect devices had been used for all PFOs with good success. The concept of opening the PFO to a maximum and corking it, so to speak, with an appropriate atrial septal defect device will be devoid of the risk of eccentric placement and incomplete coverage germane to PFO occluders. However, in longish PFO tunnels ASD occluders deploy rather awkwardly (Figure 31.30).

Pitfalls of Amplatzer PFO occluder implantation

A high quality transesophageal echocardiogram alerts to most of the potential pitfalls before the procedure. Figure 31.19 shows the case of a particularly long tunnel that required increased pull while deploying the right-sided disk to honor the Pacman sign. Such a situation may prompt the selection of a 35 mm Amplatzer PFO occluder from the beginning (Figure 31.12) and will certainly disqualify an attempt with an 18 mm Amplatzer PFO occluder.

On the other hand, even a high quality transesophageal echocardiogram may be misleading. Unless the bubble passage through the gaping PFO is clearly demonstrated, difficulties or failures to cannulate may occur. Figures 31.31–31.34 demonstrate such examples.

Figure 31.35 depicts a case where a persisting left superior vena cava was mistaken for a large atrial septal defect at a transesophageal echocardiography performed because of a cryptogenic stroke. The diagnosis was angiographically rectified during the planned atrial septal defect closure. Incidentally a PFO was found and it was successfully closed.

As with all procedures requiring venous access to the heart, local venous anomalies or thromboses may cause difficulties for the interventional cardiologist (Figure 31.36). Canulation and closure of PFO is easiest from the right femoral vein. However, it can also be accomplished from the left femoral vein or a vein of the upper half of the body.

In case it is impossible to unscrew the pusher cable from the device because the device rotates in unison with the cable, the introducer should be pushed firmly against the device, perhaps even invaginating a part of the right atrial disk while unscrewing the pusher cable. This increases friction and tends to keep the device from torquing

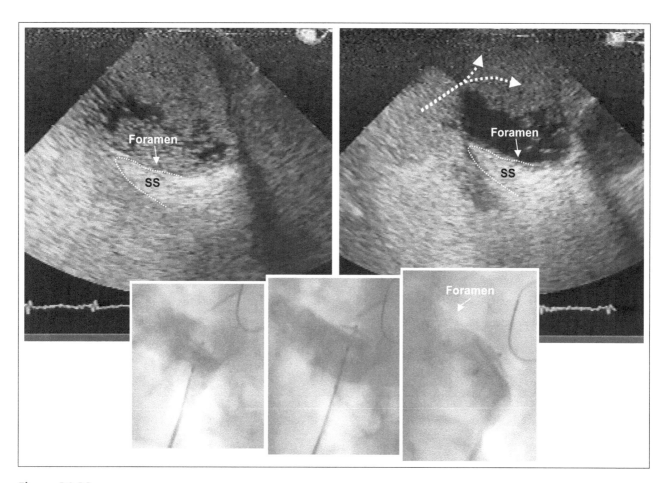

Figure 31.32

In a case similar to the one in Figure 31.31, the transesophageal bubble passage looked at first straightforward. However, when checking for the initial bubble transit it clearly indicated that the passage was through a small hole in the redundant septum primum (dotted arrows) rather than through the foramen which was tight. Luckily, the small atrial septal defect in the aneurysmatic septum primum could be cannulated and a 25 mm Amplatzer PFO occluder was inserted. The completely parallel position of the two disks (negative Pacman sign) in addition to the fact that the device appeared to be in the right atrium rather than at the level of the septum (bottom left) was explained by the fact that the hole was not the PFO but a small atrial septal defect in a redundant septal aneruysm. Shoving the device towards the left atrium proved that it was indeed at the level of the septum (bottom center). The final position showed it in the middle of the septum primum at a clear distance from the foramen (bottom right). The half circle in the right top corner of the bottom panels is a Carpentier–Edwards ring after mitral valve reconstruction. SS, septum secundum.

(Figure 31.37). If this maneuver fails, the device will have to be removed and unscrewed outside the body a quarter turn and then re-inserted.

In the rare case of loss of the device during deployment or embolization thereafter, Amplatzer devices are best caught by a Dotter basket, a wire loop, or a forceps (Figure 31.38) and brought into an easily accessible place where an attempt should be made to either capture the female plug on the right atrial disk with a catheter and reinsert the screw of the pusher cable or capture the female plug at its neck with a biotome or a gooseneck snare.[4] The latter grip may still not allow retraction of the device back into an introducer as the nipple (female screw) will arrive obliquely at the entrance of the introducer. Using a large sheath or cutting an oval sheath

endhole may help. In some cases it may only be possible to retract the device to the femoral vein (or artery), from where it will have to be removed with a cut-down.

Incidental angiographic diagnosis of PFO

Generally the most unpleasant part of diagnosis and treatment of a PFO is the initial transesophgeal echocardiography. Hence, in patients needing cardiac catheterization for another reason, patients in whom the suspicion of a PFO arises with no time for a diagnostic transesophageal echocardiogram

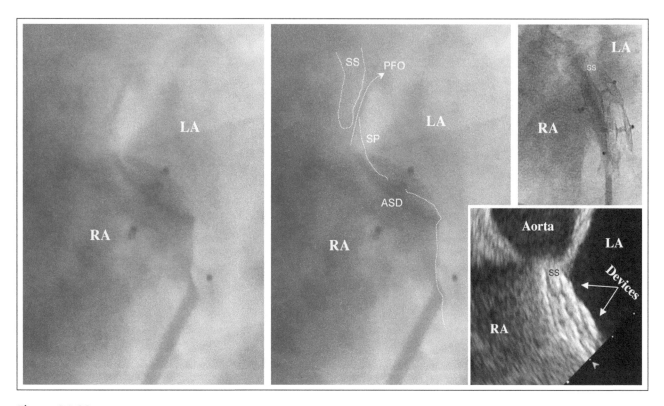

Figure 31.33
Atrial septal defect (ASD) in addition to PFO. In this patient with a true PFO the device was mistakenly placed in an unrecognized small ASD (left). The anatomy is outlined in the center panel, showing that the PFO remains open. The situation can be suspected, diagnosed, and corrected without the need for echocardiography on the basis of the parallel position of the two disks and the residual shunt to the left of the implanted device. A second 25 mm Amplatzer PFO occluder implanted through the PFO corrected the problem (right top). An 8-month follow-up transesophageal echocardiography shows the two PFO occluders, one in the ASD and the other in the PFO, and documents complete closure of both holes (right bottom). LA, left atrium; RA, right atrium; SP, septum primum; SS, septum secundum.

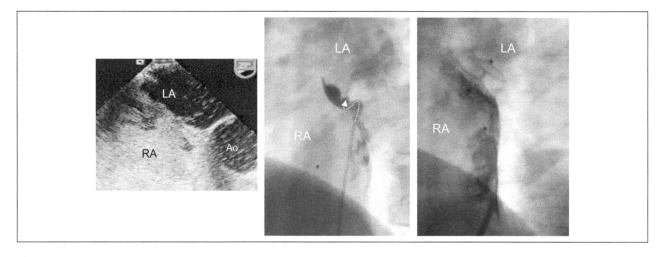

Figure 31.34
Bubble transit suggestive but not affirmative of a PFO (left). Because of difficulty in finding the passage, a dye injection into the foramen was carried out, revealing a pinhole leaving the canal perpendicularly (probably in a corner of the foramen) (center). Passage could be negotiated with a right Judkins catheter (center) and the foramen was closed with a 25 mm Amplatzer PFO occluder (right). Ao, aorta; LA, left atrium; RA, right atrium.

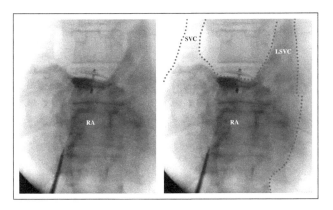

Figure 31.35
A 61-year-old woman with right heart enlargement on X-ray and a cryptogenic stroke. Transthoracic echocardiography misdiagnosed a persistent left superior vena cava (LSVC) as a 2 cm atrial septal defect. The atrial septal defect was deemed the culprit for paradoxical embolism. A bubble study was not done due to the mistakenly assumed left to right shunt which, in fact, was the venous inflow into the right atrium (RA). During attempted closure of the presumed atrial septal defect, the LSVC was recognized in addition to the normal superior vena cava. To account for the cryptogenic stroke, a PFO was looked for, found, and occluded with a 25 mm Amplatzer PFO occluder. It assumed a horizontal position due to the anomalous anatomy.

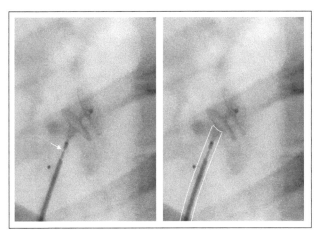

Figure 31.37
Difficulty in deployment of an 18 mm Amplatzer PFO occluder because the device kept rotating in concert with the pusher cable when trying to unscrew. By pulling part of the right disk back into the introducer (outlined in the right panel), the device could be immobilized and deployment was successful. This problem occurs more often with small devices (less friction against the tissue) and can be prevented by releasing the device a quarter turn before inserting it into the introducer. On the other hand, before advancing an Amplatzer device out of the introducer it should always be ascertained that the pusher is not already halfway unscrewed (arrow in left panel). The right picture shows the thin screw appearing between the female screw of the device and the solid part of the pusher cable.

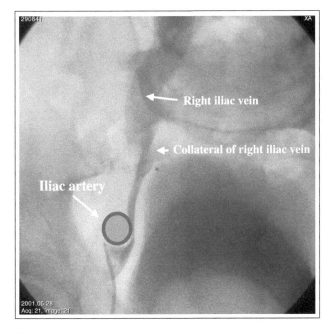

Figure 31.36
Thrombosed right iliac vein. The PFO could nonetheless be occluded by accessing the right iliac vein through a collateral. The access was further complicated by the fact that the collateral circled around a tortuous iliac artery.

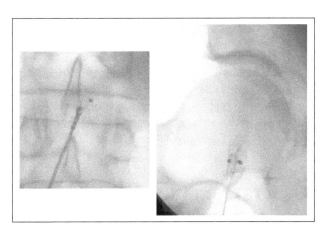

Figure 31.38
Attempt to grab an embolized Amplatzer occluder by its female plug with a biotome (left) in the descending aorta. As the grip was not strong enough to pull it back into an introducer, the device was caught between the disks with a wire loop and pulled into the femoral artery (right), from where it was removed with a cut-down.

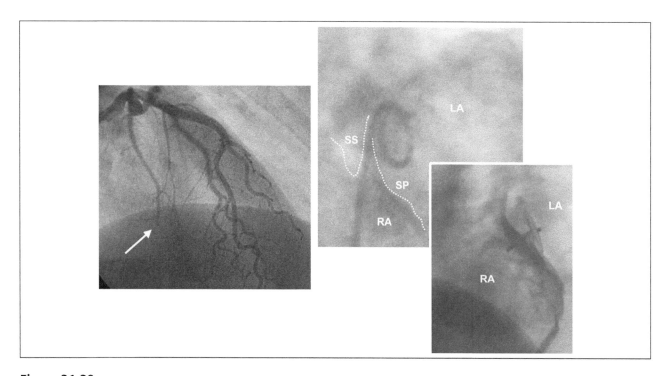

Figure 31.39
Acute myocardial infarction in a 34-year-old woman with no risk factors. The infarction was caused by an embolic occlusion of a small left circumflex coronary artery (left panel, arrow). The patient underwent emergency catheterization at 2 o'clock in the morning. The most likely reason for such a situation is a PFO. It was looked for, found, and documented with a pigtail catheter straddling it (center panel). It took about 5 minutes to occlude it with a 25 mm Amplatzer PFO occluder. The PFO closure prolonged the procedure by less than 30 minutes. LA, left atrium; RA, right atrium; SP, septum primum; SS, septum secundum.

(Figures 31.39 and 31.40), or patients either refusing transesophageal echocardiography or yielding a questionable finding, the PFO can easily be sought, documented (Figures 31.39 and 31.40), or excluded (Figure 31.41) by direct angiography.

Occasionally, angiography may have to be used to correct an erroneous diagnosis of a PFO by echocardiography (Figure 31.41). Such echocardiographic errors are due to overinterpretation of bubbles appearing late in the left atrium, shunts or normal connections in the pulmonary circulation, or shunts in other places of the interatrial septum (Figures 31.31 and 31.32). The appearance in particular of exclusively small bubbles in the left atrium occurring first after more than four heart beats is not indicative for the presence of a PFO.

General remarks

The Amplatzer PFO occluder is by a large margin the most versatile and easy to use device to close PFOs. In addition, it is less complication prone and yields better complete occlusion rates than its competitors. To occlude a PFO with an Amplatzer PFO occluder is currently the easiest therapeutic catheter intervention known to adult cardiology. This comes in handy to cope with the increasing number of patients referred for PFO closure. This trend is likely to

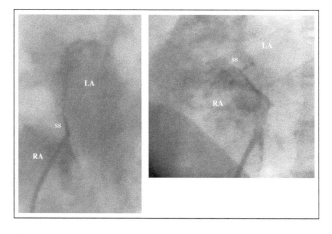

Figure 31.40
Documentation and impromptu closure of PFO suspected in a 53-year-old man referred for emergency coronary angioplasty because of an acute myocardial infarction showing an embolic occlusion of a coronary artery without atherosclerosis, which roused the suspicion of a PFO. The PFO was looked for, found, and closed during the same emergency catheterization session. The documentation occurred with a multi-purpose catheter (left panel) depicting a tunnel PFO when injecting with the tip leaning against the septum secundum (SS). A 25 mm Amplatzer PFO occluder was implanted (right panel). LA, left atrium; RA, right atrium; SS, septum secundum.

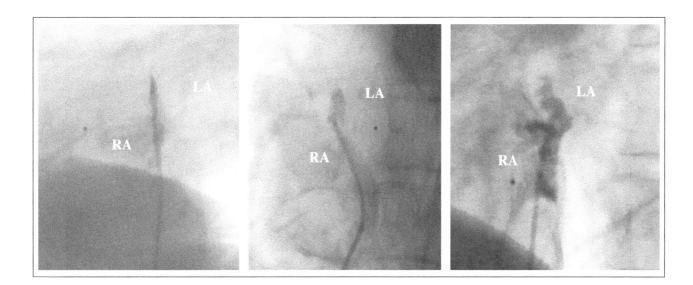

Figure 31.41
Three examples of PFOs suspected by transesophageal echocardiography but not present. A dye injection into the fossa ovalis depicts the tunnel of the PFO with no exit into the left atrium in all three cases (left: left anterior oblique projection; center and right: frontal projection). LA, left atrium; RA, right atrium.

increase further. Theoretically, about 25% of the population may have to undergo the procedure, should a PFO *per se* be considered a hazard ominous enough to warrant primary prevention with implantation of a device into the heart?[5]

References

1. Meier B. Pacman sign during device closure of the patent foramen ovale. Cathet Cardiovasc Interven 2003; 60: 221–3.

2. Krumsdorf U, Ostermayer S, Billinger K et al. Incidence and clinical course of thrombus formation on atrial septal defect and patent foramen ovale closure devices in 1,000 consecutive patients. J Am Coll Cardiol 2004; 43: 302–9.

3. Trepels T, Zeplin H, Sievert H et al. Cardiac perforation following transcatheter PFO closure. Cathet Cardiovasc Interven 2003; 58: 111–13.

4. Pfammatter JP, Meier B. Successful repositioning of an Amplatzer duct occluder immediately after inadvertent embolization in the descending aorta. Cathet Cardiovasc Interven 2003; 59: 83–5.

5. Meier B. Closure of patent foramen ovale: technique, pitfalls, complications, and follow up. Heart 2005; 91: 444–8.

32

Percutaneous closure of patent foramen ovale with the CardioSEAL®/STARFlex® Occluder

Paul Kramer

Devices

CardioSEAL® and StarFLEX® are descendants of the original Clamshell® device. Clamshell consisted of two mirror-image umbrella-like square patches of polyester connected at their hubs. The metal framework was constructed of stainless steel wires radiating from the central hub to each of the four corners of the patch with a midpoint coil in the wire rib to achieve angulation, tension, and flexibility. The fabric was sewn to the stainless steel rib skeleton. Each square patch was rotated 45° relative to its opposing counterpart. When deployed, each side of the device was concave toward the septum, and the rib coils increased the closing tension at the corners. This device suffered, however, from a high rate of wire rib fractures due to metal fatigue and/or corrosion. Clamshell® was succeeded by CardioSEAL®, which substituted MP35N alloy for the stainless steel ribs and incorporated two tandem coil hinges in each rib. Bench testing and accumulated clinical experience have confirmed a dramatic reduction in rib fracture rate. This device is the version currently available in the United States (Figure 32.1). STARFlex® represents a further modification of this technology. It consists of a CardioSEAL® and includes nitinol springs that connect the edges of the opposing sides of the device. These springs traverse the defect such that, when each side of the device is deployed, they are stretched under tension (Figure 32.2). This tension serves two purposes: (1) it draws the edges of each side of the device more firmly and securely against the septum, and (2) it causes the device to self-center, ensuring more symmetric coverage over the entrance to and exit from the patent foramen ovale (PFO). These two effects result in a higher rate of immediate and complete defect closure and in the ability to close a somewhat larger defect with a somewhat smaller device.

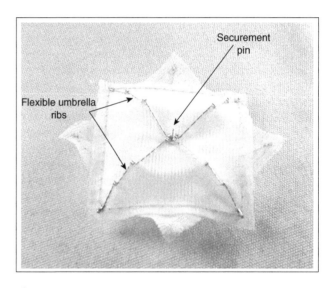

Figure 32.1
CardioSEAL device, consisting of two square patches of polyester fabric supported by umbrella ribs made of MP35N radiating from the central connecting hub to each corner. Each rib is flexible, resulting from the incorporation of two coil hinge points. Each corner exerts slight pressure across the plane which runs between the two sides of the device, helping to secure it to the interatrial septum. Note how the corners of one side of the device extend across the plane of its opposing umbrella.

Technique

In general, and from the outset, it is worth stating that percutaneous closure of PFO with CardioSEAL®/STARFlex® is a straightforward, simple, safe, and gratifying procedure to perform. However, it should be emphasized that there is a

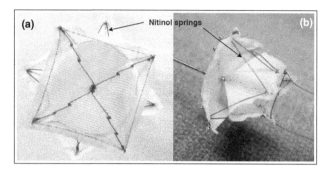

Figure 32.2
STARflex device in frontal view of left atrial side (a) and side view with left atrial umbrella partially collapsed by tension on suture (b). The nitinol springs increase the closing force against the tissue between the umbrellas and also assist in centering the device within the defect.

set of fundamental guidelines that should be followed in performing this procedure. Simplicity does not allow for oversimplification, and success is determined by outcomes rather than speed. Several critically important steps requiring little procedural time and effort can, if taken, avoid ineffective treatment and/or severe complications. The goal of percutaneous PFO closure, simply stated, is to eliminate as completely as possible the passage of blood (and potential blood-borne contaminants) from the right atrium through the interatrial septum into the systemic circulation. The objective is not merely to implant a device. The basic technique of PFO closure with CardioSEAL®/STARFlex® is described below, and technique modifications for special circumstances are discussed in the subsequent section.

Patients are positioned supine on the cath lab table as for a routine procedure. The right groin is shaved, sterilely prepared, and draped in customary fashion. If the right femoral vein cannot be used, the left side provides essentially equally effective access. The cath lab environment should be maintained similarly to an operating room for this procedure, with all personnel wearing hats and masks and minimal traffic in and out of the room. A parenteral antibiotic is administered around the time of the procedure. In our facility, 1 g of vancomycin is given intravenously over 1 hour on call to the procedure. Patients are pre-treated with aspirin and clopidogrel or ticlopidine.

Invasive echocardiography is important in performing PFO closure for multiple reasons. Such imaging can confirm the diagnosis, depict associated lesions (atrial septal 'aneurysm', Chiari network, Eustachian valve), detect thrombus trapped in the PFO (absolute contraindication to crossing the defect), and document effective closure, and it is useful in diagnosing alternative or coexisting right-to-left shunts such as pulmonary arteriovenous fistula. While transesophageal echocardiography (TEE) is an excellent imaging modality in this regard, the requirement for

additional personnel in the procedure room and the need for more intensive sedation create logistical and performance concerns. Intracardiac echocardiography (ICE) avoids these drawbacks, allowing for light conscious sedation and good patient cooperation with requests for cough or Valsalva. However, the ICE catheters are costly.

If ICE is utilized, 11 Fr and 9 Fr sheaths are placed in the right femoral vein. The 9 Fr sheath allows introduction and withdrawal of the sizing balloon catheter and is nevertheless smaller than the 10 Fr delivery sheath that replaces it for device closure. If TEE is employed, only a 9 Fr sheath is placed. The ICE catheter is advanced under fluoroscopic guidance to the right atrium and rotated toward the interatrial septum. It is then angulated to image the superior aspect of the fossa ovalis. Agitated saline is then injected via the side arm of the 9 Fr sheath, and right-to-left shunting is documented, either spontaneously or in response to cough or Valsalva. This is an important step for two reasons. First, as many as 5% of patients presenting in the cath lab for PFO closure have false positive diagnostic TEEs or transthoracic echocardiograms. The diagnosis should be confirmed before trying too vigorously to close a defect that may not exist. Secondly, the delayed appearance, e.g., four or five cycles after right atrial opacification, of robust contrast in the left atrium should alert the physician to the possibility of a pulmonary AV fistula. Depiction of a prominent Eustachian valve or Chiari network should alert the operator to the possibility of entanglement of the sizing balloon, delivery sheath, or right atrial arm of the device during deployment.

Once the presence of a PFO is confirmed, an angulated catheter (my preference is a multipurpose A curve) is advanced via the 9 Fr sheath to the right atrium. Crossing the PFO is usually straightforward. Beginning in the low right atrium (RA) with the catheter directed toward the patient's left side (3 o'clock as viewed from the patient's feet), the catheter is simultaneously advanced cephalad as it is rotated clockwise (posteriorly) about a quarter turn (to 6 o'clock). This maneuver should be performed smoothly, in one continuous motion, requiring less than one second. Repeated attempts may be necessary. The catheter should be handled gently to avoid inadvertent perforation, e.g., of the right atrial appendage. Passage into the left atrium (LA) is confirmed by monitoring the pressure waveform (LA pressure is higher and more spiked due to higher a- and v-waves and steeper x- and y-descents). Additionally, observation of the catheter well to the left of mid-line with an atrial waveform and the absence of premature ventricular contractions (PVCs) is helpful. Finally, passage beyond the cardiac silhouette into a pulmonary vein is confirmatory. If desired, the catheter can be directed into the right upper pulmonary vein from which position an angiogram can be performed. From this location, contrast streams across the left side of the interatrial septum and can depict the presence of an atrial septal 'aneurysm' or a left-to-right shunt. However,

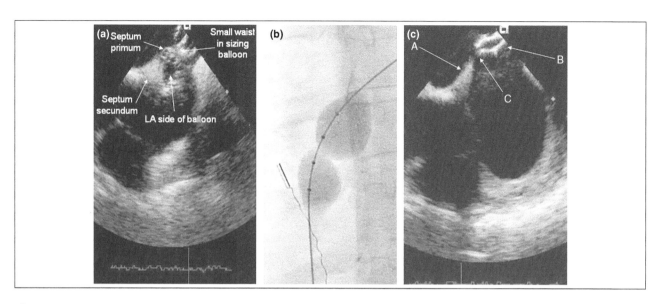

Figure 32.3

Clues to the presence and crossing of a fenestration in the septum primum. (a) Intracardiac echocardiographic image of balloon inflation in the defect. Note the delicate septum primum tissue between the small balloon waist and the septum secundum. (b) Sizing balloon inflated in defect. The small diameter of the waist, about 5 mm, should raise a suspicion that this defect is a fenestration rather than a PFO. (c) Echo image after deployment of small occluder (B) in the fenestration. Note the gap (C) between the superior extent of the occluder and the inferior edge of the septum secundum (A).

inasmuch as this information can be acquired from ICE or TEE, this step is not essential.

Once the catheter has crossed into the left atrium, anti-coagulation is achieved with a parenteral agent of choice, e.g., heparin or bivalrudin. The physician may wish to administer only a partial dose of anticoagulant if a long-tunnel PFO variant is present in case the transseptal puncture technique is opted for (see below). The catheter is directed into a left pulmonary vein, and an exchange-length (> 200 cm) 0.035–0.038 inch wire is gently advanced out the end. This does not need to be a stiff, extra support type of wire, and it should not be a hydrophilic wire in order to avoid pulmonary venous perforation. The catheter is removed over the wire, and the wire is wiped. At this point, the sheath is aspirated and flushed such that its contents are blood-tinged (pink). When introducing the balloon sizing catheter through the hemostatic valve of the 9 Fr sheath, slowly advance and withdraw the balloon in small increments to allow the pink fluid in the sheath to visibly 'milk out' trapped air in the folds of the balloon.

Balloon catheter inflation within the defect is recommended for several reasons. Originally, the purpose of this step was to measure the stretched diameter of the PFO in order to select an occluder of about twice its dimension. This sizing margin allowed for adequate coverage even with eccentric positioning of the device, although this is a smaller concern with the self-centering STARFlex®. An additional value of sizing is the finding of an unusually small defect (≤ 5 mm). Such a small dimension should alert the physician to the possibility that the initial transseptal

passage of the angulated catheter may have occurred via a small fenestration in the septum primum rather than via the PFO itself. Invasive echocardiography can reinforce this suspicion by showing that the exchange wire used for subsequent placement of the delivery sheath crosses the septum well below the level of the PFO tunnel. Simply placing a device in this location closes the small fenestration (mainly the site of a tiny left-to-right shunt) and, in the absence of utilizing invasive echocardiography, leaves the culprit defect enabling right-to-left shunting untreated. Such fenestrations exist in fewer than 5% of patients undergoing PFO closure, but, in my experience, the angulated catheter used to cross the septum always encounters and traverses the fenestration first, rather than the PFO (Figure 32.3).

The second and more important reason to inflate a sizing balloon in the defect is not to size it but to characterize it. The length of overlap of the septa varies greatly from patient to patient, and the degree of overlap defines the length of the tunnel-like pathway through the septum. Regardless of how long the tunnel appears on echocardiography, the upper edge of the septum primum is usually easily displaceable downward so that a perpendicular orientation of the interatrial communication can be created. This results from a combination of very pliable septum primum tissue and sufficient separation of the anchor points between which the upper extent of the septum primum is non-fused to the septum secundum, forming the rim of the septum primum at the exit of the defect into the left atrium. Usually, this rim is sufficiently long to enable downward displacement so that it can be aligned with the inferior edge

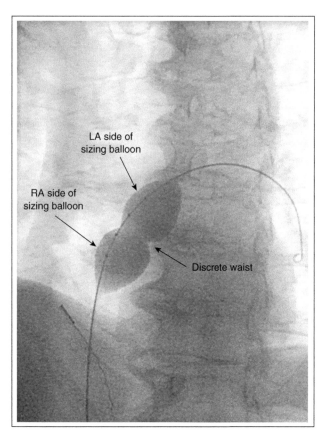

Figure 32.4

Typical appearance of sizing balloon inflated in PFO, characterized by sharply demarcated, discrete waist in the balloon. This image indicates a stretched PFO diameter of about 14mm.

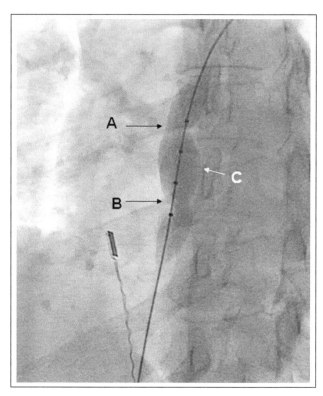

Figure 32.5

Striking example of irreducible, long-tunnel variant of PFO. (A) indicates the left atrial exit portal from the PFO, while (B) is a constriction imposed by the entrance portal. The length of the tunnel between these portals (C) is about 21 mm. Failure to recognize this anatomic variant would result in the deployment and entrapment of the left or right atrial side within the tunnel.

of the septum secundum, which is the superior limbus of the fossa ovalis. As a result, the occluder can orient perpendicularly to the plane of the interatrial septum at deployment, and the short connecting hub is sufficiently long to traverse the defect. During sizing balloon inflation, this orthogonal orientation potential is depicted by a discrete waist in the balloon as it is pressurized, even if there is a 'dog bone' appearance during initial balloon inflation (see Figure 32.4).

Sometimes, with long tunnels identified by echocardiography, only a short rim of septum primum tissue has failed to fuse with the septum secundum, creating a long tunnel with a small exit port into the left atrium. Even though septum primum tissue may be highly elastic, this short rim may not be displaceable inferiorly to the level of the superior limbus of the fossa ovalis. Such an 'irreducible tunnel' is characterized by a persistent dog bone appearance of the balloon, even when it is fully pressurized (Figure 32.5). If the length of the balloon waist (tunnel) exceeds about 8 mm, the hub of the occluder is not long enough to permit full deployment of one side of the device. This results in an unopened umbrella being constrained within the tunnel

while the opposing umbrella is deployed over the left or right atrial side of the defect (Figure 32.6). Such an outcome may be highly undesirable due to the potential for device embolization, device thrombosis, or tunnel thrombosis with subsequent thromboembolism. The finding of an irreducible tunnel longer than about 8 mm is an indication to deploy the occluder using the transseptal puncture technique (see below).

Once the PFO has been sized and characterized, the balance of the intravenous anticoagulant is given (if it had been withheld), a delivery sheath is prepared and placed, and a CardioSEAL® or STARFlex® is selected. The 10 Fr transseptal delivery sheath used for placement of these occluders mimics the shape of the distal end of the multi-purpose catheter used earlier in the procedure. All air should be evacuated from the sheath during preparation by vigorously flushing it with heparinized saline and striking the hub against the preparation table or with a hemostat during flushing. Leaving the exchange wire in place in a left pulmonary vein, the sizing balloon is withdrawn through its introducer sheath, and then the sheath itself is withdrawn. The wire is cleaned with a moist wipe, and the skin is cleansed around

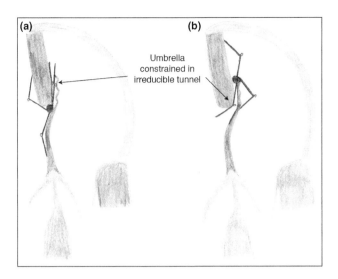

Figure 32.6
Incomplete deployment due to umbrella entrapment within irreducible tunnel. (a) diagrammatically depicts full deployment of the right atrial umbrella over the entrance to the PFO tunnel but entrapment of the left atrial side of the device. (b) demonstrates the opposite situation. When the irreducible tunnel as shown in Figure 32.5 exceeds about 8 mm in length, full opening of one side of the device can only be achieved at the expense of entrapment of its opposing side within the tunnel.

the entry site. The delivery sheath is then advanced over the wire into the left atrium. Once the tip of the sheath's dilator is judged to be well across the defect, it and the wire are held immobile while the sheath alone is advanced over them deep into the left atrium or even into the pulmonary vein. The dilator and wire are then withdrawn from the sheath in a smooth and steady movement over about 5 seconds, being careful to maintain the sheath tip in position. Some operators inject heparinized saline through the side arm of the sheath during this withdrawal to avoid pulling air into the sheath, and some recommend very slow withdrawal for the same reason. I don't feel that these precautions are necessary, but it is essential to remove any and all air that might have entered the sheath during removal of the dilator and wire. Aspirating the sheath with the hub elevated and its side arm connection directed upward and striking the hub with a flick of the finger or with a hemostat during aspiration until no bubbles appear in the side arm tubing will typically evacuate 2 to 5 ml of air. Thereafter, the sheath is flushed with about 20 ml of heparinized saline.

In ordinary circumstances, a CardioSEAL® device about 2 times, or STARFlex® device 1.6–2 times the stretched diameter of the defect is selected. The package is opened, and the device is immersed in a bowl of heparinized saline. The delivery catheter is then prepared by loosening the Tuohy–Borst adapter and the locking nut at the back end and advancing the inner catheter about 4 or 5 cm beyond

the end of the outer catheter. For the securement of a CardioSEAL®, the pin lock is released, and the locking pin is advanced 2–3 mm out of the locking pod. The catheter is then forcefully flushed with heparinized saline in order to evacuate trapped air. The Tuohy–Borst adapter is tightened, but the locking nut remains loose, permitting movement of the inner catheter relative to the outer sheath. Grasping the occluder in the left hand and the connecting end of the delivery catheter in the right, the locking pins of the device and the catheter are brought into contact by crossing them like crossed swords in a semi-orthogonal orientation. Once such contact is established, the occluder is re-oriented so that the device's locking pin aligns more parallel with the pin on the catheter. The device's pin is then slid into the locking pod and tested for entry by a gentle radial movement to confirm entrapment. Once the device pin is in the pod, the physician or an assistant withdraws the catheter's locking pin into the pod, securing the device to the catheter. The locking tab at the back end of the inner catheter is engaged, and a gentle tug on the occluder is used to confirm securement. The securement mechanism for the STARFlex® device differs in that it does not consist of overlapping ball-tipped pins within the locking pod. Rather, the ball-tipped pin on the device is grasped in a forceps which is then retracted within the pod. This arrangement allows much greater freedom of movement at the attachment point and less distortion of the device by the delivery catheter prior to device release.

After connecting the occluder to the delivery catheter, the sutures through the corners of the left atrial umbrella are pulled away from the catheter to evert and collapse this side of the device, and the introducer funnel is dropped over it. The suture is then further pulled to evert and collapse the right atrial umbrella as it enters the funnel. Continued pulling on the suture retracts the collapsed device into and to the end of the loading tube, and at this time one suture is cut. Gentle traction on one end of the cut suture enables its removal from the occluder. The protective housing around the flexible loading tube is then removed and discarded. The flushing Tuohy–Borst adapter is then connected to the loader. With the loading apparatus pointed upwards, a vigorous heparinized saline flush is used to evacuate air from the introducer system. Finally, the tip of the delivery catheter is advanced toward the occluder by gently withdrawing the inner catheter through the locking nut. The tip of the outer catheter should be advanced to 3–4 mm from the tips of the right atrial umbrella within the introducer tube and secured in this position by tightening the locking nut. This arrangement prevents the exposed inner catheter buckling during advancement of the occluder from the introducer tube into the delivery sheath.

During slow, continuous hand flushing of the introducer assembly with heparinized saline, the introducer tube is inserted through the hemostatic valve of the delivery sheath and advanced to a point of resistance. Check to make sure that the locking tab is engaged and the locking nut is tight. The delivery catheter is then advanced 20–30 cm while the delivery sheath is held stationary, advancing the occluder out of the introducer tube and well into the sheath. The introducer assembly is then withdrawn from the sheath and parked at the rear of the delivery catheter. The delivery catheter is then advanced to bring the collapsed and constrained occluder to the high inferior vena cava or low right atrium. At this point, the locking nut is loosened, and the inner catheter is advanced from the outer catheter to position the distal ends of the occluder at the tip of the delivery sheath. This maneuver serves to unmask a length of flexible inner catheter to minimize distortion of the occluder during deployment. The locking nut is retightened so that the inner catheter and its outer sheath no longer move independently. After confirming that the delivery sheath is still within the left atrium by fluoroscopy and echocardiography, the device is deployed.

With the left hand on the hub of the delivery sheath and the right hand on the delivery catheter close to its entry into the sheath, the delivery sheath is slowly withdrawn while making certain that the occluder does not move relative to bony landmarks. This usually requires a forward, advancing force on the delivery catheter to counteract the friction exerted by the delivery sheath, but the occluder should not be physically advanced relative to bony landmarks. Sheath withdrawal continues until the tip of the sheath just passes the central hub marker on fluoroscopy. At this point, the left atrial umbrella is fully unsheathed and should be able to open fully. It may be partially constrained in a pulmonary vein, and a short simultaneous withdrawal of the delivery sheath and catheter will free up the umbrellas as it disengages from the pulmonary vein and enters the left atrium. Relying now primarily on echocardiographic imaging, grasp the delivery sheath hub and the delivery catheter at the hub with one hand and slowly withdraw them together, bringing the left atrial umbrella into contact with the left side of the interatrial septum. Continue to withdraw both components together until there is palpable resistance and slight left atrial umbrella eversion. At this point, hold the delivery sheath and delivery catheter in separate hands and withdraw only the delivery sheath, being careful to maintain the same degree of tension and eversion on the left atrial umbrella. When the tip of the sheath is withdrawn beyond the tips of the right atrial umbrella, this umbrella will spring open, and any remaining tension on the delivery catheter can be released. Using ICE or TEE to confirm a proper relationship between the occluder and the septum (superior and inferior limbs on the correct sides of the septum), disengage the locking tab and advance the delivery catheter's locking pin out of the locking pod. Gently retract the delivery catheter under fluoroscopic observation to ensure full release of and disengagement from the occluder.

Once the delivery catheter is free and clear, withdraw it completely from the sheath, and then withdraw the sheath

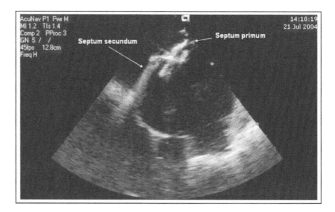

Figure 32.7
Deployed CardioSEAL® seen straddling the septa secundum and primum, giving an appearance similar to a chromosome.

into the inferior vena cava. Use echocardiography to inspect the septum and assess the final position of the occluder. Then, assess completeness of PFO closure by injecting agitated saline through the delivery sheath. Generally, complete closure of the defect is seen about 80% of the time, whereas a small residual right-to-left shunt can be seen spontaneously or with provocation in the remaining 20%. If a concerning degree of right-to-left shunt persists, wait several minutes and repeat the assessment. Usually, the shunt will diminish greatly by the end of this interval. The appearance of an optimally deployed device will resemble a chromosome, with the more superior limbs straddling the septum secundum and the more closely apposed lower limbs on either side of the thinner septum primum (see Figure 32.7). At this time, the delivery sheath, ICE catheter, and ICE introducer sheath are removed, and manual compression is used without heparin reversal to achieve hemostasis. Patients are placed at bed rest for 5 or 6 hours and discharged later in the day or the following morning.

Special circumstances

The technique described above is applicable to the vast majority of CardioSEAL®/STARFlex® implantation procedures. However, there are occasions, primarily related to anatomic considerations, when the implantation procedure requires modification. These include patients with the following: irreducible and long PFO tunnel, inferior vena cava filter, lipomatous atrial septal hypertrophy, and presence of multiple defects.

As described above, the mere presence of a long segment of overlap between septa primum and secundum does not preclude transdefect implantation of an occluder device. On the other hand, when lengthy overlap co-exists with a relatively narrow outlet into the left atrium, the superior edge of the septum primum may not be displaceable to the level of the inferior edge of the septum secundum, preventing conversion of the relatively long pathway into a short transverse track across the atrial septum. This is best detected with balloon characterization ('sizing') of the defect, when at moderate inflation pressure the balloon has the appearance of a dog bone, with bulbous ends separated by a narrower waist exceeding about 8 mm (Figure 32.4). Deployment of the occluder via the defect in such a case carries the risk that one side of the device will open fully while the other side remains collapsed within this irreducible tunnel (Figure 32.6). If the device is released in this configuration, several undesirable consequences may ensue: the device may be more prone to embolize with a transient exaggeration of the transseptal pressure gradient (e.g., cough or sneeze); the occluder might be more thrombogenic; and either the entrance to or exit from the PFO channel will be uncovered. In order to prevent such outcomes, PFO closure is performed utilizing the transseptal puncture technique. The use of invasive echocardiography assists in localizing the level of the transseptal needle just below the superior limbus of the fossa ovalis. Once the transseptal sheath is advanced into the left atrium over the needle, it is removed over an exchange wire and replaced by the 10 Fr delivery sheath. There is no need to inflate the sizing balloon in this iatrogenic defect. On average, a 28 mm device is selected and is sufficiently large to straddle the septum secundum superiorly. The left atrial umbrella acts to appose the septum primum against the secundum while the right atrial umbrella covers the entrance into the PFO. If the level of puncture is too low, this device size might not provide adequate reach of the right atrial umbrella, and the septum secundum might escape the grasp of the device, resulting in effective closure of the iatrogenic defect but a still patent foramen. Care should be exercised in puncturing high enough or, on the other hand, recognizing a slightly lower puncture, a condition easily remedied by selecting a device with a longer reach, e.g., a 33 mm occluder.

In the patient with a previously implanted inferior vena cava filter, PFO closure from a femoral venous approach is still readily performed. Most filters have large enough fenestrations, particularly at their outer margins, to allow passage of both an intracardiac echocardiography catheter and a 10 Fr delivery sheath. However, although initial passage of the sizing balloon through the filter may be feasible, withdrawal of the balloon once it has been inflated and deflated could be hazardous. Therefore, it is necessary to pass the delivery sheath through the filter *before* advancing the balloon catheter and sizing the defect. In order to do this, the multipurpose angiographic catheter is passed through a peripheral filter fenestration under fluoroscopic guidance. An exchange wire is then placed through this catheter into the right atrium or superior vena cava, and the catheter and its introducer sheath are removed. The 10 Fr sheath is then passed over the wire and steered carefully, under

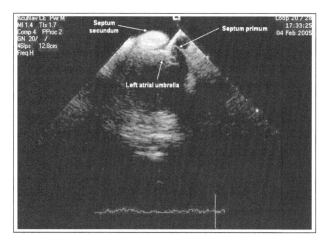

Figure 32.8
Partial device deployment in a patient with lipomatous atrial septal hypertrophy. Note that the septum secundum is unusually thickened (~12 mm). Upsizing to the next larger device size enables the superior arms of the CardioSEAL® to straddle this thickened septum.

fluoroscopy, through the filter to the level of the atrium. The multi-purpose catheter is then advanced via the sheath, through the PFO, and into the left atrium. Over an exchange wire, the balloon sizing catheter is advanced via the sheath into the defect, and defect characterization and sizing are performed. As with the conventional technique, the balloon is then deflated. At this time, the sheath can be advanced through the defect over the deflated balloon which is then withdrawn, along with the exchange wire, out of the sheath. In the alternative, the balloon catheter can be removed via the sheath while the sheath tip is still in the right atrium and replaced by the sheath's dilator to cross the defect. With either method, the balloon is withdrawn into the sheath above the level of the filter, protecting the filter from any interaction with the balloon. The occluder is then prepared, delivered, and deployed conventionally. After defect closure, the delivery catheter is removed. A straight-tipped wire is advanced though the sheath to the superior vena cava, the dilator is advanced fully into the sheath, and then the sheath, dilator, and wire are withdrawn under fluoroscopy back through the filter.

In the patient with lipomatous atrial septal hypertrophy, the septum secundum may be much thicker than normal, potentially exceeding 15 mm in thickness. This phenomenon is easily identifiable with invasive echocardiography (see Figure 32.8). The principal procedural implication of this finding is that the superior arms of the right atrial umbrella must cover a greater distance in order to sufficiently straddle the septum secundum. In order to ensure adequate reach, the next larger size of occluder should be selected. In all other respects, the closure technique is unchanged.

Finally, in the patient with a fenestrated septum primum co-existing with a PFO, initial passage of the multi-purpose catheter into the left atrium almost always occurs via a small fenestration rather than via the PFO itself. This can be suspected from several clues: the catheter (or the exchange wire placed through it) appears to pass through the body of the septum primum on invasive echocardiography rather than through the more superior PFO; color Doppler demonstrates a left-to-right shunt where the catheter or wire crosses the septum; or the stretched defect diameter is unusually small (<6 mm) (Figure 32.8). Such a crossing point is usually at least 10 mm distant from the PFO itself. In such a case, simply recrossing through the PFO and selecting an oversized occluder may not cover the co-existing defect. Therefore, a small (17 mm) occluder is deployed to cover the fenestration (and any small, immediately adjacent additional fenestrations). After release of the deployed occluder, the multi-purpose catheter is advanced through the sheath to the high right atrium, above the level of the initial device. The catheter is rotated counterclockwise to point posteriorly. Very carefully, and referring to both invasive echocardiography and fluoroscopy images, the catheter tip is repositioned to the PFO entrance using the 'back door' approach. Rather than advancing and rotating clockwise, as in the conventional method, the catheter is rotated counterclockwise and withdrawn so that it falls into the superior recess of the fossa ovalis behind and above the initially implanted occluder. It is then slowly advanced into and through the PFO, with care taken to avoid any interaction with the implanted device. Such interaction should prompt a fresh attempt to encounter the entrance to the PFO. The exchange wire is placed into a left pulmonary vein, and the balloon catheter can then be placed into the defect, again being careful not to disturb the first occluder. A low pressure, partial balloon inflation will partially distort the septum primum and, therefore, the small occluder, but this should be sufficient to determine the size of the occluder to be deployed via the PFO (Figure 32.9a and Figure 32.9b). The sheath is then advanced over the deflated balloon, again with the exercise of caution to avoid disturbing the implanted device. The left atrial umbrella is deployed conventionally, but a slightly increased retraction force against the left side of the PFO is exerted while withdrawing the sheath to release the right atrial umbrella. This extra force helps to ensure that the right atrial umbrella opens somewhat more distantly from the right side of the initial device. Once it opens, this tension is released, and the larger umbrella of the second device overlaps part of the umbrella of the initial one (Figure 32.9c and Figure 32.9d). The occluder is then released and the sheath is removed. To summarize, the two major procedure modifications in this scenario are the care in avoiding disturbing the first implant and the 'back door' approach to the PFO after the first occluder is implanted.

Complications

As with most complications that may occur during interventional cardiovascular procedures, the best way to deal with misadventures in the implantation of CardioSEAL® and STARFlex® is to avoid and prevent them. When performed with careful attention to the steps of the procedure where serious complications can occur, PFO closure with these devices can generally be accomplished in less than 25 minutes. The urge to perform the procedure as quickly as possible should not be satisfied at the expense of patient safety. Groin complications may result from arterial injury, premature ambulation, excessive anticoagulation, or combinations of these. Strict attention to anatomic landmarks and allowing for sufficient bedrest after sheath removal should prevent nearly all such complications. In advancing the ICE catheter and the angulated angiographic catheter to the right atrium, the azygous vein is frequently entered. Following the progress of these catheters fluoroscopically from the groin to the atrium will prevent inadvertent perforation of this frequently encountered vein.

Perhaps the most feared and serious complication of percutaneous PFO closure with any device is device embolization. Such an event is rare and preventable by careful attention to technique. First, when attaching the closure device to the delivery catheter, ensure firm securement by tugging on the device and also by confirming that the locking mechanism at the outside end of the delivery catheter is fully engaged. Secondly, the use of invasive echocardiography (ICE or TEE) ensures appropriate contact of the left atrial umbrella with the left side of the atrial septum and subsequent release of its opposing umbrella in the right atrium. Echocardiographic confirmation of appropriate apposition of the two sides of the device and the two sides of the atrial septum allows the safe detachment of the device without fear that it will float away. In the unlikely event that device embolism does occur, retrieval basket catheters should be readily available, and access to emergency cardiac surgery should be assured.

Invasive echocardiography enhances the safety and efficacy of percutaneous defect closure in other ways. The identification of thrombus within the PFO represents an absolute contraindication to crossing the defect. Rarely, thrombus can be seen to form on the transseptal catheter or sheath, and corrective measures need to be taken, e.g., aspiration while withdrawing the catheter/sheath back into the right atrium. When a fenestration or small atrial septal defect co-exists with a PFO, as mentioned earlier, an occluding device may be placed successfully in the septum, but it might not effectively treat the desired target of the intervention, namely, the PFO. Invasive echo enables identification of such co-existing defects and is essential in assuring successful treatment of all of them.

About 5% of patients undergoing PFO closure with CardioSEAL® or STARFlex® will develop atrial fibrillation

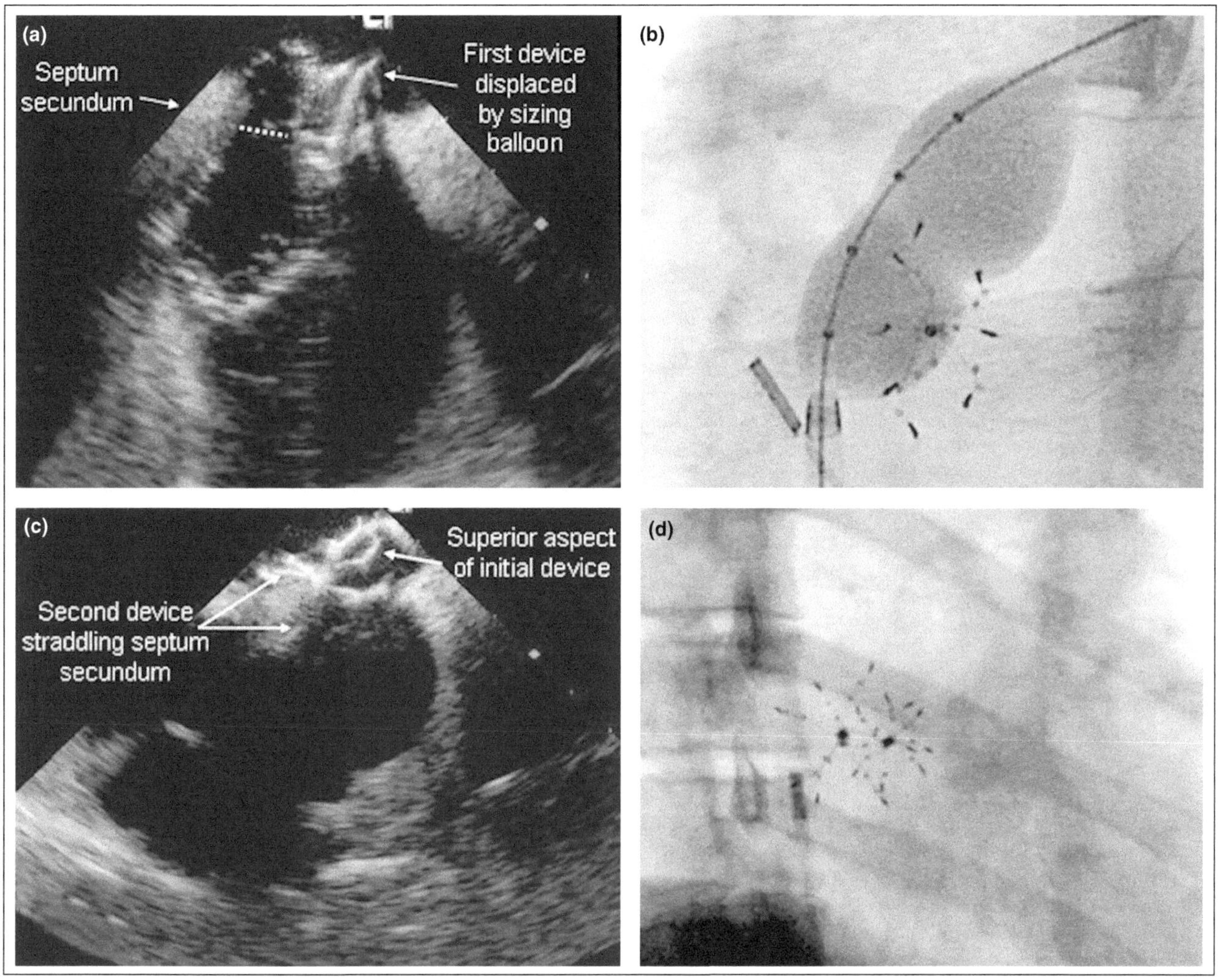

Figure 32.9
Deployment of second device in the true PFO. (a) Intracardiac echocardiographic image of the sizing balloon inflated within the PFO after deployment of the initial device in the fenestration. The device is mildly distorted by the balloon. The stretched diameter of the PFO is indicated by the dashed line. (b) Fluoroscopic image of the PFO sizing balloon inflation and mild distortion of the initial occluder. (c) Echo image of the second device deployed in the PFO, straddling the superior portion of the occluder in the fenestration inferiorly and the septum secundum superiorly. (d) Fluoroscopic image of the two deployed devices. The central connecting hubs are separated by about 9 mm.

within the first 2 months after the procedure. As with any occurrence of this arrhythmia, correcting it within the first 24–36 hours after onset is simple, whereas treatment beyond this time frame may necessitate 2 months of anticoagulation. Particular emphasis is placed upon patient education in this regard. Finally, device infection and thrombosis can occur. In order to minimize the risk of infection, the cath lab environment should be as sterile as possible. Hats and masks should be worn by all personnel in the procedure room before sterile packs are opened, and traffic into and out of the room should be minimized during the procedure. Implanting these devices should be regarded as similar to heart valve implantation. A prophylactic antibiotic should be administered, and patients should take appropriate prophylaxis for potentially bacteremic procedures performed in

the first 6 months after device placement. Finally, device thrombosis has been observed in some patients after PFO closure. The true incidence of this phenomenon is unknown. Patients should have effective antiplatelet therapy at the time of the implant procedure. This consists of aspirin initiated at least a few days and a thienopyridine at least 4 days before implantation and continued in combination for about 3 months afterwards. Protamine reversal of heparin anticoagulation should be avoided.

In summary, most of the complications discussed above are best managed by prevention rather than treatment after the fact. Scrupulous attention to proper technique and resisting the urge to 'cut corners' will avoid most serious complications and allow percutaneous closure of PFO to be a safe, effective, and highly gratifying procedure.

Suggested reading

1. Sacco RL, Ellenberg JH, Mohr JP et al. Infarcts of undetermined cause: the NINCDS Stroke Data Bank. Ann Neurol 1989; 25: 382–90.

2. Sherman DG. Prevention of cardioembolic stroke. In: Norris JW, Hachinski VC, eds. Prevention of Stroke. New York: Springer Verlag, 1991: 149–59.

3. Lechat P, Mas J-L, Lacault G et al. Prevalence of patent foramen ovale in patients with stroke. N Engl J Med 1988; 318: 1148–52.

4. Webster MW, Chacellor AM, Smith HJ et al. Patent foramen ovale in young stroke patients. Lancet 1988; 2: 11–12.

5. Hagen PT, Scholz DG, Edwards WD. Incidence and size of patent foramen ovale during the first 10 decades of life: an autopsy study of 965 normal hearts. Mayo Clin Proc 1984; 59: 17–20.

6. DeCastro S, Cartoni D, Fiorelli M et al. Morphological and functional characteristics of patent foramen ovale and their embolic implications. Stroke 2000; 31: 2407–13.

7. Overell JR, Bone I, Lees KR. Interatrial septal abnormalities and stroke. A meta-analysis of case-control studies. Neurology 2000; 55: 1172–9.

8. Mas J-L, Arquizan C, Lamy C et al. Recurrent cerebrovascular events associated with patent foramen ovale, atrial septum aneurysm, or both. N Engl J Med 2001; 345: 1740–6.

9. Cabanes L, Mas J-L, Cohen A et al. Atrial septal aneurysm and patent foramen ovale as risk factors for cryptogenic stroke in patients less than 55 years of age. A study using transesophageal echocardiography. Stroke 1993; 24: 1865–73.

10. Johnson BI. Paradoxical embolism. J Clin Pathol 1951; 4: 316–32.

11. Mas J-L. Patent foramen ovale, stroke and paradoxical embolism. Cerebrovasc Dis 1991; 1: 181–3.

12. Bogousslavsky J, Garazi S, Jeanrenaud X et al. Stroke recurrence in patients with patent foramen ovale. The Lausanne study. Neurology 1996; 46: 1301–5.

13. Homma S, DiTullio MR, Sacco RL et al. Characteristics of patent foramen ovale associated with cryptogenic stroke. A biplane transesophageal echocardiographic study. Stroke 1994; 25: 582–6.

14. Hausman D, Mugge A, Daniel WG. Identification of patent foramen ovale permitting paradoxic embolism. J Am Coll Cardiol 1995; 26: 1030–8.

15. Schuchlenz HW, Weihs W, Horner S et al. The association between the diameter of a patent foramen ovale and the risk of embolic cerebrovascular events. Am J Med 2000; 109: 456–62.

16. Albert A, Mueller HR, Hetzel A. Optimized transcranial Doppler technique for the diagnosis of cardiac right-to-left shunts. J Neroimaging 1997; 7: 159–63.

17. Anzola GP, Renaldini E, Magoni M et al. Validation of transcranial Doppler sonography in the assessment of patent foramen ovale. Cerebrovasc Dis 1995; 5: 194–8.

18. Autore C, Cartoni D, Piccininno M. Multiplane transesophageal echocardiography and stroke. Am J Cardiol 1998; 82(12A): 79G–81G.

19. Belkin RN, Pollack BD, Ruggiero ML et al. Comparison of transesophageal and transthoracic echocardiography with contrast and color flow Doppler in the detection of patent foramen ovale. Am Heart J 1994; 128: 520–5.

20. Devuyst G, Despland PA, Bogousslavsky J et al. Complementarity of contrast transcranial Doppler and contrast transesophageal echocardiography for the detection of patent foramen ovale in stroke patients. Eur Neurol 1997; 38: 21–5.

21. DiTullio M, Sacco RL, Venketasubramanian N et al. Comparison of diagnostic techniques for the detection of a patent foramen ovale in stroke patients. Stroke 1993; 24: 1020–4.

22. Mas J-L, Zuber M. Recurrent cerebrovascular events in patients with patent foramen ovale, atrial septal aneurysm, or both and cryptogenic stroke or transient ischemic attack. Am Heart J 1995; 130: 1083–8.

23. Mohr JP, Thompson JLP, Lazar RM et al. A comparison of warfarin and aspirin for the prevention of recurrent ischemic stroke. N Engl J Med 2001; 345: 1444–51.

24. Homma S, Sacco RL, DiTullio MR et al. Effect of medical treatment in stroke patients with patent foramen ovale. Patent Foramen Ovale in Cryptogenic Stroke Study. Circulation 2002; 105: 2625–31.

25. Guffi M, Bogousslavsky J, Jeanrenaud X et al. Surgical prophylaxis of recurrent stroke in patients with patent foramen ovale: a pilot study. J Thorac Cardiovasc Surg 1996; 112: 260–63.

26. Devuyst G, Bogousslavsky J, Ruchat P et al. Prognosis after stroke followed by surgical closure of patent foramen ovale: a prospective follow-up study with brain MRI and simultaneous transesophageal and transcranial Doppler ultrasound. Neurology 1996; 47: 1162–6.

27. Dearani JA, Ugurlu BS, Danielson GK et al. Surgical patent foramen ovale closure for prevention of paradoxical embolism-related cerebrovascular ischemic events. Circulation 1999; 100(Suppl II): II-171–5.

28. Ruchat P, Bogousslavsky J, Hurni M et al. Systematic surgical closure of patent foramen ovale in selected patients with cerebrovascular events due to paradoxical embolism. Early results of a preliminary study. Eur J Cardiothorac Surg 1997; 11: 824–7.

29. Hung J, Landzberg MJ, Jenkins KJ et al. Closure of patent foramen ovale for paradoxical emboli: intermediate-term risk of recurrent neurological events following transcatheter device placement. J Am Coll Cardiol 2000; 35: 1311–16.

30. Windecker S, Wahl A, Chatterjee T et al. Percutaneous closure of patent foramen ovale in patients with paradoxical embolism. Long-term risk of recurrent thromboembolic events. Circulation 2000; 101: 893–8.

31. Martin F, Sanchez PL, Doherty E et al. Percutaneous transcatheter closure of patent foramen ovale in patients with paradoxical embolism. Circulation 2002; 106: 1121–6.

32. Sommer RJ, Kramer PH, Sorenson SG et al. Closure of patent foramen ovale with the CardioSEAL septal occluder: infrequent recurrent thrombotic neurologic events. Am J Cardiol 2002; 90(Suppl 6A): 136H.

33. Zanchetta M, Rigatelli G, Onorato E. Intracardiac echocardiography and transcranial Doppler ultrasound to guide closure of patent foramen ovale. J Invas Cardiol 2003; 15: 93–6.

34. Bartel T, Konorza T, Arjumand J et al. Intracardiac echocardiography is superior to conventional monitoring for guiding device closure of interatrial communications. Circulation 2003; 107: 795–7.

35. Sievert H, Ostermayer S, Billinger K et al. Transcatheter closure of patent foramen ovale for prevention of paradoxical embolism and recurrent embolic stroke with the CardioSEAL STARFlex occluder. Am J Cardiol 2002; 90(Suppl 6A): 38H.

36. Wilmshurst PT, Nightingale S, Walsh KP et al. Effect on migraine of closure of cardiac right-to-left shunts to prevent recurrence of decompression illness or stroke or for haemodynamic reasons. Lancet 2000; 356: 1648–51.

37. Milhaud D, Bogousslavsky J, van Mell G et al. Ischemic stroke and active migraine. Neurology 2001; 57: 1805–11.

38. Konstantinides S, Geibel A, Kasper W et al. Patent foramen ovale is an important predictor of adverse outcome in patients with major pulmonary embolism. Circulation 1998; 97: 1946–51.

39. Donti A, Giardini A, Formigari R et al. Treatment of recurrent stroke and pulmonary thromboembolism with percutaneous closure of a patent foramen ovale and placement of inferior vena cava filter. Cathet Cardiovasc Interven 2003; 58: 413–15.

40. Saary MJ, Gray GW. A review of the relationship between patent foramen ovale and type II decompression sickness. Aviat Space Environ Med 2001; 72: 1113–20.

41. Bove AA. Risk of decompression sickness with patent foramen ovale. Undersea Hyperb Med 1998; 25: 175–8.

42. Knauth M, Ries S, Pohimann S et al. Cohort study of multiple brain lesions in sport divers: role of a patent foramen ovale. BMJ 1997; 314(7082): 701–5.

33

Helex occluder for occlusion of patent foramen ovale

Yves Laurent Bayard and Horst Sievert

Device

Unlike other devices, the implant is made of a single spiral-shaped nitinol wire with an expanded polytetrafluoroethylene patch attached along its length (Figure 33.1). When the nitinol wire is advanced out of the control catheter, two disks of equal size are developed. The Helex wire frame has three eyelets acting as markers and providing good visibility and positioning of the device under fluoroscopy control (Figure 33.2). There is a circular marker between the two disks of the Helex device and outside the right and left disk, respectively. A locking mechanism connects the centers of the right and the left atrial disk and thereby stabilizes the position of the Helex occluder within the atrial septum. Currently, the device is available in sizes from 15 to 35 mm (disk diameter) in 5 mm increments.

The delivery system comprises the outer delivery catheter (9 Fr), the inner control catheter for deployment or withdrawal of the occluder, and the central mandrel, which is used for steering of the device and to deploy the central locking mechanism (Figure 33.3). As a safety feature, a retention cord is attached to the tip of the control catheter and is, after looping through the right atrial eyelet, redirected to the operator through a lumen in the control catheter. Traction on this cord after final device deployment results in unlocking of the integral locking mechanism, thereby allowing for complete removal of the occluder even at this stage of the procedure. The proximal part of the delivery system ends in a y-arm hub. The proximal end of the control catheter exits from the main port of the y-arm hub and is terminated by the red retrieval cord cap. The proximal end of the mandrel exits the side port of the y-arm hub and is terminated by a clear luer.

Procedure

We recommend transesophageal echocardiography (TEE) guidance for patent foramen ovale (PFO) closure. Conscious

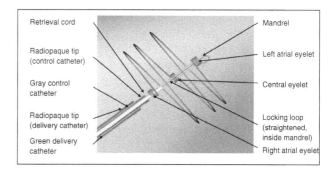

Figure 33.1
Helex septal occluder (*WL Gore & Associates, Flagstaff, AZ, USA*).

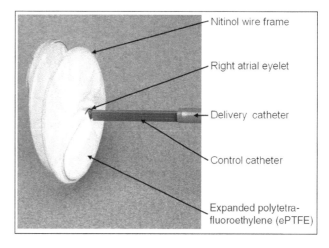

Figure 33.2
Helex septal occluder schematic.

sedation using weight-adapted propofol is initiated if the TEE probe is not tolerated well. Alternatively, intracardial echocardiography (ICE) may be used. After femoral vein access using a 9 Fr introducer sheath, 10 000 units of heparin are administered to keep the activated clotting time above 250 seconds. Before the Helex device is inserted, balloon sizing of the defect

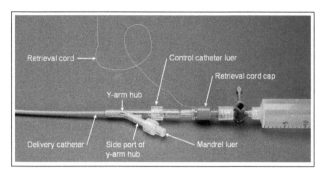

Figure 33.3
Helex septal occluder delivery system.

PFO diameter (mm)	Helex™ implant (mm)
5.0–9.0	15–20
9.5–12.5	20–25
13.0–15.5	25–35
16.0–18.5	30–35
19.0–22.0	35

Table 33.1   *Implant selection*

is performed. A stiff guidewire is advanced to the right atrium, through the PFO and into the left upper pulmonary vein. A sizing balloon (NuMED or AGA) is advanced into the left atrium and inflated with contrast dye. The pressure in the balloon should not exceed the pressure in the left atrium to avoid overstretching of the PFO. The sizing balloon is withdrawn into the PFO and the stretched diameter is measured by calibrated biplane fluoroscopy (LAO projection). When choosing the appropriate device size, the occluder-to-defect diameter ratio must be at least 1.6:1 (Table 33.1). TEE or ICE should be used to exclude thrombi and assess anatomic characteristics such as exact location of the PFO, thickness of the atrial septum, and presence of an atrial septal aneurysm (ASA).

After unpacking the Helex system, the occluder needs to be *loaded* into the green delivery catheter. This should be performed with the occluder and the distal portion of the delivery catheter submerged in heparinized saline solution. A 20 ml syringe with heparinized saline is attached to the red retrieval cord cap. After tightening of the mandrel luer and loosening of the control catheter luer, the control catheter can be flushed. When flushing is complete, the gray control catheter with the attached syringe is withdrawn until only 3 cm of the device are outside the delivery catheter. Doing so will cause the mandrel to bend slightly. At this time, the mandrel luer is loosened and the occluder is completely withdrawn into the delivery catheter by pulling the gray control catheter. The mandrel will exit the side port of the y-hub and protrude it a few centimeters. To avoid air embolism, it is important to keep the syringe with heparinized saline attached to the red retrieval cord cap at all times.

If desired, a 0.035 inch guidewire may be loaded through the guidewire port at the distal end of the delivery catheter to facilitate its transport into the left atrium. After loading of the delivery catheter into the 10 Fr introducer sheath, the syringe is removed from the red retrieval cord cap. It is important to ensure that this cap is securely attached to the control catheter as it locates the retrieval cord in position. The distal tip of the delivery catheter is equipped with a radio-opaque marker. Under fluoroscopy control and TEE guidance, it is advanced in the left atrium. If it was used, the guidewire is removed.

The left atrial disk is deployed by repeating the following steps. Fixing the delivery catheter, the gray control catheter is advanced in the left atrium until the tan mandrel luer stops against the side port of the y-hub. However, the tip of the control catheter must not touch the atrial wall. If space in the left atrium is inadequate, the control catheter should be advanced in smaller steps. Fixing the delivery and the control catheter, the mandrel is pulled back approximately 2 cm. Thus, the left atrial disk is gradually developed. The above steps are repeated until the central eyelet of the occluder exits the delivery catheter, indicating that the left atrial disk is completely deployed. To make sure it is apposed closely to the atrial septum, the tan mandrel may be slightly withdrawn.

To allow for the *right atrial disk deployment* and to bridge the PFO, the gray control catheter is fixed while the delivery catheter is pulled back gently until the mandrel luer touches the side port of the y-arm hub. The mandrel luer is tightened. The right atrial disk is now exposed by simply fixing the delivery catheter and advancing the control catheter until it stops at the y-arm hub, where the control catheter luer is then tightened.

The position and configuration of the disks should be controlled by both TEE and fluoroscopy. Both disks should be flat and close-fitting to the atrial septum, with atrial septal tissue in between them. If the position is not satisfactory at this point of the procedure, the Helex occluder may be repositioned before locking the device (see below). When the device appears well positioned, the red retrieval cord cap is removed and the mandrel luer is loosened. The locking mechanism is activated by sharply pulling the mandrel for at least 2 cm while fixing the delivery catheter in place. If the device position is not acceptable after this step, the occluder may be removed as it is still loosely attached to the control catheter via the retrieval cord (see below).

When a good device position has been achieved, the delivery system as a whole is removed from the patient. The retrieval cord will move through the control catheter hub and through the right atrial eyelet of the occluder, thereby releasing it completely.

Repositioning of the device is an option if the position is suboptimal. This is only possible prior to engaging the locking mechanism. If the occluder is already locked and its position is not acceptable, it has to be recaptured (see below). For repositioning, the red retrieval cord cap and the mandrel luer need to be tightened first. Gently pulling back the gray control catheter, the implant is completely withdrawn into the delivery catheter as it was during the initial loading procedure (see above). The delivery catheter is then repositioned within the left atrium and the device is redeployed following the above mentioned steps. If increased force is necessary during repositioning, parts of the Helex system may be damaged or kinked. In this case, we recommend completely removing the Helex system and using a new device.

Recapture of the occluder may be necessary if its position is not acceptable after lock release or if repositioning is not possible without applying increased force. The mandrel luer needs to be open. With the red retrieval cord cap removed, the retrieval cord is gently withdrawn until the control catheter meets the right atrial eyelet of the device. Now the retrieval cord cap is firmly attached and the control catheter is withdrawn, causing the device to return into the delivery catheter in its linear form. This step should be performed with caution to avoid interference of the device eyelets with the tip of the delivery sheath, which may lead to frame fracture of the occluder or ripping of the retrieval cord. If complete withdrawal of the device into the delivery catheter would require excessive force, the control catheter and the delivery catheter may be withdrawn together with parts of the device remaining out of the delivery catheter. In this case, it might be necessary to remove the whole system together with the introducer sheath. We recommend not to re-use a recaptured device.

Follow-up and medication

After PFO closure, patients are administered clopidogrel 75 mg and acetylsalicylic acid 300 mg for 6 months, respectively. Endocarditis prophylaxis is recommended for 6 months. To ensure that no thrombi form on the occluder, TEE controls should be performed 1 and 6 months post-procedure.

Complications and management

If access to the left atrium via the PFO cannot be gained, *transseptal puncture* using standard techniques can be performed. In the case of an *embolization* or malposition of the occluder after the retrieval cord has been removed, the device can be snared at any point of its frame using a loop snare. A long sheath of at least 10 Fr should be positioned nearby the occluder, allowing for complete retraction of the device. If parts of the device remain outside the long sheath, the device, snare, and sheath have to be removed as a whole. In a low percentage of patients treated with the Helex device, a wire *frame fracture* has been observed. Frame fractures usually do not require any action as they do not affect the function of the device.

Thrombus formation during follow-up is a rare complication when using the Helex device. We recommend administering clopidogrel 75 mg and acetylsalicylic acid 300 mg or low molecular weight heparin, respectively, until the thrombus has resolved. TEE controls should be performed at monthly intervals.

34

Patent foramen ovale – Premere™ PFO Closure System

Franziska Buescheck and Horst Sievert

Introduction

Percutaneous patent foramen ovale (PFO) closure has been successfully performed for many years with a low complication and recurrence rate using different devices. Many of these devices were adaptations from devices designed to close atrial septal defects (ASDs). The right and left anchor arms are rigidly connected to each other at a fixed distance. The devices also tend to be larger. Unlike an ASD, which is a hole in the interatrial septum, a PFO has a variable length tunnel that can vary from 2 mm to several millimeters. The openings of the right and left PFO can also be offset from each other. Therefore the current devices with the rigid fixed distance between the right and left anchor arms may distort the septal anatomy and, in some instances, may even cause the PFO to remain open the whole time.

Despite these drawbacks, transcatheter closure of PFO with these devices has been repeatedly shown to greatly reduce the risk of recurrent stroke from as high as 56% before closure to about 4% after closure.[1–3] Transcatheter closure of PFO with these devices has now become a standard of care for patients suffering from cryptogenic stroke.

Premere PFO Closure System

The Premere™ PFO Closure System (St Jude Medical, Maple Grove, Minnesota, USA) is a percutaneous, transcatheter, self-expanding dual-anchor arm occlusion device that is 20 or 25 mm in diameter. The anchors are made of nickel–titanium alloy (nitinol). Only the right anchor is enveloped between two layers of knitted polyester fabric. The arms are designed with a low profile and a low surface area to minimize exposure to thrombogenic surfaces and to assist in rapid endothelialization. A flexible polyester braided tether runs through the center of the anchor and holds the two anchors together. The anchors are locked together after delivery and then the tether is cut. The distance between

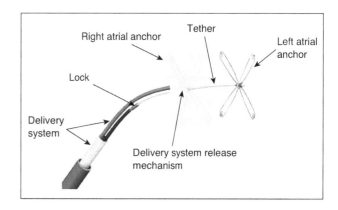

Figure 34.1
Isometric view of the implant assembly of the Premere™ Closure System.

the two anchors is variable, depending on the length of the PFO track. The schematic of the implant portion of the PFO closure device with the delivery system is depicted in Figure 34.1.

The first Premere PFO occluder was implanted on 24 November 2003 (by Prof H Sievert, Frankfurt). Since then, PFO closure using this device has been performed in over 100 patients successfully.

Device details

The Premere™ PFO Closure System consists of the implant assembly, a white delivery system (Figure 34.2a) and the cutter (Figure 34.2b). The implant assembly is supplied pre-loaded in the loading tube attached to the distal end of the delivery system.

Left atrium anchor (LAA)

Each LAA consists of four radiating arms, as shown in Figure 34.2c. A radio-opaque outer marker rivet is placed at

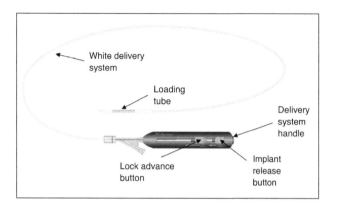

Figure 34.2a
Premere™ delivery system.

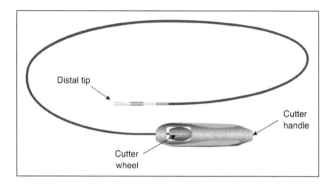

Figure 34.2b
Cutter.

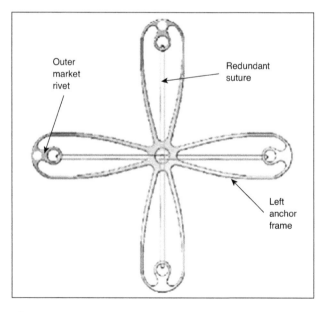

Figure 34.2c
Left anchor arm frame.

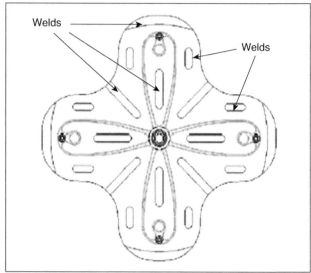

Figure 34.2d
Right anchor arm.

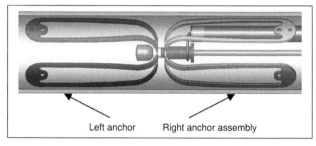

Figure 34.2e
Implant assembly in the pre-loaded state.

Right atrium anchor (RAA)

The RAA is identical to the LAA except for the right side hub marker, which is longer and has a flange to allow for retrieval if needed. In addition the nitinol anchor is enclosed within the right side covering like a sealed pouch (Figure 34.2d). The polyester material is a PET material commonly used in vascular prosthesis. The RAA rides freely on the tether in both directions for ease of advancement and retrieval.

Implant assembly

The implant assembly consists of the RAA and the LAA, flexibly fixed together by the tether. The two anchors are kept together by a mechanism that locks onto the tether on the proximal side of the RAA. The implant assembly is the only component that is a permanent implant. The implant assembly is shipped pre-loaded into the loading tube and assembled together with the delivery catheter system. A cross-section of the complete implant assembly is shown in Figure 34.2e.

the ends of each arm. At the center of the anchor is a radio-opaque left side hub which is permanently fixed to the left anchor and the tether.

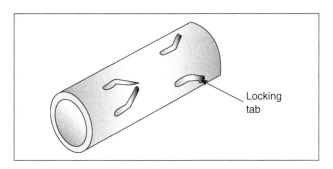

Figure 34.2f
Tether lock showing the position of the locking tab.

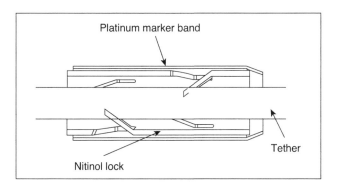

Figure 34.2g
Cross-section of tether lock (formed locking tabs).

Tether

The tether is a braided white polyester (PET) suture-like material. The tether termination engages with the left side hub marker of the LAA. Near the proximal end of the tether there is a marker to denote the position to move the tether retention clip to after deployment of the LAA. On the proximal side of the RAA the tether is trimmed after the anchors and lock placement.

Tether lock

The tether lock is made up of nitinol tubing with six tabs that protrude into the tube. The six tabs are placed on two circumferential planes with three tabs per plane. The planes are offset from each other, as shown in Figure 34.2f. The tether runs through the center of the lock and the tabs are designed to dig into the tether in one direction only (Figure 34.2g). The lock can be advanced distally but the tabs prevent it from moving proximally. For visibility the tether lock is encased within the lock marker. It is made of a platinum–iridium alloy that makes the tether lock visible under fluoroscopy.

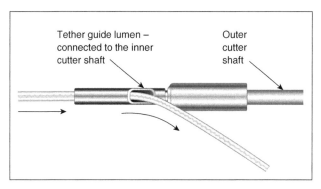

Figure 34.2h
Tether cutter distal end.

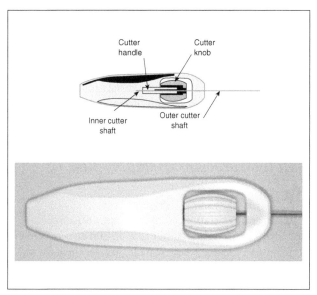

Figure 34.2i
Tether cutter hub (proximal).

Tether cutter system

The tether cutter system is advanced over the tether through the tether guide lumen after the delivery catheter system is removed. The tether cutter system is made up of an inner cutter shaft and an outer cutter shaft connected at the proximal cutter hub. The tether guide lumen is made with a cut-out window for the tether to exit and is connected to the inner cutter shaft (Figure 34.2h). To advance the outer cutter shaft, the outer cutter hub (Figure 34.2i) is rotated clockwise. As the outer cutter shaft advances forward it rotates and cuts the tether as the latter is pushed against the wall of the tether guide lumen.

Guide catheter

The guide catheter is supplied separately from the other systems. Two distal curve shapes are available to better accommodate the different anatomies of the patients. The two curves of the guide catheter are:

- 25° radius of curvature
- 45° radius of curvature.

Except for the radius of curvature of the distal tip the two guide catheters are identical. Each guide catheter consists of an obturator which is a proximal hub with a standard side arm for flushing. The schematic of the guide catheter is shown in Figure 34.2j.

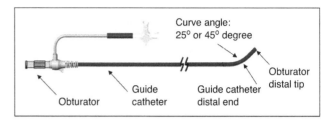

Figure 34.2j
Guide catheter and obturator.

System preparation

Fill a 20 ml syringe with heparinized saline and attach the syringe to the luer fitting on the blue Premere™ delivery sheath. Evacuate air from the delivery sheath by forcing saline from the syringe into the delivery sheath. Continue until you observe saline dripping from the distal tip. Repeat step 2 for the dilator/obturator and the Premere™ delivery system. Afterwards the Premere™ PFO Closure System is ready to use.

Implant procedure: step by step

Step 1

During the procedure administer an anticoagulant (i.e. heparin) in sufficient quantity to maintain an activated clotting time (ACT) ≥ 250 seconds. Alternatively heparin may be administered at about 100 U/kg in lieu of measuring the ACT. Prophylactic antibiotic treatment, i.e. administration of an intravenous first generation cephalosporin, is required before and after the procedure.

- Access the vascular system, place the 11 Fr introducer sheath, and load the dilator/obturator into the blue Premere delivery sheath.
- Advance the blue delivery sheath and dilator/obturator along the guidewire into the right atrium, through the PFO, and into the left atrium. *Do not advance the dilator/obturator and delivery sheath in the absence of a guidewire.*
- Remove the guidewire and ensure that the tip of the delivery sheath is in the mid-left atrium and is neither obstructed nor in contact with tissue.
- Keep the dilator/obturator hub below atrial level and ensure that blood is flowing freely out of the hub. Slowly remove the dilator/obturator as you maintain a constant column of blood out of the proximal end of the dilator/obturator.
- Open the stopcock on the delivery sheath and allow blood to flow out. Gently tap on the hub of the delivery sheath to remove any trapped air into the hub so that the air exits through the stopcock.

- Flush the delivery sheath with heparizined saline and then close the stopcock.
- Fill a 20 ml syringe with heparinized saline. Attach the syringe to the luer fitting on the white Premere™ PFO Closure System.
- While taking care to keep the loading tube in a generally horizontal orientation maintain pressure on the 20 ml syringe. Observe saline exiting the distal end of the loading tube.
- While maintaining pressure on the syringe advance the loading tube into the hub until its shoulder fits correctly against the hub of the delivery sheath (Figure 34.3).
- Transfer the implant assembly into the delivery sheath by slowly advancing the Premere™ PFO Closure System at least 5 cm into the delivery sheath. Withdraw the loading tube from the delivery sheath until it is adjacent to the proximal hub of the white delivery catheter of the delivery system. Remove the 20 ml syringe from the Premere™ PFO Closure System and verify the position of the delivery sheath in the mid-left atrium.
- Under fluoroscopic guidance advance the Premere™ implant through the blue delivery sheath until the implant is near the distal tip of the delivery sheath.
- Deploy the left atrial anchor by slowly advancing the white delivery system until the radio-opaque markers on the tips of the left atrial anchor arms expand and move away from each other (Figures 34.4 and 34.5).

It is critical to ensure that the right anchor does not exit the blue delivery sheath as you advance the left anchor. If the right atrial anchor is inadvertently deployed see the 'Retrieval' section.

Step 2

- Once the left anchor is deployed place your right hand on the mark located on the tether of the Premere™ PFO Closure System. The tether is used to maintain the tactile feel of the septum and to direct device placement.
- Apply slight tension to the tether to maintain the orientation of the left atrial anchor perpendicular to the end of the delivery sheath. Slowly retract both the delivery sheath and tether until you have seated the left anchor securely against the septal wall.

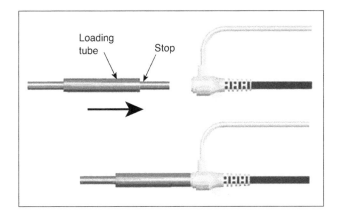

Figure 34.3a
Loading the Premere™ into the guide catheter.

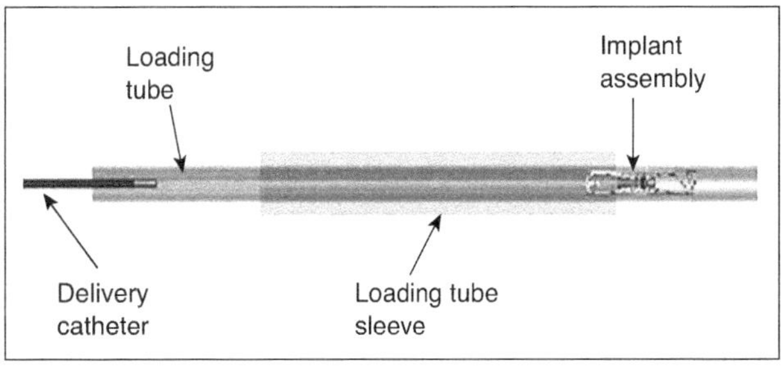

Figure 34.3b
Loading tube with the implant assembly.

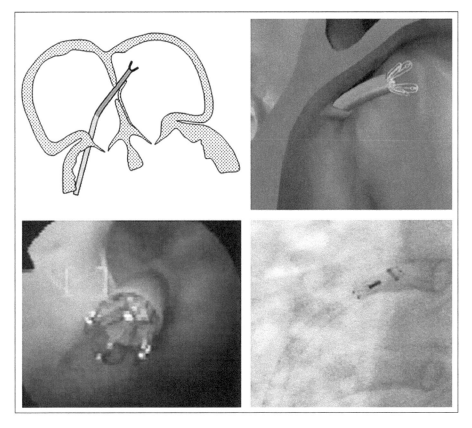

Figure 34.4
The outer delivery catheter pushes the LAA into the left atrium.

- Lightly ground the tether with your right hand.
- With your left hand continue to retract the blue delivery sheath into the mid-right atrium. As you retract the delivery sheath the white delivery system will slide back over the fixed tether (Figures 34.6 and 34.7).

Step 3

- Verify on fluoroscopy the position of the delivery sheath in the right atrium. While maintaining slight tension on the tether slowly advance the right atrial anchor out of the blue delivery sheath by advancing the white delivery system. Continue to advance the right anchor until it is seated against the septal wall of the right atrium.
- If necessary you can reposition the right anchor by retracting the white delivery system and then re-advancing it. Use tension on the tether to direct the right atrial anchor into the desired location (Figures 34.8 and 34.9).

Care should be taken to ensure that the right atrial anchor is not advanced into the PFO track. Ensure that the anchor arms are not constrained or prolapsed into the PFO tunnel. See Figure 34.10 for illustrations of incorrect placement.

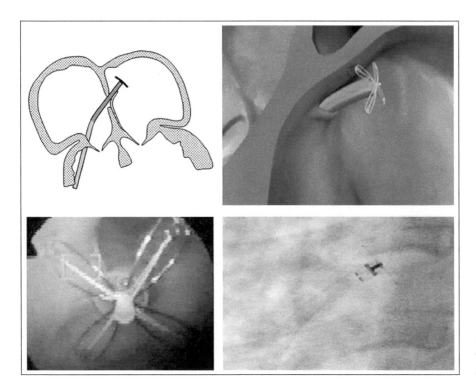

Figue 34.5
The LAA is released from the guide catheter and regains its preset shape.

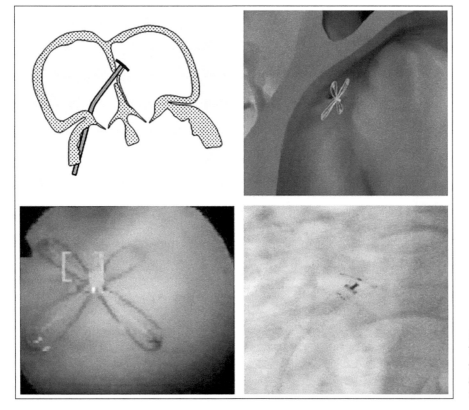

Figure 34.6
The guide catheter with the LAA in slight tension is withdrawn and the arms of the LAA draw the PFO flap towards the atrial septum.

Step 4

Loosen the Touhy–Borst on the Premere™ delivery system (Figure 34.11). Maintain tension on the tether and advance the inner delivery catheter. This movement will advance the lock mechanism. This procedure should be done under fluoroscopic guidance. Continue advancing the lock mechanism until the radio-opaque marker on the lock mechanism is adjacent to the radio-opaque marker on the right side anchor (Figure 34.12).

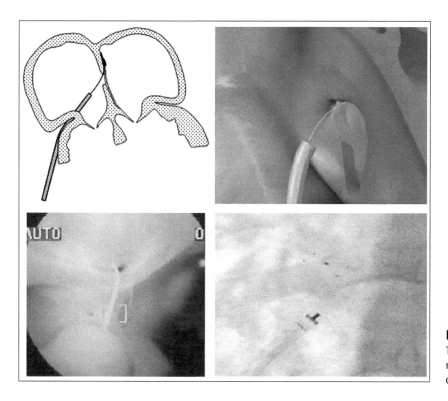

Figure 34.7
The guide catheter is withdrawn into the right atrium, and the LAA holds the PFO flap close against the atrial septum.

Step 5

Retract the Premere™ delivery system just into the tip of the guide catheter. Pull on the tether to ensure that the implant is securely in place. This should be observed under fluoroscopy at a minimum. Depress and hold the tether retention clip button and slide it proximally off the tether. Slide the delivery system proximally off the tether. Introduce the proximal end of the tether into the distal end of the cutter (Figure 34.13a). Advance the tether until it exits the cutter (Figure 34.13b). Slight rotation of the tether may be required to advance it through the proximal opening of the cutter. Maintain tension on the tether and advance the cutter into the proximal end of the guide catheter. While maintaining tension on the tether advance the cutter until the radio-opaque marker on the cutter is adjacent to the radio-opaque marker on the lock mechanism. This should be observed under fluoroscopy at a minimum.

While maintaining tension on the tether rotate the cutter wheel clockwise (typically four turns, see Figure 34.14) until the tether has been cut. This will be observed by a change in tension on the tether and typically by a change in position of the radio-opaque marker of the cutter relative to the radio-opaque marker on the lock mechanism. Rotate the cutter wheel counterclockwise to its original position and then remove the cutter and the cut tether together out of the guide catheter.

It is recommended that a right atriogram at a minimum of three orthogonal angles be performed to document the position of the implant relative to the atrial anatomy. Remove the Premere™ guide catheter (Figures 34.15–34.17).

System retrieval

In the event that the implant needs to be removed (prior to advancing the lock) the following steps should be followed. The removal process is dependent on how many steps have been performed in the procedure.

Prior to withdrawing the guide from left atrium to right atrium:

1. Align the guide catheter co-axially with the left atrial anchor and pull on the tether. The left anchor will prolapse into the distal end of the guide catheter. Pull until the radio-opaque markers on the left atrial anchor are clearly proximal of the radio-opaque marker on the guide catheter.
2. Re-insert the implant loading tube (located on the delivery system near the proximal hub) into the hemostasis valve on the hub of the Premere™ guide catheter.
3. Care should be taken to ensure that the tip of the guide catheter is unobstructed and not in contact with tissue. Slowly remove the Premere™ system from the guide catheter.

Prior to advancing the lock:

1. Remove the tether retention clip from the proximal end of the tether.
2. Unscrew the y-adapter (Figure 34.18), releasing the inner delivery catheter from the outer delivery catheter.
3. Slide the inner delivery catheter off the tether and out of the outer delivery catheter.

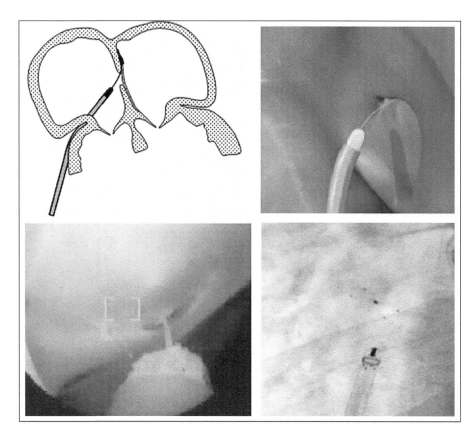

Figure 34.8
The delivery catheter system pushes the RAA out of the guide catheter into the right atrium.

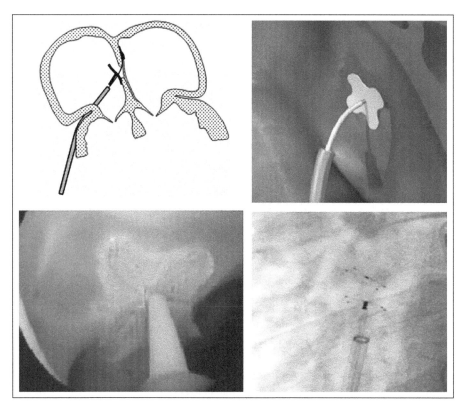

Figure 34.9
The delivery catheter system pushes the RAA against the septum secundum of the right atrium.

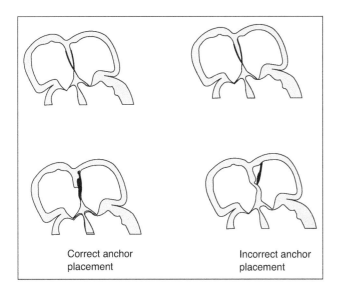

Figure 34.10
Illustration for correct and incorrect placement.

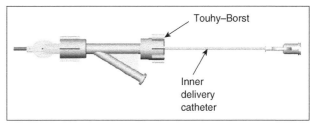

Figure 34.11
Proximal end of the delivery catheter system.

4. Load a 10 mm diameter snare (e.g. from ev3/Microvena or equivalent) over the hub and loading tube at the proximal end of the outer delivery catheter (Figure 34.19).

5. Advance the snare through the hemostasis valve on the guide catheter and down to the distal end of the delivery system.

6. Ensure that the distal end of the delivery system is in intimate contact with the hub of the right atrial anchor. The radio-opaque marker on the hub of the right atrial anchor should be adjacent to the radio-opaque shaft of the delivery system.

7. While maintaining the position of the right atrial anchor and the delivery system advance the snare onto the hub of the right atrial anchor. The radio-opaque wire of the snare should be clearly visible over the radio-opaque hub of the right atrial anchor.

8. Follow the instructions for use provided by the snare manufacturer and actuate the snare mechanism until it is very firmly down on the hub of the right atrial anchor.

9. Align the guide catheter coaxially with the right atrial anchor and withdraw the snare and delivery system. The right anchor will prolapse into the distal end of the guide catheter. Pull until the radio-opaque markers on the right atrial anchor are clearly proximal of the radio-opaque marker on the guide catheter.

10. Advance the guide catheter back through the PFO track. Maintain tension on the tether while advancing the guide.

11. Align the guide catheter coaxially with the left atrial anchor and pull on the tether. The left anchor will prolapse into the distal end of the guide catheter. Pull until the radio-opaque markers on the left atrial anchor are

clearly proximal of the radio-opaque marker on the guide catheter.

12. Re-insert the implant loading tube (located on the delivery system near the proximal hub) into the hemostasis valve in the hub of the guide catheter.

13. Care should be taken to ensure that the tip of the guide catheter is unobstructed and not in contact with tissue. Slowly remove the Premere™ system from the guide catheter.

Premere retrieval basket

The Premere™ retrieval basket is a percutaneous, transcatheter, self-expanding, retrieval device. The retrieval basket consists of a funnel-shaped mesh of braided, nitinol wire that is mechanically crimped to a stainless steel shaft. The shaft is long enough to allow the basket to be advanced out of the distal tip of the delivery sheath.

Indications for use

The retrieval basket is indicated for use in extracting a Premere™ PFO Closure System implant that has been deployed incorrectly into the right or left atrium of the heart. The retrieval basket is only required in the event that both the right and left atrial anchors have been inadvertently placed in the same atrium.

Procedure

• Prior to use attach a 20 ml syringe filled with heparinized saline solution to the luer fitting on the carrier tube. Flush the carrier tube and the retrieval basket until all of the air is evacuated out of the loading tube.

• To use the retrieval basket the Premere™ PFO Closure System delivery catheter must be removed and the tether must not have been cut. Insert the tether into the eye of the tether threading tool (Figure 34.20).

• Holding the free end of the tether, retract the tether threading tool through the retrieval basket and loading tube (Figure 34.21) until the tether threading tool and tether

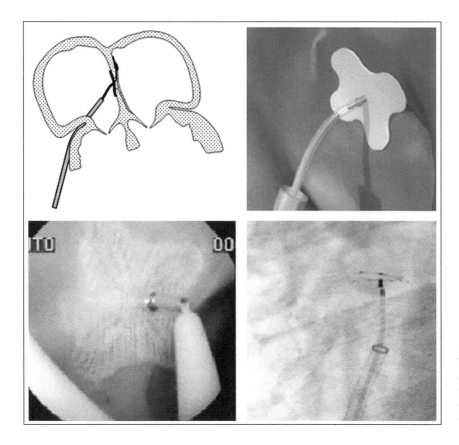

Figure 34.12
The distance between the RAA and LAA is adjusted until flush with the septum. The tether lock is advanced over the tether with the inner delivery catheter to lock the position of the LAA and RAA.

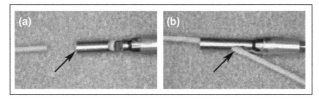

Figure 34.13
Introduce the proximal end of the tether into the distal end of the cutter (a). Advance the tether until it exits the cutter (b).

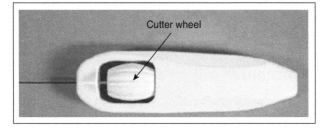

Cutter wheel

Figure 34.14
Cutter wheel.

exit the opposite side of the loading tube. Release the tether and remove and discard the tether threading tool.

- Apply tension to the proximal end of the tether and insert the loading tube into the delivery sheath. Allow adequate time for blood to completely fill the loading tube.

- Advance the retrieval basket into the delivery sheath and slide the loading tube out of the delivery sheath.
- Advance the retrieval basket to the distal tip of the delivery sheath such that the funnel extends beyond the tip of the delivery sheath and expands into the atrium (Figure 34.22).
- *The retrieval basket should be observed with fluoroscopy and ultrasound when advancing to the desired location.*
- Pull the implant assembly into the basket with the tether until it is completely seated at the bottom of the funnel-shaped basket (Figure 34.22).
- Pull both the tether and shaft of the basket together until the implant is withdrawn into the delivery sheath and completely removed.

Summary

1. Venous access is typically established via the femoral vein.
2. Based on the patient's anatomy, select the best Premere™ guide catheter curvature for crossing the PFO. If the chosen guide catheter shape is not optimal remove the guide catheter and use one with a different curvature.
3. Probe the PFO with a multi-purpose catheter and standard exchange wire or the Premere™ guide catheter.
4. Perform balloon sizing of the PFO. Document this with cine in the LAO cranial view.

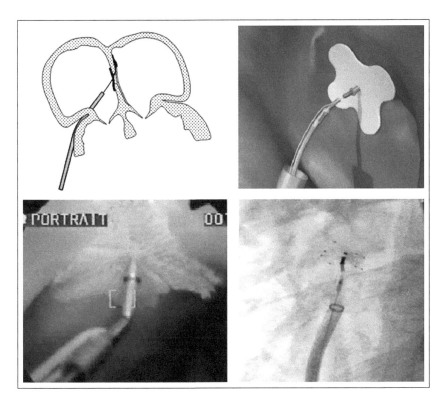

Figure 34.15
The delivery catheter system is withdrawn from the guide catheter and the tether cutter system guided to the implant site by the tether.

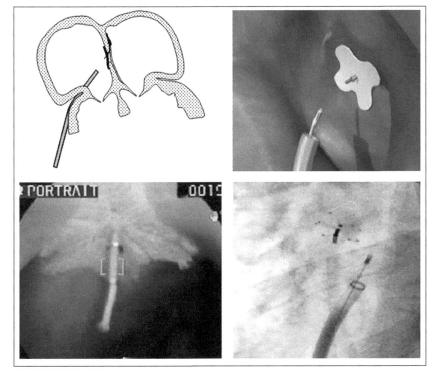

Figure 34.16
The tether is cut by the tether cutter system.

5. Guide the device by fluoroscopy and echocardiography (transesophageal echo (TEE) or intracardiac echo (ICE)) during the implantation.

6. After the guiding catheter is successfully passed into the left atrium load the Premere™ PFO Closure System and advance it to the distal tip of the guide catheter. Document proper guide placement in the left atrium and deploy the left anchor. Apply tension to the tether to verify desired seating of the left anchor to the septal tissue of the left atrium.

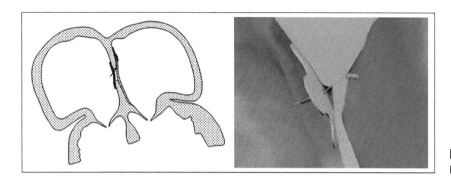

Figure 34.17
PFO closed by the implant assembly.

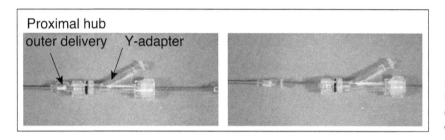

Figure 34.18
Unscrew the y-adapter releasing the inner delivery catheter from the outer delivery catheter.

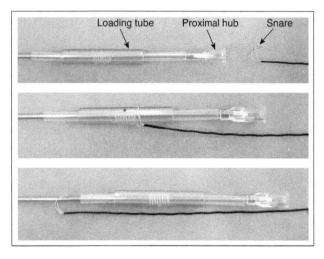

Figure 34.19
A snare is loaded over the hub and the loading tube at the proximal end of the outer delivery catheter.

7. Retract the guide catheter to the right atrium and deploy the right anchor.
8. Proceed to the next step if device placement is satisfactory. If the device placement is not satisfactory and cannot be adjusted with the Premere™ PFO Closure System retrieve the right anchor into the guide catheter with a snare and reposition it. Repeat this step until a satisfactory position is obtained.
9. Advance the lock to permanently secure the right and left anchor together. Cut the tether with the tether cutter under fluoroscopy.

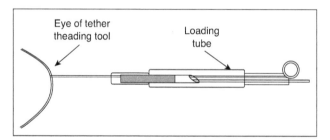

Figure 34.20
Theading tether.

10. After the device implantation is completed perform a bubble study to check for PFO closure.
11. Perform and record a right atriogram at a minimum of three orthogonal angles to document device deployment and position. Optimally silhouette the interarterial septum. TEE or ICE visualization may be taken at the physician's discretion throughout the procedure.
12. Following device deployment finally remove the Premere™ guiding catheter.

Management after implant procedure

After intervention patients are administered an endocarditis prophylaxis (e.g. cefuroxim, 1.5 g iv). Acetylsalicylic acid (100 mg pd po) and clopidogrel (75 mg pd po) are prescribed for 6 months after implantation because PFO

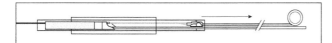

Figure 34.21
Loading tether.

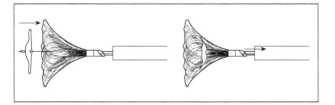

Figure 34.22
Pulling the implant into the retrieval basket.

patients obviously have a higher risk of thrombus formation. An endocarditis prophylaxis is recommended for 6 months as well. Patients were seen for follow-up visits at 2 weeks, 3 months, and 6 months post-implant. A transesophageal echo including a bubble study was required at the 2 week and 6 month follow-ups.

The Close-up trial was conducted to determine the safety of placement and effectiveness of the Premere™ device in closure of patent foramen ovale. It showed that the Premere™ device was safely implanted in all cases and provided complete closure of the PFO in 87% of the cases at 6 months. Closure rate was clearly related to the device size. The 20 mm device had a better closure rate than the 15 mm device that was only available initially. There were no serious device-related adverse events either during device implantation or during follow-up. One patient had two episodes of atrial fibrillation which had resolved by 4 months post-implant. One patient reported transient left arm weakness. He did not seek medical attention at the time, and no work-up was able to be done. This patient had no evidence of device thrombus at any evaluation and the PFO was found to be closed on echo/bubble study.

Braun et al[4] reported their results in 307 consecutive patients with symptomatic PFO using three different devices: the PFO-Star, Amplatzer PFO Occluder, and the CardioSEAL/STARFlex). They were able to implant the chosen device successfully in every case and reported peri-interventional complications in nine patients.

In a study of 66 patients Bruch et al[5] were able to successfully implant a PFO closure device in every intended patient with no complications during the procedure.

These data as well as the data from the Close-up trial indicate that closure of PFO can be successfully and safely completed.

In a study of 1000 consecutive patients Krumdorf et al[6] reported thrombus formation in 5/407 ASD patients and in 15 of 593 PFO patients at 4 weeks and 6 months after implantation. In a recent case report, Ruge et al[7] recorded a left atrial thrombus on a STARFlex device 3 years after implantation.

In the Close-Up study where transesophageal echocardiograms were performed that included a detailed examination of the left atrial anchor for evidence of thrombus no patients were found to have device-related thrombus at any time.

These data demonstrate that the Premere™ device can safely and effectively close PFO. Further studies should be undertaken to demonstrate the effectiveness of PFO closure with the Premere™ in reducing the incidence of thromboembolic events such as cryptogenic stroke.

References

1. Sievert H, Trepels T, Zadan E et al. Catheter closure of PFO for prevention of recurrent embolic stroke and TIA: acute results and follow-up in 400 patients. Am J Cardiol 2001; 88(Suppl 5A).

2. Sievert H, Ostermayer S, Billinger K et al. Transcatheter closure of PFO for prevention of paradoxical embolism and recurrent embolic stroke with the CardioSeal STARFlex occluder. Am J Cardiol 2002; 90(Suppl 6A).

3. Sommer RJ, Kramer PH, Sorensen SG et al. Closure of PFO with CardioSeal Septal Occluder: highly effective intervention. Am J Cardiol 2002; 90(Suppl 6A).

4. Braun M, Gliech V, Boscheri A et al. Transcatheter closure of patent foramen ovale (PFO) in patients with paradoxical embolism. Eur Heart J 2004; 25: 424–30.

5. Bruch L, Parsi A, Grad MO et al. Transcatheter closure of interatrial communications for secondary prevention of paradoxical embolism. Circulation 2002; 105: 2845–8.

6. Krumsdorf U, Ostermayer S, Billinger K et al. Incidence and clinical course of thrombus formation on atrial septal defect and patent foramen ovale closure devices in 1000 consecutive patients. J Am Coll Cardiol 2004; 43: 302–9.

7. Ruge H, Wildhirt SM, Libera P et al. Left atrial thrombus on atrial septal defect closure device as a source of cerebral emboli 3 years after implantation. Circulation 2005; 112: e130–1.

35

Closure of muscular VSD using the Amplatzer muscular VSD occluder

Yun-Ching Fu, Qi-Ling Cao, and Ziyad M Hijazi

Introduction

Ventricular septal defect (VSD) is the most common (approximately 20%) congenital heart disease.[1] About 10–15% of these defects are muscular VSDs located entirely within the muscular portion of the septum. The most common location is the apex, followed by the mid and anterior septum. Occasionally the defects are multiple ('Swiss cheese' VSDs). Acquired muscular VSDs are very rare and may result from postmyocardial infarction or traumatic injury to the chest.[1] Because muscular VSDs are frequently hidden within the coarse right ventricular (RV) trabeculations, they are difficult to localize through the standard surgical approach via the right atrium. Various different surgical approaches have been proposed, but still pose a remarkable challenge and carry certain morbidity and mortality.[1]

Since 1987, the Rashkind and buttoned devices have been used to close the muscular VSDs. However, these devices were originally designed for patent ductus arteriosus and atrial septal defect, respectively.[2–4] The major drawbacks of these devices were the large delivery sheaths (11 Fr) required for implantation, the complex implantation techniques, the inability to reposition and redeploy the device, interference with the mitral, tricuspid, or aortic valves, and significant residual shunts (25–60%) associated with their use. The Amplatzer muscular VSD occluder is the only device that is specifically designed for the muscular VSD. Since its initial human use in 1998[5,6] it is now the most popular and effective device to close the muscular VSD worldwide.

The device

The Amplatzer muscular VSD occluder (AGA Medical Corp., Golden Valley, Minnesota, USA) is a self-expandable double-disk device made of a nitinol wire mesh (Figure 35.1).[7–10]

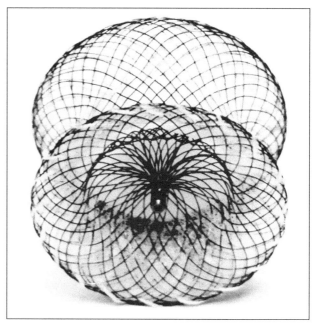

Figure 35.1
The Amplatzer muscular VSD occluder consists of three components: an LV disk, a connecting waist, and an RV disk. The connecting waist is 7 mm long and the two disks are 8 mm larger than the waist. Polyester fabric is present in both disks and the connecting waist.

The thickness of the wire is 0.004–0.005 inch. The connecting waist is 7 mm long and the left and right ventricle disks are 8 mm larger than the waist. Three Dacron polyester patches are sewn securely with polyester thread into the two disks and the waist of the device to enhance thrombosis and to achieve higher closure rates. The RV disk has a stainless steel sleeve with a female thread used to screw the delivery cable to the device. The device size corresponds to the diameter of the waist and is available in sizes ranging from

4 to 18 mm in 2 mm increments. The delivery sheaths required for deployment of these devices vary from 6 to 9 Fr (for the 4 and 6 mm the 6 Fr sheath is good; for 8–10 mm a 7 Fr delivery sheath; for 12–14 mm the 8 Fr, and for 16–18 mm the 9 Fr sheath is sufficient). The mechanism of closure involves stenting of the VSD by the device and subsequent thrombus formation within the device with eventual complete neoendothelialization.

The Amplatzer post-infarction muscular VSD occluder is slightly different from the Amplatzer muscular VSD occluder.[8–11] The connecting waist is longer (10 mm) and the two disks are bigger (10 mm larger than the waist). The device is available in sizes ranging from 16 to 24 mm in 2 mm increments, that are delivered through 8 to 12 Fr sheaths. Please refer to the chapter on Postmyocardial Infarct VSD.

Patient selection

The indications for VSD closure using the Amplatzer muscular VSD occluder include: (1) muscular VSD as demonstrated by echocardiography, and (2) symptomatic or hemodynamically significant shunt (evidence of left atrial and/or left ventricular enlargement for body surface area). Contraindications include (1) distance of less than 4 mm between the VSD and the aortic, pulmonary, mitral, and tricuspid valves, (2) pulmonary vascular resistance of greater than 8 Woods units, (3) sepsis, or (4) contraindication to antiplatelet therapy. For patients weighing more than 5 kg, the percutaneous transcatheter approach is safe and effective and has low morbidity and mortality. However, for smaller patients (less than 5 kg) or patients with other associated cardiac defects requiring concomitant surgical repair, the perventricular approach is better.

Pre-catheterization evaluation

For planning the interventional approach, echocardiographic assessment of the size, number, and location of the VSDs is of paramount importance.[1] The parasternal long axis view demonstrates anterior VSDs. The short axis view near the tips of the mitral valve is important in delineating the location of the muscular VSD. In this view, anterior defects appear between 12 and 1 o'clock; mid-muscular defects appear between 9 and 12 o'clock, and inlet defects appear between 7 and 9 o'clock. The four-chamber view at the level of the atrioventricular valves demonstrates apical, mid-muscular, and inlet defects. If the transducer is angled to the more anterior 'five-chamber view', subaortic and anterior VSDs are also delineated.

Device implantation technique

Percutaneous protocol

1. The procedure is preferably performed under general endotracheal anesthesia with continuous transesophageal echocardiographic (TEE) guidance (Figure 35.2).[1,6–10] However, for single muscular VSD, the procedure can be done safely and effectively under fluoroscopic guidance with transthoracic echocardiographic monitoring.
2. Access is obtained in the femoral artery and the femoral vein. If the VSD is mid-muscular, posterior, or apical septum, the right internal jugular vein is also accessed. If the VSD is anterior, femoral vein delivery should be good.
3. Heparin is given to keep an activated clotting time (ACT) of greater than 200 seconds at the time of device placement. We monitor the ACT every 30 minutes after the intial dose.
4. Routine right and left heart catheterization is performed to assess the degree of shunting and to evaluate the pulmonary vascular resistance.
5. Left ventriculography in the hepatoclavicular projection (35° left anterior oblique/35° cranial) is performed to define the location, size, and number of VSDs (Figure 35.3). The projection varies according to the location of the VSD. For mid-muscular/apical/posterior, the above view is good; however, for anterior muscular VSD, the view for perimembranous VSD is good (60° LAO/20° cranial).
6. The appropriate device size is chosen to be 1–2 mm larger than the VSD size as measured by TEE or left ventriculography at end-diastole.
7. A 4 or 5 Fr curved end-hole catheter (Judkins right coronary, Cobra) is used to cross the VSD from the left ventricle (LV) into either branch pulmonary artery or superior vena cava with the assistance of a 0.035 inch Terumo glide wire. When using the glide wire in a small child, extreme care has to be exercised, since perforating the ventricular septum with the wire is not a rare phenomenon! If the VSD is anterior, we cut the tip of a Judkins left coronary catheter and use it to orientate the tip to the defect. On rare occasions if the VSD cannot be crossed using the Judkins right coronary catheter, we float an endhole balloon wedge catheter and advance it to the LV cavity until it curves up to go back into the ascending aorta; with the balloon inflated, the catheter has the tendency to go through the defect. At that time, advance a wire through the catheter and follow it to the right side of the heart. We usually do not like to cross the VSD from the RV side due to the presence of trabeculations and the tendency of the sheath to be entangled by such trabeculations.

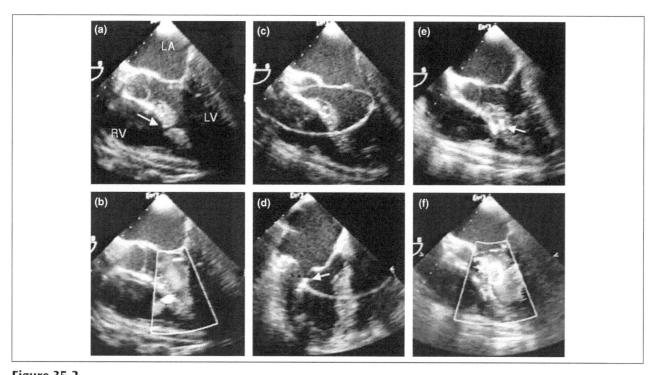

Figure 35.2

Transesophageal echocardiographic images in modified four-chamber views in a 31-year-old male patient with a 5 mm anterior muscular VSD and left-to-right shunt. (a) View demonstrates the VSD (arrow). LV, left ventricle; RV, right ventricle; LA, left atrium. (b) Similar view to (a) with color Doppler demonstrating the shunt. (c) View demonstrating the arteriovenous wire loop (from the aorta, left ventricle, VSD, right ventricle, and out the jugular vein). (d) Deployment of the LV disk of a 6 mm Amplatzer muscular VSD device in mid-LV cavity (arrow). (e) The device has been released (arrow) in the ventricular septum. Note, for an adult the connecting waist is not long enough, but it achieves closure. (f) Final image with color Doppler demonstrating good device position and no residual shunt. (See also color plate section.)

8. Once the the Terumo glide wire is across the defect into the branch pulmonary artery, we advance the catheter to follow it to that location. At that time, either you keep the Terumo or you can use another exchange length soft wire.

9. The next step is to snare the wire and exteriorize it out the vein (jugular or femoral). This is done using a gooseneck snare catheter (ev3, Plymouth, MN) with the appropriate loop diameter (for adults, we use the 20–25 mm and for children the 10–15 mm). This will establish an arteriovenous loop. Figure 35.3 demonstrates that the wire was snared out the jugular vein.

10. Over this wire, an apropriate size delivery sheath is advanced from the vein (jugular or femoral) all the way until the tip of the sheath is in the ascending aorta (Figure 35.3c). We like to keep the position of the sheath in the ascending aorta until the device reaches the tip of the sheath. After removal of the dilator from the sheath, kinking of the sheath is a problem. To overcome this problem we offer: keep a 0.018 inch Terumo glide wire inside the sheath and snared from the arterial end to keep constant tension and to facilitate passage of the device inside the sheath or use a kink resistant sheath (Arrow Flex sheath).

11. The device is loaded under a blood/saline seal in the usual fashion and attached to the delivery sheath. The device is advanced to the tip of the sheath during fluoroscopy and while looking for any evidence of air in the system.

12. We usually deploy part of the LV disk at the tip of the sheath before we start bringing the sheath back to the LV cavity. This is done mainly in cases of anterior VSD, since the sheath may jump back to the RV while it is being withdrawn back. Once the sheath is in the mid-LV cavity, the remainder of the LV disk is deployed. This can be seen easily by echocardiography. TEE or TTE is essential to make sure that the mitral valve apparatus is not entangled with the LV disk. Should this be the case, the device is recaptured or the entire assembly is pushed back inside the LV to release the anterior mitral valve leaflet.

13. The entire device assembly is withdrawn back to the septum with further retraction of the sheath to expand the waist inside the septum (Figure 35.3e).

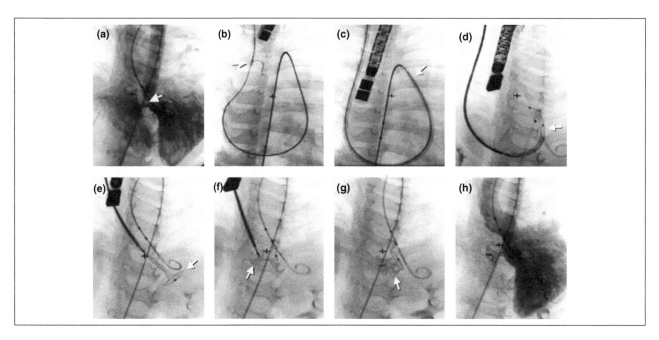

Figure 35.3
(a) Left ventriculography in the left four-chamber view demonstrating an 8 mm muscular VSD (arrow) in a 3.6-year-old boy. (b) Cine image demonstrating the snaring of the wire from the right internal jugular vein (arrow). (c) Cine image demonstrating the delivery sheath over the wire (arteriovenous loop). The sheath tip is in the ascending aorta (arrow). (d) Cine fluoroscopy during passage of a 10 mm Amplatzer muscular VSD device inside the sheath (arrow). (e) Cine fluoroscopy during deployment of the left ventricle disk (arrow) in mid-LV cavity. (f) Cine fluoroscopy during deployment of the RV disk (arrow) on the right ventricle side of the VSD. (g) Cine fluoroscopy after the device (arrow) has been released. (h) Left ventriculography after the device has been released, demonstrating good position and no residual shunt.

14. After good device position is ensured by echocardiography and left ventriculography, further retraction of the sheath to expand the RV disk is performed (Figure 35.3f).
15. After echocardiography and left ventriculography confirm good device position, the device is released by counterclockwise rotation of the cable using the pin vise. Once the device is released (Figure 35.3g), the cable should be brought inside the sheath immediately to prevent any injury from the sharp end of the cable.
16. Repeat echocardiography (Figure 35.2f) and left ventriculography (Figure 35.3h) are performed to assess the final result in terms of closure and residual shunt and to assess the function of the tricuspid, mitral, and aortic valve. If there are further defects (multiple or Swiss cheese), the same process is repeated over to close more VSDs.
17. At the end of the procedure, the ACT is checked and, if below 250 seconds, the sheaths are taken out and hemostasis is achieved. If ACT > 250 seconds, protamine sulfate can be given to reverse the heparin effect.
18. The patient stays in the hospital overnight for post-device observation and is usually discharged home the following day.

Perventricular protocol

Indications include:

1. small infant (< 5 kg) precluding safe percutaneous closure
2. patients with poor vascular access, or
3. muscular VSD associated with other defects requiring open surgical repair.[11,12]

1. The procedure is performed under general endotracheal anesthesia with continuous TEE guidance in the operating room or in the catherization laboratory. Figure 35.4 demonstrates the steps of closure.
2. After the chest and pericardium are opened by a cardiovascular surgeon, a good location for the puncture of the RV free wall is assessed by echocardiography, which should be away from any papillary muscles.
3. A 5-0 polypropelene purse-string suture is placed at the chosen location.
4. An 18 gauge needle is introduced through the chosen location into the RV cavity, pointing toward the VSD.
5. A 0.035 inch short glidewire is passed through the needle to the VSD into the LV.
6. The needle is taken out, leaving the wire in position.

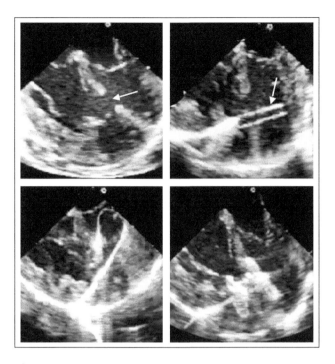

Figure 35.4

Transesophageal echocardiographic images in a 4-month-old baby with a large (7–8 mm) anterior muscular VSD who underwent closure of the VSD using the perventricular approach. Top left, four-chamber view demonstrating the VSD (arrow). Bottom left, passage of a 0.035 inch guidewire from the right ventricle free wall to the VSD to the LV cavity. Top right, the tip of a 7 Fr delivery sheath (arrow) in mid-LV cavity. Note the device is in the proximal part of the sheath being advanced to the tip. Bottom right, a 10 mm Amplatzer muscular VSD device has been deployed, but not released yet. This demonstrates good device position.

7. Over the wire, the proper size short sheath with its dilator is advanced to the LV cavity. Then the dilator is taken out. Extreme care is exercised while advancing the sheath over the wire. The dilator is sharp and could injure the LV wall if care is not taken. Once the sheath is inside the LV cavity, air should be removed to prevent any air embolism.
8. The proper size Amplatzer muscular VSD device is screwed to the delivery cable and loaded inside a smaller sheath than the one through the defect.
9. The device is then advanced inside the delivery sheath under TEE guidance until the LV disk is deployed in the LV.
10. Then the whole cable/sheath assembly is pulled toward the septum. This can be felt manually and seen by echocardiography.
11. Further retraction of the sheath deploys the connecting waist and the RV disk.
12. After echocardiography confirms the good device position, the device is released by counterclockwise rotation of the cable using the pin vise.

On rare occasions, if the VSD cannot be crossed from the RV free wall puncture, one can cross in the retrograde fashion percutaneously (as described above). The wire is advanced via the VSD to the branch pulmonary artery. Then the surgeon advances a short sheath from a puncture in the RV free wall to the main pulmonary artery. Under fluoroscopic guidance, a snare is introduced inside this sheath to the pulmonary artery. The wire which was placed in the pulmonary artery via the VSD is then snared and exteriorized out the RV free wall. Over this wire, the sheath is advanced with its dilator until the tip is in the mid-LV cavity. Once this step is achieved, the wire and dilator are removed and the remaining steps are followed as described above.

Follow-up

The follow-up protocol includes physical examination, electrocardiography, echocardiography, and chest radiography the following day, and 1 and 6 months (transthoracic echocardiography) after the procedure. Patients are routinely maintained on aspirin 3–5 mg/kg daily or equivalent antiplatelet therapy for 6 months. Patients are instructed to receive infective endocarditis prophylaxis when needed until complete closure is documented at the 6-month follow-up visit.

Possible complications

1. *Device embolization/migration.* This complication is rare, especially if the procedure is performed by an experienced operator and under cautious echocardiographic monitoring. The device can migrate to the LV, aorta, RV, or pulmonary artery. The device can be snared and retrieved percutaneously; however, a larger sheath may be needed. The presence of a cardiovascular surgeon in house is essential for device closure of a muscular VSD. Different sizes and types of sheaths and snares should be available on the premises to manage such a complication.
2. *Arrhythmia.* Ventricular arrhythmia may be encountered during catheter manipulations and device deployment, which is usually benign and transient. Conduction disturbances can be seen and complete heart block is rare. On occasions, a lidocaine drip is initiated to manage ventricular arrhythmias. The anesthesiologist managing such patients should be well versed in managing such arrhythmias.
3. *Air embolization.* Meticulous technique of catheter and wire exchanges can minimize this complication.
4. *Hemolysis.* This complication is rare and usually associated with residual shunting. The authors preferably presoak the device with the patient's own blood for about

15–20 minutes; we believe this technique can reduce residual shunt and improve immediate complete closure.

5. *Valvular regurgitation.* Tricuspid, mitral, or aortic regurgitation may occur due to impingement of the device on the valvular apparatus or subaortic septum. Therefore, echocardiographic assessment of the valvular regurgitation prior to closure and prior to device release is extremely important.

6. *Pericardial effusion.* This is a very rare complication that may result from catheter irritation or minute wire perforation during the procedure. To our knowledge, there have been no cases of tamponade or delayed pericardial effusion after 24 hours.

Results

Congenital muscular VSD

A US registry involving 14 tertiary referral centers conducted a prospective, non-randomized study of device closure of congenital muscular VSD using the Amplatzer muscular VSD occluder.[7] A total of 83 procedures (percutanous closure in 77 and perventricular closure in 6) were performed in 75 patients (median age: 1.4 years, range: 0.1–54.1 years). The median size of the VSD was 7 mm (range 3–16 mm) and in 34 of 78 (43.6%) procedures, patients had multiple VSDs (range 2–7). The device was implanted successfully in 72 of 83 (86.7%) procedures. In 17 of 83 (20.5%) procedures, multiple devices were implanted (range 2–3). Procedure-related major complications occurred in 8 of 75 (10.7%) patients, including cerebrovascular accident in 3, death in 2, device embolization in 2, and cardiac perforation in 1. Complete closure rate was 47.2% (34/72), 69.6% (32/46), and 92.3% (24/26) at 24-hour, 6-month, and 12-month follow-up. The Amplatzer muscular VSD occluder appears to be safe and effective to close the congenital muscular VSD.

Bacha et al[12] reported the multi-center experience with perventricular device closure of muscular VSDs in 12 patients (median age of 8.5 months, range 14 days to 4.3 years; median weight of 7 kg, range 3–20 kg). At a median follow-up of 12 months, all patients were asymptomatic and only 2 patients had mild residual shunts. No complications were encountered.

The authors' own personal experience with Swiss cheese VSD includes many patients who received up to nine devices to close multiple defects and achieved good results.

Summary

The Amplatzer muscular VSD occluder is the only device specifically designed for closure of the muscular VSD. It has appealing features that render it to be the most effective device for closure of the muscular VSD. In rare cases, where the VSD is very close to the apex of the heart, deployment of the RV disk may be problematic. Therefore, in such cases, we have used the Amplatzer Duct Occluder since it has no RV disk. This achieved very good closure rate and no instances of embolization.

References

1. Hijazi ZM. Device closure of ventricular septal defects. Cathet Cardiovasc Interven 2003; 60: 107–14.
2. Lock JE, Block PC, McKay RG et al. Transcatheter closure of ventricular septal defects. Circulation 1988; 78: 361–8.
3. Sideris EB, Walsh KP, Haddad JL et al. Occlusion of congenital ventricular septal defects by the buttoned device. 'Buttoned device' Clinical Trials International Register. Heart 1997; 77: 276–9.
4. Kalra GS, Verma PK, Dhall A et al. Transcatheter device closure of ventricular septal defects: immediate results and intermediate-term follow-up. Am Heart J 1999; 138: 339–44.
5. Thanopoulos BD, Tsaousis GS, Konstadopoulou GN, Zarayelyan AG. Transcatheter closure of muscular ventricular septal defects with the amplatzer ventricular septal defect occluder: initial clinical applications in children. J Am Coll Cardiol 1999; 33: 1395–9.
6. Hijazi ZM, Hakim F, Al-Fadley F et al. Transcatheter closure of single muscular ventricular septal defects using the amplatzer muscular VSD occluder: initial results and technical considerations. Cathet Cardiovasc Interven 2000; 49: 167–72.
7. Holzer R, Balzer D, Cao QL et al. Amplatzer Muscular Ventricular Septal Defect Investigators. Device closure of muscular ventricular septal defects using the Amplatzer muscular ventricular septal defect occluder: immediate and mid-term results of a U.S. registry. J Am Coll Cardiol 2004; 43: 1257–63.
8. Waight DJ, Cao QL, Hijazi ZM. Amplatzer muscular ventricular septal defect occluder. In: Rao PS, Kern MJ, eds. Catheter Based Devices for the Treatment of Non-coronary Cardiovascular Disease in Adults and Children. Philadelphia, PA: Williams and Wilkins, 2003: 245–51.
9. Chessa M, Carminati M, Cao QL et al. Transcatheter closure of congenital and acquired muscular ventricular septal defects using the Amplatzer device. J Invas Cardiol 2002; 14: 322–7.
10. Holzer R, Balzer D, Amin Z et al. Transcatheter closure of postinfarction ventricular septal defects using the new Amplatzer muscular VSD occluder: results of a U.S. Registry. Cathet Cardiovasc Interven 2004; 61: 196–201.
11. Bacha EA, Cao QL, Starr JP et al. Perventricular device closure of muscular ventricular septal defects on the beating heart: technique and results. J Thorac Cardiovasc Surg 2003; 126: 1718–23.
12. Bacha EA, Cao QL, Galantowicz ME et al. Multicenter experience with perventricular device closure of muscular ventricular septal defects. Pediatr Cardiol 2005; 26: 169–75.

36

Transcatheter closure of muscular ventricular septal defects: tips regarding CardioSEAL double umbrella technique

Michael Landzberg

Introduction

Transcatheter closure of muscular ventricular septal defects (VSDs) first achieved practical potential with the improvement in design of double umbrella closure devices. These double umbrella device modifications subsequently led to the first and only transcatheter device approval to date by the FDA for ventricular septal defect closure (CardioSEAL device). The original Lock Clamshell Occluder (CR Bard, Boston, MA) consisted of two opposing, self-expanding umbrellas, scaffolded by single spring-loaded stainless steel arms and covered in a Dacron meshwork. The original design allowed for operator and device strategies that

1. maximized device apposition to the septal surfaces with least stress placed on the myocardium and device
2. provided greatest potential to conform to defect anatomy, with least distortion of surrounding myocardium
3. lessened interference with adjacent structures
4. allowed for post-deployment device auto-adjustment
5. increased the potential for complete closure, and decreased the time to accomplish such
6. increased MRI compatibility, and
7. lessened the use of potentially corrosive metallic components with the goal of increased biocompatibility and bioabsorption.

Device design progressed to Clamshell I and II (CR Bard, Boston, MA), and then CardioSEAL and its CardioSEAL–STARFlex modifications (NMT Medical, Inc., Boston, MA), led to the incorporation of MP35N alloy for the umbrella arms, and an internally suspended self-adjusting nitinol microspring meshwork, accomplishing many of these goals. Increased bioabsorption has been recently achieved in Biostar (NMT Medical, Inc., Boston, MA) modification of CardioSEAL, with the ultimate projection of a 100% bioabsorbable double umbrella device, with properties otherwise undifferentiated from those listed above.

Double umbrella closure registries, retrospective reviews and prospective studies, most notably for use in closure of muscular ventricular septal defects,[1] have contributed to models of device and closure safety and outcome assessment that have set standards for similar devices and interventions. Likewise, through such continuous review, application and technique have been modified to achieve improvement in patient outcomes. These modifications are highlighted below, and the reader is referred to earlier references and texts for outlining of the basic principles serving as foundation for double umbrella VSD closure.[2,3]

Patient selection

As with all device-based VSD closures, patients should have hemodynamically significant, complex VSDs that based on (1) defect characteristics (in particular location, involvement of previously placed patch components, intramural nature, concomitant additional VSDs) or (2) patient characteristics (in particular, co-morbid medical issues), cannot be closed with standard risk by a standard transatrial or transarterial technique. In particular for double umbrella devices, a 10 Fr or greater sheath is used for deployment, mandating sufficient patient size to accommodate such (typically > 10 kg, but devices have been deployed safely in infants as small as 6 kg).

Catheter crossing through the VSD

With the exception of transposed ventricles, we maintain the suggestion of crossing the VSD from the systemic to subpulmonary ventricle, to allow passage of and ultimately guide the catheter course through the greatest unobstructed portion of the defect without interference from adjacent muscle bundles or accessory tissue. At times, this is best accomplished by passage through the defect of a balloon-tipped catheter, either under its own guidance via the current flow, or with forced extrusion over a stiffened guide or tip-deflecting wire. Subsequent passage of the balloon-tipped catheter to the pulmonary artery best allows for ultimate formation of an arteriovenous loop without undermining of tricuspid valve attachments, which can easily occur with a subpulmonary to systemic ventricular defect crossing, solitary wire defect crossing, or formation of the arteriovenous loop either in the right atrium or subpulmonary ventricle. We have found that the use of preshaped (coronary) catheters as a guide for wire snares allows for faster and more efficient wire manipulations.

The approach to the systemic ventricular septum can be either anterograde across the semilunar valve or via the transseptal approach. We have found the latter to be of particular use in hemodynamically unstable patients, in particular with low cardiac output syndromes or with increasing age, due to less potential for compromising the semilunar valve function.

On increasing numbers of occasions, hybrid use of transcatheter device deployment in the operating amphitheater, with either direct visualization with/without videoscopic surveillance, transmyocardial echocardiography, or fluoroscopy, has led to novel transatrial or direct transventricular sheath entry and approach and access to the most central portions of the VSD.

Stabilizaton of the arteriovenous loop

Use of a stiffened arteriovenous loop, as outlined above, allows for delicate and precise anatomic understanding and localization, as well as subsequent delivery system and device positioning. However, such a stiffened guide can place considerable tension on the atrioventricular and/or semilunar valve and attachments, and can distort intracardiac structures and compromise cardiac output, both transiently and permanently. Constant attention to multi-planar assessment of such is requisite to avoid these outcomes. Similarly, even hydrophilic wires have the potential to traumatize intracardiac structures. Therefore, when feasible, the looping guidewire should optimally be covered by catheters when portions of it move over intracardiac structures.

Choice of venous exit of arteriovenous loop

Use of either internal jugular or femoral venous access for recovery of the venous arm of the arteriovenous loop has been proposed, based upon defect location and anatomy of contiguous structures. In general, extrusion of the venous guidewire end from the internal jugular vein is preferred for ultimate delivery to defects that are more posteriorly (or, at times, apically) located, so as to minimize curves within the guiding sheaths that may impede ultimate passage. (As well, deployment of a device in a more apical defect may at times require a transseptal approach and distal arm deployment in the subpulmonary ventricle, so as to ensure an optimal approach to the defect with least tightening of the guidesheath curvature.) The approach to all other defects typically allows for wire extrusion via the femoral vein. When deploying a device from a neck vessel venous entry, operators should take greater caution, given the change in hand–eye coordination that occurs in this position. The increasing current use of braided sheaths may eventually alter many of these concerns.

Anatomic VSD definition

Potentially the single most important aspect of both safe and effective device-based VSD closure is detailed anatomic understanding of the defect. While echocardiographic assessment assists in such, we have found fluoroscopic and angiographic assessment additive and critical to implantation success. Multiple advancements have been suggested to optimize such definition, and include (1) localized angiography, either over modified pigtail or over-the-wire angiographic catheters, within the defect and its confines, (2) use of camera angles tailored to VSD location and configuration, and (3) pulling an endhole catheter, with the balloon tip filled with dilute contrast, to the defect margins (assisting in estimation of the proximity to adjacent structures) and through the defect (in part sizing, and in part localizing the narrowest defect portions). Sufficient angiography so as to assess not only the defect, but the surrounding ventricular tissue, should be performed, so as to determine the best approach that will allow maximal expansion of the device's arms so as to conform best to defect and contiguous structure anatomy.

Device–defect approach

Devices are typically chosen to be 1.5–2.2× maximal balloon or angiographic size (currently available in 23 mm, 28 mm, and 33 mm sizes of CardioSEAL, and similar sizes plus an additional 17 mm device for the CardioSEAL-STARFlex modification). Approach, by the delivery sheath system, to allow distal umbrella expansion on either the subaortic or subpulmonary ventricule, should be determined by a combination of assessment of

- VSD size
- VSD angulation and location
- distance to adjacent structures or ventricular surfaces

- goal to ensure maximal arm expansion over the high pressure end of the defect
- potential to decrease tightness of the curvatures of the guide sheath.

Delivery sheath angulation

When deploying subaortic ventricular arms initially within a defect localized in the ventricular outflow (approaching and/or including membranous localization), placement of the guide sheath in the subaortic ventricular apex, rather than in the ascending aorta or subaortic ventricular outflow, may be optimal. This can be accomplished by placement of a balloon-tipped or pre-shaped catheter through the guide sheath, angulated to the ventricular apex. By doing such, optimal arm apposition without encroaching on semilunar valve tissue may be facilitated.

At times, regardless of care in the choice of approach, defect anatomy may force a catheter approach course that contains tight bends. Steam-guided pre-shaping of the delivery sheath, or the use of braided sheaths, may facilitate delivery system passage without sheath kinking.

Delivery system tension

Every device and every delivery system, regardless of manufacturer, stores some degree of torque and tension obtained during sheath and delivery system passage. Care to consider these degrees of tension, and their release during device manipulation, assists in optimal device placement. This may be encountered when retracting a guide and expecting device 'unsheathing', only to recognize that a particular curvature in the guide has been shifted. This may create increased torque and pressure on the delivery system, altering release and potential to shift within the defect and intracardiac structures. Care to restore a neutral curvature with a push–pull coordination between the sheath and delivery system can assist in these considerations.

Sheath/delivery system device tension after proximal arm delivery

After device delivery, but before release from the delivery system sheath, undue tension can be placed on the device, jeopardizing the success of implantation. This consideration is amplified in the double umbrella model of devices as contrasted to center-stem, more-solid devices, yet is a byproduct of specific device features that otherwise serve as theoretic advantages of the double umbrellas. These devices

allow for sufficient arm and material contact so as to promote endothelialization and fibrous tissue coverage, yet minimize tissue tension and stress. Hence, until firmly incorporated into the ventricular and septal walls, these devices are more easily dislodged by incidental less calculated movements. It is recommended that all movements be timely, yet observed in multiple planes, and that least traction be placed on all delivery system components. This can be facilitated by retracting several centimeters of the stiffer, delivery system cover over the central wire delivery system core prior to initiating device unsheathing, allowing the more subtle core to have greater freedom, and to minimize tension on the partially released device.

Arm expansion

On rare occasions, ventricular anatomy permits incomplete arm expansion within ventricular trabeculations or imbedded directly within ventricular muscle. Retraction of these arms within the guiding sheath, and subsequent re-angulation and unsheathing, are typically suggested, though on occasion when such occurs with the proximal umbrella, the multi-planar approach by the sheath to the expanded umbrella may allow for more complete arm expansion.

Assessment of residual defect flow

While it is typical for patients to have near immediate hemodynamic improvement after device implant in muscular VSD, it is also not uncommon to recognize residual transdefect flow, the majority of which tends to occur through the device fabric prior to its endothelialization and formation of a fibrous covering.

Anticoagulation

While pre- and post-procedural antiplatelet therapy is mandated, only peri-procedural anticoagulant therapy is typically utilized, with prompt discontinuation of such post-procedure.

Team coordination

Coordinated non-fluoroscopic imaging and peri-procedural anesthesia, and intensive care planning and support are a central aspect of patient success surrounding VSD closure. Continuous and coordinated communication amongst all team members is stressed.

Patient and family communication

While technical and procedural success with double umbrella closure of muscular VSDs is extremely high,[1] most patients present with a considerable recognized risk for morbidity. Family and patient discussions regarding such potential are typically welcomed, and facilitate peri-procedural care.

For many of the reasons discussed above, double umbrella devices remain a cornerstone for muscular VSD closure. We look forward, with anticipation, to results and technical advancements achieved with newer generation devices.

References

1. Knauth AL, Lock JE, Perry SB et al. Transcatheter device closure of congenital and postoperative residual ventricular septal defects. Circulation 2004; 110: 501–7.
2. Bridges ND, Perry SB, Keane JF et al. Preoperative transcatheter closure of congenital muscular ventricular septal defects. N Engl J Med 1991; 324: 1312–17.
3. Kumar K, Lock JE, Geva T. Apical muscular ventricular septal defects between the left ventricle and the right ventricular infundibulum: diagnostic and interventional considerations. Circulation 1997; 95: 1207–13.

37

Closure of perimembranous VSD using the Amplatzer membranous VSD occluder

Yun-Ching Fu, Qi-Ling Cao, and Ziyad M Hijazi

Introduction

Ventricular septal defect (VSD) is the most common (approximately 20%) congenital heart disease.[1] About 70% of these defects are perimembranous (PmVSD), involving the membranous septum and the adjacent area of muscular septum. Since 1987, devices (Rashkind and button' devices) that were originally designed to close the patent ductus arteriosus or atrial septal defects have been used to close the PmVSD.[2–6] The major drawbacks of these devices were the large delivery sheaths (11 Fr) required, the complex implantation techniques, the inability to reposition and redeploy the devices, the potential interference with the aortic and tricuspid valves, and the significant residual shunts associated with them (25–60%). The Amplatzer membranous VSD occluder was the only device that was specifically designed for the PmVSD. In 2002, Hijazi et al reported the initial human use in six patients with complete closure in all and the absence of any significant complications.[7] Now it is the most popular device to close the PmVSD worldwide.

The device and delivery system

The Amplatzer membranous VSD occluder (AGA Medical Corp., Golden Valley, Minnesota, USA) is an eccentric self-expandable double-disk device made of a nitinol wire mesh (Figure 37.1).[7] The thickness of the wire is 0.003–0.005 inch. The device length corresponds to the waist diameter (1.5 mm) of the device. The aortic end of the left ventricle (LV) disk is 0.5 mm larger than the waist and the opposite end is 5.5 mm larger than the waist. The right ventricle (RV) disk is 2 mm larger than the waist. There is a platinum marker positioned in the LV disk. This marker is important to confirm good device position. The screw in the device has a flat part that should align on the flat part of the capsule located at the end of the pusher catheter (Figure 37.2). The

device is currently available in sizes ranging from 4 to 18 mm in 2 mm increments. The delivery system consists of a sheath, dilator, pusher catheter, cable, loader, and a pin vise. The sheath is braided to prevent kinking and has a tight curve (Mullins type) to allow positioning of the sheath tip into the LV apex. The sheath is available in 7 Fr (for 4 and 6 mm), 8 Fr (for 8 and 10 mm), and 9 Fr (for 12–18 mm) sizes. The cable is fed through the pusher catheter, then this assembly is fed through the hub of the side arm provided with the system and, once the pusher catheter and cable go through the hub, the entire assembly is passed through the loader. Note, the loader hub should be connected to the hub of the side arm. Then the microscrew of the cable is screwed into the proper size device in the usual fashion (male/female mechanism). With the help of an assistant, the flat part of the microscrew is aligned with the flat part of the capsule that is located at the end of the pusher catheter. Once the two flat parts are engaged, the pin vise is securely tightened to the cable at the end of the hub of the pusher catheter. This will prevent premature disengagement of the two flat parts. Then the device is loaded under a water or blood seal inside the loader. The side arm is flushed with saline or blood to reduce the risk of air embolism. The device is not loaded inside the loader until one is ready to deploy the device inside the LV. The presence of the two flat parts (microscrew and capsule) ensures correct device deployment. This is indicated by the smaller LV disk being toward the aorta and the larger disk towards the patient's feet. This is identified by fluoroscopy by the presence of the platinum marker in the LV disk orientated towards the patient's feet.

Patient selection

Patients with moderate size, somewhat restrictive PmVSDs that can be managed medically are considered candidates for device closure once the patient's weight is over 8 kg. The presence of left ventricle and/or left atrial volume overload,

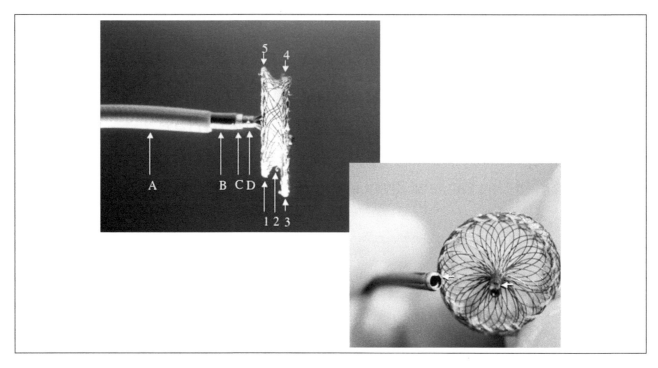

Figure 37.1
Left, lateral view of the Amplatzer membranous VSD occluder attached to its delivery system. The aortic end of the LV disk (designated by number 4) is 0.5 mm larger than the waist, and the opposite end (3) is 5.5 mm larger than the waist. The RV disk (1 and 5) is 2 mm larger than the waist. The connecting waist is 1.5 mm long (2). The screw of the device (D) is screwed into the cable. The cable is inside the pusher catheter (B) with the capsule at the end (C) and the delivery sheath (A). Right, the two flat parts of the screw and the capsule should align with each other to ensure the proper position of this asymmetric device.

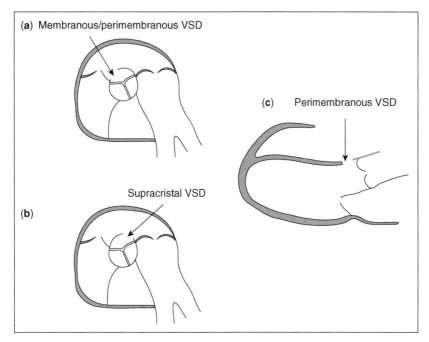

Figure 37.2
(a) and (b) Schematic representation of a short axis parasternal view by the transthoracic echocardiographic view demonstrating the types of perimembranous/membranous (a) and supracristal (b) VSDs. (c) Parasternal long axis view demonstrating perimembranous VSD. Note, only perimembranous and membranous VSDs are amenable for device closure.

as documented by transthoracic echocardiography (TTE), cardiomegaly on chest radiograph, and repeat infective endocarditis, are criteria for the use of the device to close these defects. The presence of a 2 mm or more rim of tissue between the aortic valve and the defect is also considered a prerequisite for device closure. However, measurement of such a distance can be subjective. TTE plays an essential role in delineating the exact location of the VSD. This, in turn, is important for selection of patients for device closure. The left parasternal long axis view demonstrates perimembranous defects. In this view, if the transducer is angled towards the patient's left shoulder to a plane parallel to the right ventricle outflow tract, defects in the subpulmonary region 'supracristal' can be seen well. The short axis view at the semilunar valve plane is probably the best view to delineate the exact location of the VSD (Figure 37.3). Defects seen between 7 and 9 o'clock are termed perimembranous, defects seen between 9 and 12 o'clock are termed membranous, and defects seen between 12 and 1 o'clock are termed supracristal or subpulmonary. Only perimembranous and membranous defects are eligible for device closure. Supracristal defects are not appropriate for device closure. Furthermore, other contraindications to the use of this device include: the presence of aortic valve prolapse, left ventricle to right atrial shunt (Gerbode defect), sepsis, inability to tolerate antiplatelet agents, and the presence of complex congenital heart defects requiring surgical repair.

Device implantation technique

1. Prior to the procedure: patients are asked to take aspirin 81 mg (children) or 325 mg (adults) 48 hours prior to the procedure. This is continued daily for 6 months after closure.
2. If the imaging windows are good, the procedure can be done under TTE guidance with mild sedation; otherwise, transesophageal echocardiography (TEE) under general anesthesia can be used. Figures 37.3 and 37.4 demonstrate the steps of closure by TEE and cine fluoroscopy.[1,7–12] Alternatively, in centers where intracardiac echocardiography (ICE) is available, the procedure can be performed using this technology (see chapter 4).
3. Access is obtained in the right femoral artery (4–5 Fr sheath) and the right femoral vein (7–9 Fr sheath).
4. Heparin is given to keep an activated clotting time (ACT) greater than 200 seconds at the time of device placement. We monitor ACT every 30 minutes.
5. Routine right and left heart catheterization is performed to assess the degree of shunting and to evaluate pulmonary vascular resistance.
6. Left ventriculography in the long axial oblique view (60° left anterior oblique/20° cranial) is performed to define the location and size of the VSD. In our laboratory, we use solely single plane for the entire procedure.
7. At this point, echocardiography (TTE/TEE/ICE) is used to assess the location and size of the VSD. The best TEE views are the short axis view (between 0 and 30°) and the longitudinal view (between 90 and 120°), to evaluate the presence or absence of aortic valve insufficiency and to measure the distance between the valve and the superior

margin of the defect. The tricuspid and mitral valves are also visualized to look for any regurgitation prior to device deployment. Also, while looking at the AV valves, it is important to make comments about whether the VSD extends to the inlet septum or not. Once all of the above is achieved, then a suitable device 1–2 mm larger than the defect is chosen. Since there are no calibration issues with echocardiography, we rely mainly on this imaging modality to choose the device size.

8. With the camera in the same projection as the angiogram, a 4 or 5 Fr Judkins right coronary catheter of appropriate curve is used to cross the VSD from the LV side. We use a curved 0.035 inch Terumo glide wire to help cross the VSD. In about 70% of the patients, the wire goes to either branch pulmonary artery and in the remainder to the superior vena cava. The catheter is advanced over the wire until it reaches that location.
9. The Terumo glide wire is removed and the noodle wire (AGA Medical) is advanced inside the catheter until it exits the tip. The camera can now be moved to straight projection.
10. The noodle wire is snared using a gooseneck snare (ev3, Plymouth, MN) and exteriorized out the right femoral vein. This establishes an arteriovenous wire loop from femoral artery to femoral vein. In adults, it is best to use a 20–25 mm snare loop and in children, 10–15 mm will be sufficient. At this point, the shape of the loop on frontal projection is important. The loop has to be straight without kinks at all. Echocardiography is used to assess the tricuspid valve for regurgitation. If the loop is passing through the valve, regurgitation should be minimal; however, if the loop is passing through chordae or leaflets, the regurgitation is greater and this should give a warning sign that when the sheath is advanced, resistance will be felt.
11. The camera is moved now to the same projection as the angiogram. Over the noodle wire, an appropriate size delivery sheath is advanced from the femoral vein all the way until the tip of the sheath is in the ascending aorta. Now, the Judkins right coronary catheter is advanced over the arterial end of the wire until the catheter tip touches the dilator of the sheath.
12. Slowly draw back the dilator to the inferior vena cava. Then withdraw back the sheath itself with slight counterclockwise rotation until the tip of the sheath is just above the aortic valve. A frozen image from the angiogram on a different monitor should help the operator to tell the position of the VSD and the aortic valve. Also, echocardiography can tell where the tip of the sheath is in relation to the aortic valve. The Judkins catheter is now advanced until it touches the tip of the sheath. The operator now pushes the noodle wire while fixing the catheter. This will help push the sheath into the LV apex. Once the sheath is in the LV apex, the Judkins catheter is advanced until it touches the tip of

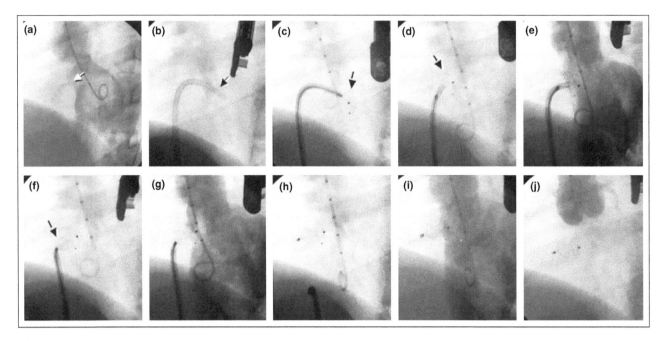

Figure 37.3

(a) Left ventriculography in the left anterior oblique view demonstrating an 8 mm perimembranous VSD (arrow) in a 34-year-old patient. (b) Cine image demonstrating the position of the delivery sheath (arrow) in the LV apex. (c) Cine fluoroscopy image during deployment of the left ventricle disk (arrow) of a 10 mm Amplatzer membranous VSD device in the LV mid-cavity. (d) Cine image after the LV disk (arrow) was brought close to the ventricular septum. Note, the platinum marker is orientated correctly towards the patient's feet. (e) Left ventriculography demonstrating good position of the LV disk at the septum. (f) Cine image immediately after the right ventricle disk (arrow) has been deployed. (g) Left ventriculography demonstrating good device position before its release. (h) Cine image after the device has been released. Note, the platinum marker is pointed towards the patient's feet, indicating good device position. (i) Final left ventriculography indicating good device position and no residual shunt. (j) Ascending aortogram after device release demonstrating no aortic insufficiency and good distance between the device and aortic valve leaflets.

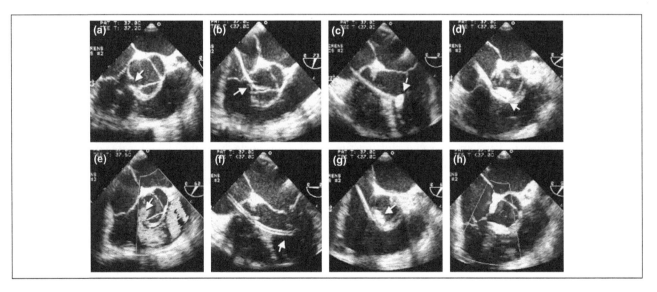

Figure 37.4

Transesophageal echocardiographic images of a 34-year-old male patient with an 8 mm perimembranous VSD. (a) and (b) Short axis view without and with color Doppler at the subaortic level demonstrating the defect (arrow) with left to right shunt (arrow). (c) Short axis view demonstrating passage of the wire forming an arteriovenous loop (wire is passing from the aorta through the VSD to the right atrium). (d) Four-chamber view showing the delivery sheath in the left ventricular apex. (e) The left ventricle disk is deployed. (f) Short axis view showing good position of the LV disk (arrow) in short axis view. (g) Short axis view showing the two disks of the device in good position (arrow). (h) Short axis view with color Doppler mapping showing no residual shunt with a trivial tricuspid regurgitation. (See also color plate section.)

the sheath. Then the wire is removed from the Judkins. Care has to be exercised while pulling the wire out the Judkins. We advance the dilator of the sheath until it is just outside the tip of the sheath; with the Judkins touching the dilator, the wire can be removed easily without the fear of pulling the sheath out the LV to the ascending aorta. Once the wire is out, the Judkins is removed and a pigtail catheter is advanced from the femoral artery to the LV apex. This is used for angiography during various steps of device deployment. The dilator of the sheath is now removed.

13. At this point, we perform an angiogram from the sheath using a 20–30 ml syringe. We first draw saline and then layer 10 ml of contrast at its bottom. The purpose of this angiogram is to make sure that the sheath has crossed the actual defect and not a fenestration and also this angiogram can be used now as a road map for further device deployment.

14. Now, with the help of an assistant, the proper device size is attached to the cable as described above. When the loader is attached to the hub it clicks, indicating secure attachment. The pusher catheter is then advanced until the device reaches the tip of the sheath in the LV apex. One can see the platinum marker at this point. Make sure the tip of the sheath is in the mid-LV cavity, away from the wall and mitral valve.

15. Deploy the LV disk by gentle and slow withdrawal of the sheath over the pusher catheter. Remember, the entire waist length is 1.5 mm, so the movement has to be extremely careful, otherwise, the entire device is deployed. Cine fluoroscopy and echocardiography are used liberally to monitor this step. At this point, the platinum marker is checked and should be pointing towards the patient's feet. If the platinum marker is not in the correct orientation, the entire device is deployed in the LV. Immediately, once this is done, the platinum marker rotates to the correct position. Then recapture the RV disk and waist.

16. The entire assembly (device/pusher catheter/cable) is withdrawn back to the septum. This can be seen by angiography in the LV and by echocardiography.

17. Once the LV disk is confirmed to be in good position by the angiogram and echocardiography, the connecting waist and RV disk are deployed in one motion by fixing the pusher catheter/cable assembly and sliding the sheath back over the assembly. This can be seen by echocardiography and repeat LV angiogram. One cannot overemphasize the importance of echocardiography and the interaction between the echocardiographer and the interventionalist. The echocardiographer has to make sure that there is one disk at each side of the ventricular septum. This is best seen in the two views which were used to assess the defect at the beginning of the case (short axis and longitudinal views). By angiography, if the device is in the proper position, the LV disk

will opacify significantly and the waist and the RV disk will have much less contrast through them.

18. Once good device position is confirmed, the next step is to detach the flat part of the microscrew of the device from the flat part of the capsule of the pusher catheter. This is done by releasing the pin vise and bringing it back a few millimeters. Then fix the cable and slide the pusher catheter over the cable back a few millimeters. This can be seen on cine fluoroscopy.

19. The final step is to release the device by counterclockwise rotation of the pin vise. Once the device is released, the cable should be immediately brought inside the sheath to prevent any injury from the sharp end of the cable to any cardiac structure.

20. Repeat echocardiography and left ventriculography are performed to assess the final result in terms of closure and residual shunt and to assess the function of the tricuspid, mitral, and aortic valves. An ascending aorta angiogram can also be done if there is any concern about aortic insufficiency. One has to be extremely careful removing the pigtail catheter from the LV to the ascending aorta. We use the Terumo wire to remove the catheter from the LV into the aorta. Advance the Terumo until it exits the tip of the pigtail catheter, keep advancing wire into the LV while pulling the catheter over the wire until the catheter is in the ascending aorta.

21. At the end of the procedure, check the ACT and, if less than 250 seconds, sheaths can be removed without reversing the heparin.

22. The patient stays in the hospital overnight for postdevice observation and is usually discharged home the following day.

23. Prior to discharge, a physical examination, a TTE, an EKG, and a chest radiograph are performed to assess the device and to look for any potential complication.

Follow-up

The follow-up protocol includes physical examination, electrocardiography, echocardiography, and chest radiography at 6 weeks and 6 months, and yearly thereafter. Patients are routinely maintained on aspirin 3–5 mg/kg or 321 mg for adults daily or equivalent antiplatelet therapy for 6 months. Patients are instructed to receive infective endocarditis prophylaxis when needed until complete closure is documented at the 6-month follow-up visit.

Possible complications

1. *Device embolization/migration.* This complication is rare, especially if the procedure is performed by an experienced operator. The device can migrate to the LV,

aorta, RV, or pulmonary artery. The device can be snared and retrieved percutaneously; however, a larger sheath may be needed. The presence of a cardiovascular surgeon in house is essential for device closure of membranous VSD. When the device is snared, a long sheath should be very close to the device prior to removing it from the body. This is done to minimize any trauma to vital structures. A useful tool to keep in the catheter laboratory is the En Snare (Hatch Medical, LLC. Duluth, GA).

2. *Arrhythmias.* Ventricular arrhythmia may be encountered during catheter manipulations and device deployment. It is usually benign and transient. The anesthesiologist should be familiar with ventricular arrhythmias and their management.

3. *Heart block.* This is the worst complication after device closure of PmVSD that we encountered. Fortunately, it is rare (1–2%). However, in some cases this complication was not encountered in the hospital, but a few days after discharge. The exact mechanism is not well understood. If a patient presents with complete heart block and adequate ventricular escape rate, observation and treatment with steroids may reverse this block. Our policy is not to rush and implant a permanent pacemaker until after at least one week of hospitalization and treatment with high dose steroids and high dose aspirin (up to 80 mg/kg per day). We have succeeded in avoiding pacemaker implantation in two patients who presented with complete heart block a few days after device implantation. Both patients were treated successfully with high dose steroids and high dose aspirin and were discharged home in sinus rhythm. Both patients are a few months from the procedure and continue to be in sinus rhythm.

4. *Air embolization.* Meticulous technique of catheter and wire exchanges should minimize this complication.

5. *Hemolysis.* This complication is rare and usually associated with residual shunting. We prefer to pre-soak the device with the patient's own blood for about 15–20 minutes to enhance clotting. If hemolysis is significant, the patient may require transfusion. We believe that with time, the shunt will cease and the hemolysis will disappear.

6. *Valvular regurgitation.* Tricuspid, mitral, or aortic regurgitation may occur due to impingement of the device on the valvular apparatus or subaortic septum. Therefore, echocardiographic assessment of the valvular regurgitation prior to closure and prior to device release is extremely important.

7. *Pericardial effusion.* This is a very rare complication that may result from catheter irritation or minute wire perforation during the procedure. To our knowledge, there have been no cases of tamponade or delayed pericardial effusion after 24 hours. Furthermore, we have not encountered any case of device erosion.

Results

Hijazi et al[7] reported their initial use in six patients in 2002 resulting in complete closure in all and absence of significant complications. After that, several centers in a small series reported similar encouraging results of initial complete closure rates of 90–92%.[8–11] A multi-center clinical trial in the United States from October 2003 to August 2004 enrolled a total of 35 patients with median age of 7.7 years (1.2–54.4 years) and median weight of 25 kg (8.3–110 kg).[12] The median Qp/Qs ratio was 1.8 (range 1–4) and the median VSD size as assessed by echocardiography was 7 mm (4–15 mm). The attempt to place a device was successful in 32 patients (91%). The median device size used was 10 mm (6–16 mm). The complete closure rates by echocardiography at 10 minutes (transesophageal/intracardiac), 24 hours, 1 month, and 6 months (transthoracic) were 47% (15/32), 63% (20/32), 78% (25/32), and 96% (27/28), respectively. The median fluoroscopy time was 36 minutes (14–191 minutes) and the median total procedure time was 121 minutes (67–276 minutes). Three patients (8.6%) had serious adverse events of complete heart block (one patient), peri-hepatic bleeding (one patient), and rupture of tricuspid valve chordae tendineae (one patient). No other patient encountered serious adverse events during the follow-up. Based on these this data, the phase II study is ongoing in the United States.

In another study, VSD with aneurysm formation was noted in 45.7% (16/35) of patients.[12] Two of them had multiple fenestrations. The results revealed that the presence of an aneurysm did not prevent device closure. If the aneurysm was big and the opening was solitary, the device could be accommodated within the aneurysmal sac, away from the aortic valve, thereby preventing AR. In most situations, the device was placed in the usual septal position.

A recently published report of an international registry of 100 patients who underwent an attempt at device closure. The attempt was successful in 93 patients. Of those, there was complete closure in 58.1% immediately after the procedure that increased to 83.6% at 6 months follow-up. 29% of the patients had complications, however, the majority of such complications were transient and only 4 patients developed complete heart block. Only 2/4 patients required placement of a pacemaker.[13]

Summary

So, in summary, the Amplatzer membranous VSD occluder is the only device specifically designed for closure of PmVSD and the high closure rates achieved with this device are due to the mechanism of closure (stenting the defect with the waist). This is one of the reasons that it can achieve a better complete closure rate than other devices (90–100% vs 25–60%).[1–12]

Acknowledgement

The authors wish to thank Dr Ra-id Abdulla, University of Chicago, for providing Figure 37.2.

References

1. Hijazi ZM. Device closure of ventricular septal defects. Cathet Cardiovasc Interven 2003; 60: 107–14.
2. Lock JE, Block PC, McKay RG et al. Transcatheter closure of ventricular septal defects. Circulation 1988; 78: 361–8.
3. Rigby ML, Redington AN. Primary transcatheter umbrella closure of perimembranous ventricular septal defect. Br Heart J 1994; 72: 368–71.
4. Sideris EB, Walsh KP, Haddad JL et al. Occlusion of congenital ventricular septal defects by the buttoned device. 'Buttoned device' Clinical Trials International Register. Heart 1997; 77: 276–9.
5. Kalra GS, Verma PK, Dhall A et al. Transcatheter device closure of ventricular septal defects: immediate results and intermediate-term follow-up. Am Heart J 1999; 138: 339–44.
6. Vogel M, Rigby ML, Shore D. Perforation of the right aortic valve cusp: complication of ventricular septal defect closure with a modified Rashkind umbrella. Pediatr Cardiol 1996; 17: 416–18.
7. Hijazi ZM, Hakim F, Haweleh AA et al. Catheter closure of perimembranous ventricular septal defects using the new Amplatzer membranous VSD occluder: initial clinical experience. Cathet Cardiovasc Interven 2002; 56: 508–15.
8. Bass JL, Kalra GS, Arora R et al. Initial human experience with the Amplatzer perimembranous ventricular septal occluder device. Cathet Cardiovasc Interven 2003; 58: 238–45.
9. Thanopoulos BD, Tsaousis GS, Karanasios E et al. Transcatheter closure of perimembranous ventricular septal defects with the Amplatzer asymmetric ventricular septal defect occluder: preliminary experience in children. Heart 2003; 89: 918–22.
10. Pedra CA, Pedra SR, Esteves CA et al. Percutaneous closure of perimembranous ventricular septal defects with the Amplatzer device: technical and morphological considerations. Cathet Cardiovasc Interven 2004; 61: 403–10.
11. Pawelec-Wojtalik M, Masura J, Siwinska A et al. Transcatheter closure of perimembranous ventricular septal defect using an Amplatzer occluder – early results. Kardiol Pol 2004; 61: 31–40.
12. Fu YC, Bass J, Amin Z et al. Transcatheter closure of perimembranous ventricular septal defects using the new Amplatzer membranous VSD occluder: result of the U.S. phase I trial. J Am Coll Cardiol 2006; 47: 319–25.
13. Holzer R, de Giovanni J, Walsh KP, et al. Transcatheter closure of perimembranous ventricular septal defects using the Amplatzer Membranous VSD Occluder: Immediate and Midterm results of an international registry. Cathet Cardiovasc Interven 2006; 68: 620–28.

38

Closure of VSDs – PFM coil

Trong-Phi Lê

Introduction

Transcatheter closure of selected perimembranous and muscular ventricular septal defects (VSDs) using various devices is gaining increasing acceptance in the pediatric cardiology community.[1–8] Even though transcatheter closure avoids the inherent risk of cardiopulmonary bypass, surgical closure remains the therapy of choice for VSDs. Any new procedure will be measured against this gold standard. In order for an interventional procedure to be accepted as an alternative therapeutic choice, its outcome must be at least comparable to surgical results with regard to its efficacy and safety.

The wide range of VSD sizes and morphologies requires a closure system which can be easily adapted to different types of VSDs. Although the Amplatzer VSD occluder (AVSO, AGA Medical, Golden Valley, MN) is currently the most commonly used device for transcatheter VSD closure, alternative devices are still needed. Conical-shaped nitinol coils could be one of the solutions to this dilemma.

The rim of the VSD closed by an AVSO remains under continuous pressure due to the 'stenting philosophy' of this device. If an oversized device is placed in a large VSD, the neighboring conduction system could be compressed over time and could cause heart block, and it is also possible that the neighboring tissue will eventually erode due to the continuous stretching caused by the device. This may explain the late onset of complete AV block, as described in the literature.[1–4]

In contrast to the Amplatzer device and others, the nitinol Nitocclud coil is more flexible.[9] It adapts itself to the shape of the VSD and does not cause additional pressure on the margins of the septum. This mechanism could lead to irritation of the neighboring conduction system and varying degrees of AV block. The implanted coil does not significantly reinforce the septum, as occurs when a more rigid metal mesh disk is deployed. Additionally, the coil delivery system is much softer and more flexible than the delivery systems of other occluder devices. The deployment procedure in general is less traumatic.

Because of the nitinol (or NiTi – a nickel–titanium alloy) manufacturing constraints, it is not yet possible to construct stable coils with a distal loop diameter larger than 18 mm. Therefore, only VSDs with diameters of less than 8 mm are amenable to device closure with the Nitocclud coils. To date, 45 VSDs have been closed with the Nit-Occlud coil (PFM, Cologne, Germany). Although these coils were specifically designed for occlusion of persistent ductus arteriosus (PDA), 82% of the VSDs were completely occluded 6 months after implantation. No rhythm disturbances or valve dysfunction have been seen on short and medium term follow-up. A new Nit-Occlud coil device has been specifically designed for the occlusion of VSDs. This Nit-Occlud VSD device is stiffer than the PDA coils and is covered with Dacron fibers at its distal end to promote early defect closure. With this device, the occlusion rate within 4 weeks of implantation was 96% in 44 patients. On follow-up evaluation, there was no evidence of device embolization, valve dysfunction, endocarditis, hemolysis, arrhythmias, or other conduction problems.

Device and delivery system

Similar to the PDA coil, the Nit-Occlud VSD device is made of nitinol coils shaped in a cone-in-cone configuration (Figure 38.1a). The device has been modified by adding additional larger reinforced coil loops on both the left and the right ventricular ends of the coil. More importantly, polyester fibers have been added to the left ventricular cone (Figure 38.1b). Fibers are placed between the tightly spaced primary coils of the device, much like the synthetic fibers in a standard Cook Gianturco coil. Several prototype devices have been manufactured, the smallest being the 10 mm × 6 mm and the largest being the 18 mm × 8 mm device. The device nomenclature refers to the sizes of the largest diameter of the left ventricular coil, followed by the largest diameter of the right ventricular coil. For example, the 14 × 8 device has a

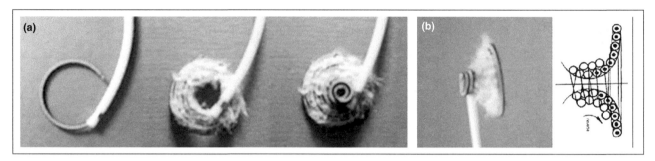

Figure 38.1
(a) The first distal and proximal loops are free from fibers, the remaining loops are covered with Dacron fibers down to the smallest central loop. (b) Lateral and cross-sectional imaging of a PFM nitinol coil: the distal cone is reinforced, the proximal cone is smaller and reversed (cone-in-cone shape).

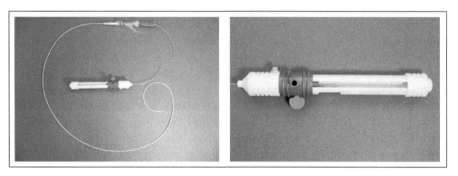

Figure 38.2
The complete system consists of a 6 Fr delivery catheter with pre-mounted coil, pusher, and handle. The handle has a safety clip and release ring. To activate the coil detachment mechanism, the release ring is pulled back after removal of the safety clip.

maximum left ventricular coil diameter of 14 mm and a maximum right ventricular coil diameter of 8 mm. The smallest loop of the coil is 2.5 mm. The coil is currently produced in four different sizes (distal loop diameter of 10, 12, 14, and 18 mm) and is pre-mounted on a 6 Fr delivery catheter. Therefore a 6 Fr kink-resistant long sheath is needed for the implantation.

Due to the asymetric cone-in-cone design and the fact that the distal loops of the coil are stiffer with larger loop diameters, all implantations must be performed from the venous side. A hemostatic Y-connector is attached to the proximal end of the delivery catheter to allow for flushing the system. The tip of the delivery catheter has a radio-opaque marker. The pusher is labeled with two markers. When the first marker reaches the Y-connector, the coil is fully deployed except for the last two proximal loops. These loops will still be in a stretched configuration in the delivery catheter. When the second marker reaches the Y-connector, all loops have been expelled from the delivery system (Figure 38.2).

Angiography

Whenever possible, the VSD should be measured accurately by angiography. The pressure difference across the VSD, combined with the continuous left-to-right shunting across it, gives the VSD a conical shape. Additionally,

perimembranous VSDs are often associated with aneurysmal septal rims of different shapes and sizes. The effective diameter of the VSD is the measurement taken from the right ventricular side. The larger VSD diameter is commonly seen from the left ventricular side. If necessary, repeat injections with different angulations (left anterior oblique (LAO) 30 to 60°; cranial 20 to 30°) are recommended until the defect is fully profiled.

Device selection

The distal diameter of the chosen coil should be at least double the size of the effective diameter of the VSD measured on the right ventricular side and about 1–2 mm larger than the VSD diameter from its left ventricular opening. Estimation of the VSD size is more difficult when the defect is associated with an aneurysmal septum, especially in the setting of complex shaped VSDs with more than one opening into the right ventricle. In this case only the left ventricular diameter of the aneurysm is used when selecting coils. Closure of a perimembranous VSD with a well developed aneurysm does not require a rim to the aortic valve. The selected coil should fit into the aneurysm without protruding into the left ventricular outflow tract. Post-implantation angiography and echocardiography are used to ensure that there is no interference with or distortion of the aortic valve.

Patient selection

Patients weighing over 5 kg with clinical and echocardiographic diagnosis of a muscular or perimembranous VSD, with an effective diameter of less than 7 mm, qualify for this procedure. The pulmonary vascular resistance should not be elevated above 4 Wood units. In the case of perimembranous VSDs, the distance from the cranial rim of the VSD to the aortic valve should exceed 4 mm. If the perimembranous VSD has a well developed aneurysm, a rim of less than 4 mm may be acceptable.

Patients should be heparinized with a bolus of 100 units/kg. The active clotting time should be maintained at 200 to 250 seconds throughout the procedure. After successful implantation of the coil, 200 units/kg of intravenous heparin are administered over a period of 24 hours. The first of three doses of cephalosporin is administered intravenously immediately prior to implantation at a dose of 30–50 mg/kg. The second and third doses are given at 8 and 16 hours, respectively, after implantation.

Post-catheter management

The patient is usually allowed to recover from general anesthesia in the catheterization laboratory and transferred to the recovery room for routine clinical observation. An ECG and a transthoracic echocardiogram are obtained within 12 hours of implantation. The patient is discharged home the following day at the earliest. The patient is given aspirin (2–3 mg/kg per day, maximum 100 mg) for the next 6 months and advised to avoid contact sports for one month. Endocarditis prophylaxis should be continued for 6 months or until complete occlusion is documented. The first follow-up with physical examination, ECG, and transthoracic echocardiography (TTE) is performed one week after discharge. Subsequent follow-up visits are scheduled at 1 month, 6 months, and yearly thereafter.

The implantation procedure

Access to the femoral artery and the femoral vein is obtained with a 4 Fr or 5 Fr sheath in the artery and a 7 Fr sheath in the vein. Standard right and left heart catheterization with baseline hemodynamic data are recorded. A left ventricular angiogram is also routinely performed in the long axial view. The largest dimension of the defect is measured. The VSD is crossed retrogradely using a 4 Fr Judkins right coronary catheter (Cordis, Miami, FL) or an Amplatz right coronary catheter with the aid of a 0.035 inch Terumo 260 cm long exchange guidewire with a J curve. The Terumo wire should cross the VSD with a slightly cranial orientation in order to be positioned into the pulmonary artery. This orientation is important in order to avoid entering the area of the moderator band. To ensure subsequent free passage of the delivery sheath across the tricuspid valve, a 6 Fr end hole Berman catheter (Arrow, Reading, PA) is initially used to reach the pulmonary artery. It is then exchanged for a 5 Fr end hole catheter for the snaring maneuver.

The Terumo exchange wire is snared in the pulmonary artery and exteriorized out of the femoral vein to establish an arteriovenous guidewire circuit. The arterial catheter is advanced across the VSD over the wire and positioned in the upper part of the inferior vena cava. The 6 Fr or 7 Fr long sheath (ArrowFlex, Arrow or Flexor, Cook) with its dilator is advanced from the femoral vein until the tip of the dilator touches the tip of the catheter already positioned in the inferior vena cava. The arteriovenous loop is tightened by pulling the guidewire on both sides of the system and fixing its position at the hub of the arterial catheter and the long sheath using surgical clamps. The long sheath is advanced from the femoral vein to the ascending aorta across the VSD by gently pulling on the arterial catheter and pushing the venous sheath. Once the long sheath reaches the ascending aorta, the arterial catheter is replaced by a pigtail catheter over the guidewire. The dilator of the long sheath and the guidewire are then removed to break the guidewire circuit.

Prior to introducing the coil delivery catheter, the long sheath must be aspirated and flushed to ensure no thrombi are inadvertently pushed into the patient's circulation. It is worthwhile mentioning that the coil delivery catheter is 10 mm longer than the long sheath and hence its tip will protrude by this amount into the circulation. Apart from the last two loops, all the other loops of the coil are deployed in the ascending aorta. Thereafter, the entire system (i.e., delivery catheter and long sheath) is gently pulled back across the aortic valve and positioned into the left ventricular outflow tract. When the coil is pulled back into the VSD, it usually adapts itself to the configuration of the defect (Figures 38.3–38.5).

When the deployed loops are well anchored in the VSD, the remaining two loops can be positioned on the right ventricular side of the defect. The deployment is performed in the following way: the delivery catheter is pulled back slowly from the left ventricle into the right ventricle, while the remaining loops are simultaneously pushed out. During this maneuver, it is of paramount importance that the tip of the long sheath remains close to the VSD entrance from the right ventricular side. Doing so helps to avoid any interference or entangling of the coil with the tricuspid valve.

It is possible that after passing the aortic valve, the coil may not form its expected shape. In such cases, it is recommended that the coil be pulled back into the delivery catheter in close proximity to the ventricular septum. A second attempt to deploy the coils should be made close to the septum.

Jugular venous access is recommended for occlusion of muscular VSDs. If the defect cannot be crossed from the right ventricle, a guidewire circuit must be established.

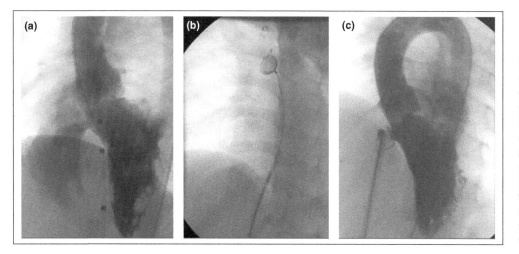

Figure 38.3
(a) Angiogram of the left ventricle in LAO projection to visualize the VSD in its best profile. (b) The coil is configured in the ascending aorta. The coil is placed in the VSD after passage through the aortic valve. (c) The coil is completely configured with two loops on the right ventricular side of the VSD.

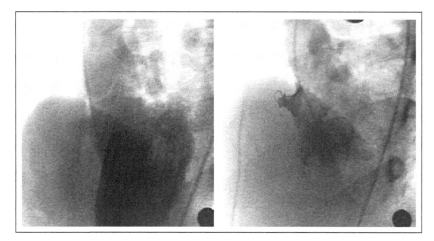

Figure 38.4
Coil implanted in a perimembranous VSD with a flat profile.

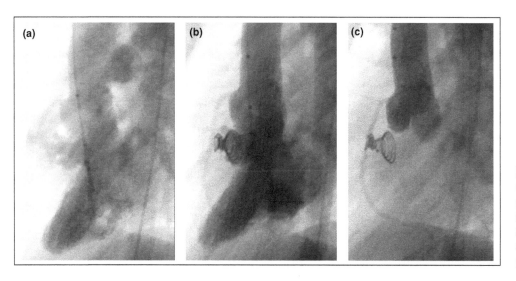

Figure 38.5
Coil implanted in a perimembranous VSD with a well developed aneurysm (a) Angiogram of LV (b) and ascending aorta (AAO) post-implantation (c).

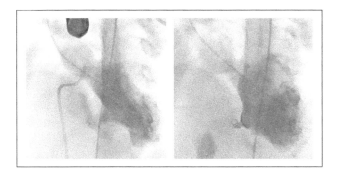

Figure 38.6
Coil implanted in a muscular VSD.

While positioning the coil in a muscular VSD, the tip of both the delivery catheter and the long sheath should be in close proximity to the ventricular septum (Figure 38.6). When delivering the coils, the loops must be kept far away from the mitral valve apparatus. If the coil has formed optimal configuration, the next steps are performed as for the membranous VSDs.

Occasionally during positioning of the coil across the VSD, too many loops are delivered on the right ventricular side. These additional loops could interfere with the tricuspid valve apparatus and may lead to residual shunting. This is best dealt with by pulling the coil back into the delivery catheter whilst simultaneously pushing the delivery catheter across the VSD back into the left ventricular outflow tract. The implantation can then be re-attempted.

If the delivery catheter cannot be advanced into the left ventricular outflow tract, the coil must be retrieved via the catheter. If it is not possible to pull the coil completely back into the delivery catheter, it should be pulled back along with the delivery catheter inside the long sheath.

If the coil is prematurely released from the delivery system while it is in a suboptimal position, it does not usually embolize into the right ventricle, as the distal loops will hold it in position. In this case, the VSD should be recrossed in a retrograde fashion and a new guidewire circuit is re-established. A long sheath is carefully positioned next to the proximal end of the coil. Next, a snare catheter is also advanced along the long sheath with the guidance of the wire circuit. The coil is snared from its right ventricular end and then pulled back into the long sheath (Figure 38.7). It is essential that during this maneuver, the coil is not positioned too deep into the right ventricle, as it could become entangled with the tricuspid valve apparatus.

A poorly positioned coil in the VSD can also be dealt with by snaring it at its distal end and pulling the coil back into the descending aorta. With the help of a larger arterial long sheath, the coil can be safely retrieved. Alternatively, after accessing the contralateral femoral artery, a guidewire circuit can be established as described before. A long sheath is then positioned from the venous side across the VSD into the descending aorta. The coil can then be retrieved with a snare transvenously.

If a significant residual shunt is still present 6 months after implantation, a second coil can be deployed across the first one in the same manner as described above. Usually positioning of the second coil is much easier than the first one, as the first coil guides the second into position (Figure 38.8).

Hints

- Open the snare in the main pulmonary artery before advancing the wire. Crossing the VSD with the wire and catheter and establishing the AV circuit should be conducted as smoothly as possible. The AV circuit should have a smooth course inside the right ventricle. Difficulty in advancing the sheath over the guidewire is likely to be caused by the wire crossing the tricuspid valve tensor apparatus or the wire getting entangled in the moderator band. Highlight the position of the aortic valve in patients with perimembranous VSDs immediately before coil deployment.
- Pull the pigtail catheter back in the descending aorta (DAO) to avoid interference with the coil during coil exposure.
- Keep the tip of the delivery catheter approximately 10 mm apart from the tip of the long sheath when pulling the configured coil from the ascending aorta back into the left ventricle.

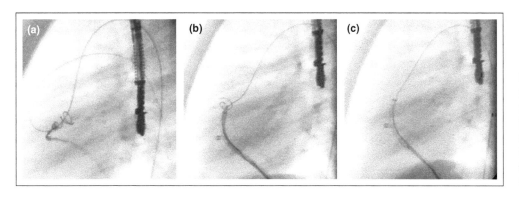

Figure 38.7
Removal of an improperly deployed coil using a snare. Snaring of the proximal end of the coil (a). Coil being pulled back into long sheath (b). Coil completely retrieved (c).

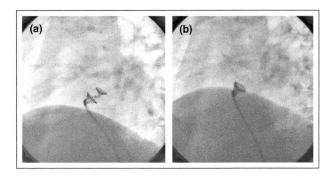

Figure 38.8
Coil-in-coil technique for closure of residual shunt (a). Second coil being configured in first coil in a cone-in-cone shape (b).

References

1. Carminati M. Transcatheter treatment of congenital and postinfarction ventricular septal defects: preliminary Results of a European Multicenter Study. 8th International Workshop on Catheter Interventions in Congenital and Structural Heart Disease, Frankfurt, Germany 16–19 June 2005.

2. Thanopoulos BD, Rigby ML. Outcome of transcatheter closure of muscular ventricular septal defects with the Amplatzer ventricular septal defect occluder. Heart 2005; 91: 513–16.

3. Arora R, Trehan V, Thakur AK et al. Transcatheter closure of congenital muscular ventricular septal defect. J Interven Cardiol 2004; 17: 109–15.

4. Holzer R, Balzer D, Cao QL et al. Amplatzer Muscular Ventricular Septal Defect Investigators. Device closure of muscular ventricular septal defects using the Amplatzer muscular ventricular septal defect occluder: immediate and mid-term results of a U.S. registry. J Am Coll Cardiol 2004; 43: 1257–63.

5. Pedra CA, Pedra SR, Esteves CA et al. Percutaneous closure of perimembranous ventricular septal defects with the Amplatzer device: technical and morphological considerations. Cathet Cardiovasc Interven 2004; 61: 403–10.

6. Arora R, Trehan V, Kumar A et al. Transcatheter closure of congenital ventricular septal defects: experience with various devices. J Interven Cardiol 2003; 16: 83–91.

7. Bass JL, Kalra GS, Arora R et al. Initial human experience with the Amplatzer perimembranous ventricular septal occluder device. Cathet Cardiovasc Interven 2003; 58: 238–45.

8. Hijazi ZM, Hakim F, Haweleh AA et al. Catheter closure of perimembranous ventricular septal defects using the new Amplatzer membranous VSD occluder: initial clinical experience. Cathet Cardiovasc Interven 2002; 56: 508–15.

9. Lê TP, Freudenthal F, Sievert H et al. Transcatheter occlusion of subaortic ventricular septal defect using a nitinol coil (NitOcclud): Initial clinical results. Circulation 2001; 104: II593.

39

Amplatzer™ post-myocardial infarction VSD occluder

Kevin P Walsh and Patricia Campbell

Transcatheter closure of post-myocardial infarction ventricular septal defects (PMIVSDs) remains challenging because of the infrequency and severely ill nature of the patients referred. The GUSTO-1 investigators found that in the era of thrombolysis only 0.2% of acute myocardial infarctions are complicated by a VSD compared to 1 to 2% in the pre-thrombolytic era.[1,2] Furthermore, the patients referred for transcatheter closure have usually been turned down for surgery because of severe co-morbidity, established cardiogenic shock, or advanced age. This sets the stage for a severely ill patient undergoing a relatively rarely performed procedure as an emergency. Patients turned down for surgery because of age rather than condition may do well with the transcatheter technique.

PMIVSDs are not discrete holes but rather represent ruptures in a necrotic lake or aneurysm of myocardium.[3] The defect is therefore more akin to a tear (Figure 39.1), with the potential for further expansion, and can be very large or multiple. Many centers approach these problems by using a 'trial of life' and only considering patients for surgery or transcatheter intervention if they survive for 3 or 4 weeks. This approach will produce better results for the treatment but not necessarily better results for the pool of patients presenting, many of whom will have died or become inoperable in the intervening time. The 30-day mortality for patients treated surgically in the GUSTO-1 trial was 47% versus 94% for those who were treated medically.[1]

A residual/recurrent post-surgical VSD occurs in about 10–40% of the survivors of surgery for acute PMIVSD, depending on the surgical technique used.[4] Mortality associated with a second surgical procedure to repair a recurrent PMIVSD has been reported to be as high as 31%.[5] Patients with residual or recurrent defects are clearly natural survivors, both from the MI and the surgical repair of the VSD. Furthermore, the tissue surrounding the VSD is likely to be firm and relatively static in size. This group of patients does well with device closure, which avoids the need for a redo open-heart procedure. While other devices such as the Lock Clamshell device[6–8] have been used to close post-infarct VSDs, this chapter deals with the Amplatzer occluders.[9–14]

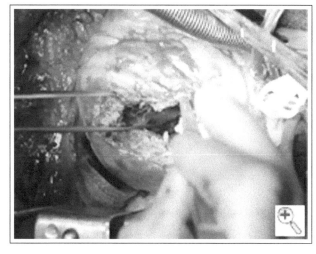

Figure 39.1
Ruptured interventricular septum. A ragged perforation (forceps holding it open) seen at the time of surgical repair. (See also color plate section.)

Patient selection

Patients are selected for the procedure on the basis of imaging, clinical condition, and institutional experience. Institutions without experience in device occlusion technology are likely to opt for surgical management. Patients with residual or recurrent defects are 'natural survivors', have defects with established firm margins, and make ideal cases for a transcatheter approach. Patients in the early acute phase are much more difficult to select for either surgery or device closure. There is the dilemma as to how to obtain the best result for the patient versus the best results for the technique or operator.[15] The introduction of Web published cardiac surgical results in the United Kingdom has increased the number of surgical turn-downs and consequent referral for consideration of device closure. Survivors of a 'trial of life' are likely to do well with any technique, but the overall results for patients with acute PMIVSD will remain poor. We should probably turn down patients for device closure who are moribund despite an

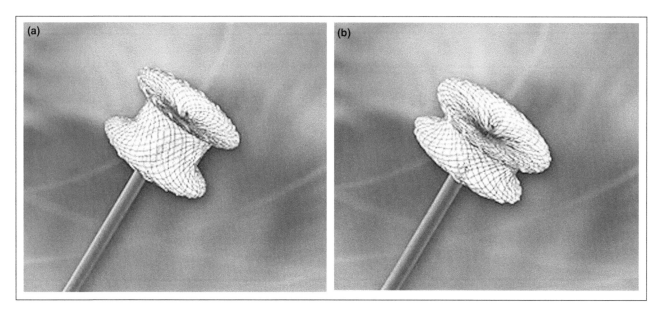

Figure 39.2
Amplatzer muscular ventricular septal defect (VSD) occluder. The device has three components: a left ventricular disk, a connecting waist, and a right ventricular disk. The post-infarct muscular VSD occluder (a) has a 10 mm long waist, compared to 7 mm for the congenital muscular VSD device (b).

intra-aortic balloon pump (IABP) and inotropes, and also those where the defect is too large. Early surgery should be considered for acutely presenting large defects where surgery with stabilization on cardiopulmonary bypass and infarct exclusion may currently offer better results. This may well change with the introduction of larger diameter and less porous devices with better delivery systems. Patients who are in good condition at the time of referral and/or who can be stabilized with an intra-aortic balloon pump and who have a moderate sized defect (<2 cm) are good candidates for device closure. Stenting of the infarct-related artery at the time of IABP insertion is considered by some to be helpful.

Technique of device closure

Devices

Amplatzer ASD devices and congenital muscular VSD devices have been used for PMIVSD patients; however, these devices may not conform well to the thicker interventricular septum in adults and thereby permit significant residual shunting. A specific Amplatzer PMIVSD device has been developed to deal with this issue. This device is similar to the congenital muscular VSD device in being shaped like a drum with rims made from a 0.005 inch nitinol self-expanding wire mesh with the disks and waist filled with polyester

patches sewn on with polyester thread. The PMIVSD has a longer waist of 10 mm (Figure 39.2a) compared to 7 mm in the MVSD device (Figure 39.2b). The PMIVSD device is available with waist diameters from 16 to 24 mm in 2 mm increments and can be delivered through 9 to 10 Fr long sheaths (Table 39.1). However, the largest size currently available (24 mm) is too small for some of the defects encountered, particularly if a degree of further expansion of the defect is to be allowed for. The porosity of the device is also of concern as significant residual shunting can continue for a number of weeks after implantation. In addition to a hemodynamic burden, hemolysis through the device may occur which will compromise an already severely ill patient. *Pre-clotting* the device in 20 ml of the patient's unheparinized blood may help to diminish significant early shunting.

Imaging

Echocardiography both before and during the implantation is the most important imaging modality. Imaging of these defects in large adults is more difficult than that of congenital muscular VSDs in smaller children. Transesophageal echocardiography can be helpful, but usually requires general anesthesia which patients in cardiogenic shock may tolerate poorly. Transgastric views are particularly useful for delineating the defect (Figure 39.3). *It is important to visualize the maximum LV, septal, and RV orifices of the intended*

Table 39.1 *Amplatzer post-infarct muscular VSD occluder*

Code	Waist diameter (mm)	RV disk (mm)	LV disk (mm)	Waist length (mm)	Sheath size (Fr)
9-VSDMUSC-PI-016	16	22	24	10	9
9-VSDMUSC-PI-018	18	24	26	10	9
9-VSDMUSC-PI-020	20	26	28	10	10
9-VSDMUSC-PI-022	22	28	30	10	10
9-VSDMUSC-PI-024	24	30	32	10	10

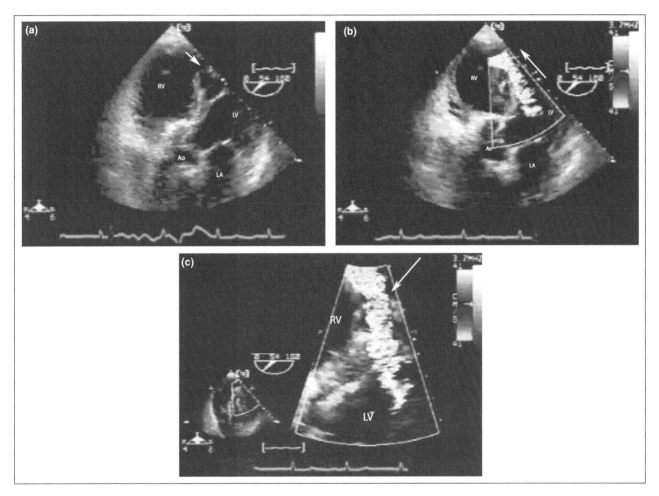

Figure 39.3

Transesophageal echocardiographic (TEE) images of an acute post-infarct ventricular septal defect (VSD). The transgastric view (a) shows the ragged margins of the ruptured (arrow) septum. Color-flow mapping (b) shows a high velocity flow exiting the tunnel-like VSD (arrows) (c). RV, right ventricle; LV, left ventricle; LA, left atrium; Ao, Aorta. (See also color plate section.)

defect and to see the guidewire crossing these (Figure 39.4). Otherwise, particularly in patients with multiple defects, the device will end up in an adjacent unimportant defect, that in addition to producing significant residual shunting may impede a second device from completely closing the important defect. Transesophageal echocardiography does not always provide good images of very apical defects and it may be better to use transthoracic imaging. Angiography allows for a crude assessment of the amount of shunting of dye before and after device implantation. It can be the sole imaging modality for patients with single defects, particularly if the defect is well profiled.

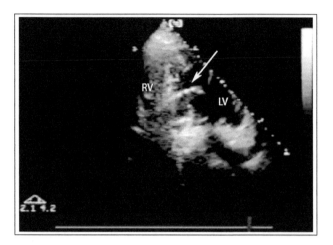

Figure 39.4
Transthoracic echocardiographic image of guidewire passage through a post-infarct ventricular septal defect (VSD). The arrow shows a Terumo guidewire crossing an acute post-infarct VSD from right to left. Transthoracic imaging confirmed that the wire had passed through the major orifices of the VSD. The right ventricular approach was used in this particular patient to introduce a 24 mm post-MI VSD device without the need for an arterio-venous guidewire loop. LV, left ventricle; RV; right ventricle.

Arterio-venous guidewire circuit

The most common method used has been to cross the defect via the left ventricle and create an arterio-venous guidewire circuit. The left ventricle can be entered through the aortic (retrograde arterial) or mitral valves (transseptal). A right coronary or balloon wedge catheter is used to cross the defect, often with the aid of a torque wire (Terumo Corporation, Japan; or Storq, Cordis J&J, USA) (Figure 39.5a). A 6 Fr JR4 and exchange length angled Terumo guidewire is usually the initial catheter/wire combination chosen. The wire will often be directed to the pulmonary artery, from where it can be snared (Figure 39.5b) and pulled out to the jugular or femoral vein. We usually use an Amplatzer 25 mm diameter gooseneck snare (Microvena). The guidewire course that allows the straightest introduction of the long sheath is chosen. This is usually the jugular vein, but may be the femoral vein for anterior defects. It is helpful to use a wedge balloon catheter (7 Fr Monitoring (non-thermodilution) Swan–Ganz catheter, Edwards) from the jugular vein to enter the pulmonary artery and pass an exchange wire to introduce the snare catheter, in order to avoid looping the wire around a chord or papillary muscle of the tricuspid valve when the guidewire circuit is created. An AGA exchange Ropewire can be very helpful as it is very unlikely to kink. The defect can then be balloon sized over the wire (Figure 39.5c), which also ensures that the guidewire is not trapped around a chord.

The appropriate long sheath (9 Fr for 16 and 18 mm PMIVSD devices, 10 Fr for 20 to 24 mm devices) and dilator

are then introduced over the wire (Figure 39.5d). When the tip of the dilator meets the tip of the arterial catheter, the long sheath and arterial catheter are advanced and withdrawn respectively using a 'kissing' technique. The dilator usually passes into the left ventricle without too much difficulty. The sheath often requires some encouragement by either holding the guidewire circuit taut or often, more usefully, just peeling the sheath over the dilator. It is a mistake to 'overintroduce' the long sheath into the left ventricle, as the sheath will buckle when the dilator and wire are removed. After removal of the dilator and de-airing of the long sheath, the guidewire is partly withdrawn via the artery to about the level of the tricuspid valve. The sheath is then clamped, with rubber shods or an artery clamp over gauze, and the device introduced and passed down to the level of the guidewire and then advanced while the guidewire is withdrawn. Once the device is at the tip of the sheath the echo is checked to ensure that the device does not open inside the mitral tension apparatus. The deployment is monitored mainly on echo (Figure 39.5e,f). The RV disk may need time to fully configure. If the lips of the device are tilted into the defect then the sheath can be advanced back over the device to recapture it and redeploy it. Echocardiography (Figure 39.5g) and angiography are then used to check its final position prior to release. After release any residual shunting should be through the device; however, at this stage it may become apparent that there are other significant defects that require further implants. It is usually better to go on and implant the additional devices during the same session.

While this technique is usually successful, it remains very cumbersome and time consuming. Kinking of the long sheath can be sufficient to prevent device delivery and necessitates starting again as the A-V guidewire loop will have been withdrawn by then (Figure 39.6). Leaving a 0.014 or 0.018 inch guidewire through the sheath after the dilator and AV wire loop has been withdrawn may help to avoid kinking (Figure 39.7). When the sheath develops a kink as the device is being advanced then simply withdrawing the sheath while the device is advanced may be enough to get the device through the kinked area. Braided sheaths may also prevent kinking but the Arrowflex sheath has a polyurethane inner coating, which creates tremendous frictional resistance to the passage of the nitinol device. This can be got around by backloading the device into the usual AGA long delivery sheath and advancing the entire unit inside an Arrowflex sheath 2 Fr sizes larger. The standard Cook blue sheaths with radio-opaque marker bands, although not braided, kink much less frequently than the standard AGA sheaths. A 12 Fr blue Cook sheath can be used to deliver a 24 mm PMIVSD device backloaded in a 10 Fr AGA long sheath. Cook also manufactures Flexor sheaths which are braided and have a Teflon inner lining that permits easy advancement of the device. I have found these sheaths to be of great help during these procedures. The new AGA braided Torq Vue sheaths for atrial septal defect

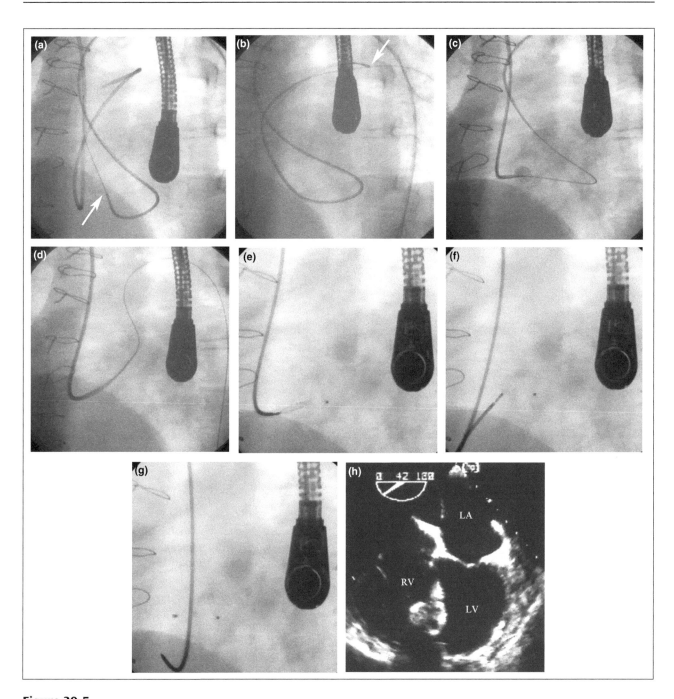

Figure 39.5

Transcatheter closure of a residual post-infarct ventricular septal defect (VSD). The defect is crossed via the retrograde arterial approach. Using an El-Gamal catheter a torque wire (arrow) has been directed from the left ventricle through the VSD and into the right ventricular outflow tract. The exchange length guidewire is then snared out (arrow) from the pulmonary artery using an Amplatzer gooseneck snare. A 7 Fr monitoring Swan–Ganz catheter has been passed over the created arterio-venous (A-V) guidewire loop and dye used to inflate the balloon to size the defect (c). The long delivery sheath is then passed from the right internal jugular vein over the A-V guidewire loop into the left ventricle (d). The left ventricular disk (e) followed by the right ventricular disk (f) is deployed and then the device is unscrewed from the delivery cable (g). Transesophageal echo shows the device to be well seated on the ventricular septum (h). LA, left atrium; LV, left ventricle; RV; right ventricle.

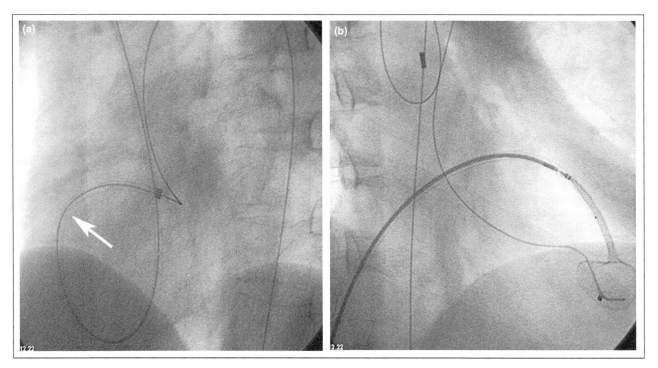

Figure 39.6
Sheath kinking. The long sheath has been introduced from the right internal jugular vein over an arterio-venous guidewire loop in a patient with an acute post-infarct ventricular septal defect (VSD). The arrow points to the kink in the sheath which developed after removal of the long dilator from the delivery sheath. Recrossing the VSD and snaring out the femoral vein has produced a much gentler angle on the sheath and avoided kinking of the sheath (b) in this patient with an anterior VSD.

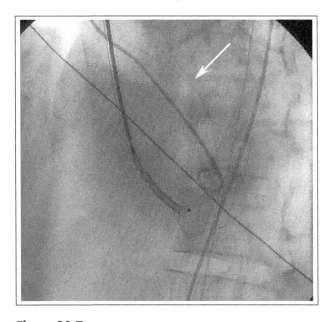

Figure 39.7
Sheath re-inforcement. A 0.014 inch coronary guidewire (arrow) has been passed into the long sheath and the device loaded and passed alongside it and opened in the left ventricle.

devices are large enough to deliver the post-MI VSD device and should markedly reduce the incidence of sheath kinking and considerably simplify the procedure.

Right ventricular approach

The technique of using a retrograde arterial approach to cross the defect, create an arterio-venous guidewire loop, and then introduce the delivery sheath transvenously is cumbersome. In order to simplify the technique we have sometimes adopted the approach of crossing the maximum RV orifice of the defect with a catheter (Rt Coronary, Multipurpose) and/or Terumo guidewire, usually introduced from the right internal jugular vein (Figure 39.8a and b). The guidewire is then directed out through the aortic valve, followed by the catheter, and the guidewire is passed down the descending aorta or into the subclavian artery. The Terumo wire is exchanged for a normal Teflon-coated J-tipped guidewire. A long sheath and dilator are then hand curved to match the guidewire curve and passed over the wire into the left ventricle. Device introduction and deployment then proceeds as before. If the long sheath should fall back or kink then an 8 Fr Rt Coronary guide catheter inside the long sheath can be

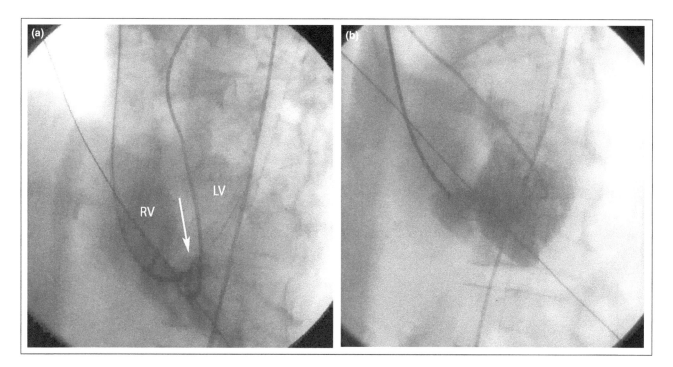

Figure 39.8
Right ventricular approach. The arrow shows the Terumo guidewire passing through the VSD (a). The catheter was introduced from the right internal jugular vein and passed into the right ventricle. The right ventricular approach was used in this particular patient to introduce a 24 mm post-MI VSD device (b) without the need for an arterio-venous guidewire loop. LV, left ventricle; RV, right ventricle.

used to recross the VSD from the RV and pass the sheath back into the LV for a further attempt.

Clinical experience

We attempted transcatheter closure in 18 patients with PMIVSDs, 12 native (within 5 weeks of myocardial infarction) and 6 with residual defects after surgical repair of PMIVSDs. There were 13 male and 5 female patients who ranged in age from 50 to 86 years. The transvenous route was used in all patients to implant 8 Amplatzer ASD devices, 4 MVSD devices, and 7 PMIVSD devices. Two patients each received 2 devices. Device sizes ranged from 10 to 26 mm.

One patient died during introduction of a 12 Fr sheath and in another patient a 24 mm PMIVSD device pulled through repeatedly and he died 8 hours later. Five patients had complete closure, 9 patients had trivial or small residual leaks, and 3 patients had a large residual leak. One woman with a small VSD associated with an inferior MI, very poor LV function, and rheumatic mitral stenosis died 12 hours later despite complete closure of her defect.

Of the three patients with large residual leaks, one died and two received a second device, with one of these two patients crossing over to surgery. The patient who died was a woman with a large anterior VSD who died 3 days later with continuous shunting through her 28 mm ASD device. Her RCA had been dissected at the time of PTCA. A second device (both 14 mm muscular VSD devices) was implanted in 2 patients with abatement of the large residual shunt in one patient and a continuing large residual shunt in the other. The latter patient underwent successful surgical repair of a 5 cm diameter VSD 4 weeks after his MI.

Complications consisted of 1 transient CHB, 3 episodes of VF arrest, avulsion of the tricuspid septal leaflet in 1 patient, and hemolysis in 1 patient. Eight out of 12 patients with AMI survived to hospital discharge and one of these died 2 months later with continuing heart failure despite a small residual shunt. All 6 of the post-surgical residual PMIVSD group are alive and clinically improved, although the patient with avulsion of his septal TV leaflet did develop right heart failure which responded to diuretics.

Analysis of failures

The most frequent cause of failure was related to limitations in the device and delivery system. *Device porosity* was probably related to one patient's cross-over to surgery (Figure 39.9)

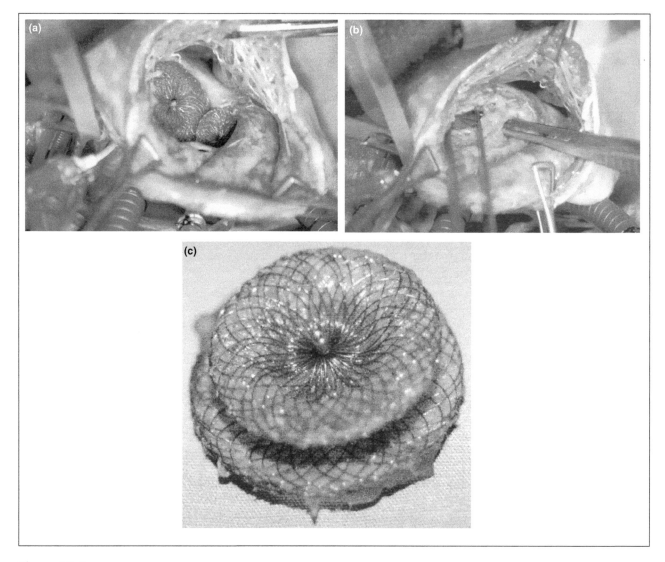

Figure 39.9
Cross-over to surgery. An interoperative photograph via the left ventriculotomy shows the previously placed 20 mm atrial septal defect and 14 mm congenital muscular devices (a). Neither device appears to have developed much 'endothelialization'. After device removal two well circumscribed VSDs can be seen with surgical forceps inside each of them (b). The relatively incomplete 'endothelialization' can be seen on the right ventricular aspect of the congenital muscular device (c).

and another patient's death; both of these patients had ASD devices which are clearly likely to have trouble resisting the high pressure left to right shunt coming from the left ventricle. Hemolysis through a muscular VSD device in a post-operative patient, which later resolved, was a potential failure. The 'endothelialization' of large devices in humans is probably quite a slow process occurring from the outside in. High velocity shunting through the mesh and fabric of the device will further retard this process.

Limitation of device sizes was the reason for failure to implant in one patient in whom a 24 mm PMIVSD device repeatedly

pulled through. The same patient also had significant *sheath kinking* as a reason for additional procedural difficulties. *Poor delivery systems* resulted in prolonged procedures in many patients, mainly due to sheath kinking with inability to advance the device and having to start all over. Tricuspid valve damage occurred in one patient because of an inability to get the long sheath through the VSD without extreme traction (at the surgeon's request) on the arterio-venous guidewire loop. A further patient died when a 12 Fr sheath was passed into the right ventricle; this may well have been due to damage to the tricuspid valve, but no post-mortem was obtained.

Conclusions

Transcatheter closure of VSD post-MI is probably the treatment of choice for recurrent post-infarction VSD following patch repair. Primary catheter closure of VSD following acute myocardial infarction is an evolving technique that may avoid surgery or serve as a bridge to subsequent elective lower risk surgery. The results in patients with acute VSDs should improve with larger diameter, less porous devices, simpler delivery techniques, and clearer imaging. Selection of patients who are not in cardiogenic shock at the time of referral and who have survived for a couple of weeks after developing the VSD should further improve results. However, while this approach is good for the technique, it may not necessarily produce the best results for the entire group of patients presenting with post-MI VSD. An earlier aggressive approach may salvage more patients, particularly in centers where a policy of 'trial of life' is also adopted by the surgical team. To this end, the availability of less porous, larger diameter devices coupled with improved delivery systems is urgently required.

References

1. Crenshaw BS, Granger CB, Birnbaum Y et al. Risk factors, angiographic patterns, and outcomes in patients with ventricular septal defect complicating acute myocardial infarction. GUSTO-I Trial Investigators. Circulation 2000; 101: 27–32.

2. Held AC, Cole PL, Lipton B et al. Rupture of the interventricular septum complicating acute myocardial infarction: a multicenter analysis of clinical findings and outcome. Am Heart J 1988; 116: 1330–6.

3. Edwards BS, Edwards WD, Edwards JE. Ventricular septal rupture complicating acute myocardial infarction: identification of simple and complex types in 53 autopsied hearts. Am J Cardiol 1984; 54: 1201–5.

4. Killen DA, Piehler JM, Borkon AM et al. Early repair of postinfarction ventricular septal rupture. Ann Thorac Surg 1997; 63: 138–42.

5. Deja MA, Szostek J, Widenka K et al. Post infarction ventricular septal defect – can we do better? Eur J Cardiothorac Surg 2000; 18: 194–201.

6. Lock JE, Block PC, Mc Kay RG et al. Transcatheter closure of ventricular septal defects. Circulation 1988; 78: 361–8.

7. Landzberg MJ, Lock JE. Transcatheter management of ventricular septal rupture after myocardial infarction. Semin Thorac Cardiovasc Surg 1998; 10: 128–32.

8. Pienvicht P, Piemonte TC. Percutaneous closure of post-myocardial infarction ventricular septal defect with the CardioSEAL septal occluder implant. Cathet Cardiovasc Interven 2001; 54: 490–4.

9. Lee EM, Roberts DH, Walsh KP. Transcatheter closure of a residual post-myocardial infarction ventricular septal defect with the Amplatzer septal occluder. Heart 1998; 80: 522–4.

10. Demkow M, Ruzyllo W, Konka M et al. Staged transcatheter closure of chronic post-infarction ventricular septal defects with the Amplatzer septal occluder. Int J Cardiovasc Interven 2001; 4: 43–6.

11. Rodes Cabau J, Figueras J, Pena C et al. Communication interventricular postinfarto de miocardio tratada en fase aguda mediante cierre percutaneo con el dispositivo Amplatzer. Rev Esp Cardiol 2003; 56: 623–5.

12. Mullasari AS, Umesan Ch V, Krishan U et al. Transcatheter closure of post-myocardial infarction ventricular septal defect with Amplatzer septal occluder. Cathet Cardiovasc Interven 2001; 54: 484–7.

13. Szkutnik M, Bialkowski J, Kusa J et al. Post-infarction ventricular septal defect closure with Amplatzer occluders. Eur J Cardiothorac Surg 2003; 23: 323–7.

14. Goldstein JA, Casserly IP, Balzer DT et al. Transcatheter closure of recurrent post-myocardial infarction septal defects utilizing the Amplatzer post-infarction VSD device: a case series. Cathet Cardiovasc Interven 2003; 59: 238–43.

15. Topaz O. The enigma of optimal treatment for acute ventricular septal rupture. Am J Cardiol 2003; 92: 419–20.

40

Transcatheter closure of post-myocardial infarction muscular ventricular septal rupture: tips regarding CardioSEAL double umbrella technique

Michael Landzberg

Introduction

Repair of post-myocardial infarction (post-MI) ventricular septal (VS) rupture remains a 'most precarious of all' intervention within the spectrum of transcatheter (as well as any form of) closures of muscular VS defects. Surgical success, despite published improvement in outcomes by patch-exclusion techniques in limited centers, remains extremely limited.[1–3] Patient hemodynamic status, acute decompensation of non-cardiovascular system health (in particular renal and hepatic function), accompanying ventricular necrosis, and ventricular arrhythmic instability all combine not only to make the procedural technique complex, but to add, as well, to the marked tenuousness of patient stability.

To date, reports of device-based post-MI septal rupture closure remain anecdotal, with little intermediate- or long-term definition of outcome, thus making suggestions of 'optimal technique' of limited utility. As such ultimately become better defined as per outcomes assessments, certain concepts, nonetheless, suggest that double umbrella devices will sustain a sentinel role in their application to this indication. The reader is referred to chapter 36 regarding double umbrella closure of congenital muscular VS defects for additional specific discussion of the concepts outlined below.

Patient selection

For patients with post-MI VS rupture, timing of intervention is one of the key aspects of potential for intermediate- and longer-term success. Undue delay typically leads to a multi-organ, unrecoverable morbid spiral. Typically, maximal hemodynamic stabilization with inotropy and systemic pharmacologic or physical afterload reduction, as well as assessment of infectious potentials, requires up to 24 hours from presentation. Intervention rarely should occur after this timing, and mandates a '24/7' co-ordination of catheterization laboratory, as well as pediatric and adult anesthesia, intensive care, and nursing staffs.

Arteriovenous looping

Defect crossing with least potential for tissue obstruction of maximal defect for catheter passage nearly always requires systemic to pulmonary ventricular passage. We tend to favor a transseptal defect approach in this setting, due to the not infrequent prior implantation of a transarterial intra-aortic balloon pump, as well as the tendency to create some degree of compromising semilunar valve regurgitation if a retrograde transarterial approach is utilized. Particular attention to loop formation in a fashion that allows minimal potential for atrio-ventricular valve, semilunar valve, or intracardiac distortion is critical to minimize worsening of already low systemic cardiac output.

Defect localization

Defects are classically serpiginous 'ruptures', rather than smoothly defined passages. The subpulmonary and subaortic ventricular septal exits (or even free-wall exit) may be distant from each other. Defects may be of variable 'tunnel' length. Due to these considerations, particular attention to anatomic detail and proximity to adjacent structures is required. Localized angiography, in multi-planar projections specific to defect location, appears additive, even with supporting echocardiography or concern of renal dysfunction. Given a relatively consistent sizing at catheterization laboratory presentation of necrotic ruptured segments, as well as a recognized subsequent pathologic course, we tend not to balloon size such defects, with concern of worsening tissue dehiscence or permitting rupture extension throughout the septum or free walls.

Device–defect approach and sheath angulation

Specific double umbrella device characteristics suggest potential for its use as an optimal choice to permit defect approach and reduction. A low profile with concomitant double-hinged arm retraction to allow tissue–device adherence with minimal device–tissue stress and strain, independent arm flexion to allow unique device conformations, and auto-adjusting inner-spring mechanisms appear to all combine to provide 'least-harm' potential of nearly all of the existing defect closure devices purported for this application. Nonetheless, particular care in the approach of guiding the sheath to the necrotic septum and surrounding septum and free wall (with similar potential for unrecognized but existing necrosis and rupture if undue stress is placed on them) is required. Most laboratories that have performed more than several such procedures have unfortunately been home to occurrence of free wall rupture complicating attempted closure of a VS rupture after MI. Minimal sheath, wire, and device interaction with surrounding structures (either of a direct nature or through tension caused by wire and sheath looping) is recommended.

Implantation of double umbrella devices of maximal available size is typically recommended. This allows for greatest coverage of myocardium at risk for pressure-induced necrosis and subsequent potential defect expansion. With CardioSEAL (as with center-stem, more solid devices without potential to adjust days after implant), it is not unusual to require additional device implantation in the post-procedural 72–144 hours, as further necrosis modifies the original defect size and anatomic configuration. With maximal sizing of CardioSEAL STARFlex and subsequent

modified devices, concerns regarding the need for additional devices may be lessened.

The potential for hybrid use of transcatheter device deployment, either alongside percutaneous coronary interventions or in the operating amphitheater during coronary revascularizaton, remains anecdotal, with insufficient data available to guide alteration of technique.

Anticoagulation

Most rapid elimination of anticoagulation may be difficult in post-MI patients in low output requiring inotropic support, though such is still emphasized, combined with vigorous antiplatelet therapy.

Above all, these suggestions do not stand alone, and should be taken in concert with those listed, in detail, regarding double umbrella closure of other muscular VS defects. Post-MI VS rupture transcatheter closure results in appropriate centers of combined pediatric and adult expertise with support systems in place for such. It appears to rival the best of surgical outcomes and may be an optimal therapeutic choice, either in concert with or stand alone from coronary revascularization. We continue to await orchestrated trials with defined patient outcomes prior to more detailed recommendations regarding use of any such devices in this setting.

References

1. Birnbaum Y, Fishbein MC, Blanche C, Siegel RJ. Ventricular septal rupture after acute myocardial infarction. N Engl J Med 2002; 347: 1426–32.
2. Menon V, Webb JG, Hillis JD et al. Outcome and profile of ventricular septal rupture with cardiogenic shock after myocardial infarction: a report from the SHOCK Trial Registry. SHould we emergently revascularize Occluded Coronaries in cardiogenic shocK? J Am Coll Cardiol 2000; 36(Suppl A): 1110–16.
3. Crenshaw BS, Granger CB, Birnbaum Y et al. Risk factors, angiographic patterns, and outcomes in patients with ventricular septal defect complicating acute myocardial infarction. GUSTO-I (Global Utilization of Streptokinase and TPA for Occluded Coronary Arteries) Trial Investigators. Circulation 2000; 101: 27–32.

Section VIII

Aorto–pulmonary shunts

41

PDA occlusion with the Amplatzer devices

Mazeni Alwi

Isolated patent ductus arteriosus (PDA) is one of the commoner congenital heart lesions comprising approximately 10% of congenital heart disease.[1] Most patients are asymptomatic as the PDA tends to be small or moderate in size (< 3.5–4.0 mm). Diagnosis is suspected on the presence of continuous murmur. Large PDAs may present with high output cardiac failure, frequent chest infections, and failure to thrive. Bounding pulses and a continuous murmur are characteristic, though with the development of pulmonary hypertension the diastolic component of the murmur may disappear and the second heart sound may become loud. The diagnosis of PDA, and the evaluation of its size and hemodynamic impact, is easily made by two-dimensional (2D) and Doppler echocardiography.

Those with significant left to right shunt manifest features of left heart volume overload, i.e., dilatation of left atrium, left ventricle (LV). Doppler is helpful in assessing pulmonary artery pressure, but accurate direct measurement is an integral part of the closure procedure. It is recommended that all PDAs be closed to prevent infective endocarditis, relieve heart failure symptoms, and prevent progression to irreversible pulmonary vascular disease. Opinion is divided with regard to the small, silent PDA which is defined as a duct identified echocardiographically but without a typical continuous murmur.

Small PDAs (< 2.5–3.0 mm) can be easily closed with Gianturco or Cook detachable (Flipper) coils with minimal complications and excellent results.[2,3] Those with a significant shunt from a large PDA, i.e., patients who are symptomatic and with obvious evidence of LV volume overload and pulmonary hypertension, are generally not good candidates for PDA closure with coils because of the technical difficulty in achieving a stable position of the coils and the attendant complication of embolization. The large number of coils required for effective closure can also deform and obstruct adjacent structures such as the left pulmonary artery and descending aorta. Until fairly recently, surgical ligation was the most appropriate treatment for such large ducts.

The Amplatzer Ductal Occluder or ADO (AGA Medical, Golden Valley, MN), first introduced in 1997, shares the modular design features of the Amplatzer Septal Occluder,

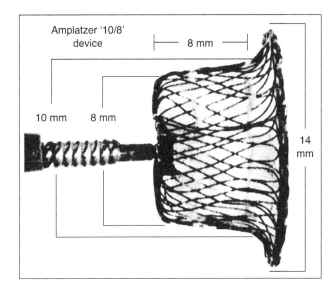

Figure 41.1
The Amplatzer Duct Occluder device. In this example of a 10/8 mm device, the '10' refers to the aortic end of the device, and '8' refers to the pulmonary end. The retention disk on the aortic end is 4 mm larger in diameter than the aortic end's diameter.

i.e., retrievability for repositioning or change to a more appropriate sized device before release. It was initially developed in a canine model with encouraging results.[4] The ADO has made transcatheter closure of moderate to large PDA a safe and efficacious procedure.[5–9]

The cylindrical, slightly tapered device has a thin retention disk 4 mm larger in diameter than its body to ensure secure positioning in the ductal ampulla. The polyester fibers sewn into the device induce thrombosis and rapid complete occlusion. Platinum marker bands are applied to the wire ends and are laser welded. A stainless steel sleeve with a female thread is then welded to the marker band (Figure 41.1). The delivery system consists of a delivery cable with a male thread to which the device is screwed, a loading device, a long Mullins type delivery sheath, and a pin vise to unscrew and release the device. The designation of device sizes 6/4 mm, 8/6 mm, 10/8 mm, etc., refers to the body of the device. The first number denotes the larger distal (aortic) end of the device at the retention disk whereas the second number, which is always 2 mm smaller, denotes the size of the proximal (pulmonary) end where the stainless steel sleeve for screwing onto the cable is located in its recess. It is important to remember that the retention disk at the distal (aortic) end of the device is always 4 mm larger in diameter than the larger of the quoted sizes. For example, the aortic retention disk on a 6/4 mm device is 10 mm in diameter. The device sizes available are in increments of 2 mm, with a range from 5/4 mm to 16/14 mm. The smallest two sizes are 7 mm in length and the remainder are 8 mm.[5]

Patient selection, hemodynamics, and angiographic evaluation

Patients with small PDAs – asymptomatic patients with no clinical, ECG, chest X-ray, and echo evidence of left heart volume overload – may be treated effectively by coil occlusion. For symptomatic infants who weigh less than 5 kg with severe failure to thrive and heart failure due to a large PDA, surgical ligation is the most appropriate treatment. Interventional treatment for these infants is likely to require a relatively large device, and the risk of protrusion of the retention disk into the aortic lumen causing obstruction precludes its use. Additionally the passage of a large and stiff delivery sheath and dilator through the heart may compromise patient hemodynamics by splinting open the tricuspid valve, inducing tricuspid regurgitation. The tight radius imposed on the curve of the delivery sheath because of the small antero-posterior (AP) diameter of the thorax may also result in kinking when the device is being advanced.

We would recommend a weight limit of 5 kg for infants with significant symptoms. However, in patients who are only mildly symptomatic it is preferable, where possible, to perform the procedure when they attain 7–8 kg in weight. Rarely, adult patients are referred late with advanced pulmonary vascular disease and this clinical problem is dealt with in the later part of this section.

Procedure

Policies vary with regard to the use of general anesthesia (GA) in different institutions. It is recommended that the procedure is done under GA in infants and small children if at all possible. Both the femoral artery and vein of usually the right groin are cannulated using a 4 Fr sheath in the artery and a 5 or 6 Fr sheath for the vein. For the initial hemodynamic evaluation, a 5–6 Fr diagnostic catheter (NIH or multi-purpose) is used for pressure and oximetry studies. A 4 Fr pigtail is used for left heart study and aortography.

Ductal morphology

After the hemodynamic study has been completed, an aortogram using the pigtail catheter is performed with the 'pigtail' of the catheter at the level of or slightly above the PDA ampulla. The lateral projection is the most useful and, if a biplane system is available, the other projection can be straight frontal or with some right anterior oblique (30°). The great majority of isolated PDAs arise in the distal arch/proximal descending aorta, just beyond and opposite the origin of the left subclavian artery. They tend to be short, conical-shaped structures rather than long and tube like. The aortic end is a wide ampulla whereas the narrowest part is where it inserts to the superior aspect of the main pulmonary artery close to the origin of the left pulmonary artery. The PDA runs in a posterior–anterior, and slightly inferior–superior, leftward direction from the aorta to the pulmonary artery. The important measurements are the diameter of the ampulla, the length of the PDA, and, most importantly, its narrowest diameter for selection of the appropriate device size. In a PDA with a large shunt, a large volume of contrast of 2 ml/kg over 1 second may be needed to outline the PDA morphology well. Occasionally having a large Mullins sheath across the PDA during aortography may be useful in outlining the ductus, particularly in adult patients. Balloon sizing techniques have occasionally been employed to accurately outline the PDA in adults.[10] On the lateral projection, the narrowest part of the PDA is usually seen overlapping with the tracheal air column and this serves as a useful landmark at the time of deployment. The short conical ductus is most suited for the ADO. This is designated as type A ductus in the Krichenko angiographic classification.[11] Further subgrouping according to where the narrowest diameter is in relation to tracheal air column (A1, A2, A3) is superfluous. A small number of isolated PDAs have a less typical morphology, chiefly the long tubular ductus with or without a constriction at the pulmonary insertion (types C and E, respectively, in the Krichenko classification) and even less common is the window type short ductus with virtually no ampulla (type B). The long tubular ductus requires some modification of technique or choice of device. In adult patients with large PDA, although the morphology is usually the typical conical type, the actual ductal length may be far in excess of device length, rendering the ADO unsuitable.

Selection of device size and long sheath

For the great majority of PDAs, especially those with a conical shape, the device size selected (the pulmonary end) should be at least 2 mm larger than the narrowest PDA diameter. For example, if the narrowest PDA diameter is 3.6 mm, an 8/6 mm device should be selected. In practice the sizes used are overwhelmingly 8/6 mm and 10/8 mm, taking into consideration that many ducts measuring less than 2.5–3.0 mm are closed with coils as a matter of policy. However the '2 mm rule' may not be applicable to the larger ducts. For instance, in an adult patient with a 7 mm PDA, the 12/10 mm device may easily slip through into the pulmonary artery as the ratio between the retention disk diameter and the distal device diameter becomes increasingly smaller with increasing device size (the retention disk is always 4 mm bigger than the distal device diameter, regardless of size). In such large PDAs, one or two sizes bigger may need to be chosen. Another factor for failure of implantation is the relatively longer PDA in adult patients whereas the device length remains 8 mm even in the largest size available (see below). For the 8/6 mm device, a 7 Fr long sheath is recommended and 8 Fr for the 10/8 mm device to facilitate easy advancement during device delivery.

Implantation of device

Once the measurements of the duct from the descending aortogram have been made and a device size selected, a 5 Fr or 6 Fr multi-purpose catheter is advanced from the venous side through the PDA and into the descending aorta. This catheter is exchanged for the delivery sheath and dilator over a 0.035 inch exchange guidewire. The dilator is then removed, leaving the sheath in the descending aorta.

To load the device, the delivery cable is passed through a short cannulation sheath ('loading pod') with a side port 1 Fr size smaller than the delivery sheath. The device is screwed onto the tip of the delivery cable and pulled into the loading pod. The side port allows easy flushing of the loaded device within the sheath. The loading pod is introduced into the delivery sheath and the cable is then pushed to advance the device. To prevent inadvertent unscrewing, rotation of the cable should be avoided when the device is being advanced.

Under fluoroscopy, the device is advanced by pushing the delivery cable until it reaches the tip of the delivery sheath in the descending aorta. The sheath is gently withdrawn to deploy the retention disk only, following which the cable and delivery sheath are pulled as one unit under lateral fluoroscopy until the retention disk is against the ductal ampulla. This can be observed by fluoroscopy using the tracheal air column as landmark from the diagnostic aortogram previously or felt as a tugging sensation in synchrony with the aortic pulsation. Once the position has been affirmed based on the location of the narrowest diameter in relation to the tracheal air column, the cylindrical portion of the device is deployed by retracting the delivery sheath while applying slight tension on the cable.

An aortogram is then performed to verify correct positioning of the device. This is evident by the retention disk being well apposed to the ampulla and a slight waist seen in the middle portion of the device induced by constriction at the narrowest part of the PDA. If the position is satisfactory,

the device is then released by screwing the plastic vise on the delivery cable and rotating it counterclockwise as indicated by the arrow on the vise. It is common to see residual shunt through the device, sometimes described as 'foaming' on the immediate post-implantation aortogram. This is acceptable and it is usually unnecessary to repeat the aortogram 5–10 minutes later to document complete closure. However, if a definite jet is seen, usually above the body of the device, this indicates that the device is not 'stenting' the narrowest part of the PDA either due to inappropriate device size or incorrect positioning. In the case of unusual PDA morphology, the ADO may not be the suitable device to use (see below). In this case, the device should be recaptured into the sheath by pulling on the cable while fixing the delivery sheath with the other hand and the steps repeated or a more suitable device selected.

Problems and complications
Small infants with a large PDA

The indication to close a PDA in small infants is the presence of significant 'cardiac failure' symptoms and failure to thrive due to a relatively large ductus. In these infants the forced passage of a stiff delivery sheath and dilator in the right ventricular outflow tract (RVOT) may cause hemodynamic compromise. Tracking the sheath–dilator ensemble over an extra stiff exchange guidewire may smoothen the passage by reducing the pressure against the RVOT as the sheath is being maneuvered. In these infants the long sheath forms a tight curvature as it conforms to the RVOT, main pulmonary artery, and descending aorta. The sheath may kink as the device is advanced at the RVOT level as the stiffer cable conforms less to the curvature than the device, causing its tip to push against the wall of the sheath. This may be overcome by using a kink-resistant sheath 2 Fr larger or alternatively the curvature of the delivery sheath can be reduced by placing its tip at the level of the ductal ampulla instead of lower in the descending aorta (Figure 41.2).

As noted above, in these symptomatic infants a relatively large device is often required, usually 8/6 mm or 10/8 mm. The large retention disk may sit against the aortic wall rather than on the rim of the ductal ampulla causing a mild gradient. This mild hemodynamic problem is, however, transient and becomes insignificant with somatic growth (Figure 41.2d). In general, problems and complications are commoner in children weighing less than 10 kg.[12]

Undersizing and embolization to pulmonary artery

Embolization of the ADO is rare. In the typical PDA morphology this may be due to undersizing the device or

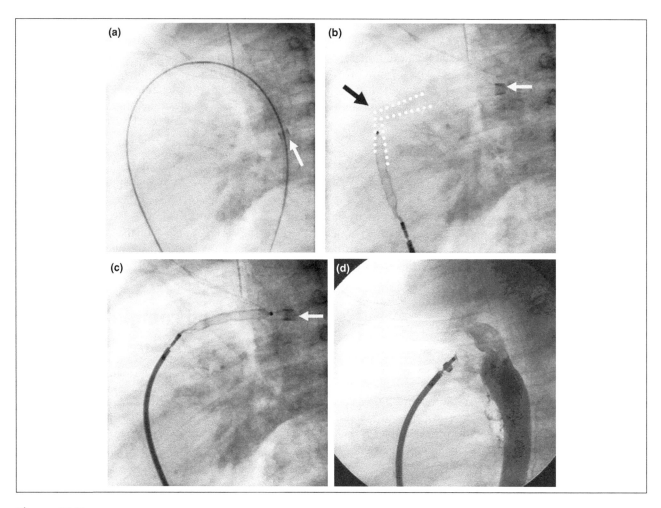

Figure 41.2
5.2 kg infant with 4.5 mm PDA. (a) Tight curvature of delivery sheath with its tip (white arrow) in the descending aorta. (b) Kinking of delivery sheath (black arrow). (c) Curvature of delivery sheath is reduced by placing its tip at the level of the ductal ampulla to prevent kinking. (d) Upper rim of retention disk (8/6 mm device) protrudes into the aorta causing a 10 mm gradient.

positioning the device too deep within the ductus before its release. Ideally in the conical-shaped PDA the retention disk should be seated within the ampulla rim. When the device is pulled too deep, which may be partly due to undersizing, a 'bump' caused by the retention disk is seen on the top part of the PDA. Although complete occlusion is achieved in the laboratory, the device may embolize later, probably due to a 'milking' action of the ductal wall (Figure 41.3). It is safer to reposition the device and if the same appearance caused by the retention disk is seen, a device one size bigger is probably more appropriate (Figure 41.4).

An embolized ADO device into the pulmonary artery is difficult to retrieve because the sleeve housing female screw thread is located in a recess. However, the device can be easily removed at the time of surgical ligation.

Long tubular PDAs

Ducts that are long and tubular may or may not have a constriction at the site of pulmonary insertion. Those with a definite constriction do not pose a major problem as the device may be pulled deep into the ductus before release. The device will be elongated and the retention disk will not configure fully due to the limited space, but embolization to the pulmonary artery is not likely to occur because of the constriction (Figure 41.5).

However, the long, large tubular ductus without a definite constriction may not be suitable for closure with an ADO because the device is relatively short (7 or 8 mm) and only has one retention disk. As illustrated in Figure 41.6, if the retention disk is correctly positioned on the rim of the

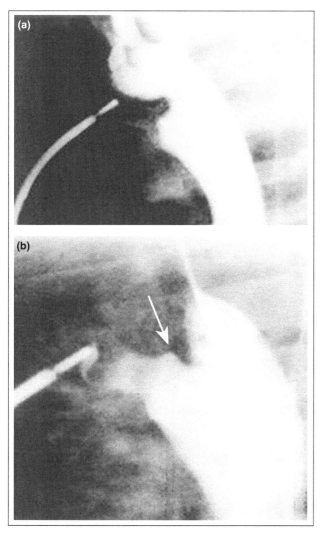

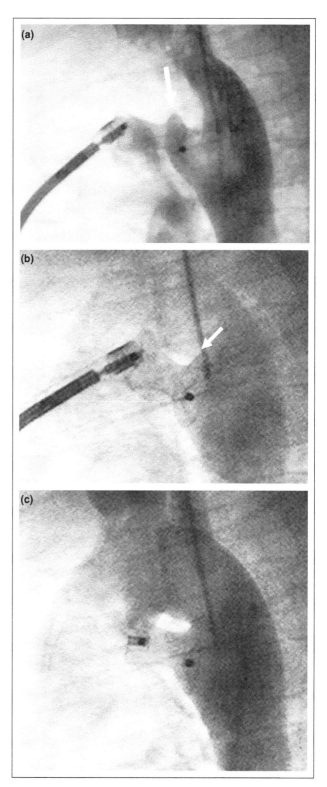

Figure 41.3

(a) Retention disk of the device seated on the rim of the ductal ampulla. The ductus is completely occluded and the device is not likely to embolize. (b) A completely occluded ductus but the device is too small, causing the retention disk to be pulled deep into the ductus, resulting in a 'bump' (arrow) on the upper wall. This device embolized to the right pulmonary artery after 24 hours.

ductal orifice, the proximal (pulmonary) end of the device is still well within the long PDA. Releasing the device in this position will likely cause embolization to the descending aorta or protrusion of the retention disk into the aorta, causing a significant gradient.[13] On the other hand, pulling the device too deep to bring the proximal end into the main pulmonary artery will likely cause embolization to the right side in the absence of a definite constriction. In this uncommon type of PDA, a device like the AMVO (Amplatzer muscular VSD occluder), though equally short, has two retention disks and has the advantage of ensuring stable

Figure 41.4

(a) The narrowest part of the PDA is well stented by the device but the 'bump' (arrow) indicates that the retention disk has been pulled too deep into the ductus. (b) and (c) The device was recaptured and repositioned with the retention disk correctly seated in the ampulla.

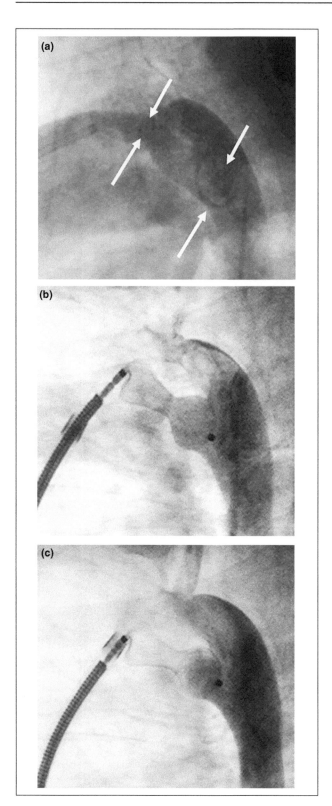

Figure 41.5
(a) Long tubular ductus with constriction at the pulmonary end; length 17 mm, aortic end diameter 8 mm, pulmonary end 4.2 mm. (b) and (c) 8/6 mm device pulled deep into the tubular ductus. The retention disk does not reconfigure fully due to limited space, but the ductus is completely occluded and the device does not protrude into the aorta.

positioning and reduces the risk of embolization. The Amplatzer Septal Occluder (ASO), having similar features, may also be used, but the 'connecting waist' or body of the device is shorter (4 mm). Apart from the large, long tubular ductus without constriction, the double disk device is also appropriate for the short, window type PDA with no ampulla. In this case the ASO is more suitable as its short waist would conform to the PDA length.[10]

If an ADO embolizes to the descending aorta it is probably unwise to remove it percutaneously through the femoral artery. For reasons mentioned above, it would be extremely difficult to catch by a snare the stainless steel sleeve housing the female screw threads. It is perhaps safer to snare the body of the device and push it back to the level of the ductal ampulla and remove it surgically with the PDA ligated at the same time. However aortic embolization and successful retrieval using a snare from the venous side have been described.[8]

Large PDA in adults

A large PDA in adult patients, although typically conical in shape, tends to be longer than the ADO length. Such large PDAs may be successfully closed with the largest of the ADO devices.[14] However, to have the proximal (pulmonary) end correctly positioned may result in the device being pulled too deep into the ductus. The retention disk thus 'stents' the PDA instead of the body of the device, causing a residual jet above it (Figure 41.7). There is the likelihood of embolization to the pulmonary artery when the device is released in this position. In this situation, a device with two retention disks like the amplatzer muscular VSD occluder (AMVO) would be more suitable.

Large PDA with advanced pulmonary vascular disease

Occasionally an adult patient may present symptomatically with severe pulmonary hypertension due to a large PDA. The PDA may not be apparent on clinical and echo examination, and only diagnosed at cardiac catheterization in the course of evaluation of pulmonary hypertension. The hemodynamic data at this stage would normally reveal advanced pulmonary vascular disease with pulmonary artery/aorta (PA:Ao) pressure ratio > 0.8 and pulmonary/systemic blood flow (Qp:Qs) ratio < 1.5:1. Surgical ligation is usually considered inappropriate. It is our institutional practice to subject the patient to trial closure with either an ASO or AMVO, where the device is deployed but not released. The patient is then stressed with dobutamine to achieve maximum heart rate while observing the hemodynamics – recording of blood gases, and aortic and pulmonary artery (PA) pressures. If they remain stable and the PA pressure does not exceed the systemic, the patient is further observed

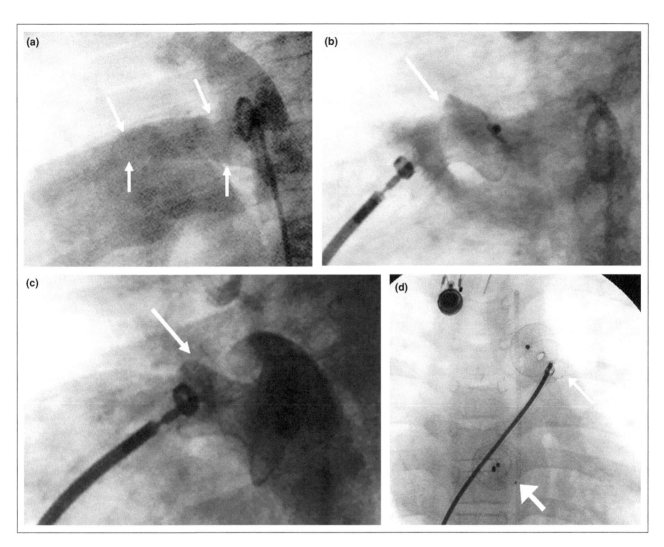

Figure 41.6
(a) Large, long tubular ductus with no constriction at the pulmonary end; length 18 mm, aortic end diameter 12 mm, pulmonary end 7 mm. (b) 12/10 mm device properly 'stents' the pulmonary end of the ductus but as the device is 8 mm in length, the retention disk is inevitably pulled deep into the PDA, as indicated by the 'bump' (arrow). The device will likely embolize to the pulmonary artery if released. (c) The device is repositioned to have the retention disk seated in the ampulla, but the pulmonary end of the ductus is not stented because the device is too short. Likelihood of embolization to the descending aorta if released. (d) Amplatzer Septal Occuluder device implanted to close this PDA (small arrow). A membranous VSD was closed prior to the PDA (large arrow).

in the intensive care unit with the cable remaining attached to the device. The patient is kept immobile under full sedation and the hemodynamics are closely monitored for 48–72 hours. If the hemodynamics and blood gases deteriorate the device is recaptured into the sheath and removed. Otherwise it is released permanently and the patient maintained on vasodilators for a long period.

Conclusion

The ADO has made transcatheter closure of moderate and large PDAs a generally safe and effective procedure. It is particularly suited to the conical-shaped duct, which is the commonest morphologic type of PDA. Its use should be limited to patients above 5 kg, as in such small, severely symptomatic infants, hemodynamic compromise may be encountered with the passage of the stiff sheath and dilator, with the additional hazard that the relatively large device may partially obstruct the aorta. For the less common ductal morphology where the PDA is long, tubular, and has no definite constriction at the pulmonary end, the relatively short ADO with only one retention disk may not be the most suitable device. The same limitation may apply in typical conical-shaped but large PDAs in adult patients because of its relative length. In both situations, the AMVO is the more suitable device. For the short window type PDA with no ampulla, the ASO is more suitable.

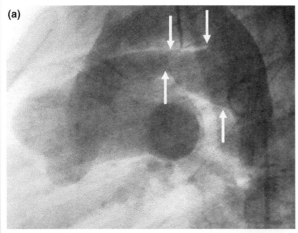

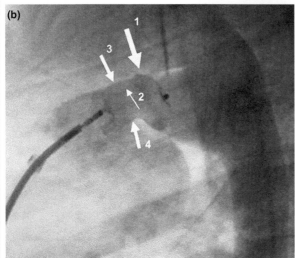

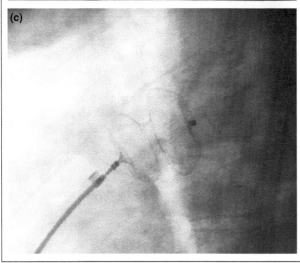

The management of adult patients with advanced pulmonary vascular disease due to a large PDA is controversial. Trial closure with ASO or AMVO and observing the hemodynamic response for up to 72 hours may have a role in this small number of patients.

References

1. Benson LN, Cowan KN. The arterial duct: its presence and patency. In: Anderson RH, Baker EJ, Macartney FJ et al, eds. Paediatric Cardiology, 2nd edition. London: Churchil Livingstone, 2002: 1405–59.
2. Hijazi ZM, Geggel RL. Results of anterograde transcatheter closure of patent ductus arteriosus using single or multiple Gianturco coils. Am J Cardiol 1994; 74: 925–9.
3. Tometzki AJP, Arnold R, Peart I et al. Transcatheter occlusion of the patent ductus arteriosus with Cook detachable coils. Heart 1996; 76: 531–4.
4. Sharafuddin MJ, Gu X, Titus JL et al. Experimental evaluation of a new self expanding patent ductus arteriosus occluder in a canine model. J Vasc Interven Radiol 1996; 7: 877–87.
5. Masura J, Walsh KP, Thanopoulous B et al. Catheter closure of moderate-large sized patent ductus arteriosus using the new Amplatzer duct occluder: immediate and short-term results. J Am Coll Cardiol 1998; 31: 878–82.
6. Bilkis AA, Alwi M, Hasri S et al. The Amplatzer duct occluder: experience in 209 patients. J Am Coll Cardiol 2001; 37: 258–61.
7. Thanopoulos BD, Hakim FA, Hiari A et al. Further experience with transcatheter closure of the patent ductus arteriosus using the Amplatzer duct occluder. J Am Coll Cardiol 2000; 35: 1016–21.
8. Faella HJ, Hijazi ZM. Closure of the patent ductus arteriosus with the Amplatzer PDA device: immediate results of the international clinical trial. Cathet Cardiovasc Interven 2000; 51: 50–4.
9. Pass RH, Hijazi ZM, Hsu DT et al. Multicenter USA Amplatzer patent ductus arteriosus occlusion device trial. J Am Coll Cardiol 2004; 44: 513–19.
10. Pedra CA, Sanches SA, Fontes VF. Percutaneous occlusion of the patent ductus arteriosus with the Amplatzer device for atrial septal defect. J Invas Cardiol 2003; 15(7): 413–17.
11. Krichenko A, Benson LN, Burrows P et al. Angiographic classification of the isolated, persistently patent ductus arteriosus and implications for percutaneous occlusion. Am J Cardiol 1989; 67: 877–80.
12. Ata JA, Arfi AM, Hussain A et al. The efficacy and safety of the Amplatzer ductal occluder in young children and infants. Cardiol Young 2005; 15: 279–85.
13. Duke C, Chan KC. Aortic obstruction caused by device occlusion of patent arterial duct. Heart 1999; 82(1): 109–11.
14. Kanter JP, Hellenbrand WE, Pass RH. Transcatheter closure of a very large patent ductus arteriosus in a pregnant woman at 22 weeks of gestation. Cathet Cardiovasc Interven 2004; 61(1): 140–3.

Figure 41.7
(a) Adult with a large conical PDA, ampulla 17 mm, narrowest diameter 7.1 mm, and length 16 mm. (b) PDA is partly 'stented' by the retention disk of ADO seen as 'bump' (thick arrow) (1)), leaving a large gap between the upper margin of the body of the device (thin arrow (2)) and upper wall of the duct (arrow (3)). Lower wall of the duct is appropriately 'stented' by the body of the ADO device (arrow (4)). (c) ASO device implanted.

42

Patent ductus arteriosus: coil occlusion

R Krishna Kumar

Introduction

Gianturco coils were originally developed for the closure of undesirable vessels in the late 1970s.[1] They have been used successfully in a variety of situations by interventional radiologists and later by pediatric cardiologists.[2,3] Initial reports of the use of Gianturco coils for the patent ductus arteriosus (PDA) were published in the early 1990s.[4] Coil occlusion is now almost universally established as a simple, safe, and effective technique for occlusion of the small PDA, which measures less than 2 or 3 mm in diameter at its narrowest point (which is usually at the site of insertion of the duct into the pulmonary artery).[5,6]

Coil occlusion of larger ducts is technically more challenging because of a greater tendency for coil embolization.[7] Various technical modifications have been suggested to reduce the risk of embolization of these coils. They include the use of detachable coils,[8] deployment of thicker (0.052 inch) coils,[9] simultaneous deployment of two or more coils,[10] snare-assisted delivery,[11] and bioptome-assisted delivery.[12–14] Occlusive devices such as the Amplatzer Duct Occluder (ADO) overcome many limitations of the coils for closure of large PDAs and allow for better control and safety. Most institutions now prefer occlusive devices for PDAs that are > 3 mm.[15,16] These devices are, however, considerably more expensive than coils and in many developing countries device closure costs substantially more than surgical closure. The bioptome-assisted coil occlusion technique has emerged as a less expensive alternative to the ADO.[13,14] With careful attention to case selection and technique it is possible to coil occlude the majority of ducts. Furthermore, in specific instances, such as in selected small infants, coil occlusion may have an advantage over the ADO. This chapter will describe case selection strategies and the coil occlusion techniques in detail for small as well as large ducts.

Anatomy

The PDA is typically shaped like an asymmetric, truncated cone with considerable variations in its size, shape, and attachment to the aorta (Figure 42.1). The narrowest part of the duct is typically close to the pulmonary arterial end of the duct. This is perhaps because of the tendency of the duct to close from its pulmonary artery (PA) end early after birth. Variations in the size of the ampulla often determine suitability for coil occlusion.[17] The ampulla in the majority of ducts is large enough to accommodate coils of appropriate size for occluding the PA end. In some instances, however, the ampulla is shallow (Figures 42.1 and 42.2) Rarely, it is absent altogether. The broader aortic end of the ampulla typically originates from the leftward aspect of the aorta. There are variations such as the duct ampulla being situated entirely to the left of the aorta (Figure 42.2). Such ducts are typically profiled in the right anterior view of the aortogram and may be completely overlapped by the aorta in the left lateral view. Some ducts, particularly the ones seen in early infancy, are tubular (Figure 42.1h). These ducts may be constricted in the middle and, in rare instances, towards the aortic end (Figure 42.2).

Pathophysiology

Unless the pulmonary vascular resistance is considerably elevated, the PDA shunts continuously from aorta to PA. The duct size and relative resistances of the systemic and pulmonary artery circuits determine the extent of flow reversal that occurs in the proximal descending aorta (Figure 42.3, see color plate section). From the standpoint of coil occlusion the flow reversal is a useful phenomenon because it can be used for angiographic definition (see below) and for deposition of the coils. The hemodynamic and, therefore,

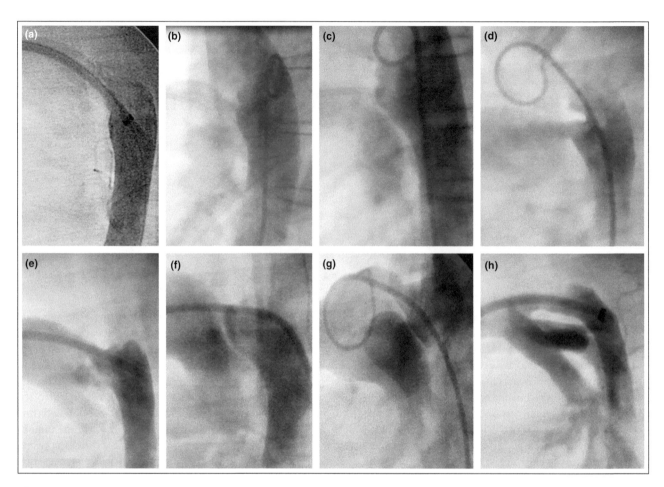

Figure 42.1
Angiograms obtained from eight patients are shown to illustrate the wide variety encountered with anatomy of the ampulla of the PDA. The angiograms are arranged according to the size of the ampulla from the most shallow (a) to the relatively generous (e, f, and g). (h) Example of a tubular duct.

clinical significance of the duct is determined by size, length (longer ducts are likely to offer greater resistance to flows), and age at presentation.

Clinical symptoms and indication for treatment

Moderate or large ducts often require attention in infancy because of symptoms of heart failure, frequent respiratory infections, and failure to thrive. The size of the duct needs to be viewed in the context of the weight and the age of the patient. A 2 mm duct can result in major hemodynamic consequences in a preterm infant weighing 2 kg or less, whereas a 4 mm duct can result in no symptoms in a 40 kg adolescent. Hemodynamically significant ducts (moderate

or large) often have symptoms, wide pulse pressure, active praecordial pulsations, and a loud continuous or systolic murmur. These ducts require closure early in infancy.

Hemodynamically insignificant or small ducts result in no symptoms. They are typically referred because of detection of a continuous or systolic murmur on routine evaluation. Such ducts need not be closed in infancy. The only indication to close these is for the prevention of endarteritis.[18] The timing and indications for closure of small ducts are controversial.[19] Most pediatric cardiologists would hesitate to close clinically silent ducts picked up by Doppler in spite of isolated case reports of ductal endarteritis in patients with a silent PDA.[20] Some pediatric cardiologists require the presence of a continuous murmur as a minimum to recommend closure. By these criteria, ducts that are very small and result only in a systolic murmur would not therefore qualify for coil closure.

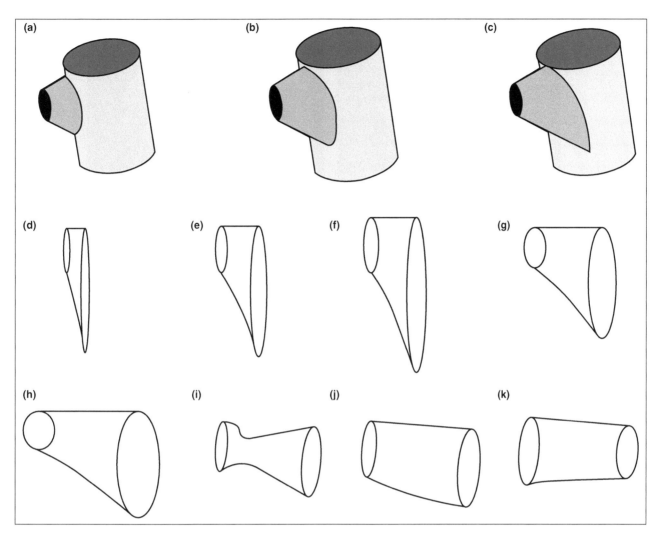

Figure 42.2

Representation of duct anatomy. The patent ductus arteriosus is in the shape of an asymmetric truncated cone. The variations in the attachment to the aorta are shown on the top panels (a–c). In (a) the duct arises from the anterior aspect of the aorta. In (c) the duct arises substantially from the leftward aspect of the aorta. Such ducts are better profiled in the right anterior oblique view. The lower panels (d–k) show representations of the ampulla. Tubular ducts are often constricted in the middle (g) or rarely towards the aortic end (k). The last example is not suited for coil occlusion.

Pre-catheter assessment (Table 42.1)

Clinical evaluation, chest X-ray, and ECG

A good clinical evaluation provides valuable clues on the likely size of the duct and pulmonary blood flow. Increased praecordial activity, bounding pulses, and grade III or louder murmur all suggest that the duct is likely to be large with a significant left to right shunt. The chest X-ray in these patients may reveal increased pulmonary blood flow and cardiac enlargement, and ECG reveals prominent left ventricular forces with prominent q waves in lateral chest leads. Clinical, X-ray, and ECG features of elevated pulmonary vascular resistance (Table 49.1) may preclude the possibility of coil occlusion.

Echocardiography

A detailed echocardiographic evaluation of the duct anatomy and physiology is a must for all patients undergoing coil occlusion. Excellent definition of anatomy is feasible in almost all infants and children and in many adults as well,

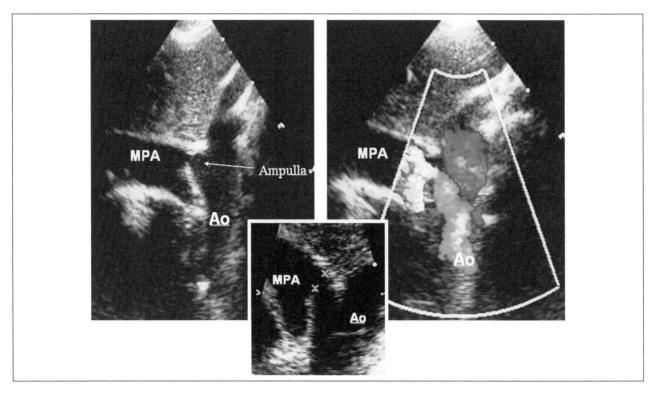

Figure 42.3

Echo definition of the patent ductus arteriosus. This is a high left parasternal view (ductal view) obtained in an infant. The duct insertion as well as the ampulla is clearly defined. Measurement of the duct insertion site is made in the magnified view (bottom insert). Note the retrograde flow of blood in the color Doppler picture (right). MPA, main pulmonary artery; Ao, aorta. (See also color plate section.)

although in many adults it may not be possible to obtain adequate views of the duct.[20] The duct diameter should be measured in a high parasternal long axial view at the point of entry into the pulmonary artery (Figures 42.3 and 42.4). The measurement must be made using the zoomed 2D echocardiographic image (Figure 42.3) and not the width of the color Doppler jet. Subtle adjustments in the transducer position and angulations are required for precise definition of the PDA at its pulmonary artery insertion. Since this measurement varies with different phases of the cardiac cycle, the maximum diameter at pulmonary artery insertion should be measured. Repeated measurements may have to be made and the most concordant measurement should be reported. The ductal ampulla is often defined in the high parasternal long axial or in the suprasternal long axis view (Figure 42.5). The ductal ampulla is considered adequate if its maximal dimension along the long axis is greater than twice the measured ductal diameter (Figure 42.5). Essentially, one needs to visualize whether a coil that is large enough to occlude the duct can occupy the ampulla without protrusion into the aorta. It is a good idea to plan the strategy for coil occlusion based on the echocardiographic anatomy (Figure 42.5).

Echocardiography provides many clues about the physiologic significance of the duct. A large duct with increased pulmonary blood flow is suggested by a left atrial and left ventricular enlargement and flow reversal in the descending thoracic and abdominal aorta. The Doppler gradients across

such a duct at end diastole are typically low (< 30 mmHg). In our experience, peak systolic Doppler gradients do not correlate well with duct size. Elevation in pulmonary vascular resistance is suggested by low velocities in both directions across the PDA together with absence of flow reversal in the descending aorta. These ducts are typically very large and coil occlusion is often not an acceptable option.

In addition to evaluation of the PDA, origins of the branch pulmonary arteries should be carefully inspected for stenosis at their origins. Any internal inconsistencies between duct size estimation and hemodynamic correlates (above) should prompt re-assessment of size through repeat measurements. For example, if the duct is measured as 2 mm in a child who has a large shunt that is clinically obvious with echocardiographic features of a large shunt, there is a distinct possibility of an error in the measurement.

Case selection

The decision on the closure strategy for PDA is determined by the following considerations:

1. duct size at its narrowest point (usually at PA insertion)
2. size of the ampulla
3. shape of the ampulla
4. age and weight of the patient.

Table 42.1 *Pre-catheter assessment of hemodynamic significance of patent ductus arteriosus*

Clinical, EKG , X-ray and echo features	Small duct	Large duct with large left to right shunt	Large duct with elevated pulmonary vascular resistance
Clinical assessment			
Pulse pressure	Normal	Wide	Normal
Precordium	Normal	Pulsatile, thrill of PDA murmur	Palpable pulmonary artery pulsations and P2
Second heart sound			
Murmur	Normal Continuous, (<3/6)	Paradoxical Continuous (<3/6) eddy sounds, apical mid-diastolic murmur	Single, loud P2 None or short systolic murmur
EKG	Normal	LV forces, 'q' in lateral chest leads	Right ventricular hypertrophy
Chest X-ray			
Heart size, contour	Normal	Enlarged, prominent LV and aorta	Normal heart size, PA prominence.
Lung vasculature	Normal	Increased	Prominent hilar vessels, peripheral pruning
Oxygen saturation and blood gas	Normal	Normal	Lower limb desaturation or low PO_2
Echocardiography			
Chamber enlargement	Mild LA, LV enlargement	Significant LA and LV enlargement	LA and LV often normal, RA and RV may be enlarged
Doppler flow across duct	Continuous with diastolic gradients >30 mmHg	Entirely left to right, low diastolic gradients (<300 mmHg)	Bidirectional, right to left during systole, left to right in diastole
Descending aortic flow	Normal or minimal flow reversal in diastole	Prominent flow reversal in diastole	Normal

For coil occlusion to be successful the coil diameters typically have to be greater than or equal to twice the smallest diameter of the duct, and the ampulla on the aortic aspect of the duct should be large enough to accommodate the coil(s) (maximum dimension ≥ twice the smallest duct diameter). A conical or funnel-shaped ampulla is best suited for coil occlusion because it allows the coil loops to pack themselves without protrusion into the aorta. Fortunately, the vast majority of ducts have this shape. Tubular ducts have a relatively small diameter at the aortic end. This may prevent some of the coil loops from entering the ampulla as the coil(s) are pulled towards the pulmonary arterial end.

The age and weight of the patient determine the diameter of the descending aorta, which needs to be large enough for the coils to form without straightening up. The maximum size of the delivery system is also determined by the age and weight of the patient. Based on these considerations, the following 'rules of thumb' can be used as approximate guides:

Adults and older children (>15 kg). It is possible to coil occlude most ducts <5 mm in adults and older children and

the size of the ampulla is seldom a major consideration. The ADO is a better option for ducts >5 mm in diameter, but coil occlusion can be attempted in institutions where costs matter. Ducts greater than 8 mm in diameter are by and large unsuitable for coil occlusion and should undergo closure using the ADO, irrespective of the size of the ampulla.

Infants and young children (5–15 kg). Ducts that are greater than 5 mm in diameter are often difficult to coil occlude irrespective of the size of the ampulla. Ducts that are 3 mm or smaller can be coil occluded even when the ampulla is small. For ducts that are 3–5 mm in diameter, the size of the ampulla matters (Figure 42.4). The maximum diameter of the ampulla should be ≥ twice the smallest duct diameter. The ADO usually works well as an alternative to coils for this category of patients except in the occasional child with a very large duct (>8 mm).

Small infants (<5 kg). This is a challenging subset of patients. In these patients, coils are often a better alternative to the conventional ADO since they do not protrude into the aorta. An important additional consideration is the size

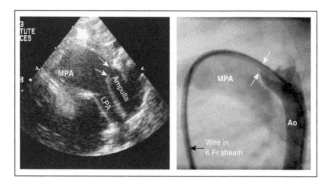

Figure 42.4
The frame on the left shows a 2D echocardiography frame (high parasternal view). An angiographic frame from the same patient in the lateral view (right frame) has been obtained by hand injection through the long sheath placed across the duct. White arrows show the pulmonary artery end of the duct. LPA, left pulmonary artery; MPA, main pulmonary artery; Ao, aorta.

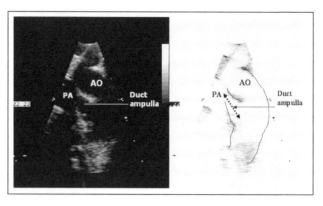

Figure 42.5
Suprasternal view of the duct ampulla. The frame on the left is an echo frame showing the duct ampulla. The pulmonary artery end of the duct may not be profiled in this view. The frame on the right is a cartoon from the same echo image. The line with arrows at its ends shows the long axis of the ampulla. Ao, aorta; PA, pulmonary artery.

of the descending aorta. In general, it is difficult to deploy coils larger than 8 mm in diameter. Therefore, ducts larger than 4 mm in diameter are usually not suited for coil occlusion irrespective of the size of the ampulla. For ducts smaller than 4 mm, the same rules (above) apply.

Very small infants and preterm newborns (<2 kg). Here the size of the delivery system is an additional concern. Typically only 4 Fr delivery systems can be used. Such systems allow a single 0.052 inch coil or two 0.038 inch coils. Coil diameters of 6 mm or more often cannot be used because of the size of the descending aorta. In these babies, ducts >3 mm in diameter should undergo surgery.

Anesthesia

Conscious sedation is usually adequate for all patients, except small infants or those with compromised airways, such as in Trisomy 21. For patients less than 10 years, intravenous ketamine can be used. Additional sedation if required can be provided using midazolam. For patients over 10 years in age, a combination of pentazocine and promethazine is preferred in our institution. Midazolam is used for additional sedation if required. However, many institutions prefer general anesthesia.

Access

For infants and young children with good echocardiographic windows arterial access may not be required at all. A venous access with a 5 or 6 Fr introducer is usually adequate initially and arterial access need not be obtained.[21]

After coil occlusion, it is usually possible to evaluate the results through echocardiography in the catheterization laboratory. The advantages of avoiding arterial access include avoiding heparin and thereby potentially accelerating occlusion of the duct, and elimination of inherent risks of arterial puncture such as bleeding and femoral artery thrombosis. If additional coils have to be delivered, it is necessary to obtain arterial access. For this purpose, a 4 Fr introducer sheath is sufficient.

Antibiotic prophylaxis

We prefer to use a single dose of a second-generation cephalosporin (cephazolin) soon after access is obtained.

Hardware

The hardware requirements for PDA coil closure using the techniques described in this chapter are listed in Table 42.2.

Hemodynamic evaluations

Pressure measurements from the right atrium (RA), right ventricle (RV), and individual branch pulmonary arteries should be recorded. The pressure in the main pulmonary artery (MPA) often tends to be spuriously high if the catheter tip is close to the duct orifice. The descending aortic pressure should be recorded after the duct is crossed. For calculation of flows and resistances, it is necessary to obtain oxygen saturations from the superior vena cava (SVC), branch

Table 42.2   *Hardware requirements for coil occlusion of patent ductus arteriosus*

Hardware item	Purpose
0.038 inch coils, 4 mm, 5 mm, 6 mm, 8 mm diameters	Smaller ducts, tubular ducts, additional coils
0.052 inch coils, 6 mm, 8 mm, 10 mm, 12 mm, 15 mm diameters	Larger ducts (> 3 mm)
Jackson detachable coils with delivery wire (5–8 mm in diameter)	For operators who prefer controlled release coils for small ducts
Multi-purpose catheter 5 Fr	Crossing the duct initially, free coil delivery
0.038 inch straight tip, Teflon coated wire	Crossing the duct initially, free coil delivery
0.038 inch glide wire	Recrossing the duct for additional coil delivery
Right coronary catheter, 4 Fr, JR 4	Delivering additional coils from the arterial route
Balkan contralateral sheath (Cook) 5.5 Fr, 6 Fr, 45 cm long	Well suited for infants and small children
Mullins sheaths, 7, 8, and 9 Fr	Older children with large ducts, 7 Fr can be used for selected infants and smaller children (> 5 kg)
Bioptomes (120 cm long), 3 and 5 Fr	3 Fr bioptome can be passed via a 4 Fr sheath and is well suited for very small infants (< 3 kg), for all other situations the 5 Fr bioptome is adequate
Amplatz gooseneck snares, 5, 10 mm	Coil retrieval
Vascular retrieval forceps (3 Fr)	Coil retrieval

pulmonary artery, and descending aorta. Again, oxygen saturations from the MPA are spuriously high and thus shunt quantification in the presence of a duct is often inaccurate.

If the pulmonary vascular resistance is elevated and there are doubts as to whether the PDA closure would reverse the pulmonary artery hypertension, it may be wise to balloon occlude the duct and measure the pulmonary artery pressures. Balloon occlusion can be accomplished by a balloon endhole catheter (a 7 Fr Swan–Ganz catheter is well suited for this purpose) passed from the venous route into the aorta. The inflated balloon is then pulled back into the duct. This may necessitate an additional venous access. Alternatively, the balloon catheter may be passed via a larger long sheath and the PA pressure can be measured from the side arm of the sheath. The systemic arterial pressure should be measured simultaneously and arterial access is therefore needed. It is also useful to obtain blood gas samples from the ascending and descending aorta. Large ducts (> 10 mm) may require balloon occlusion catheters. Such ducts are seldom suited for coil occlusion. Few data are currently available on how balloon occlusion data can be interpreted in hypertensive ducts. From our preliminary experience with 20 patients who had hypertensive ducts, it appears that a decline in PA mean and PA diastolic pressures to less than 25% of the baseline appears to predict a good long-term outcome after duct closure.

Angiography

Aortography for profiling the PDA

If arterial access is obtained, a conventional aortogram in the left lateral view and 45° right anterior oblique (RAO) views with the pigtail catheter in the proximal descending aorta positioned just distal to the ampulla usually allow

reasonable definition of the PDA (Figure 42.6). The use of a marker pigtail allows for accurate measurements of the PA end of the duct. Large volumes (1–2 ml/kg) at the maximum possible flow rates recommended for the catheter ($\cong$18 ml/s) should be used. If the pulmonary arterial end of the duct is not profiled using the conventional aortogram, the pigtail catheter may be passed across the duct and placed in the proximal descending aorta just beyond the ampulla. Rarely, temporary balloon occlusion of the descending aorta may allow better definition of the PA insertion.

Angiography when arterial access is not obtained

In our institution, we do not routinely obtain arterial access for coil occlusion of PDA in infants and small children.[15] It is still possible to obtain a satisfactory angiographic profile of the PDA without arterial access using the techniques outlined below.

Angiography before free coil delivery in small ducts

A 5 Fr multi-purpose catheter is used to cross the duct from the main pulmonary artery with the help of the straight end of a 0.038 inch guidewire. Crossing the duct is usually straightforward. Rarely, difficulty may be encountered if the duct inserts on the superior aspect of the MPA. The duct is profiled in the left lateral view with the tip of the catheter positioned within the ductal ampulla or the proximal descending aorta (Figure 42.7). The retrograde blood flow into the pulmonary artery (Figure 42.3) and proximal descending thoracic aorta often allows definition of the pulmonary artery insertion of the duct and the ampulla.

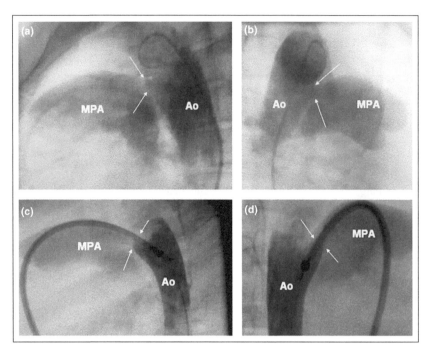

Figure 42.6
Angiograms from selected ducts. Panels (a) and (b) are from an older patient with a relatively shallow duct. Panels (c) and (d) are from an infant. (a) Left lateral view of an aortogram. The ampulla is better profiled in this view as compared to (b). In the second example, the ampulla appears larger in the right anterior oblique (RAO) view (d) as compared to the left lateral view (c).

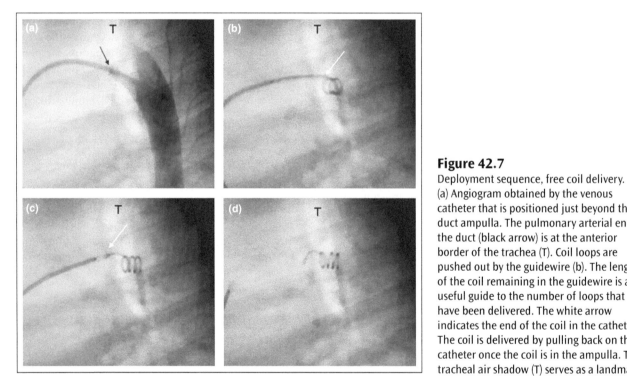

Figure 42.7
Deployment sequence, free coil delivery. (a) Angiogram obtained by the venous catheter that is positioned just beyond the duct ampulla. The pulmonary arterial end of the duct (black arrow) is at the anterior border of the trachea (T). Coil loops are pushed out by the guidewire (b). The length of the coil remaining in the guidewire is a useful guide to the number of loops that have been delivered. The white arrow indicates the end of the coil in the catheter. The coil is delivered by pulling back on the catheter once the coil is in the ampulla. The tracheal air shadow (T) serves as a landmark.

In patients with very small ducts, where the catheter completely occludes the duct, the injection has to be made in the duct ampulla close to the pulmonary artery insertion. The relation of the ductal ampulla and its pulmonary artery insertion to the tracheal air shadow should be noted. This injection may be repeated in the 45° RAO view if the ampulla overlaps the aorta.

Angiography before bioptome-assisted coil delivery

After obtaining baseline hemodynamic information, a long sheath passed via the femoral vein is positioned across the PDA in the descending aorta over a 0.038 inch guidewire (Figure 42.6c,d). Guidelines for selecting the size of the long

Table 42.3   *Coil combination and sheath sizes for bioptome-assisted occlusion of patent arterial ducts > 2.5 mm*

Duct size (mm)	Suggested coil combination[a]	Minimum size of the long sheath (Fr)
2.5–3	Two 0.038 inch 6 mm–6 cm coils or a single 0.052 inch 6 mm–6 cm coil	4[b]
3–3.5	Two 0.038 inch 8 mm–8 cm coils or a single 0.052 inch 8 mm–8 cm coil	4[b]
3.5–4	A combination of one 0.052 inch 8 mm–8 cm coil with one 0.038 inch 8 mm–8 cm coil	5.5
4–4.5	Two 0.052 inch 8 mm–8 cm coils	7
4.5–5	Three 0.052 inch 8 mm–8 cm coils or one 10 mm, 10 cm with two 8 mm–8 cm coils	8
5–6	Four coils: two 0.052 inch, 12 mm–15 cm coils, and two 0.052 inch, 10 mm–10 cm coils	9
6–8	Five coils: two 0.052 inch, 15 mm–15 cm coils, two 0.052 inch ,12 mm–15 cm coils, one 0.052 inch 10 mm–10 cm coil	9
>8	Usually not suited for coil occlusion	

[a]Coil lengths have not been specified, usually coil lengths (in cm) that are same as the coil diameters (in mm) are adequate. For PDAs with a shallow ampulla in infants and small children, however, coil turns have to be cut to ensure that the coil turns fit into the ampulla.
[b]3 Fr bioptome will need to be used if a 4 Fr sheath is to be used. For all other situations a 5 Fr bioptome is adequate.

sheath are shown in Table 42.3. The 45 cm Balkin contralateral introducer sheath (Cook Inc., Bloomington, IN) can be used for the PDA in infants and small children. This sheath has a shape that is well suited for the PDA and comes in sizes from 5.5 to 7 Fr. For small infants (<3 kg) with ducts <3.5 mm, a 4 Fr long sheath (>25 cm long, Cook) can be used (Table 42.3). When two or more 0.052 inch coils are to be simultaneously delivered, a 7 Fr contralateral or 8–9 Fr Mullins sheath (Cook Inc.) is used (Table 42.3). Once the sheath is in the descending aorta, the dilator of the long sheath is removed. With the guidewire in place, the sheath is withdrawn until the aortic end of the duct ampulla. A hand injection of 5–10 ml of contrast into the sheath in the lateral and 45° RAO views usually allows excellent definition of the duct ampulla and measurement of the duct diameter at pulmonary insertion (Figure 42.6).

Measurements

The maximum diameter of the pulmonary artery (PA) end of the PDA should be measured. The lateral view is usually better suited for this purpose. The diameter of the pulmonary arterial end of the duct varies with the cardiac cycle and the largest diameter should be identified through careful frame-by-frame evaluation.

Ductal spasm

Ductal spasm is not infrequent in infants and may be provoked by attempts to cross it, although on occasion it may occur spontaneously. This may be a justification for aortography routinely in all patients prior to coil occlusion, especially if accurate echocardiographic measurements are not available. Figure 42.8 shows an example of ductal spasm. In our institution, we prefer to use the echocardiographic measurement of the duct size to guide the choice of coil diameter unless the angiographic measurement is larger.

Deployment technique

Free coil delivery (Figure 42.7)

This is essentially applicable for the small duct (<2.5 mm in diameter). A Gianturco coil (Cook Inc., Bloomington, IN) with a diameter of at least twice the measured duct diameter is chosen. Typically, this is a 5 mm diameter coil. The length of the coil is determined by the size of the ampulla. Shorter coils, such as 3–4 cm long, are chosen for patients with a relatively shallow ampulla to prevent coil loops from protruding into the aortic lumen. We prefer coil deployment from the venous route as it allows better control of coil deployment than the arterial route (Figure 42.7). The technique for arterial delivery of coils is described below in the section on 'delivery of additional coils.'

The duct is crossed from the pulmonary artery using a 5 Fr multi-purpose catheter. After the catheter is advanced into the descending aorta, it should be flushed to clear the contrast in it. The coil is introduced into the catheter and advanced to its tip. Between one and a half to two turns of the coil are released into the descending aorta. The coil/catheter assembly is then pulled together as one unit to the mouth of the ampulla using the tracheal air shadow as the visual landmark for the position of the ampulla and pulmonary arterial insertion. Pulsatile flow in the aorta causes oscillatory movement of the coil turns in the descending aorta. As the coil is pulled towards the pulmonary end of the ductal ampulla, abrupt cessation of oscillations of the coil occurs and this can be used as an indicator that the coil is positioned in the duct ampulla. At this point additional turns of the coil should be delivered. The catheter should then be pulled back into the pulmonary artery when less than half a turn remains in the catheter. The coil should be released by gently pulling back the catheter into the MPA (Figure 42.7). Three minutes after successful release of the coil, echocardiography should be performed with color flow imaging in the high parasternal view for assessment of

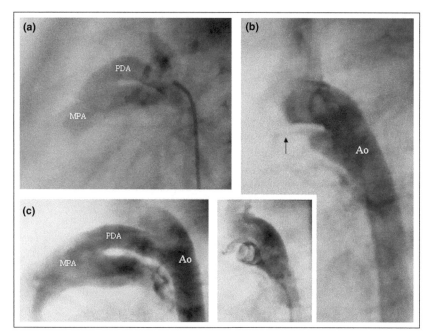

Figure 42.8
These images show an example of transient but dramatic spasm of a large patent arterial duct in an 8-month-old infant. (a) Lateral angiogram showing the large tubular patent arterial duct (PDA), opacifying main pulmonary artery (MPA), and its branches. (b) Aortogram showing the duct to be severely constricted in the middle (black arrow) and non-opacification of the MPA. (c) Repeat angiogram showing completely opened up arterial duct. The duct was coil occluded (insert).

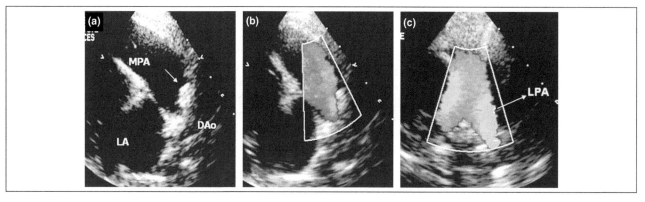

Figure 42.9
Echocardiographic assessment after free coil delivery. (a) High parasternal view of a duct after coil occlusion. (b) The color Doppler picture in the same view. (c) Short-axis view with the same transducer position. It is important to demonstrate a laminar flow in the origin of the left pulmonary artery (LPA). (See also color plate section.)

residual flow across the duct as well as turbulence at the origin of the left pulmonary artery (Figure 42.9). If there is a clearly defined color jet of residual flow at 3 minutes, additional coils (see below) may need to be delivered. For patients with small, poorly defined residual color flow, imaging can be repeated on the table every few minutes. If the flow shows a tendency to diminish over the next 10 minutes, catheters may be removed.

Detachable coils

To decrease the incidence of coil embolization, the controlled-release modified Jackson detachable coils (Cook PDA coils) are a useful but more expensive alternative to free coils for small ducts. The spring coil (similar in shape and size to the Gianturco coils) has a central lumen through which the delivery wire or mandrill is passed. Interlocking screws between the spring coil and the delivery wire help in holding the coil until the correct position is achieved in the duct. The delivery wire is introduced into the sleeve housing the coil and rotated clockwise until the screw locks with the coil. The coil is deployed in a manner identical to that of free coils but by withdrawal of the mandrill, which allows coil loops to form. The coil is released by unscrewing the wire (counterclockwise rotation) once the position is deemed satisfactory.[8]

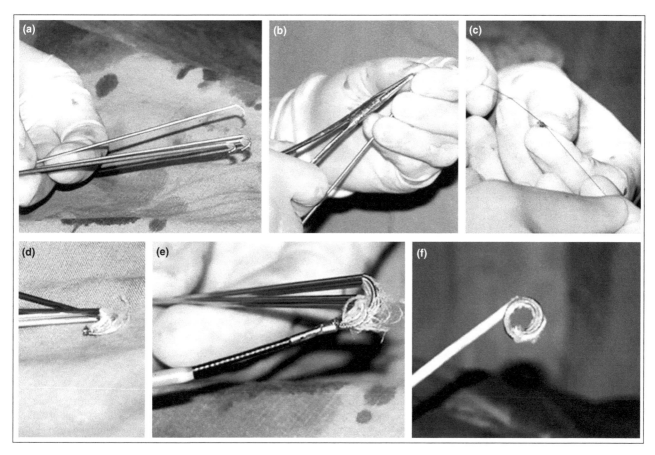

Figure 42.10

Coil preparation for bioptome-assisted coil occlusion. This sequence shows the preparation of four coils for simultaneous deployment in a 6 mm duct. The deployment sequence is shown in Figure 42.12. A small segment of each coil is brought out of the steel tubing (a). The ends of the coil are stretched out using a hemostat (b). The stretched out ends are secured together using a 3-0 prolene suture (c and d). A 5 Fr bioptome is passed through a short (8 Fr) introducer (e); the secured end of the coil is held by the jaws of the bioptome and pulled into the introducer (f).

Bioptome-assisted coil delivery

Coil selection (Table 42.3)

Gianturco coils (Cook Inc.) with diameters at least twice the measured duct diameters at the PA end are chosen. We prefer to use the echocardiographic measurement to guide coil selection unless the duct diameter by angiography is larger than the echo measurement. It is preferable to use simultaneously delivered multiple coils for ducts that measure more than 3–3.5 mm in diameter. This usually results in a higher immediate occlusion rate. For ducts >3.5 mm in diameter, one or more 0.052 inch coils should be used. For ducts >4.5 mm in diameter, it may be necessary to deliver up to three coils simultaneously, and for ducts >6 mm in diameter, four coils may have to be delivered simultaneously. Ducts >8 mm in diameter are best closed by the ADO. Suggested coil diameters and coil combinations for various duct sizes are shown in Table 42.3.

Coil preparation (Figure 42.10)

Coils are housed in steel tubing with a black sleeve at one of its ends. The coil is pushed out by a wire introduced from the end with the black sleeve. The round ball at the tip of the coil that emerges from the tube is stretched out by about 2 mm using a hemostat. If multiple coils are used, the stretched-out ends are secured together using a 3-0 prolene suture. A 5 Fr 120 cm long bioptome (Cook, Inc.) is passed via a short introducer sheath (one size smaller than the long sheath used for deployment of the coils in the PDA). The secured end of the coils is grasped by the bioptome. It is important to ensure that the coil is firmly held by the jaws of the bioptome. The coils are then pulled into the short sheath by the bioptome. The short sheath essentially serves as an introducer for delivering the coils into the long sheath that is previously positioned across the duct. If it is anticipated that coil turns would not fit into the ampulla, between one-half and two coil turns should be cut with a scissor. The cut end of the coil should be inspected for sharp edges and a few more millimeters of the coil can be

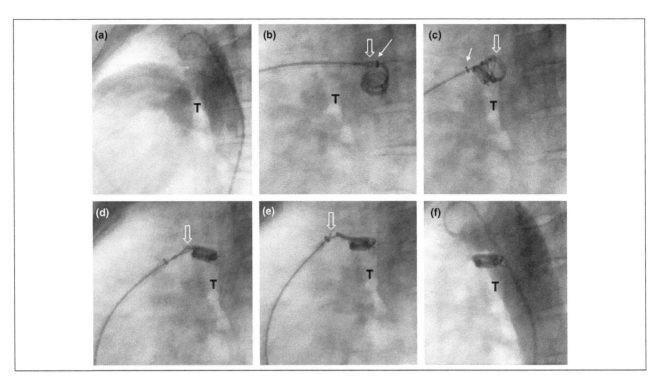

Figure 42.11
Bioptome-assisted simultaneous deployment of multiple coils. (a) Aortogram in the left lateral view. The duct measures 6 mm. Fousr coils (two 12 mm 0.052 inch coils and two 8 mm 0.038 inch coils) are simultaneously held by a 5 Fr bioptome and brought out of a 9 Fr long sheath placed across the duct in the descending aorta (b). The block arrow points at the jaws of the bioptome and the smaller arrow indicates the tip of the sheath. The assembly is pulled back until the tip of the sheath is in the MPA. This is recognized by a decline in pressure in the side-arm of the long sheath. This event coincides with the coils moving into the ampulla. The coils start to compact at this stage (c). The bioptome is then gently pulled into the MPA (d) and the jaws of the bioptome are opened after a small length (< half a turn) of coil protrudes into the MPA (e). (f) Angiogram obtained 3 minutes after release. The tracheal air shadow (T) serves as an additional guide for the coil positioning.

cut to ensure smoothness. Cutting off the end of the coil is often necessary in infants.

Deployment of coils (Figure 42.11)

The coils are delivered via the long sheath all the way and one to two loops are extruded out of the tip of the sheath in the descending thoracic aorta. The side arm of the sheath should be connected to the pressure transducer. The entire assembly is pulled back towards the pulmonary artery until the sheath tip is just beyond the duct ampulla. Coils are almost entirely brought out of the sheath. Typically the retrograde flow across the duct pushes the entire coil mass into the ampulla. There is an abrupt cessation of oscillatory movements together with compaction of the coils as they enter the duct ampulla. All coil turns should compact in the ampulla. This is sometimes difficult to ensure when coil diameters are very large or when more than four coils are simultaneously delivered. The tracheal air shadow serves as an additional landmark to guide the coil placement. The

relationship of the tracheal air shadow to the duct ampulla and the pulmonary arterial end of the duct is previously identified in the ductal angiogram. Once the coils compact in the ampulla, the sheath is slowly pulled back until the pressure recorded from the side-arm of the sheath declines, indicating that the tip of the sheath is now in the pulmonary artery. At this point, the bioptome is slowly pulled back until a small part of the coil protrudes into the pulmonary artery. Some resistance is felt at this stage. There is further compaction of the coil turns in the ampulla. Efforts should be made, as far as possible, to leave less than half a turn to protrude into the pulmonary artery. Contrast injection through the side arm can be made to ensure that the coils are correctly positioned and there is free flow into the branch pulmonary arteries. The jaw of the bioptome should be released soon after a satisfactory position is obtained. Attempts to hold the coils for longer periods should be avoided because this often results in one or more coil turns being inadvertently pulled into the pulmonary artery. In the event that the coils are too small for the duct, one or more turns or the entire coil mass can be pulled into the pulmonary artery by

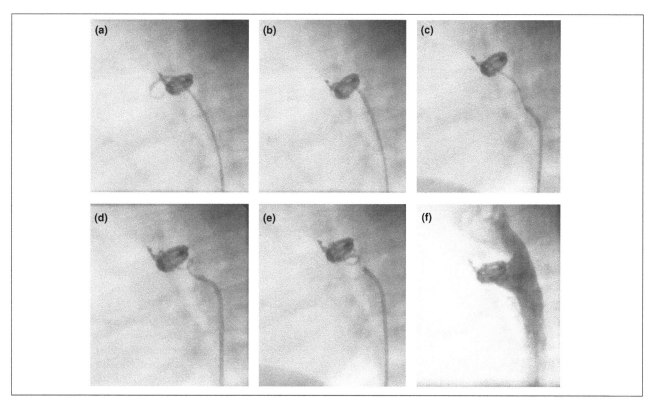

Figure 42.12

Deployment sequence for additional coil via the arterial route. Half a turn of the coil is brought out of the catheter in the pulmonary artery (a). The catheter is pulled back until it is flush with the rest of the coils (b). The catheter is then slowly withdrawn, keeping a constant length of the coil loop in the pulmonary arterial end of the duct (c). Once a sufficient length of the coil is exposed (enough to form one or more loops), the assembly is advanced into the ampulla (d) and the rest of the coil is delivered (e). The final angiogram is shown in (f).

the bioptome. The coils can be withdrawn into the sheath and redeployed after addition of another larger coil to the coil mass. An echocardiogram or aortogram (if arterial access was obtained) should be performed after 3 minutes. Additional 0.038 inch coils are delivered if a well defined jet of residual flow was demonstrable by either color Doppler or angiography (see below). Small diffuse whiffs of flow often disappear over the next 12–24 hours.

Delivery of additional coils (Figure 42.12)

Delivery of additional coils is contemplated whenever there is an unacceptable amount of residual flow (a clearly defined color jet on Doppler, or filling of the entire MPA on angiography). It is advisable to obtain arterial access if the duct needs to be recrossed. A 4 Fr introducer sheath can be used for this purpose. Heparin needs to be administered at this stage. The duct is crossed from the arterial end using a 0.035 inch glide wire (Terumo or Roadrunner, Cook) and a 4 Fr right coronary catheter. The regular Teflon-coated

guidewire should not be used because of the possibility of the Dacron fibers of the previously deployed coils getting entangled with the wire. Once the wire is across the duct, the catheter should be gently advanced over the wire. Some resistance is usually encountered when the catheter crosses the previously deployed coils. The catheter position should be confirmed through pressure measurement or contrast injection. Irrespective of the initial size of the duct, additional coils should be 5 mm in diameter. The length of the coil is determined by the size of the ampulla. In general, 5 cm long coils work well as additional coils in most situations. The technique of coil delivery from the arterial route is different from the venous route. Half a turn of the coil is brought out of the tip of the 4 Fr catheter positioned in the MPA across the duct. The catheter is slowly pulled back until the protruding half turn reaches the PA end of the duct. The coil is then delivered by slowly withdrawing the catheter while keeping the guidewire in the catheter in close contact with the coil. Catheter withdrawal tends to pull the protruding coil out of the MPA and guidewire advancement may result in excessive coil protrusion. Coil delivery has to be accomplished in small steps, ensuring at all times that the coil length protruding out into the MPA is kept constant at

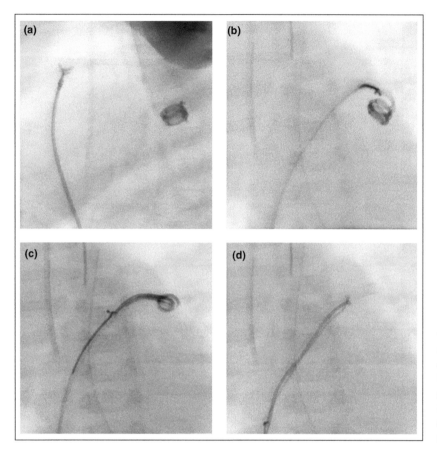

Figure 42.13
Retrieval sequence after embolization into the left pulmonary artery. Two coils were used to close a large duct in an infant. These coils embolized as soon as the jaws of the bioptome were opened into the LPA (a). The sutured ends of the coils have been grasped by a snare (b) and withdrawn into a long sheath in the proximal left pulmonary artery (c and d).

half a turn until a substantial length of coil is exposed out of the catheter. Advancing the catheter towards the ampulla usually results in formation of coil turns that should be positioned in the ampulla. Hand injections of contrast 3 minutes after coil delivery should be made to assess residual flows.

Troubleshooting

Difficulty in crossing the duct from the pulmonary arterial end

This is relatively uncommon. Difficulties may be occasionally encountered in adult patients and in ducts inserting onto the proximal MPA on its superior aspect. These ducts may be crossed from the aortic end using a right coronary or multi-purpose catheter. A guidewire can be passed through this catheter and its tip can be held with a snare passed from the venous catheter. The venous catheter is simply advanced through the PDA while holding the wire tip.

Unsatisfactory coil position in the PDA

This may result from excessive deployment of the coil turns in either the aortic or pulmonary end of the PDA. With

excessive deployment at the aortic end, aortic embolization is likely, especially if the coil turns oscillate with pulsatile aortic flows. Rarely the coil turns may protrude into the aorta sufficiently to result in a gradient in the descending aorta. Excessive coil turns in the pulmonary artery may result in stenosis of the left pulmonary artery at its origin. If the coil position is deemed unsatisfactory, the coils should be retrieved (below) and redeployed.

Embolization to the branch pulmonary arteries (Figure 42.13)

Typically, this happens soon after coil release. The dislodged coils usually embolize to the proximal right or left pulmonary arteries if they are large and if multiple coils are used. Single coils usually embolize distally to smaller branches. There is no need to panic because hemodynamic instability does not usually result from the event. The long sheath should be retained in the MPA. A 4 Fr multi-purpose catheter or the 4 Fr snare catheter should be passed via the long sheath and positioned near the embolized coil mass with the help of a glide wire. Small contrast injections in multiple views allow precise determination of the vessel into which the coil has embolized. An Amplatz gooseneck snare (5 mm for children and small vessel embolization, 10 mm for other situations) should be used to grasp the coil

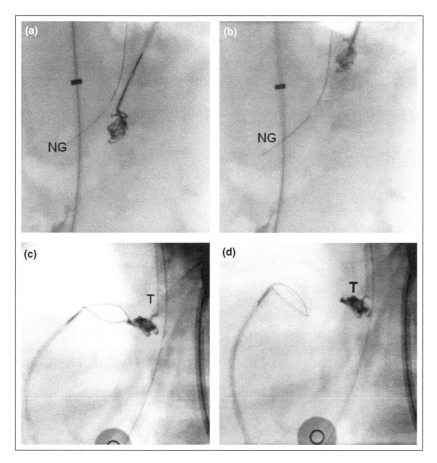

Figure 42.14
Retrieval sequence after embolization into the descending aorta. The snare catheter is introduced via the femoral vein and advanced into the descending aorta via the duct. The sutured end of the coil is grasped by the snare (a) and withdrawn (b) until the coil mass is firmly anchored in the duct ampulla (c). The snare is released after ensuring a secure position (d). NG, nasogastric tube; T, tracheal air shadow.

tip. When multiple coils have been used for PDA closure, it is important to hold the coils at the sutured end. The coils must be captured into the long sheath in the pulmonary artery because it is important to prevent the coil mass from being entangled in the tricuspid valve tensor apparatus.

Embolization to the descending thoracic aorta (Figure 42.14)

When coil(s) embolize into the aorta, the duct should be immediately recrossed with a 5 Fr multi-purpose catheter or snare catheter. A 10 mm Amplatz gooseneck snare (Microvena, MN) should be used to hold the end of the coil(s) and the same coil(s) can be deployed in the duct once again as the catheter is pulled back towards the MPA.

Loss of grip on the coil mass

The jaws of the bioptome may sometimes lose their grip on the coil mass when coils are being pulled back into the long sheath after an initial unsatisfactory deployment. A variable part of the coil remains in the sheath. Attempts to recapture the coils with the bioptome are unlikely to succeed and the coils may get pushed out of the sheath. Similarly, attempts

to snare the coils also may not work because the snare loop may not open inside the sheath. A 3 Fr vascular retrieval forceps (Cook) works well in this situation. The tip of the vascular retrieval forceps has a short (3 cm), soft guidewire that can be positioned adjacent to the coil tip in the sheath. The jaws of the forceps open adequately enough to grasp the coil tip and retrieve the coil mass.

Inability to release the coil after the bioptome jaws are opened

Occasionally the coil tip remains in the jaws after they are opened. The coils can be released by slow rotation of the bioptome with the jaws open. Alternatively, advancing the long sheath to the jaws of the bioptome helps in the release of the coil.

Hemolysis from residual flow

Hemolysis is a rare but serious complication of coil occlusion.[22–24] For hemolysis to occur, there often has to be clearly defined residual flow at the end of the procedure together with an audible murmur. Of 992 patients who underwent PDA coil occlusion at our institution since 1998, 7 patients (age 6 weeks to 64 years) developed overt hemolysis. All had large ducts and residual flows after the procedure. The occurrence of hemolysis correlated significantly with both age and duct size. Hemolysis was associated with a fall in hemoglobin of 3–6 g/100 ml (3 patients), jaundice (3), and renal failure (1). Hemolysis subsided spontaneously in 2 patients and additional coils had to be deployed in 3 patients. Once hemolysis is established, it is often difficult to eliminate flows and many additional coils may be required. It is therefore important to be aggressive and early intervention should be considered, if residual flows are significant. In our series, one 6-week-old infant continued to have significant flow and ongoing hemolysis after three additional coils were deployed in two sittings. The hemolysis in this infant only resolved after exchange transfusion.

Post-procedure management

The patient may be sent home 6–8 hours after the procedure once recovery from sedation or anesthesia is complete, especially if arterial access has not been used.[19] For children in whom arterial access has been obtained, we choose to keep them overnight. We consider it mandatory to obtain an echocardiogram just prior to discharge for residual flows across the PDA, LPA turbulence, and aortic flows and ventricular function. A small fraction of patients develop varying degrees of left ventricular dysfunction immediately after duct closure. We suggest antibiotic prophylaxis for endocarditis 6 months after the procedure. We recommend follow-up echocardiography 3 months after the procedure and yearly thereafter.

Long term concerns

Compatibility with magnetic resonance (MR) imaging

The conventional stainless steel coils are not MR compatible and likely to produce artifacts during imaging. Most manufacturers have started to make coils using materials that are MR compatible. The 0.052 inch coils are still made of stainless steel. This is an important limitation that needs to be overcome by manufacturers in the future.

Stenosis of the left pulmonary artery origin

It is important, particularly in infants, to avoid excess coil protrusion into the left pulmonary artery. Both after initial deployment and during follow-up the LPA flows should be carefully evaluated by color Doppler.

Residual flows and recanalization

Residual flows at 24 hours may occasionally persist. In addition, a small proportion of completely occluded ducts (0.3% in our experience) may re-canalize. The indication for repeat coil occlusion is not clear. We recommend coil occlusion if a murmur is audible.

Acknowledgements

The author wishes to acknowledge Dr BRJ Kannan, Dr SR Anil, Dr K Sivakumar, and Dr Balu Vaidyanathan for their inputs that have helped refine the technique; Arun and the catheter laboratory staff for their assistance with illustrations; and Dr Prakash Kamath for reviewing the manuscript.

References

1. Anderson JH, Wallace S, Gianturco C. Transcatheter intravascular coil occlusion of experimental arteriovenous fistulas. Am J Roentgenol 1977; 129: 795–8.
2. Fuhrman BP, Bass JL, Castaneda-Zuniga W et al. Coil embolization of congenital thoracic vascular anomalies in infants and children. Circulation 1984; 70: 285–9.
3. O'Halpin D, Legge D, MacErlean DP. Therapeutic arterial embolisation: report of five years' experience. Clin Radiol 1984; 35: 85–93.
4. Lloyd TR, Fedderly R, Mendelsohn AM, et al. Transcatheter occlusion of patent ductus arteriosus with Gianturco coils. Circulation 1993; 88: 1412–20.
5. Magee AG, Huggon IC, Seed PT et al. Association for European Cardiology Transcatheter coil occlusion of the arterial duct; results of the European Registry. Eur Heart J 2001; 22: 1817–21.
6. Hijazi ZM, Geggel RL. Results of antegrade transcatheter closure of patent ductus arteriosus using single or multiple Gianturco coils. Am J Cardiol 1994; 74: 925–9.
7. Hijazi ZM, Geggel RL. Transcatheter closure of large patent ductus arteriosus (> or = 4 mm) with multiple Gianturco coils. Heart 1996; 76: 536–40.
8. Tometzki AJP, Arnold R, Peart N et al. Transcatheter closure of patent ductus arteriosus with Cook detachable coils. Heart 1996; 76: 531–5.
9. Owada CY, Teitel DF, Moore P. Evaluation of Gianturco coils for closure of large (> or = 3.5 mm) patent ductus arteriosus. J Am Coll Cardiol 1997; 30: 856–62.
10. De Wolf D, Verhaaren H, Matthys D. Simultaneous delivery of two patent arterial duct coils via one venous sheath. Heart 1997; 78: 201–2.
11. Sommer RJ, Gutirrez A, Lai WW, Mullins CE. Use of preformed nitinol snare to improve transcatheter coil delivery in occlusion of patent ductus arteriosus. Am J Cardiol 1994; 74: 834–9.
12. Grifka RG, Jones TK. Transcatheter closure of large PDA using 0.052 inch Gianturco coils: controlled delivery using a bioptome catheter through a 4 French sheath. Cathet Cardiovasc Interven 2000; 49: 301–6.
13. Kumar RK, Krishnan MN, Venugopal K et al. Bioptome-assisted simultaneous delivery of multiple coils for closure of the large PDA. Cathet Cardiovasc Interven 2001; 54: 95–100.
14. Kumar RK, Anil SR, Philip A, Sivakumar K. Bioptome-assisted coil occlusion of moderate–large patent arterial ducts in infants and small children. Cathet Cardiovasc Interven 2004; 62: 266–71.

15. Masura J, Walsh KP, Thanapoulos B et al. Catheter closure of moderate to large-sized patent ductus arteriosus using the new Amplatzer duct occluder: immediate and short-tern results. J Am Coll Cardiol 1998; 31: 878–82.

16. Grifka RG, Vincent JA, Nihill MR et al. Transcatheter patent ductus arteriosus closure in an infant using the Gianturco– Grifka vascular occlusion device. Am J Cardiol 1996; 78: 721–3.

17. Krichenko A, Benson LN, Burrows P et al. Angiographic classification of the isolated, persistently patent ductus arteriosus and implications for percutaneous catheter occlusion. Am J Cardiol 1989; 63: 877–80.

18. Sadiq M, Latif F, Ur-Rehman A. Analysis of infective endarteritis in patent ductus arteriosus. Am J Cardiol 2004; 93: 513–15.

19. Thilen U, Astrom-Olsson K. Does the risk of infective endarteritis justify routine patent ductus arteriosus closure? Eur Heart J 1997; 18: 364–6.

20. Ozkokeli M, Ates M, Uslu N, Akcar M. Pulmonary and aortic valve endocarditis in an adult patient with silent patent ductus arteriosus. Jpn Heart J 2004; 45: 1057–61.

21. Anil SR, Sivakumar K, Kumar K. Coil occlusion of the small patent ductus arteriosus without arterial access. Cardiol Young 2002; 12: 51–6.

22. Anil SR, Sivakumar K, Philip A et al. Management strategies for hemolysis after transcatheter closure of the patent arterial duct. Cathet Cardiovasc Interven 2003; 59: 538–43.

23. Perez Rodriguez MJ, Quero Jimenez MC, Herraiz Sarachaga I et al. Intravascular hemolysis following percutaneous occlusion of the ductus arteriosus. Rev Esp Cardiol 1999; 52: 449–50.

24. Henry G, Danilowicz D, Verma R. Severe hemolysis following partial coil-occlusion of patent ductus arteriosus. Cathet Cardiovasc Diagn 1996; 39: 410–12.

43

Aorto-pulmonary window

Ramesh Arora

Introduction

Aortopulmonary window (APW) is an abnormal communication between the ascending aorta and the main pulmonary artery, just above two normally formed semilunar valves. It is the rarest of the four types of septal defects and accounts for approximately 0.15% of all congenital cardiac defects.[1] Just one or two neonates present with this problem in a given year.[2] It may occur as an isolated lesion but is more commonly associated with other cardiovascular anomalies such as transposition of great arteries, tetralogy of Fallot, and interrupted aortic arch.[3,4] Complex APW accounts for about 25% of all patients.

APW causes a significant systemic to pulmonary artery shunt at the arterial level similar to a large patent ductus arteriosus leading to congestive heart failure, failure to thrive, and the development of pulmonary artery hypertension.[5] The prognosis of uncorrected aortopulmonary window is poor, with 40% of the infants dying during the first year of life. A substantial proportion of survivors die from congestive heart failure in childhood. Closure is indicated at the time of diagnosis to prevent the development of irreversible pulmonary vascular disease. However, owing to the rarity of this entity, reports on treatment and outcome are limited to a relatively small group of patients.[4,6]

Today, most centers agree that surgical treatment of APW should be performed as early as possible after birth.[7] If the diagnosis is made later in life, operability is determined by assessment of pulmonary arterial resistance during cardiac catheterization,[3,4,6] however, at an older age even in the presence of reversible pulmonary vascular resistance, repair of APW may not alter the development of severe pulmonary vascular disease later in life.[4]

Since the first successful repair of APW by Gross in 1952,[8] several surgical techniques have been used, from less invasive simple ligation or division without cardiopulmonary bypass to patch closure of the defect through great vessels under direct vision using cardiopulmonary bypass and arresting the heart. In the past, without echocardiography, simple ligation/division of APW carried a relatively high complication rate (recanalization, bleeding, pulmonary artery narrowing) due to inadequate pre-operative definition of the defect morphology, combined with necessary dissection around the APW that led to a high risk of entering the defect and bleeding.[4] At present, division of APW is reserved for the simple types of relatively small size defect located at a safe distance from the branch pulmonary arteries and semilunar valves. With the introduction of occlusion devices, it may be possible to close such a defect by transcatheter closure, attempted for the first time for a residual defect by Stamato et al.[9]

An APW is the result of malformation in the division of the aorto-pulmonary trunk during embryogenesis. This defect can also show various sizes and locations. Several classifications have been proposed based on the pathologic[10] and angiographic anatomy,[11] but these have been modified by Ho and associates[12] to be more useful for interventional cardiologists considering transcatheter device closure of this defect. They kept the basic terminology from Mori and associates,[11] with additional description:[12]

Type I. These are proximal defects located between the ascending aorta and the main pulmonary artery, just above the sinus of Valsalva a few millimeters above the semilunar valves, i.e., having little inferior rim separating the APW from the semilunar valves. Genetically these are due to incomplete septation of the aorto-pulmonary trunk.

Type II. Distal defects are located in the uppermost portion of the ascending aorta and the origin of the right pulmonary artery, having a well formed inferior rim but little superior rim. These are due to abnormal migration of the sixth aortic arch.

Type III. Total defects are called confluent defects with little superior and inferior rims. They are the result of unequal septation of the aorto-pulmonary trunk or truncus arteriosus.

Type IV. Intermediate defects with adequate superior and inferior rims are the ones most suitable for possible device closure.

Two-dimensional (2D) and color Doppler echocardiography have facilitated the diagnosis. In transthoracic studies, communication between the aorta and pulmonary artery

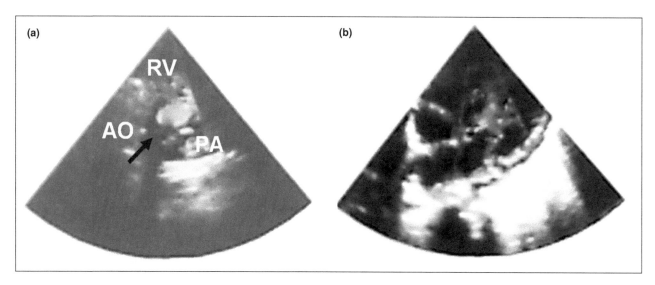

Figure 43.1
Two-dimensional echo and Doppler color flow imaging in the high parasternal short-axis view in a 2-year-old with severe pulmonary artery hypertension. (a) Showing APW defect with low velocity color flow; (b) after oxygen inhalation – high velocity color flow (arrow). AO, aorta; PA, pulmonary artery; RV, right ventricle. (See also color plate section.)

can be best visualized in the high parasternal short-axis views with cranial angulation.[13] Not only the size and the location but its relationship to the surrounding structures such as pulmonary valve, origin of the right pulmonary artery, and left coronary artery can be assessed. Moreover, the pressures in the pulmonary artery can be estimated. However, if the operator is not alert to the possibility of APW, the findings may be misinterpreted.[14] The high pulmonary artery pressure and pulmonary vascular resistance results in a low velocity flow across the defect, which is difficult to detect with color flow imaging. Exposing the patient to high fractional concentration of oxygen in a hood for several minutes may decrease pulmonary vascular resistance and thereby increase left to right shunting, which leads to a better Doppler signal (Figure 43.1). With the availability of these anatomic and physiologic parameters of APW by non-invasive techniques, the feasibility of non-surgical closure can be decided. Cardiac catheterization should be performed only if the morphology cannot otherwise be defined or transcatheter closure is to be attempted.

Materials and methods: transcatheter closure

Inclusion criteria

The various concerns about the procedure of transcatheter closure in APW are the complexity and the applicability in selected groups as anatomic delineation in relation to semilunar valves and coronary/pulmonary arteries is essential. The selection criteria will vary depending upon the choice and availability of the particular device in an institution. For the choice of the Amplatzer duct occluder, which has retention skirts of only 2 mm on either side, the guidelines are:[15]

1. Location of the defect in the middle of the two great arteries at least 5 mm from the origin of the left coronary artery and the right and left main pulmonary arteries.
2. Distance from the center of the defect to the ostium of the left coronary artery and the origin of the right pulmonary > 50% of the required device size.
3. No anomalous origin of the right or left pulmonary arteries from the aorta.

Procedure

After informed consent, cardiac catheterization is performed under light sedation and local anesthesia. By the percutaneous Seldinger approach, the right femoral vein and artery are cannulated with hemostatic sheaths. Unfractionated heparin 80–100 units/kg is administered intravenously. Pressure data and blood samples for oximetry are obtained from all right and left heart chambers. The pulmonary to systemic flow ratio is calculated. Aortic root angiography in the shallow left anterior oblique (20 to 30°) view with cranial angulation (about 15°) and in the shallow right anterior oblique (10°) view is performed using a pigtail catheter to define the defect (Figure 43.2). The angiographic size of the

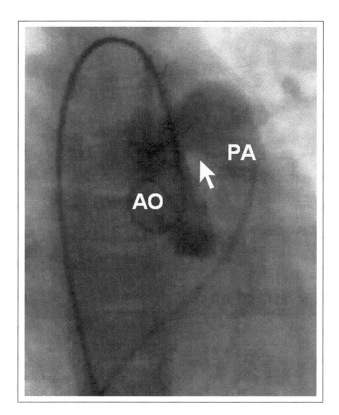

Figure 43.2
Aortogram in the right anterior oblique projection showing APW (arrow). AO, aorta; PA, pulmonary artery.

defect and its distance from the origin of the left main coronary artery as well as from the pulmonary valve and bifurcation of the pulmonary trunk are evaluated. The defect is crossed via the retrograde route from the ascending aorta. A 5–6 Fr right coronary (Judkins or Amplatz right coronary AR1) catheter is advanced from the right femoral artery to the ascending aorta up to the opening of the defect, which is then crossed with a 0.035 inch, 260 cm long Terumo wire or Bentson wire (Cook, Bloomington, Indiana, USA). The wire is further advanced from the pulmonary artery into the right ventricle and across the tricuspid valve, through the right atrium into the superior vena cava. If it does not take this route easily, then it is snared in the pulmonary artery. The endhole catheter is then advanced over the guidewire. This wire is then exchanged with a J-tipped 0.035 inch, 260 cm long guidewire. A 10 mm gooseneck snare (Microvena, White Bearlake, Minnesota, USA) is introduced into the right femoral vein and the wire from the superior vena cava is snared and exteriorized out through the femoral vein, establishing an arterio-venous guidewire circuit. As an alternative, the antegrade venous route can be used to cross the defect from the pulmonary trunk, although a more stable position is obtained by crossing from the aortic side and maintaining an arterio-venous monorail system.

Sizing of the defect

The sizing of the defect can be done from the angiographic jet or by using the balloon occlusion[16] or static balloon technique.[17]

Occlusion technique. An endhole balloon-tipped catheter with a central lumen diameter of 0.038 inch (6 or 7 Fr wedge pressure Swan–Ganz catheter) is passed antegradely from the femoral vein across the defect over the wire into the ascending aorta. The balloon is inflated with dilute contrast agent to a size bigger than the defect. The inflated balloon is pulled slowly back to the opening in the ascending aorta. By applying gentle traction on the balloon catheter and slow deflation, the catheter is withdrawn slowly until it pops through the defect. To judge the temporary occlusion of the defect by the balloon, angiography is performed with a pigtail catheter in the ascending aorta and by concomitant color Doppler echocardiography. The pigtail catheter can be passed alongside the guidewire in the femoral artery hemostatic sheath. The deflated balloon is then withdrawn, keeping in the syringe the measured amount of contrast. The size of the inflated balloon can be measured from fluoroscopic frame of digital imaging system with online quantitative analysis and also by inflating the exteriorized balloon with the same amount of contrast on the measuring plate to obtain the size of the defect.

Static technique. An Amplatzer sizing balloon is passed from the femoral vein over the wire and is positioned across the defect. The balloon is inflated to 1 to 1.5 atm to avoid stretching the defect. There may at times be technical difficulty in maintaining the position because of the high flow in the aorta.

Selection of the device

Of the devices used for occlusion of patent ductus arteriosus, the Amplatzer duct occluder or muscular ventricular septal defect occluder 2–3 mm larger than the measured defect should be selected as the first choice.[18,19]

Deployment of the device

After removing the hemostatic sheath from the femoral vein, an appropriate sized Mullins sheath of 6 to 8 Fr is passed over the wire through the APW and its tip is positioned in the descending aorta. The selected device loaded on to the delivery cable is then advanced to the tip of the Mullins sheath. The retention disk is then opened in the aorta and the entire assembly is withdrawn to the opening of the defect under fluoroscopic and echocardiographic (transthoracic or transesophageal) guidance. Aortography is performed to confirm the occlusion status and also the position of the device in

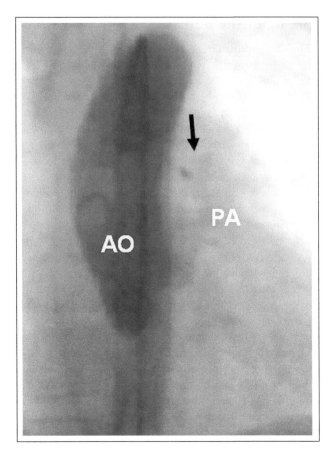

Figure 43.3
Aortogram in the AP projection showing the Amplatzer Ductal Occluder device in position and complete occlusion (arrow). AO, aorta; PA, pulmonary artery.

relation to the left coronary artery ostium. Keeping steady traction on the delivery cable, the whole device is opened by carefully withdrawing the Mullins sheath. Correct position of the device is confirmed and, if all the findings are satisfactory, the device is released (Figure. 43.3). Antiplatelet agents such as clopidogrel and aspirin 75 mg daily are given for 6 months.

Antibiotic prophylaxis

All patients should receive antibiotics prior to the procedure and two doses at an 8-hour interval.

Follow-up

Re-evaluation is performed after 1 month and thereafter every 6 months. A detailed clinical and echocardiographic (2D, continuous wave Doppler, and color flow imaging) assessment is performed on each visit to assess for a residual shunt, stenosis of the pulmonary artery, thrombus formation, and embolization of the device.

Therapeutic results

In the absence of associated anomalies which are not suitable for percutaneous treatment, transcatheter closure of an APW of suitable anatomy is feasible.[17,20,21] There are only a few case reports in the literature as the majority of the isolated defects are large and also do not have adequate rims on either side. Using a modified umbrella occluder system, Stamato et al[9] described the first transcatheter closure of an APW in a 3-year-old child who had a residual shunt following surgery, avoiding the need for a second thoracotomy with its associated higher morbidity and mortality. Encouraged by this, Tulloh and Rigby[20] attempted closure of a native defect in a 6 month 8 kg child with a 3 mm APW using a 12 mm Rashkind umbrella device. After non-availability of the Rashkind device, Jureidini et al[21] reported the use of a buttoned device for the closure of APW in an adult. All these defects were small and complete occlusion was achieved without any complication. After the Amplatzer Duct Occluder became available, with its encouraging results for closure of patent ductus arteriosus, Richens and Wilson[22] closed a residual APW. Subsequently, Naik et al[17] demonstrated two cases with isolated native defects. In the first case, with a defect size of 3.7 mm on echocardiography, an Amplatzer Duct Occluder of 6/4 mm resulted in complete occlusion. In the second case, in which the defect was 6 mm on 2D echocardiography, balloon sizing was done. With a stretched diameter of 7 mm, an Amplatzer Duct Occluder (ADO) of 10/8 mm was selected but, by gentle traction, the device was pulled through the defect. Because of the non-availability of the larger ADO at that time, an Amplatzer Septal Occluder of 14 mm (with 7 mm margins on each side) was attempted, which did not encroach on the important surrounding structures. All these patients received aspirin therapy for 6 months and the short term follow-up results have been satisfactory without embolization, residual shunt, or infective endarteritis.

Discussion

The use of various occlusion devices for the closure of a patent ductus arteriosus is well established and all morphologic types at any age can be attempted with high success rates and limited complications compared with surgical closure.[18,23] However, most infants presenting with an APW require early correction by the time of diagnosis.[4] The evolution of surgical techniques and results of the surgical correction over a 40-year period have revealed a steady decline in mortality from 37% to almost 0% with the changes in the current diagnostic techniques and the operative approaches.[4] The age at the time of repair has decreased to where most children are treated in the neonatal period. This has improved the results with regard to complications from pulmonary artery hypertension. No doubt the use of echocardiography for early diagnosis and prompt surgical intervention with patch closure under cardiopulmonary bypass has led to optimal early and long term results, but the inherent risk of morbidity from thoracotomy and cardiopulmonary bypass still remains.[24] In addition, operative scar, blood transfusion, psychologic trauma, acceptability, special wards including post-operative care, and long hospital stay for recovery are also of great concern. With the availability of better occlusion devices and delivery systems, the applicability in suitable anatomic APW has been attempted as an alternative therapeutic modality.[17,20,21]

The experience with transcatheter closure of APW is limited as this is a rare congenital cardiac malformation with almost 50% having associated lesions. The defect is small in only 10% of cases with adequate superior and inferior rims as well as a reasonable distance from the other important structures such as the ostium of the left coronary artery, both semilunar valves, and the origin of the right pulmonary artery.[25] What is actually the adequate distance is not described in numeric terms in any of the reported cases of transcatheter closure, although Jureidini et al[21] clearly delineated the anatomic details on angiography showing the APW was located in the anterior left aspect of the proximal ascending aorta 14 mm away from the left coronary artery and it communicated with the pulmonary trunk 25 mm away from both structures.[21] The optimum distance would depend on the size of the defect as well as the type of occluder. This situation is similar to the perimembranous ventricular septal defect. All these measurements should be accurately defined by detailed transthoracic echocardiography in the high parasternal short-axis view[13] and then confirmed on angiography. Balloon sizing of the defect using a static technique is technically difficult and not very accurate.[17] The occlusion approach may be more useful in assessing the size and relationship to other anatomic structures before selection of the device.

There are many embolization devices available but the ADO has several desirable characteristics such as simplicity of use, ability to recapture and reposition the device, high (>95%) complete closure rates, and the requirement of relatively small introducer sheaths.[18] To occlude the defect effectively the device must completely fill the defect, hence oversizing by 2–3 mm is recommended. The APW resembles type B patent ductus arteriosus, also called a window defect, so most of the 8 mm axial length of the ADO will lie within the pulmonary trunk. One must carefully look for any pulmonary artery stenosis. In the presence of pulmonary artery hypertension, as in PDA, it is better to use the Amplatzer muscular ventricular septal defect occluder with retention disks on both sides of the defect to prevent embolization.[19] Immediately following deployment of the device, high velocity blood flow can potentially produce mechanical fragmentation of erythrocytes and intravascular hemolysis, but residual shunting through the Amplatzer device usually disappears by the next day and rarely results in clinically significant hemolysis.[18]

Conclusion

At present, APW can be diagnosed early in life with the help of 2D, Doppler, and color Doppler flow echocardiography. Both morphology and hemodynamic parameters can be assessed with reasonable accuracy. Most infants with large defects having inadequate surrounding rims and associated anomalies will require conventional surgical repair under cardiopulmonary bypass. However, when the defect is isolated, at an appropriate distance from the semilunar valves and not associated with an anomalous origin of the right or left pulmonary arteries from the ascending aorta, transcatheter closure of APW is feasible and has been shown to be safe and effective.

References

1. Tiraboschi R, Salmone G, Crupi G et al. Aorto-pulmonary window in the first year of life: report on 11 surgical cases. Ann Thorac Surg 1988; 46: 438–41.

2. Castaneda AR, Jonas RA, Mayer JE, Hanley FL. Cardiac Surgery of the Neonate and Infant. Philadelphia, PA: WB Saunders Company, 1994: 295–300.

3. McElhinney DB, Reddy MV, Tworetzky W et al. Early and late results after repair of aorto-pulmonary septal defect and associated anomalies in infants <6 months of age. Am J Cardiol 1998; 81: 195–201.

4. Backer CL, Mavroudis C. Surgical management of aorto-pulmonary window: a 40 year experience. Eur J Cardiovasc Surg 2002; 21: 773–9.

5. Rowe RD. Aorto-pulmonary septal defect. In: Keith JD, Rowe RD, Vlad P, eds. Heart Disease in Infancy and Childhood, 3rd edition. New York: McMillan, 1978.

6. Tkebuchava T, Von Segesser LK, Vogt PR et al. Congenital aorto-pulmonary window: diagnosis, surgical technique and long term results. Eur J Cardiothorac Surg 1997; 11: 293–7.

7. Erez E, Dagan O, Georghiou GP et al. Surgical management of aorto-pulmonary window and associated lesions. Ann Thorac Surg 2004; 77: 484–7.

8. Gross RE. Surgical closure of an aortic septal defect. Circulation 1952; 5: 858–63.

9. Stamato T, Benson LN, Smallhorn JF, Freedom RM. Transcatheter closure of an aorto-pulmonary window with a modified double umbrella occluder system. Cathet Cardiovasc Diagn 1995; 35: 165–7.

10. Kutsche LM, Van Microp LHS. Anatomy and pathogenesis of aorto-pulmonary septal defect. Am J Cardiol 1987; 59: 443–7.

11. Mori K, Ando M, Takao A et al. Distal type of aorto-pulmonary window: report of 4 cases. Br Heart J 1978; 40: 681–9.

12. Ho SY, Gerhs LM, Anderson C et al. The morphology of aorto-pulmonary window with regard to their classification and morphogenesis. Cardiol Young 1994; 4: 146–55.

13. Balaji S, Burch M, Sullivan ID. Accuracy of cross-sectional echocardiography in diagnosis of aorto-pulmonary window. Am J Cardiol 1991; 67: 650–3.

14. DiBella I, Gladstone DJ. Surgical management of aorto-pulmonary window. Ann Thorac Surg 1998; 65: 768–70.

15. Arora R, Trehan V, Kumar A et al. Transcatheter closure of congenital ventricular septal defect: experience with various devices. J Interven Cardiol 2003; 16: 83–91.

16. Arora R, Trehan V, Rangashetty UMC et al. Transcatheter closure of ruptured sinus of valsalva. J Interven Cardiol 2004; 17: 53–8.

17. Naik GD, Chandra SV, Shenoy A et al. Transcatheter closure of aorto-pulmonary window using Amplatzer device. Cathet Cardiovasc Interven 2003; 59: 402–5.

18. Faella HJ, Hijazi ZM. Closure of the patent ductus arteriosus with the Amplatzer PDA device: immediate results of the international clinical trial. Cathet Cardiovasc Interven 2000; 51: 50–4.

19. Demkow M, Ruzyllo W, Siudalska H, Kepka C. Transcatheter closure of a 16mm hypertensive patent ductus arteriosus with the Amplatzer muscular VSD occluder. Cathet Cardiovasc Interven 2001; 52: 359–62.

20. Tulloh RM, Rigby ML. Transcatheter umbrella closure of aorto-pulmonary window. Heart 1997; 77: 479–80.

21. Jureidini SB, Spadaro JJ, Rao PS. Successful transcatheter closure with buttoned device of aorto-pulmonary window in an adult. Am J Cardiol 1998; 81: 371–2.

22. Richen T, Wilson N. Amplatzer device closure of a residual aorto-pulmonary window. Cathet Cardiovasc Diagn 2000; 50: 431–3.

23. Arora R, Singh S, Kalra GS. Patent ductus arteriosus: catheter closure in the adult patient. J Interven Cardiol 2001; 14: 255–9.

24. Galal MO, Wobst A, Halees Z et al. Perioperative complications following surgical closure of atrial septal defects type II in 232 patients – a baseline study. Eur Heart J 1994; 124: 172–5.

25. Neufeld HN, Lester RG, Adam P Jr et al. Aorto-pulmonary septal defect. Am J Cardiol 1962; 9: 12–16.

Section IX

Fistulas

44

Systemic arterio-venous fistulas

Grazyna Brzezinska-Rajszys

Introduction

Systemic arterio-venous fistulas are a group of vascular anomalies characterized by abnormal communications between systemic arteries and veins without normal capillary development. This situation results in shunting of blood from the high pressure arterial to the low pressure venous system. This abnormal circuit steals blood from the normal capillary bed and can result in tissue ischemia. Increased flow in the afferent artery and efferent vein causes dilatation, thickening, and tortuosity of the vessels. Depending on the shunt volume, it may cause right ventricular volume overload and decrease of the peripheral vascular resistance, leading to increased stroke volume and cardiac output. Such hemodynamics can lead to heart failure.

Systemic arterio-venous fistulas may be congenital or acquired, resulting from injury or infection. Congenital systemic arterio-venous fistulas are relatively rare lesions, the majority of which do not present with symptoms until adult life. They may become progressively larger throughout childhood, but occasionally spontaneous thrombosis and closure may occur. These fistulas may be found in the brain, spinal cord, and the liver, but may occur anywhere in the body.

Clinical manifestations of systemic arterio-venous fistulas depend on their location, pathophysiology, and hemodynamic effects, and on the size, number, and nature of the vessels within the lesions. In infants and children, large systemic arterio-venous fistulas involving the brain or liver can present with congestive heart failure.

Embolization is an accepted primary therapeutic approach in the majority of systemic arterio-venous fistulas, sometimes needing to be combined with surgery. The optimal technique of embolization depends on the type of vascular connection to be occluded and the specific defect and the preference of the operator for the type of equipment. Generally, vascular embolization may be undertaken:

- To occlude the entire arterial tree in part or all of an organ – frequently for management of diseased organs prior to their surgical removal. It requires microvascular embolization techniques (using very small particles or solutions).
- To occlude only the large arterial branches – for example vessels feeding an arterio-venous malformation. It requires different embolization techniques and the use of different coils, devices, and material such as gelfoam, ivalon, or a combination of these.
- To occlude a vessel at a very localized point – for example major aorto-pulmonary collaterals, patent ductus arteriosus. Precisely localized interruption of vascular flow using coil embolization or device closure techniques are the most commonly used in the practice of the pediatric interventional cardiologist.

The decision concerning embolization of a fistula should be taken by clinicians responsible for the patients and who refer their patients for therapy to interventionists. Due to a lack of formal guidelines for the interventional standards, embolization of different arterio-venous malformations is performed in different countries by interventionists from different specialities. The interventional cardiologists perform embolization of systemic arterio-venous fistulas more commonly in pediatric patients, especially in centers where cardiologists share catheterization theaters with radiologists. In such situations, co-operation between pediatric cardiologists and radiologists is mandatory to achieve good results. From a technical point of view, embolization can be performed by specialists familiar with interventional procedures and with the available embolization materials, and who have an understanding of the clinical indications for these procedures. It should be stressed that, due to the complexity of the intracranial arterio-venous malformations, their embolization is most commonly performed by interventional radiologists, interventional neuroradiologists, or neurosurgeons. Some of these procedures may necessitate a joint interventional–surgical approach (e.g., transtorcular approach to close intracranial arterio-venous malformations).

Neurologic manifestations of the intracranial arterio-venous malformations may appear at any age, but only when the damage they cause to the brain or spinal cord reaches a critical level. This damage occurs by reducing the amount of oxygen delivered to neural tissues, by causing bleeding into surrounding tissue, and by compressing parts of the brain or spinal cord. Detailed analysis of the angio-architecture of malformation is imperative for planning the appropriate treatment. The diagnosis is based on ultrasound, computed tomography, and magnetic resonance imaging studies.

Endovascular therapy is the standard care for aneurysms of the great vein of Galen, dural arterio-venous malformations in different locations, and other intracranial and spinal arterio-venous malformations.[1]

Types of arterio-venous fistulas

The vein of Galen aneurysm is characterized by the presence of a dilated mid-line deep venous structure, fed by abnormal arterio-venous communications. Vein of Galen malformations have been variably referred to as 'aneurysms of the vein of Galen', 'arteriovenous aneurysms of the vein of Galen', 'vein of Galen aneurysmal malformations', and 'vein of Galen malformations'. The nomenclature is imprecise as the dilated venous structure characteristic of these malformations has been demonstrated to represent the embryonic median prosencephalic vein, and not the vein of Galen.[2]

Several systems of classification have been used to describe malformations of the vein of Galen.[3–5] These malformations should be differentiated from the vein of Galen aneurysmal dilatation, which represents dilatation of a normally formed vein of Galen, secondary to outflow obstruction.[5] Correct diagnosis is important to the treatment that should be applied.

The vein of Galen aneurysm is a rare congenital abnormality (1% of all intracranial vascular malformations) that can cause severe morbidity and mortality, particularly in neonates, but also in infants and older children.[6] It represents 30% of vascular malformations presenting in the pediatric age group and is the most common cerebrovascular arterio-venous malformation presenting with cardiac manifestation.[7] The clinical presentation depends on the age of the patient and the severity of the lesion.[8] Whilst *in utero*, cerebral arterio-venous malformations can be detected, but cardiac failure may be absent. Cardiac failure is related to the co-existing low resistance cerebral and placental circulations. After birth, with the exclusion of the low resistance placental circulation, flow is directed toward the cerebral malformation.[9–11] The cerebral circulation may have 80% or more of the cardiac output, resulting in a large left to right shunt and severe congestive heart failure in neonates. The shunt through the malformation increases the pulmonary

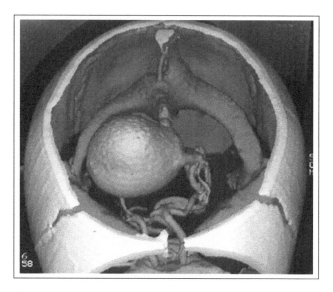

Figure 44.1
Vein of Galen aneurysm, spiral computed tomography, 3D reconstruction.

flow and may cause pulmonary hypertension. Increased systemic venous return to the right atrium promotes right to left shunt through the foramen ovale. In most patients, right to left shunt also occurs at the level of the ductus arteriosus. These shunts may cause cyanosis in these patients. A large shunt significantly reduces the diastolic pressure within the aorta, causing reduced coronary artery flow. This, combined with increased cardiac output, reduces the subendocardial blood flow and promotes myocardial ischemia.[12,13]

Hydrocephalus, seizures, subarachnoid hemorrhage, or venous congestion of the scalp and facial veins are clinical symptoms that occur later in infancy. Older children are more likely to present with mild cardiac failure, hydrocephalus, headache, or focal neurologic signs. Neurologic deterioration is due to a steal phenomenon resulting in insufficient brain perfusion and compression by an aneurysm on brain tissue.[14,15]

Malformations can be detected with two-dimensional (2D) combined with color Doppler cranial ultrasound techniques. Computed tomography and magnetic resonance demonstrate the nature and location of intracerebral arterio-venous malformations, morphology of the dural sinuses, and associated pathology such as ventriculomegaly, ischemic infarction[16,17] (Figure 44.1). Selective arteriography is the 'gold standard' which is required to provide precise information about the anatomy of the malformation necessary for planning the most effective therapy[18] (Figure 44.2). Manifestation of the vein of Galen aneurysm may give a clue in a chest X-ray showing cardiomegaly with right heart dilation, increased pulmonary vascularity, retrosternal fullness, and retropharyngeal soft tissue thickening due

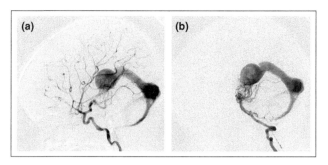

Figure 44.2
Vein of Galen aneurysm, Internal carotid arteriogram, lateral projection (a) and vertebral arteriogram, lateral projection (b).

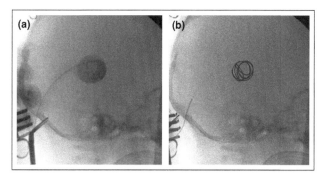

Figure 44.3
Vein of Galen aneurysm, transtorcular approach. Angiography (a); coil embolization (b).

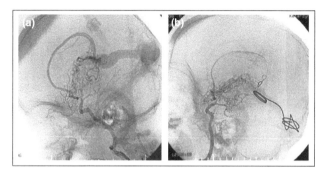

Figure 44.4
Vein of Galen aneurysm, embolization. Internal carotid arteriogram before (a) and after coil embolization (b). Coils were introduced using the transfemoral arterial and transtorcular approach.

to dilatation of the ascending aorta and brachiocephalic vessels, on echocardiography showing normal heart anatomy, dilated hyperdynamic cardiac chambers with increased run-off to the upper half of the body, abnormal dilatation of the superior vena cava, ascending aorta, aortic arch, and brachiocephalic vessels, on a Doppler study showing retrograde diastolic steal in the descending aorta with the continuous forward flow in the aortic arch and brachiocephalic vessels, and on contract echocardiography showing recirculation of microbubbles from the left side of the heart to the superior vena cava.

Surgery is associated with fatal outcome in 80–100% of cases. The results have improved over recent years with endovascular management in infants and children, but mortality and morbidity remain high in the neonatal group, with mortality ranging from 23 to 75% and morbidity from 21 to 88% in different series.[19–22] Morbidity can be reduced by selecting patients with no evidence of cerebral parenchymal damage or severe multi-system failure. In patients with persistent cardiac failure (mostly neonates), urgent endovascular treatment should be performed directed toward correcting the cardiac failure and cerebral ischemia. The transfemoral arterial, venous, or sonographically guided transtorcular approach should be used.[6,8,23–26] The transtorcular approach is convenient as it is a direct route and allows the use of larger coils. In neonates, puncture of the torcular is performed with an open 20-gauge needle and a 4 Fr catheter placed in the falcine sinus using the Seldinger technique (Figure 44.3).

There are encouraging results for modern endovascular embolization treatment of patients with aneurysm of the vein of Galen (Figure 44.4). After multiple stages of the embolization procedure using multiple embolization strategies, the cardiac symptoms resolved and improved in over 90% of cases and mortality reached 9%.[8,27–29] Although embolization may be effective in controlling the shunt and the congestive heart failure, it may not always completely obliterate the lesion. After embolization, surgical excision may be performed later in more stable patients. The major

risk of the interventional procedure includes intraventricular bleeding and inadvertent occlusion of an uninvolved vessel. Close follow-up with serial cranial ultrasound and color Doppler techniques, magnetic resonance, or computed tomography is important to demonstrate progressive thrombosis of malformations after embolotherapy.

Arterio-venous malformations of the liver are an important group of systemic arterio-venous fistulas. A variety of vascular lesions arises within the liver. Hepatic hemangiomas or hemangio-endotheliomas are benign vascular tumors, that may be part of multi-nodular hemangiomatosis of the liver. The syndrome consists of hepatomegaly, congestive heart failure, and cutaneous hemangioma and is associated with consumptive coagulopathy, thrombocytopenia, and liver dysfunction. More than 50% of the total cardiac output may be shunted through the liver, causing congestive heart failure, which is often the dominant clinical and prognostic feature in patients with hepatic hemangio-endotheliomas.[30–33] The hepatic hemangiomas involute in many cases, but those presenting with congestive heart failure have a poor prognosis. Hepatic arterio-venous malformations may be single,

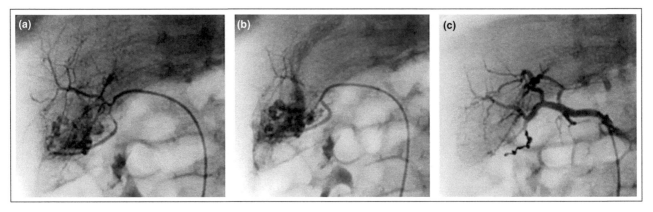

Figure 44.5
Occlusion of hepatic arterio-venous malformations localized in the right lobe of the liver (V and VI segments) presenting with congestive heart failure. Selective arteriography to feeding vessel of malformation: (a) arterial phase; (b) venous phase; (c) arterio-venous fistulas occluded with microcoils (Hilal Embolization Microcoils, Cook Europe).

multiple, or diffuse, with a large spectrum of diameters ranging from a few millimeters to several centimeters. Hepatic arterio-venous malformations presenting with congestive heart failure contain the direct arterio-venous fistulas between the hepatic arteries and hepatic veins.

The diagnosis of hepatic arterio-venous malformations is confirmed by hepatic ultrasonography, computed tomography, and magnetic resonance imaging. Aortography and selective arteriography are necessary if arterial embolization or surgical intervention is considered (Figure 44.5).

The treatment depends on the anatomy of the malformation and its hemodynamic effects. Different embolization techniques using different materials (e.g., coils, radiolabeled polyvinyl alcohol particles, or a combination of different materials) have been used to embolize hepatic arterio-venous fistulas.[31–34] Prednisone in combination with anticongestive therapy may be an effective treatment for diffuse hemangiomas. Surgical resection is reserved for localized tumors. It should be stressed that a combination of all treatment modalities may need to be applied in some patients. In some cases with diffuse arterio-venous malformations and significant symptomatology, liver transplantation is the only therapeutic option. Hepatic arterio-venous malformations are relatively common and often asymptomatic in hereditary hemorrhagic telangiectasia.

Hereditary hemorrhagic telangiectasia (Osler–Weber–Rendu syndrome) is a genetic vascular disorder with autosomal dominant inheritance and an estimated frequency of 1–2:100 000. It is characterized by telangiectasias, arterio-venous fistulas, and aneurysms and may involve skin, mucosa, and blood vessels of the liver, lungs, and central nervous system.[35] Hepatic arterio-venous malformations occur in approximately 30% of patients, pulmonary in 15–20%, and central nervous system in less than 10%. There is a strong association between pulmonary arterio-venous malformations and

hereditary hemorrhagic telangiectasia. Between 40 and 70% of patients with pulmonary arterio-venous malformations have hereditary hemorrhagic telangiectasia. Treatment depends on the clinical symptoms and percutaneous embolization techniques play an important role in the treatment of these malformations.[32,34,36] Arterial embolotherapy of hepatic arterio-venous fistulas can improve the clinical condition of patients with heart failure, but transplantation remains the treatment of choice for hepatic arterio-venous malformations with significant symptoms.

Miscellaneous arterio-venous malformations, congenital and acquired, can occur anywhere in the body. In the developing embryo, there are multiple communications between arteries and veins. Persistence of these channels may be the basis for congenital arterio-venous fistulas. Different locations of congenital systemic arterio-venous fistulas are reported mostly as case reports, e.g., the common carotid artery and internal jugular vein, between the descending aorta and the superior vena cava, the azygos vein, and the innominate vein, between the ascending aorta and the superior vena cava – very uncommon[37–40] (Figure 44.6). The majority of peripheral fistulas occur as a result of trauma. These acquired arterio-venous fistulas usually occur in sites where an artery and vein, that are side-by-side, are damaged. These occur mostly in the legs or arms.[41] The healing process results in the two vessels becoming linked. A second group of acquired fistulas are iatrogenic, such as after cannulation of vessels with different catheters and cannulas, after surgery.[42–44] After cardiac catheterization, arterio-venous fistulas may occur as a complication of the arterial puncture in the leg or arm.[45] The clinical significance of all types of systemic arterio-venous fistulas is an indication for treatment, which should be based on the detailed analysis of the anatomy of the fistula. When a systemic arterio-venous fistula is associated with heart disease, it should be treated during cardiac catheterization by the cardiologists.

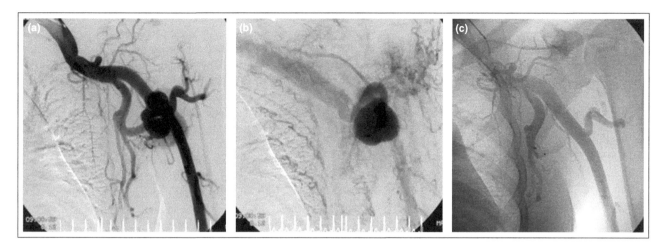

Figure 44.6
Congenital arterio-venous fistula between the axillary artery branch (subscapular artery) and axillary vein occluded with the Amplatzer PDA Plug (AGA Medical Corporation). Subclavian arteriogram: (a) arterial phase; (b) venous phase; (c) arteriogram after occlusion.

Occlusion of systemic arterio-venous fistulas

All therapeutic decisions should be made on a case-by-case basis. For a particular lesion, the optimal closure technique is best determined by considering its anatomy in the context of the specific goals of the occlusion. Vessel occlusion may be achieved using a variety of transcatheter methods including coil embolization (e.g., different types of Gianturco coils, detachable coils, microcoils), device closure (e.g., the Amplatzer Duct Occluder, Amplatzer Vascular Plug), gelfoam embolization, particulate embolization, liquid agent embolization (absolute ethanol, ivalon, agents containing cyanoacrylate monomers). The choice of occlusion material can be critical for embolization. Systemic arterio-venous fistulas are mostly occluded with coils and devices.

Coils

Coils are available in wire diameters from 0.018 to 0.052 inch and extruded diameter from 2 to 20 mm, of almost any length, different shapes, and materials. Controlled release coils can also be used.

The Gianturco coils (Cook Europe) are made from stainless steel wire with Dacron fibers attached to increase their thrombogenicity.

A detachable coil-delivery system using the same type of coils is also available (e.g., Flipper detachable embolization coil, Cook Europe). This can result in more control during the coil placement. The proximal end of the detachable coil locks into the delivery cable. With the delivery cable the coil is pushed out of the appropriately positioned endhole guiding catheter. When the extruded coil is in a satisfactory position, it can be unlocked and released from the delivery

cable. If the position is unsatisfactory before its final release, the coil can be simply removed by withdrawing the delivery cable with the coil still attached. The detachable coil is particularly useful when there is a high risk of inappropriate coil positioning or its inadvertent migration during deployment, either because of difficult vessel anatomy or because the site of occlusion is particularly critical.

Hilal Embolization Microcoils (Cook Europe) are platinum coils (0.018 inch) with spaced synthetic fibers. They are available in different shapes and lengths. These coils are delivered through 3 Fr delivery catheters (e.g., Microferret, Cook Europe) passed through a guiding catheter with inner diameter of 0.038 inch to selectively occlude very tortuous vessels.

Fibered Platinum Coils (Boston Scientific, Inc.) are available in a simple helical shape made of 0.035 inch wire and complex cloverleaf shapes made of 0.018 inch wire that are sold with a system of coil pushers and delivery tracker microcatheters, which fit in the lumen of any catheter with an inner diameter of 0.038 inch. The larger catheter is used as a guiding catheter.

Guglielmi Detachable Coils (GDC) (Boston Scientific, Inc.) are coils with different 2D and complex 3D shapes. The system consists of a soft platinum coil soldered to a stainless steel delivery wire. When the coil is positioned correctly, a 1 mA current is delivered to dissolve by electrolysis the delivery wire attachment point proximal to the platinum coil. At the same time, the positively charged platinum theoretically induces thrombosis of negatively charged blood elements (white and red blood cells, platelets, and fibrinogen). Once electrolysis occurs, the delivery wire can be removed, leaving the coil in place.

TruFill DCS Orbit Detachable Coil (Cordis, Inc.) has a spherically coiled shape with a maximum diameter of 20 mm and a length of 30 cm.

Devices

The Amplatzer Vascular Plug (AGA Medical Corporation) is a self-expandable, cylindrical device made from nitinol wire mesh and is indicated for arterial and venous embolization in the peripheral vasculature. It is available in sizes from 4 to 16 mm in 2 mm increments. The plug is secured at both ends with platinum marker bands. A stainless steel microscrew is welded to one of the platinum marker bands, which allows attachment to the delivery cable. The plug is pre-loaded in a loader and delivered through 5, 6, or 8 Fr guiding catheters.

The Amplatzer Duct Occluder (AGA Medical Corporation) is another type of self-expandable device made from a nitinol wire mesh with polyester fabric sewn into the occluder to induce thrombosis. The conical shape of the device with retention skirt was produced for occlusion of patent ductus arteriosus, but this device is very effective in the closure of different vessels including systemic arterio-venous fistulas.

Covered stents are not typical embolization materials, but some mostly post-traumatic fistulous communications between big arteries and veins can be treated with balloon-expandable or self-expandable covered stents implanted into the artery.

Technique of embolization

Use of anesthesia depends on the age of the patient, the complexity of the procedure, and the local preferences. Intracranial, spinal malformation, and procedures performed in younger patients should be occluded under general anesthesia. Antibiotics are administered in intravenous doses. Embolization can be performed by the retrograde arterial approach but the transvenous approach has also been used. The choice depends on the lesion. As a rule, the approach should provide the straightest and least complicated course to the systemic arterio-venous fistula. Usually femoral artery access is used. Occasionally other arteries can be used for the arterial approach. For a transvenous approach, the femoral vein is the most frequently used access. Venous or arterial access can also be used for the introduction of balloon catheters for temporary occlusion of the flow through the fistula. This can be helpful during embolization of high flow fistulas with coils or other solid material.

An appropriate diameter (usually 5–7 Fr) introducer sheath is used. It should provide access to a wide range of catheters, which might be needed for embolization. Anticoagulation with heparin, 100 international units per kg, is usually used. From the arterial approach, an angiographic catheter (multi-purpose or pigtail) is used for angiography to show the location of the fistula and its relation to the main vessels. With the multi-purpose catheter advanced into the branch of the artery feeding the lesion, further selective angiography is performed. Different projections such as anterior-posterior, lateral, oblique and axial, and magnified views are helpful in delineating the exact anatomy of the fistula. Embolization is performed after identification and selective catheterization of the feeding branch with the delivery catheter. The inner diameter of the delivery catheter should be equal to or at most only slightly larger than the coil diameter. If the delivery catheter has a lumen which is too large for the coil, then the guidewire may wedge itself inside the coil and it may be difficult to advance the coil inside the catheter. Easy passage of the wire through the tip of the delivery catheter should be checked before insertion of the coil. The 0.018 inch and 0.025 inch coils can be delivered through 3 Fr catheters and 0.035 inch and 0.038 inch coils through 4 Fr catheters.

If the lesion is accessed by the delivery guiding catheter, than steel coils are deployed through it. The embolization material should be positioned in the vessels feeding the arterio-venous fistula, within the fistula, or a combination of these. The size of the coil should be 10–30% larger than the vessel diameter. A smaller coil will not cause complete occlusion, while a larger coil straightens out and may extend beyond the site of embolization. Coils are pre-loaded in a stainless steel or plastic tube. The coils are passed from the tube into a delivery catheter using an appropriate sized guidewire. When extruded from the catheter, the coil forms to its stated size and shape.

For simple helical coils, the length of the coil and its diameter determine the number of loops. The extruded intravascular coil is thrombogenic. After implantation of the coils, occlusion of the vessel occurs as the result of thrombus formation and its subsequent organization. If the lesion is peripherally located and follows a tortuous course, a co-axial microcatheter system is used to reach the appropriate site. Some microcatheters, such as Tracker (Boston Scientific, Inc.) or Microferret (Cook Europe) and a compatible guidewire, can be introduced through a guiding catheter with an inner diameter of 0.038 inch. Complex helical fibered platinum coils or other microcoils are then deployed, depending on the size of the vessel to be occluded. Intermittent check angiography is done with hand injections approximately 5 minutes after deployment of each coil to look for the degree of occlusion, any inadvertent non-target embolization, additional feeding vessels, and to check the catheter position for the subsequent coil deployment. Temporary occlusion of the flow by a balloon catheter can help with occlusion. If satisfactory occlusion is not achieved with coils, this may be combined with injection of gelatine sponge (Gelfoam, Upjohn Co.). Gelfoam particles are mixed with contrast and saline and injected slowly by hand, so that there is no reflux into the adjacent normal vessels.

Systemic arterio-venous fistulas may have multiple feeding vessels and so, after the occlusion of the main vessel, additional feeding arteries should be sought and occluded.

The catheter occlusion technique may require many coils to occlude the solitary malformation. Usually several coils have to be tightly packed in order to achieve complete occlusion, especially if there is a high flow in a vessel. In general, the first coil should be the largest to prevent distal embolization.

The feeding vessels can be embolized with the new Amplatzer Vascular Plugs or the Amplatzer Duct Occluder. The choice between coils or devices is dependent on the anatomy of the fistula as well as on the experience and preferences of the operator. Plugs can be delivered through a guiding catheter with an inner diameter of 0.056–0.088 inch depending on the plug diameter and a duct occluder needs a long 5–6 Fr sheath.

Complications

Inadvertent migration of the embolization material is the commonest complication. When this occurs, embolization material moves distally into the arterial tree, in most instances to the distal pulmonary arteries. Such materials as coils or devices are relatively easily removed with vascular retrieval techniques.

Hemolysis is a serious complication occurring only in cases of significant residual flow. This complication should be treated with additional embolization, if it is impossible to remove previously used material to exchange it for a different one.

After the procedure

Patients may experience post-embolization syndrome, with transient fever, pain, and leukocytosis, which is usually self-limiting and treated symptomatically. Ultrasonography with Doppler study, spiral computed tomography, and/or magnetic resonance should document the result of embolization prior to or soon after the patient is discharged from hospital. The follow-up protocol of patients with intracranial malformation should be discussed with neurosurgeons.

References

1. Humphreys RP, Hoffman HJ, Drake JM et al. Choices in the 1990s for the management of pediatric cerebral arteriovenous malformations. Pediatr Neurosurg 1996; 25: 277–85.
2. Gupta AK, Varma DR. Vein of Galen malformations: review. Neurol India 2004; 52: 43–53.
3. Berenstein A, Lasjaunias P. Arteriovenous fistulas of the brain. In: Berenstein A, Lasjavnias P. Surgical Neuroangiography 4. Endovascular Treatment of Cerebral Lesions. Berlin: Springer-Verlag, 1992: 267–317.
4. Garcia-Monaco R, Lasjaunias P, Berenstein A. Therapeutic management of vein of Galen aneurysmal malformations. In: Vinuela F, Halbach VV, Dion JE, eds. Interventional Neuroradiology: Endovascular Therapy of the Central Nervous System. New York: Raven Press, 1992: 113–27.
5. Lasjaunias P, Terbrugge K, Piske R et al. Vein of Galen dilatation: anatomo-clinical forms and endovascular treatment. Fourteen cases explored and/or treated between 1983 and 1986. Neurochirugie 1987; 33: 315–33.
6. Casasco A, Lylyk P, Hodes JE et al. Percutaneous transvenous catheterization and embolization of vein of Galen aneurysms. Neurosurgery 1991; 28: 260–6.
7. Pellegrino PA, Milanesi O, Saia OS, Carollo C. Congestive heart failure secondary to cerebral arterio-venous fistula. Childs Nerv Syst 1987; 3: 141–4.
8. Jones BV, Ball WS, Tomsick TA et al. Vein of Galen aneurysmal malformation: diagnosis and treatment of 13 children with extended clinical follow-up. Am J Neuroradiol 2002; 23: 1717–24.
9. Vintzileos AM, Eisenfeld LI, Campbell WA et al. Prenatal ultrasonic diagnosis of arteriovenous malformation of the vein of Galen. Am J Perinatol 1986; 3: 209–11.
10. Reiter AA, Huhta JC, Carpenter RJ Jr, Segall GK, Hawkins EP. Prenatal diagnosis of arteriovenous malformation of the vein of Galen. J Clin Ultrasound 1986; 14: 623–8.
11. Rodesch G, Hui F, Alvarez H et al. Prognosis of antenatally diagnosed vein of Galen aneurysmal malformations. Childs Nerv Syst 1994; 10: 79–83.
12. Cumming GR. Circulation in neonates with intracranial arteriovenous fistula and cardiac failure. Am J Cardiol 1980; 45: 1019–24.
13. Garcia-Monaco R, de Victor D, Mann C et al. Congestive cardiac manifestations from cerebrocranial arteriovenous shunts: endovascular management in 30 children. Childs Nerv Syst 1991; 7: 48–52.
14. Bhattacharya JJ, Thammaroj J. Vein of Galen malformations. J Neurol Neurosurg Psychiatr 2003; 74: 142–4.
15. Zerah M, Garcia-Monaco R, Rodesh G et al. Hydrodynamics in vein of Galen malformations. Childs Nerv Syst 1992; 8: 111–17.
16. Seidenwurm D, Berenstein A, Hyman A. Vein of Galen malformation: correlation of clinical presentation, arteriography and MR imaging. Am J Neuroradiol 1991; 12: 347–54.
17. Lasjaunias P, Garcia-Monaco R, Rodesch G et al. Vein of Galen malformation: endovascular management of 43 cases. Childs Nerv Syst 1991; 7: 360–7.
18. Horowitz MB, Jungreis CA, Quisling RG, Pollack I. Vein of Galen aneurysms: a review and current perspective. Am J Neuroradiol 1994; 15: 1486–96.
19. Johnston IH, Whittle IR, Besser M, Morgan MK. Vein of Galen malformation: diagnosis and management. Neurosurgery 1987; 20: 747–58.
20. Hoffmann HJ, Chuang S, Hendrick EB, Humphreys RP. Aneurysms of the vein of Galen: experience at the Hospital for Sick Children, Toronto. J Neurosurg 1982; 57: 316–22.
21. Lasjaunias P, Rodesch G, Terbrugge K et al. Vein of Galen aneurysmal malformations. Report of 36 cases managed between 1982 and 1988. Acta Neurochir 1989; 99: 26–37.
22. Brunelle F. Arteriovenous malformation of the vein of Galen in children. Pediatr Radiol 1997; 27: 501–13.
23. Dowd CF, Halbach VV, Barnwell SL et al. Transfemoral venous embolization of vein of Galen malformations. Am J Neuroradiol 1990; 11: 643–8.
24. Mickle JP. The transtorcular embolization of vein of Galen aneurysms and update on the use of this technique in twenty four patients. In: Marlin AE, ed. Concepts in Pediatric Neurosurgery Karger: Basel, 1991: 69–78.
25. Lylyk P, Vineula F, Dion JE et al. Therapeutic alternatives for vein of Galen vascular malformation. J Neurosurg 1993; 78: 438–45.
26. Halbach VV, Dowd CF, Higashida RT et al. Endovascular treatment of mural type vein of Galen malformations. J Neurosurg 1998; 89: 74–80.

27. Mitchell PJ, Rosenfield JV, Dargaville P. Endovascular management of vein of Galen aneurysmal malformations presenting in the neonatal period. Am J Neuroradiol 2001; 22: 1403–9.

28. Lasjaunias P, Alvarez H, Rodesch G et al. Aneurysmal malformations of the vein of Galen. Follow up of 120 children treated between 1984 and 1994. Interven Neuroradiol 1996; 2: 15–26.

29. Lasjaunias P, Hui F, Zerah M et al. Cerebral arteriovenous malformations in children. Management of 179 consecutive cases and review of the literature. Childs Nerv Syst 1995; 11: 66–79.

30. Boon LM, Burrows PE, Paltiel HJ et al. Hepatic vascular anomalies in infancy: a twenty-seven-year experience. J Pediatr 1996; 129: 346–54.

31. Stanley P, Grinnell VS, Stanton RE et al. Therapeutic embolization of infantile hepatic hemangioma with polyvinyl alcohol. Am J Roentgenol 1983; 141: 1047–51.

32. Whiting JH Jr, Morton KA, Datz FL et al. Embolization of hepatic arteriovenous malformations using radiolabeled and nonradiolabeled polyvinyl alcohol sponge in a patient with hereditary hemorrhagic telangiectasia: case report. J Nucl Med 1992; 33: 260–2.

33. Subramanyan R, Narayan R, Costa DD et al. Transcatheter coil occlusion of hepatic arteriovenous malformation in a neonate. Ind Heart J 2001; 53: 782–4.

34. Derauf BJ, Hunter DW, Sirr SA et al. Peripheral embolization of diffuse hepatic arteriovenous malformations in a patient with hereditary hemorrhagic telangiectasia. Cardiovasc Interven Radiol 1987; 10: 80–3.

35. Abdalla SA, Geisthoff UW, Bonneau D et al. Visceral manifestations in hereditary haemorrhagic telangiectasia type 2. J Med Genet 2003; 40: 494–502.

36. Stockx L, Raat H, Caerts B et al. Transcatheter embolization of hepatic arteriovenous fistulas in Rendu–Osler–Weber disease: a case report and review of the literature. Eur Radiol 1999; 9: 1434–7.

37. Gutierrez FR, Monaco MP, Hartmann AF, McKnight RC. Congenital arteriovenous malformations between brachiocephalic arteries and systemic veins. Chest 1987; 92: 897–9.

38. Romero M, Pan M, Suarez de Lezo J et al. Congenital fistula between the left subclavian artery and the innominate vein. A rare cause of intractable insufficiency in the newborn infant. Rev Esp Cardiol 1988; 41: 630–2.

39. Oomman A, Mao R, Krishnan P et al. Congenital aortocaval fistula to the superior vena cava. Ann Thorac Surg 2001; 72: 911–13.

40. Soler P, Mehta AV, Garcia OL et al. Congenital systemic arteriovenous fistula between the descending aorta, azygos vein, and superior vena cava. Chest 1981; 80: 647–9.

41. Ramsay DW, McAuliffe W. Traumatic pseudoaneurysm and high flow arteriovenous fistula involving internal jugular vein and common carotid artery. Treatment with covered stent and embolization. Australas Radiol 2003; 47: 177–80.

42. Droll KP, Lossing AG. Carotid–jugular arteriovenous fistula: case report of an iatrogenic complication following internal jugular vein catheterization. J Clin Anesth 2004; 16: 127–9.

43. Uchida Y, Kawano H, Koide Y et al. Arteriovenous fistula of internal thoracic vessels. Intern Med 2003; 42: 987–90.

44. Thiel R, Bircks W. Arteriovenous fistulas after median sternotomy – report of 2 cases and review of the literature. Thorac Cardiovasc Surg 1990; 38: 195–7.

45. Onal B, Kosar S, Gumus T et al. Postcatheterization femoral arteriovenous fistulas: endovascular treatment with stent-grafts. Cardiovasc Interven Radiol 2004; 27: 453–8.

45

Pulmonary arterio-venous fistulas

John F Reidy

Anatomy and pathophysiology

Pulmonary arteriovenous fistulas (PAVFs) or pulmonary arteriovenous malformations (PAVMs) are now usually classified either as simple or complex based on the angiographic findings[1] (Figure 45.1). Simple PAVMs are more common (80%) and have a single feeding artery and vein which is usually larger with a non-septated aneurysmal sac. Complex PAVMs have multiple feeding arteries.[1] The malformation then is cirsoid with multiple septations and there can be more than one draining vein. PAVMs may be solitary or multiple, which occurs more commonly when they are associated with hereditary hemorrhagic telangiectasia (HHT).[2] If PAVMs are of significant size then significant right to left shunting will occur, which is associated with desaturation, hypoxia, and polycythemia.[3]

Clinical symptoms and indication for treatment

PAVMs can occur at any age but often present in adult life. Earlier and in children they may present with dyspnea and fatigue, which may have been present for many years undiagnosed. Cyanosis and polycythemia may be noted.[4] Some cases may present with a cerebrovascular accident (CVA), which may be due to thrombosis secondary to the associated polycythemia or alternatively may be due to paradoxical embolism consequent on venous thrombosis (Figure 45.2). Even in the absence of any known clinical CVA an occult CVA may have occurred so it makes sense to do a baseline head CT scan prior to any embolization procedure. Occasionally PAVMs are noted as an incidental finding on a routine chest X-ray. In all symptomatic PAVMs treatment is indicated. Very small PAVMs, especially in older patients, can probably be left safely, but any PAVM with a feeding artery diameter greater than 3 mm on CT should be treated.

Embolization procedures have for some years now been regarded as the treatment of choice, with surgery reserved

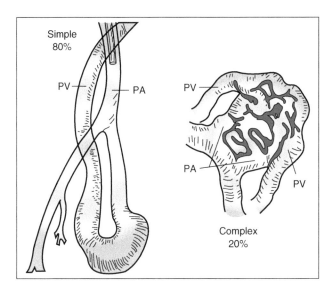

Figure 45.1
Angiographic classification of PAVMs. PA, pulmonary artery; PV, pulmonary vein.

for large or very complex cases. Recent improvements in embolization techniques and a greater range of devices have extended the range of embolization even further.

Up until 1977 the only treatment available for PAVMs was surgery. This was an effective treatment but, aside from a significant morbidity, it was associated with a mortality of about 4–5%. Multiple PAVMs presented a particular problem, especially when they involved both lungs. The first reported case of PAVM embolization was in 1977. The first cases used detachable coils but there was then a period when detachable balloons were favored, particularly for larger malformations. Detachable balloons have now been superseded by improved coil devices and controlled release coils.[5]

The diagnosis of PAVMs does not usually present a problem.[3,4] Usually a CT scan will have been obtained (Figure 45.2). This will provide useful information regarding the size of the malformation and the feeding artery as well as

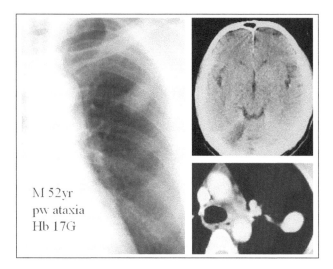

Figure 45.2
Presentation of a simple single large PAVM in an adult. The chest X-ray is very suggestive but the CT confirms the diagnosis. The brain scan shows a cerebellar infarct.

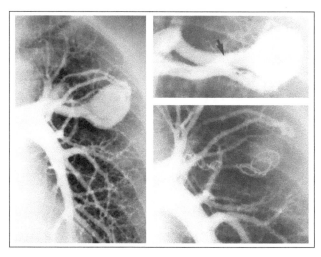

Figure 45.3
Same patient as in Figure 45.2. A selective injection into the left pulmonary artery (LPA) (early arterial) shows a single feeding artery. A superselective injection shows the PAVM more clearly with a mass of coils just beyond a small branch to normal lung parenchyma (black arrow). Even despite this the flow was such that a second procedure was necessary to effect occlusion.

identifying multiple malformations, particularly when there are smaller ones seen at the lung bases. The quality of images obtained now with multi-slice CT scanners is such that the same detail available on conventional pulmonary angiography can be achieved.

Particularly when there are multiple PAVMs it is useful to have baseline blood gas measurements so that the overall effect of treatment can be monitored. It is also important when there are multiple PVMs to warn patients or parents that more than one session of embolization may be required.

Pulmonary angiography

This is carried out using a femoral vein approach. Infants and children will clearly need a general anesthetic, but this is not necessary for adults. The aim of the pulmonary angiography is to confirm the presence and location of the PAVMs and to clearly demonstrate the feeding artery or arteries supplying it.[4] Normally selective right and left pulmonary arteriograms will be performed using a pigtail catheter, but then more detailed angiograms will be needed with a curved multi-purpose catheter. More detailed and more selective arteriograms are then needed focusing on the malformation and its feeding artery until a selective injection is made directly into the feeding artery, in the case of a simple PVAM, or one of the arteries in the complex lesions. As the same catheter will then be needed for the embolization procedure it is important that this has only an endhole with no side holes. More commonly, malformations are situated in the lower lobes and sometimes it may

prove quite difficult to identify the feeding artery. Using an angled hydrophilic guidewire can prove particularly useful in this situation. The aim is to have the catheter positioned in the feeding artery in a view where the angulation shows the length of the artery to best advantage. Magnified views are important and it is not necessary to have subtraction images. To have the catheter in a good and stable position for a subsequent embolization a 6 Fr catheter is a good size and, to give it stability, the use of a long sheath with the tip in the main pulmonary artery is advantageous. One of the concerns about embolizing PAVMs and having catheters directly into the malformation is that any embolic particles will pass immediately into the systemic circulation, so giving some systemic heparinization is felt to reduce this risk.

Embolization procedure

In the commonest form of PAVM (simple type) with a single feeding artery the aim should be to occlude this artery immediately before it enters the aneurysmal part of the PAVM (Figure 45.3). Embolizing more proximally would occlude branches to normal lung parenchyma and possibly result in some pulmonary infarction. It is important to assess the diameter of the feeding artery as this must not be bigger than the diameter of the coil. If the diameter of the extruded coil was less than that of the feeding artery the coil could then pass with the high flow into the non-septated aneurysmal part of the AVM and then into the single draining vein, which is usually larger than the feeding artery.

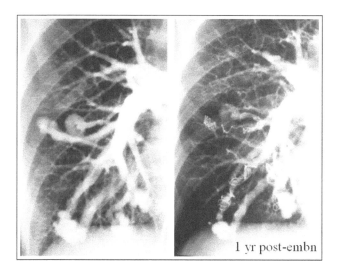

1 yr post-embn

Figure 45.4
Multiple simple PAVMs. Note that the embolization of the largest one has coils spread out along the feeding artery and this has not effected occlusion.

This could produce systemic embolism with potentially catastrophic consequences. Thus it is very important that the tip of the catheter is precisely placed and in a stable position and that this is checked immediately before delivering any coils. A long floppy-tipped guidewire should be used to push out and deliver the coils. The aim of coil embolization is to produce a localized mass or nest of coils immediately proximal to the malformation that will produce a critical mass and thus effect occlusion of the artery. If the coil diameter is significantly larger than the diameter of the artery it could then end up being extended along the length of the vessel and would not then occlude the artery[6,7] (Figure 45.4).

Initially standard coils were pushed out of the tip of the catheter with a guidewire. Once the coil emerged at the tip of the catheter there was little control on the placement. There are now available controlled-release coils (W Cook).[5] The advantage of these coils is that they can be fully deployed but they are still attached to the pusher wire and then are only detached if the position is satisfactory. Currently the largest diameter of these devices is 12 mm. When aiming to achieve a localized nest of coils, the most critical coil to be placed is the first coil or anchor coil. Once this is satisfactorily placed it is possible to place further coils next to it, usually of a slightly smaller size. If the feeding artery to the PAVM is of large size and with a short neck, a further technique to effect occlusion is to pass the catheter into the aneurysmal sac and to then deploy large diameter coils (e.g. 20 mm) directly into it. These will then prevent any coils in the distal artery migrating through the malformation sac. Very large PAVMs may present a particular problem as the right to left shunt will be very large and there are particular concerns regarding systemic embolism. Good

long term results have been reported, but in such cases a second embolization procedure is sometimes necessary.[8] New devices such as the vascular plug (AGA Medical Corporation) can be a very effective and safe means of effecting occlusion.[9] The largest device available has a diameter of 16 mm and requires an 8 Fr catheter for its deployment. As with the controlled-release coils, these have a release mechanism so the device is not finally detached from its delivery cable until its position is satisfactory.

As pulmonary embolization will usually follow on from pulmonary arteriography it is essential that a good selection of embolization coils and devices is available as it is sometimes necessary to adapt the embolization technique depending on the detailed anatomy found. After completion of the embolization procedure with coils it is important to demonstrate on check arteriography that the feeding artery is occluded or severely restricted. Anything less than this is likely not to effect a permanent occlusion. It is also important to check that there are not other and smaller feeding arteries as sometimes there may be a small accessory artery.

Complications and their avoidance

If marked polycythemia is a feature of the PAVM then venesection to reduce the hemoglobin level has been advocated, to reduce the risk of spontaneous thrombosis. The most serious complication that is unique to the embolization of PAVMs is systemic or paradoxic embolism. This is more likely to occur in the more common simple PAVMs. With correct sizing of coils and controlled-release devices this should be minimized. The other concern relates to the use of large endhole only catheters and the possibility of micro air embolism. When the catheter has been carefully positioned using a guidewire and the guidewire is removed it is sometimes difficult to get good back flow on the catheter due to the tip being up against the arterial wall. There is then a risk that small amounts of air can be introduced. An effective means of avoiding this is to have the end of the catheter and guidewire in a bowl of water prior to removal of the guidewire. This will prevent any possible air getting into the system so that if aspiration of blood is not possible then this will not be a problem.

By identifying and selectively catheterizing the feeding artery to a PAVM and embolizing immediately proximal to the malformation then the PAVM should be occluded with little or no loss of normal parenchyma. Even with such a careful approach there is the likelihood of a small amount of normal lung being infarcted and this may then result in some pleuritic chest pain. Such pain usually lasts only a few days and is associated with full recovery.

A particular problem occurs when there are multiple and diffuse PAVMs[10] (Figure 45.5). In such cases embolizing all

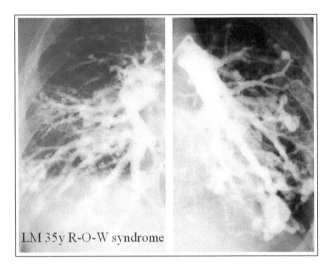

Figure 45.5
Multiple PAVMs in an adult with hereditary hemorrhagic telangiectasia. In this situation cure is impossible as embolizing the PAVMs is going to result in loss of normal lung parenchyma. The best to be hoped for is palliation and an improvement in oxygen saturation after multiple procedures.

the lesions is not possible and the aim should be to embolize the clearcut localized PAVMs. If a small PAVM is coming off the same branch as normal parenchyma then this is probably best left alone.

Post-procedure and follow-up

It should only be necessary for patients to spend one to two nights in hospital following embolization procedures. Pleuritic chest pain may keep the patient in for longer. The best way of following up these patients is with a follow-up CT scan with contrast. This will confirm exclusion of the PAVMs.

References

1. White RI Jr, Mitchell SE, Barth KH. Angioarchitecture of pulmonary arteriovenous malformations: an important consideration before embolotherapy. AJR 1983; 140: 681–6.
2. Marianeschi SM, McElhinney DB, Reddy VM. Pulmonary arteriovenous malformations in and out of the setting of congenital heart disease. Ann Thorac Surg 1998; 66(2): 688–91.
3. Gossage JR, Kanj G. Pulmonary arteriovenous malformations. A state of the art review. Am J Resp Crit Care Med 1998; 158(2): 643–61.
4. White RI Jr, Pollak JS, Wirth JA. Pulmonary arteriovenous malformations: diagnosis and transcatheter embolotherapy. J Vasc Interven Radiol 1996; 7(6): 787–904.
5. Coley SC, Jackson JE. Endovascular occlusion with a new mechanical detachable coil. AJR 1998; 171: 1075–9.
6. Sagara K, Miyazono N, Inoue H. Recanalization after coil embolotherapy of pulmonary arteriovenous malformations: study of long-term outcome and mechanism for recanalization. AJR 1998; 170: 727–30.
7. Milic A, Chan RP, Cohen JH. Reperfusion of pulmonary arteriovenous malformations after embolotherapy. J Vasc Interven Radiol 2005; 16(12): 1675–83.
8. Lee DW, White RI Jr., Egglin TK. Embolotherapy of large pulmonary arteriovenous malformations: long-term results. Ann Thorac Surg 1997; 64: 930–40.
9. Hill SL, Hijazi ZM, Hellenbrand WE. Evaluation of the AMPLATZER vascular plug for embolization of peripheral vascular malformations associated with congenital heart disease. Cathet Cardiovasc Interven 2006; 67(1): 113–19.
10. Pollak JS, Saluja S, Thabet A. Clinical and anatomic outcomes after embolotherapy of pulmonary arteriovenous malformations. J Vasc Interven Radiol 2006; 17(1): 34–5.

46

Transcatheter closure of coronary artery fistulas

Shakeel A Qureshi

Introduction

Coronary artery fistulas are connections between one or more of the coronary arteries and a cardiac chamber or great vessel. They are rare but are the commonest hemodynamically significant coronary artery abnormality, and usually occur in isolation.[1] Although usually congenital, they have been noted after cardiac surgery, such as valve replacement, coronary artery bypass grafting, and after repeated myocardial biopsies in cardiac transplantation.[2,3]

The fistula tends to be a dilated, long, and tortuous artery taking a course around the heart before terminating in a chamber or a vessel. It may drain from a main coronary artery or one or several branches of a coronary artery to a cardiac chamber or into a nearby vessel. Multiple feeding arteries to a single coronary artery fistula may exist.[2] More than 55% of the fistulas originate from the right coronary artery, with the left anterior descending coronary artery being the next most frequently involved.[4] Over 90% of the fistulas from either coronary artery drain to the right side of the heart. The remainder drain to either the left atrium or the left ventricle.[5] The sites of drainage in the right heart include the right atrium, vena cavae, right ventricle, or the pulmonary trunk. Multiple fistulas between the three major coronary arteries and the left ventricle have also been reported.[6]

Pathophysiology

When the coronary artery fistulas drain to the right side of the heart, the volume load is increased to the right heart as well as the pulmonary vascular bed, the left atrium, and the left ventricle. When the fistula drains into the left atrium or the left ventricle, there is volume overloading of these chambers but no increase in the pulmonary blood flow.

Clinical features

Although the majority of the fistulas are congenital, they do not usually cause symptoms or complications in the first two decades, especially if they are small. After this age, the frequency of both symptoms and complications increases.[7] The complications include 'steal' from the adjacent myocardium, thrombosis and embolism, cardiac failure, atrial fibrillation, rupture, endocarditis/endarteritis, and arrhythmias.[1,4,8,9] Thrombosis within the fistula, whilst rare, may cause acute myocardial infarction, paroxysmal atrial fibrillation, and ventricular arrhythmias.[10] Spontaneous rupture of the aneurysmal fistula causing hemopericardium has also been reported.[11]

Some fistulas may be large in the neonatal period, but others may increase in size over time. They vary from short and direct connections of a coronary artery with a chamber or a large vessel to complex aneurysmal cavities, in which blood may stagnate, clot, and calcify. The largest shunts tend to occur in those fistulas in which the coronary artery connects to the right side of the heart rather than the left heart chambers.

The majority of the patients are asymptomatic. Symptoms, when present, include exercise intolerance because of dyspnea, angina, and arrhythmias. Patients with large left-to-right shunts may have symptoms of congestive cardiac failure, especially in infancy and occasionally in the neonatal period.[12] Some patients may have angina and electrocardiographic evidence of myocardial ischemia.[2] Angina may occur because of a 'steal phenomenon'.[13] The commonest presentation is with detection of an asymptomatic continuous murmur over the praecordium. The murmur is heard over the mid-chest rather than below the left clavicle and typically peaks in mid-diastole rather than systole, as occurs when the murmur originates from the arterial duct.

Investigations

The electrocardiogram and chest X-ray are unlikely to help in the diagnosis. The electrocardiogram may show the effects of left ventricular volume overload and ischemic changes. However, in the presence of a normal electrocardiogram, if the patient is old enough to exercise on the treadmill with electrocardiographic monitoring, then ischemic ST-segment changes may become apparent.[13] Generally the chest X-ray is normal, but occasionally moderate cardiomegaly may be present.

Selective coronary angiography of both the coronary arteries is essential for confirming the diagnosis, the detailed anatomy of the fistula, and the presence of multiple fistulas. However, this should only be performed when definitive treatment such as an interventional procedure is planned. During such an intervention, a preliminary aortic root angiogram in a 'laid-back view' helps in determining which coronary artery to selectively catheterize.[14] Coronary angiography in several planes assumes great importance and should be performed in the same views as in adults. These views include right anterior oblique, straight antero-posterior, left anterior oblique, left anterior oblique with caudo-cranial angulation, and left lateral projections.

Treatment

The indications for treatment of coronary artery fistulas include the presence of a large or increasing left to right shunt, evidence of left ventricular volume overload, myocardial ischemia, left ventricular dysfunction, congestive cardiac failure, and prevention of endocarditis/endarteritis.

Surgery of coronary artery fistulas is associated with a low morbidity and mortality rate ranging from 0 to 6%.[15,16] Myocardial infarction has been reported in less than 5% of cases and there is a low but significant risk of persistence or recurrence of the fistula.[17] Over the last decade or so, trans-catheter closure of coronary artery fistulas has emerged as an effective and safe alternative to surgery, so, when available, it should be considered the treatment of choice.[2,18,19]

The aim of catheter closure is to occlude the fistulous artery as distally as possible or as close to its termination point as possible, avoiding any possibility of occluding branches to the normal myocardium. If, however, embolization is effected too distally, the embolization device could pass inadvertently beyond the fistula into the draining vessel or chamber and into the pulmonary circulation. Thus, it is important that whichever technique is used, the occlusion is effected at a very precise point. In practice, this involves the use of different types of embolization materials, such as detachable balloons, stainless steel coils, or platinum micro-coils.[2,19–23] The technique employed is influenced by several factors including the age of the patient, the morphology of the feeding arteries, their size and degree of tortuosity, and the location of the fistulous connection.

Equipment

The availability of a wide variety of equipment in the catheterization laboratory is essential for transcatheter closure of the fistula (Figure 46.1). This includes a selection of non-tapered catheters, Berman or Swan–Ganz balloon catheters, 3 Fr Tracker or Ferret catheters, a variety of floppy or superfloppy coronary guidewires of 0.014 inch caliber, a range of different types and sizes of coils (conventional Gianturco coils and controlled-release coils), detachable balloons, and a variety of umbrella type devices, which are used to close atrial septal defects or patent arterial ducts.

The choice of the equipment and the technique to be used depend on the tortuosity of the fistula vessels, the presence of a high flow in the fistula, aneurysmal dilation of the feeding vessel, and the point of intended occlusion. Other factors influencing the choice include the age and size of the patient, the catheter size that can be used in the patient, the size of the vessel to be occluded, and the tortuosity of the catheter course to reach the intended point of occlusion. For example, if the access artery is small, then a technique needing smaller sheaths and catheters is chosen. If the target vessel to be occluded is large, a large device that fits in the smallest guiding catheter or sheath is chosen. If the route to the target vessel is tortuous, then superfloppy guidewires and Tracker or Ferret catheters are preferable. If there is a high flow through the target vessel, then the stop–flow technique is used, in which a balloon inflated proximally stops the blood flow through the fistula. In all of the considerations, because of the need for precise occlusion, a potentially reversible technique is preferred.

Technique

Generally, access is obtained via both the femoral arteries and a femoral vein, in which 5 Fr sheaths are inserted. Both the femoral arteries are cannulated as, through one of the catheters, coils are deployed whilst check angiograms can be performed through a catheter from the other femoral artery. Alternatively, a balloon catheter can be inflated through the second arterial access to aid in coil deployment. Judkins left and right coronary catheters are used for selective angiography and, subsequently, a balloon catheter (Berman or Swan–Ganz) is passed and the balloon inflated with contrast or carbon dioxide to temporarily occlude the vessel. The balloon is kept inflated for 5–10 minutes and evidence of ischemia is sought.

If there are no ischemic changes, then a guiding coronary catheter appropriate for the coronary artery is positioned in the artery. If the fistula drainage point is fairly proximal and has a fairly straight course, then with the help of a 0.035 inch standard guidewire advanced into the fistula, the catheter can be passed to the point of intended occlusion. Through this catheter either Gianturco or Cook-PDA coils can be used to achieve occlusion. Stainless steel Gianturco coils of 0.038 inch caliber have been widely used and require standard non-tapered catheters of 5 or 6 Fr size for

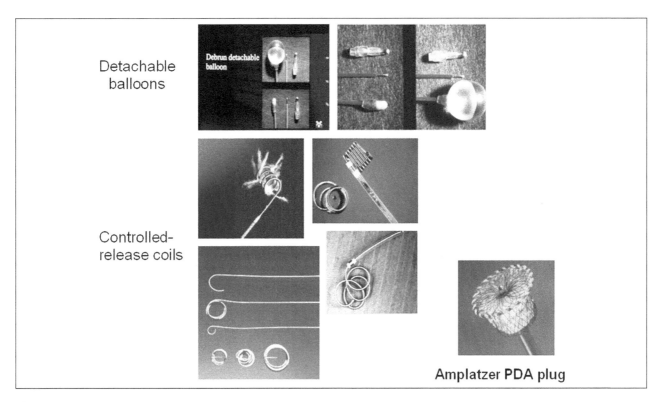

Figure 46.1
A variety of equipment for use in embolization.

the delivery of the coils (Figure 46.2). The size of the coil should be up to 30% larger than the vessel diameter, and in particular the drainage point, so that the coil does not pass through and embolize inadvertently. If this method is used, the first coil is the important one as, once this is in the correct position, different sizes of coils can be deployed subsequently to form a tight nest, which will promote occlusion. Positioning such catheters satisfactorily in a distal location in a coronary artery fistula may be both difficult and hazardous. The tortuosity of the fistula may prevent attempts at passing these larger catheters distally into the coronary artery. Therefore, this method may be used safely only in those patients in whom the fistulas have a short, relatively less tortuous course and in whom there may be aneurysmal dilation present in the fistulous vessel.

In those patients in whom the fistulous vessel is tortuous with multiple bends needing to be negotiated, or when the guiding catheter cannot reach the point of occlusion or when there is a high flow, it may be more appropriate to use controlled-release platinum micro coils of 0.018 inch caliber, which can be deployed using a co-axial 3 Fr Tracker or Ferret catheter passed through the guiding catheter. Such catheters, when used with superfloppy, steerable 0.014 inch coronary guidewires, can be manipulated through tortuous arteries into very distal locations and through them interlocking-detachable coils (IDC) or detachable coil system (DCS) coils

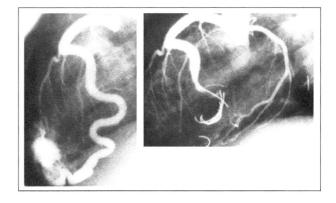

Figure 46.2
A fistula between the diagonal branch of the left anterior descending coronary artery and the right ventricle. The vessel is moderately tortuous and has been closed with Gianturco coils.

can be used (Figure 46.3a–d). These coils have controlled-release mechanisms and so make the procedure reversible and more controlled. If there is a high flow, then temporary balloon occlusion will be needed during the deployment of the coils (Figure 46.4).[24,25] Multiple coils can be deployed serially through these catheters. When negotiating these catheters, it is important to use a torque device to manipulate the guidewire around the various curves in the fistula.

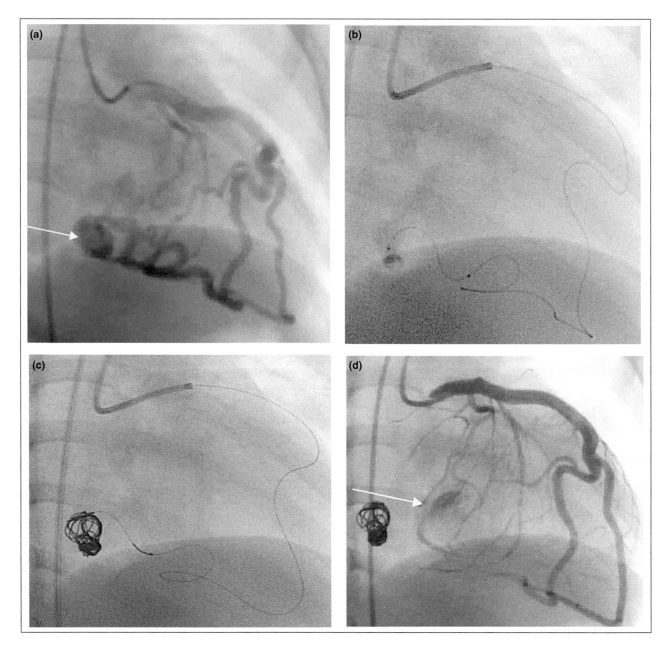

Figure 46.3
(a) A fistula between a branch of the left anterior descending coronary artery and the right ventricle. There are possibly two feeding vessels with a very tortuous course. The arrow points to the presence of an aneurysm at the point of entry into the right ventricle. (b) The Tracker catheter has been passed through the guiding catheter around the tortuous course into the aneurysm at the point of occlusion. (c) A nest of controlled-release coils packed into the aneurysm. (d) Complete occlusion of the main fistulous vessels, but now there is a tiny residual fistula from another vessel draining into the left ventricle (arrow).

A short distance of the guidewire is passed, followed by gentle and gradual movement forwards of the 3 Fr catheter, until this catheter has reached the point of occlusion. By gentle manipulation, it is surprising how relatively easily the curves can be negotiated and how far distally into the fistula the 3 Fr catheter can be passed. It is important to use a Tuohy–Borst adapter connected to the guiding catheter as well as the 3 Fr catheter for prevention of gradual blood loss.

The coil will then need to be passed through the hemostatic valve using an introducer provided with the coil.

Very high flow fistulous arteries present a particular problem because there will be a tendency for the coils to be pushed by the coronary blood flow into the right heart circulation. This potential practical difficulty can be overcome by using temporary occlusion of the proximal fistulous artery with a Berman balloon occlusion catheter, which

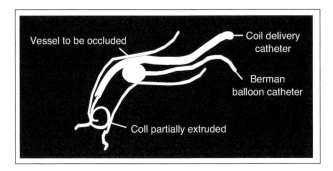

Figure 46.4
Diagrammatic illustration of the stop–flow technique using a balloon catheter.

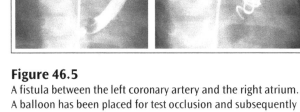

Figure 46.5
A fistula between the left coronary artery and the right atrium. A balloon has been placed for test occlusion and subsequently Gianturco coils have been deployed, resulting in complete occlusion of the fistula.

arrests the blood flow in the vessel. Whilst the balloon is kept inflated, several coils can be deployed to form a nest before deflating the balloon.[24] This technique has allowed an occluding mass of these coils to be safely and satisfactorily positioned to achieve complete occlusion (Figure 46.5).

A high flow artery can be difficult to occlude, so a mass of platinum coils is necessary. Availability of controlled-release coils has made the procedure more practical and safe. These coils can be positioned and withdrawn back into the catheter, if the final position is not satisfactory. The coils are not fibered and this results in very little resistance to passage through the microcatheters around the many curves that are normally encountered. However, the disadvantage of these coils is that thrombosis takes a considerably longer time than for the fibered coils.

If the fistula morphology is such that it can be accessed easily from the right side of the heart and when there is a large aneurysmal fistula near the drainage point into the right side of the heart (most often such fistulas drain into the right atrium), then this may be suitable for occlusion with an Amplatzer Duct Occluder or atrial septal occluder device.[12,26] The fistula vessel needs to be large, have easy and straight access from the right heart, even if an arteriovenous guidewire circuit is needed, and allow a guiding sheath to be passed into the vessel before deploying a device. In such cases, either femoral venous or internal jugular venous access is required over an arteriovenous guidewire circuit (Figure 46.6a–c). Creation of a circuit facilitates the passage of an appropriate sheath over the guidewire.

Detachable balloons have been deployed in the past as they can be floated out with the arterial flow and achieve immediate occlusion, which is reversible until the balloon is detached.[20,23] They are, however, complex to use and require large caliber, non-tapered introducer catheters (6–8 Fr). This presents a limitation to their use in infants and young children. Early deflation and premature detachment of these balloons are further problems and so they are rarely used.

After occluding the main fistulous vessel, it is imperative to repeat selective coronary angiography in both the coronary arteries as on occasions a second branch feeding the fistula may be visualized, which may then need to be occluded at the same procedure.

With transcatheter techniques, complete occlusion of the fistula may be achieved in >95% of the patients. The main complications (albeit of low frequency) encountered include either premature deflation (in the case of detachable balloons), inadvertent coil embolization (Figure 46.7a,b), transient T-wave changes, transient bundle branch block, and myocardial infarction (Figure 46.8). Some of the inadvertent embolizations may occur as a result of high flow in the large fistulas or with the selection of undersized coils.[24]

Discussion

A majority of coronary artery fistulas are asymptomatic in the early years. However, when large, they can cause symptoms of congestive cardiac failure or angina. This may be the cause at the extremes of life, in infants or middle aged or older adults. Coronary fistulas have been detected prenatally too, in which case, because of a large left to right shunt, they may cause congestive cardiac failure soon after birth.[27] If the congestive cardiac failure cannot be controlled, transcatheter closure may be needed early after birth.[12] If fistulas are detected in infancy and are asymptomatic, conservative management is appropriate as, very rarely, spontaneous closure of a small fistula has been reported.[28] Even if the fistula does not close, the older the patient, the fewer the technical complications encountered when the catheter procedure is attempted. Some authors recommend closure even in the absence of symptoms on the grounds that, with increasing age, the incidence of complications increases.[7]

As these fistulas are infrequently encountered, most operators will only deal with a small number of cases of coronary artery fistulas each year. The aim of the catheter

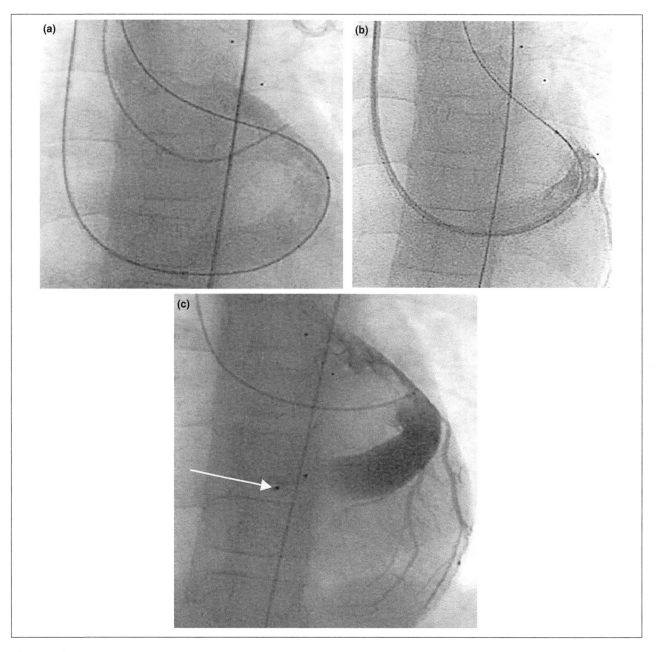

Figure 46.6

(a) A large fistula between the circumflex coronary artery and the right atrium. This fistulous vessel has been approached from the right internal jugular vein and an arteriovenous guidewire circuit has been established. (b) A sheath has been passed from the internal jugular vein into the dilated fistulous vessel, with improved filling of the native coronary artery. (c) An angiogram after implantation of an Amplatzer Duct Occluder (arrow) resulting in complete occlusion of the fistula and improved filling of the native coronary arteries.

procedure should be to achieve complete occlusion at as distal a location as possible in the fistulous vessel and this can be achieved with meticulous attention to the details of the technique. Specialized techniques and equipment are needed for catheter closure of these fistulas. Occasionally a combination of techniques is required, but the procedure has become easier with the availability of controlled-release platinum coils and the range of Amplatzer occluders, and any complexity of the fistulous vessel can be treated. The main complication is inadvertent embolization of the devices. However, even if any of these devices embolize, they can be retrieved by snares.

Conclusions

Excellent results can be achieved by the transcatheter embolization techniques to treat coronary artery fistulas.

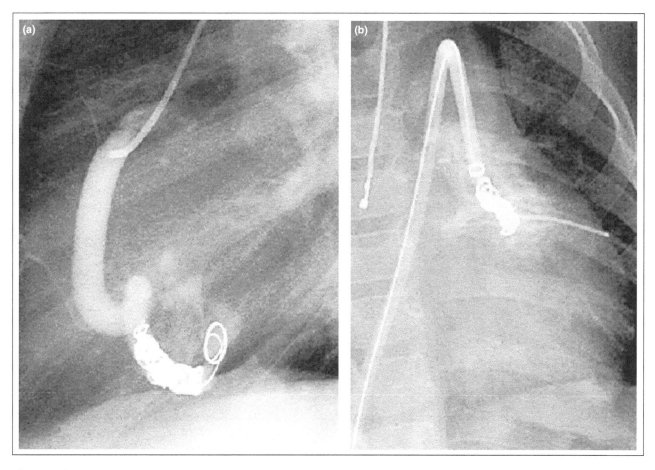

Figure 46.7
(a) A nest of coils released in the right coronary artery to right ventricle fistula, resulting in near complete occlusion. (b) The coils have embolized to the left pulmonary artery. A sheath has been placed close to the coils for retrieval with a snare catheter.

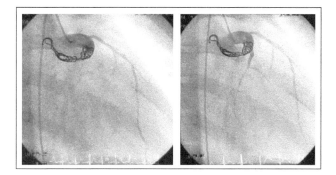

Figure 46.8
Coils implanted into a branch of the circumflex coronary artery (fistula between this and the right atrium) have produced complete occlusion of the main circumflex coronary artery. After thrombolysis with alteplase, there is now a patent circumflex coronary artery.

Furthermore, the technique of catheter closure allows a further arterial feeding vessel to be discovered by selective coronary angiography at the end of the procedure and, if such a dual supply is noted, this vessel can also be occluded.

It is vital to select an embolization technique suitable for the size and location of the fistula. A wide range of equipment should be available to cope with the great variety of fistulas as well as possible complications of the techniques. Nowadays, no patient should be referred for surgical ligation unless transcatheter closure has been considered.

References

1. Wilde P, Watt I. Congenital coronary artery fistulae: six new cases with a collective review. Clin Radiol 1980; 31: 301–11.
2. Reidy JF, Anjos RT, Qureshi SA et al. Transcatheter embolization in the treatment of coronary artery fistulas. J Am Coll Cardiol 1991; 18: 187–92.
3. Somers JM, Verney GI. Coronary cameral fistulae following heart transplantation. Clin Radiol 1991; 44: 419–21.
4. McNamara JJ, Gross RE. Congenital coronary artery fistula. Surgery 1969; 65: 59–69.
5. Levin DC, Fellows KE, Abrams HL. Hemodynamically significant primary anomalies of the coronary arteries. Circulation 1978; 58: 25–34.
6. Black IW, Loo CK, Allan RM. Multiple coronary artery–left ventricular fistulae: clinical, angiographic, and pathologic findings. Eur J Cardiothorac Surg 1991; 23: 133–5.

7. Liberthson RR, Sagar K, Berkoben JP et al. Congenital coronary arteriovenous fistula: report of 13 patients, review of the literature and delineation of management. Circulation 1979; 59: 849–54.

8. Alkhulaifi AM, Horner SM, Pugsley WB, Swanton RH. Coronary artery fistulas presenting with bacterial endocarditis. Ann Thorac Surg 1995; 60: 202–4.

9. Skimming JW, Walls JT. Congenital coronary artery fistula suggesting a 'steal phenomenon' in a neonate. Pediatr Cardiol 1993; 14: 174–5.

10. Ramo OJ, Totterman KJ, Harjula AL. Thrombosed coronary artery fistula as a cause of paroxysmal atrial fibrillation and ventricular arrhythmia. Cardiovasc Surg 1994; 2: 720–2.

11. Bauer HH, Allmendinger PD, Flaherty J et al. Congenital coronary arteriovenous fistula: spontaneous rupture and cardiac tamponade. Ann Thorac Surg 1996; 62: 1521–3.

12. Khan MD, Qureshi SA, Rosenthal E, Sharland GK. Neonatal transcatheter occlusion of a large coronary artery fistula with Amplatzer duct occluder. Cathet Cardiovasc Interven 2003; 60: 282–6.

13. Oshiro K, Shimabukuro M, Nakada Y et al. Multiple coronary LV fistulas: demonstration of coronary steal phenomenon by stress thallium scintigraphy and exercise hemodynamics. Am Heart J 1990; 120: 217–19.

14. Hofbeck M, Wild F, Singer H. Improved visualisation of a coronary artery fistula by the 'laid-back' aortogram. Br Heart J 1993; 70: 272–3.

15. Mavroudis C, Backer CL, Rocchini AP et al. Coronary artery fistulas in infants and children: a surgical review and discussion of coil embolization. Ann Thorac Surg 1997; 63: 1235–42.

16. Rittenhouse EA, Doty DB, Ehrenhaft JL. Congenital coronary artery–cardiac chamber fistula. Ann Thorac Surg 1975; 20: 468–85.

17. Kirklin JW, Barrat-Boyes BG. Cardiac Surgery, New York: John Wiley, 1987; 945–55.

18. Reidy JF, Jones ODH, Tynan MJ et al. Embolization procedures in congenital heart disease. Br Heart J 1985; 54: 184–92.

19. Perry SB, Rome J, Keane JF et al. Transcatheter closure of coronary artery fistulas. J Am Coll Cardiol 1992; 20: 205–9.

20. Reidy JF, Sowton E, Ross DN. Transcatheter occlusion of coronary to bronchial anastomosis by detachable balloon combined with coronary angioplasty at the same procedure. Br Heart J 1983; 49: 284–7.

21. Van den Brand M, Pieterman H, Suryapranata H, Bogers AJ. Closure of a coronary fistula with a transcatheter implantable coil. European J Cardiothorac Surg 1992; 25: 223–6.

22. De Wolf D, Terriere M, De Wilde P, Reidy JF. Embolization of a coronary fistula with a controlled delivery platinum coil in a 2-year old. Pediatr Cardiol 1994; 15: 308–10.

23. Skimming JW, Gessner IH, Victorica BE, Mickle JP. Percutaneous transcatheter occlusion of coronary artery fistulas using detachable balloons. Pediatr Cardiol 1995; 16: 38–41.

24. Qureshi SA, Reidy JF, Alwi MB et al. Use of interlocking detachable coils in embolization of coronary arteriovenous fistulas. Am J Cardiol 1996; 78: 110–13.

25. Quek SC, Wong J, Tay JS et al. Transcatheter embolization of coronary artery fistula with controlled release coils. J Paediatr Child Health 1996; 32: 542–4.

26. Sadiq M, Wilkinson JL, Qureshi SA. Successful occlusion of coronary arteriovenous fistula using an Amplatzer duct occluder. Cardiol Young 2001; 11: 84–7.

27. Sharland GK, Tynan M, Qureshi SA. Prenatal detection and progression of right coronary artery to right ventricle fistula. Heart 1996; 76: 79–81.

28. Muthusamy R, Gupta G, Ahmed RA et al. Fistula between a branch of left anterior descending coronary artery and pulmonary artery with spontaneous closure. Eur Heart J 1990; 11: 954–6.

Section X

Obstructions

47

Obstructions of the inferior and superior vena cava

Marc Gewillig

Anatomy and pathophysiology

Obstruction of caval veins is rare, and usually iatrogenic. Any surgical procedure involving the caval veins, including cannulation for bypass, may be complicated with caval vein obstruction. It was a common complication of the Mustard operation during early and long term follow-up, with restrictive venous pathways in the majority of the patients.[1,2] It has been described after a Senning type procedure, after a Glenn shunt or other cavopulmonary connections, after transplantation with structure of the anastomosis,[3] or after repair of abnormal pulmonary venous return with subdivision of the superior caval vein (SCV).

Multiple pacing leads or other long term catheters may lead to progressive narrowing, especially during growth of the patient. Thrombosis of a caval vein may occur after endothelial damage during traumatic puncture for central lines, after a long period of low cardiac output with hypertonic IV fluids, after recurrent and long term central venous lines,[4] and infections. Any hyperthrombotic state may exacerbate this problem (protein C or S, antithrombin 3, Leiden factor).

Congenital membranous obstruction of the inferior caval vein (ICV) at the junction with the right atrium has been described.[5] An obstructed inferior caval vein may present as Budd–Chiari syndrome.

External compression by a tumor (lung cancer, lymphoma), aneurysmal dilation of the ascending aorta, pseudoaneurysm of a venous coronary graft,[6] goiter, mediastinal fibrosis, constrictive pericarditis, bile duct distension, polycystic kidneys, hydatid cyst, and hematoma after blunt liver trauma have been reported. Vasculitis such as Behçet disease may lead to shrinkage and obstruction of the caval veins.[7]

Clinical symptoms, indications for treatment, and alternatives

Clinical symptoms depend on the onset and the rate of obstruction, the development of collateral flow and the function or patency of the other caval vein.

Obstruction of the SCV may result in superior caval vein syndrome: congestion, swelling and cyanosis of the head and the upper limbs, headache or cerebral venous hypertension, (pre)syncope, cough, and airway obstruction. Pemberton's sign involves jugular vein distension in the upright position, which progresses to cyanosis and facial edema while keeping both arms elevated. Retrograde congestion of the thoracic duct may lead to leakage of chyle into the gut (resulting in protein-losing enteropathy), into the pleural or pericardial space (chylothorax[8] or chylopericardium), or into the bronchial tree (plastic bronchitis).

Obstruction of the ICV may lead to abdominal congestion, chronic hepatic congestion leading to fibrosis, varices, exercise intolerance, fatigue or swelling of the legs, renal insufficiency with proteinuria,[9] or Budd–Chiari syndrome.[10,11]

If inflow to the heart is severely limited from all sides, this will result in decreased cardiac output, which can be very difficult to detect clinically. Tachycardia or exercise may then result in vertigo, syncope, or sudden death.

Alternative treatment from interventional catheterization depends on the etiology: mass resection or debulking, thrombolysis, anticoagulation, treatment with anti-inflammatory, antibiotic, or oncologic drugs, or radiation treatment may result in fast relief.

History of the procedure

For a long time surgery has been the therapy of choice for caval vein obstruction; it is, however, less well tolerated and has a significant morbidity. Stents have changed the treatment strategies enormously. The technique has evolved from bail-out for significant stenosis or obstruction, to electively altering flows to the heart. Currently percutaneous Fontan completion with rerouting of the ICV to the SCV or hemi-Fontan is being evaluated.

Pre-catheter imaging/assessment and indications

A high clinical suspicion for caval venous obstruction is mandatory in patients with previous caval vein surgery. Because of the sharp angles of Mustard patches when entering the pericardium, a subtotal obstruction can easily be missed with echocardiography. Similarly, Fontan conduits may be difficult to visualize. Even good clinicians may clinically miss obstruction of major caval veins, as this will not always result in retrograde congestion, but in low flow cardiac output.

Prior to the catheterization, the interventionalist should know which vessels are open and can be punctured, and whether a thrombus in the SCV or ICV is present. All information can usually be obtained with an echocardiogram. If a recent thrombus is present, thrombolysis should be given followed by anticoagulation, as any manipulation near or through the thrombus may cause multiple (paradoxic) embolizations.

Anesthesia/supporting imaging

Interventions of the SCV or ICV can best be approached from the ipsilateral femoral and/or jugular vein. After cannulation, an angiogram through the sheath should be performed to exclude thrombi. If the caval vein is completely obstructed, both the femoral and/or jugular vein should be cannulated, as this will allow the interventionalist to visualize the 'target' from both ends; occasionally this may reveal 'hidden' hypoplastic but patent pathways.

Stenting the ICV has been reported to be performed under echographic guidance only from centers with no or limited access to radiographic equipment,[12] and is not recommended.

Protocol of hemodynamic assessment

Gradients across obstructions can be obtained, but because of the collateral circulation with low flow and low cardiac output, the clinical significance of a stenosis can be severely underestimated.

Angiography catheter selection

Good angiographic visualization in standard perpendicular planes proximal and distal to the stenosis/obstruction is important. If the vessel is no longer patent, the lesion should be approached from both ends (cannulation of groin and neck veins). This will allow accurate determination of the length of the obstruction and the desired diameter of the final stent.

Catheter/wire interchange for delivery of balloon/stent/device

After visualization of the obstruction (whether total or subtotal), a wire must be positioned across the lesion. If the caval vein is still patent, this is usually easy. If a segment has thrombosed or is atretic, a new channel must be made.

Frequently a small vein may partially bridge the thrombosed distance; this vein should be probed with a thin wire such as a 0.018 inch Terumo wire or a 0.014 inch non-kinkable coronary wire (PT2), followed by a thin catheter or tracker system (Micro catheter system: 0.021 inch hydrophobic wire in a 2.7 Fr co-axial catheter system, used through a 4 Fr vertebral catheter with a 0.035 inch lumen). A final segment can be completely obliterated, making a new route necessary. The most common technique involves puncturing with a straightened Brockenbrough needle within a 6 or 8 Fr dilator and transseptal sheath. It is important to determine the cannulation point (groin or neck) from which the puncture will be easiest. Preference will be given to the side which allows a straight route. When puncturing from one end, it is wise to provide a target at the other side: deployment of a 5 or 10 mm snare perpendicular to the needle provides a vessel-centered and radio-opaque marker; it also allows snaring and exteriorizing of the wire once grabbed, creating a veno-venous loop (Figure 47.1). Alternatively, a new route can be made with radiofrequency ablation or laser ablation.

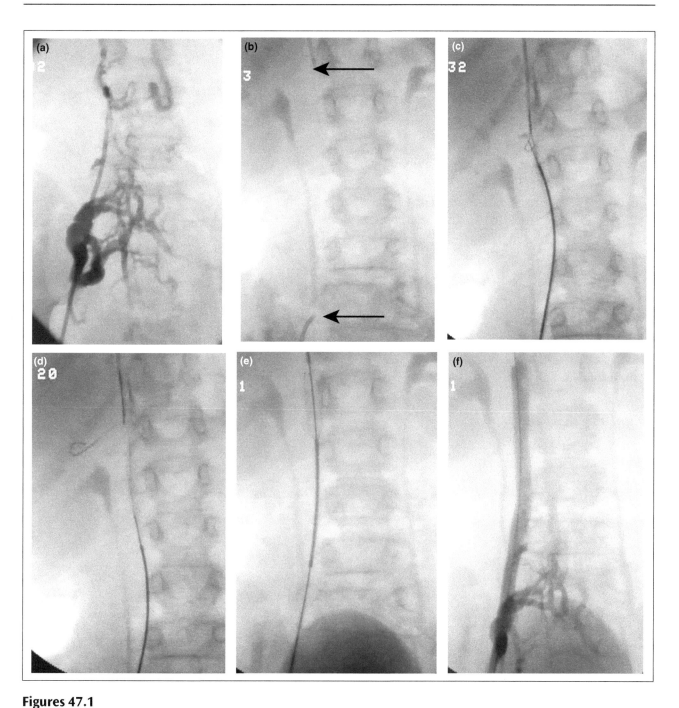

Figures 47.1

(a) 10-year-old patient with obstruction of inferior caval vein between the iliac vein and insertion of renal veins. (b) Shows the distance to cover between the catheter in the iliac vein and the catheter from the jugular vein down to the obstruction (arrows). (c) A 10 mm snare was used as target for the Brockenbrough needle within a 6 Fr long sheath. (d) A 0.014 inch wire was inserted through the Brockenbrough needle and grasped by the snare. (e) Partial opening of a 10/80 SMART Cordis self-expandable stent, which was lengthened with a 10/60 SMART Cordis stent. (f) Final result after balloon dilation with an 8 mm balloon; good patency and run-off were documented 3 years after this procedure.

Once the lesion is crossed, an extra stiff wire should be used, to give optimal support and steering of the balloon during deployment. Balloon dilation alone may give good relief,[13] however, with frequent early recurrence of stenosis.[14,15] Most interventionalists therefore will currently prefer stent implantation. Pre-dilation with small balloons may be indicated in order to get the stent or delivery system in place across the obstruction. Pre-dilation with large

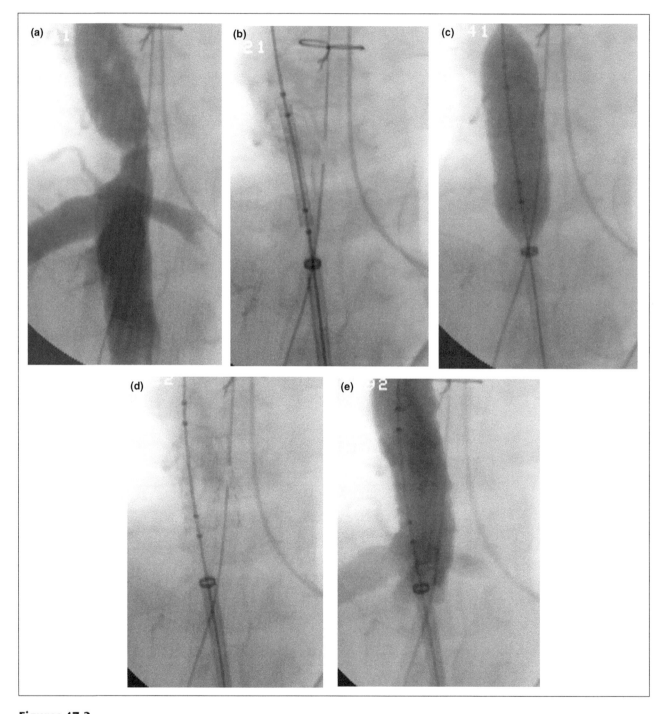

Figures 47.2

(a) 4-year-old patient 1 hour after TCPC (total cavo pulmonary connection) Fontan completion: a significant stenosis at the caudal junction of the inferior caval vein with an 18 mm Goretex conduit is demonstrated. (b) A 25 mm Genesis stent (Johnson & Johnson) mounted on a 14 mm BIB (balloon in balloon, Numed Inc., Huntington, New York, USA) is positioned through an 11 Fr long Mullins sheath (Cook). (c) Full inflation of outer BIB balloon. (d) Stent well deployed. (e) Cavogram through the sheath demonstrating good relief of the stenosis. This stent was fully expanded up to 18 mm 6 months later.

balloons may allow assessment of the contours of the stenotic site, the stretchability, and the recoil; however, it may cause the subsequent stent to have less grip on the wall.

A choice must be made from different types of stents: self-expanding or balloon-expandable stents.

A self-expanding stent is more flexible, it will continuously push radially to reach its nominal value, and it will re-expand after external compression (resuscitation, blunt thoracic trauma). A self-expanding stent is limited in maximal diameter, and cannot be dilated beyond a nominal value. Such a stent is good for long lesions but not ideal for short discrete lesions, such as obstruction in Mustard repair.[16]

Balloon-expandable stents have a high radial strength and are ideal for short lesions (Figure 47.2). An external force may deform such stents, thereby decreasing or obliterating the lumen.

Both types of stents are available with a covering (graft stents). Covered stents are indicated if rupture to an adjacent cavity/vessel is likely or has occurred, such as the pulmonary pathway (in Mustard with patch leak, rupture to pleura), or if an endothelial reaction or tumoral invasion is likely.

Multiple case reports or small series can be found in the world literature.[17–30]

Post-deployment protocol

Angiography post-deployment of the stent must be made prior to removal of the wire by injection through the sheath, or via a multi-track catheter (NUMED). If extravasation of contrast is observed, a covered stent can still be positioned and deployed. If blood loss is significant, gentle balloon occlusion may temporarily obliterate the tear while preparing the covered stent.

Pitfalls, problems, and complications

Dilation of the caval veins may be complicated by rupture into the pleura with hemothorax, tear extending into the pericardium with tamponade, tear into the pulmonary venous pathway allowing right-to-left or left-to-right shunting, tear into the ascending aorta, compression or damage of phrenic or vagal nerves, compression or elongation of the sinus node artery with loss of stable sinus rhythm, compression of the thoracic duct, or compression of the ureter.

Caval veins can significantly stretch and may show some contractility/peristalsis; this may lead to stent migration within minutes or hours after deployment, and embolization to the right ventricle or into the pulmonary artery. Self-expanding stents can be recaptured with a snare at one end, and refolded into a big sheath;[31] balloon-expandable stents are much more difficult to retrieve, and should be parked or expanded and left safe somewhere in the circulatory system, or retrieved surgically.

Recurrent stenosis or thrombosis may occur and appropriate anticoagulation should be given. However, large stents in large veins in patients with good cardiac output have a low tendency to thrombose. When in doubt it is safer to give anti-aggregation or anticoagulation, at least early

after the procedure, allowing the endothelium to cover most of the bare metal.

During long term follow-up a stent may fracture, or may be compressed by blunt external trauma such as resuscitation or a car accident. Radiographic control in two perpendicular dimensions will easily reveal this complication.

When deployed next to pacing wires, the pacing lead may be subject to concentrated movements in one limited region, resulting in metal fatigue and lead fracture; damage to the insulation may cause a current leak of the pacemaker leads, with dysfunction of the pacing system.

References

1. Moons P, Gewillig M, Sluysmans T et al. Long term outcome up to 30 years after the Mustard or Senning operation: a nationwide multicenter study in Belgium. Heart 2004; 90: 307–13.
2. Michel-Behnke I, Hagel KJ, Bauer J, Schranz D. Superior caval venous syndrome after atrial switch procedure: relief of complete venous obstruction by gradual angioplasty and placement of stents. Cardiol Young 1998; 8(4): 443–8.
3. Jayakumar A, Hsu DT, Hellenbrand WE, Pass RH. Endovascular stent placement for venous obstruction after cardiac transplantation in children and young adults. Cathet Cardiovasc Interven 2002; 56: 383–6.
4. O'Mahony M, Skehan S, Gallagher C. Percutaneous stenting of the superior vena cava syndrome in a patient with cystic fibrosis. Ir Med J 2005; 98(3): 85–6.
5. Gandhi S, Pigula F. Congenital membranous obstruction of the inferior caval vein. Ann Thorac Surg 2004; 78: 1849.
6. Kavanagh E, Hargaden G, Flanagan F, Murray J. CT of a ruptured vein graft pseudoaneurysm: an unusual cause of superior vena cava obstruction. Am J Radiology 2004; 183: 1239–40.
7. Ousehal A, Abdelouafi A, Thrombati, Kadiri R. Thrombosis of the superior vena cava in Behcet's disease. A propos de 1 cas. J Radiol 1992; 73: 383–88.
8. Rao PS, Wilson AD. Chylothorax, an unusual complication of baffle obstruction following Mustard operation: succesful treatment with balloon angioplasty. Am Heart J 1992; 123(1): 244–8.
9. Stecker MS, Casciani T, Kwo PY, Lalka SG. Percutaneous stent placement as treatment of renal vein obstruction due to inferior vena caval thrombosis. Cardiovasc Interven Radiol 2005; 8: [Epub].
10. Sanchez-Recalde A, Sobrino N, Galeote G et al. [Budd–Chiari syndrome with complete occlusion of the inferior vena cava: percutaneous recanalization by angioplasty and stenting.] Rev Esp Cardiol 2004; 57(11): 1121–3.
11. Han SW, Kim GW, Lee J et al. Successful treatment with stent angioplasty for Budd–Chiari syndrome in Behcet's disease. Rheumatol Int 2005; 25(3): 234–7.
12. Zhang C, Fu L, Zhang G et al. Long-term effect of stent placement in 115 patients with Budd–Chiari syndrome. World J Gastroenterol 2003; 9: 2587–91.
13. Berg A, Norgard G, Greve G. Hemoptisis as a late complication of a Mustard operation treated by balloon dilation of a superior caval venous obstruction. Cardiol Young 2002; 12: 298–301.
14. Lock JE, Bass JL, Castaneda W et al. Dilation angioplasty of congenital or operative narrowings of venous channels. Circulation 1984; 70: 457–64.
15. Abdulhamed JM, al Yousef S, Khan MA, Mullins C. Balloon dilatation of complete obstruction of the superior vena cava after Mustard operation for transposition of great arteries. Br Heart J 1994; 72(5): 482–5.
16. Brown S, Eyskens B, Mertens L et al. Self expandable stents for relief of venous baffle obstruction after the Mustard operation. Heart 1998; 79: 230–3.

17. Ing FF, Mullins CE, Grifka RG et al. Stent dilation of superior vena cava and innominate vein obstructions permits transvenous pacing lead implantation. Pacing Clin Electrophysiol 1998; 21(8): 1517–30.

18. MacLellan-Tobert SG, Cetta F, Hagler DJ. Use of intravascular stents for superior vena caval obstruction after the Mustard operation. Mayo Clin Proc 1996; 71(11): 1071–6.

19. Castelli P, Caronno R, Piffaretti G et al. Endovascular treatment for superior vena cava obstruction in Behcet disease. J Vasc Surg 2005; 41: 548–51.

20. Bansal N, Deshpande S. Novel use of Brockenbrough needle in relieving membranous obstruction of the inferior vena cava. Heart 2005; 91: e38.

21. Ward CJ, Mullins CE, Nihill MR. Use of intravascular stents in systemic venous and systemic venous baffle obstructions: short term follow-up results. Circulation 1995; 91: 2948–54.

22. Trerotola SO, Lund GB, Samphilipo MA et al. Palmaz stent in the treatment of central venous stenosis: safety and efficacy of dilation. Radiology 1994; 190: 379–85.

23. Stavropoulos GP, Hamilton I. Severe superior vena caval syndrome after the Mustard repair in a patient with persistent left superior vena cava. Eur J Cardiothorac Surg 1994; 8(1): 48–50.

24. Ro PS, Hill SL, Cheatham JP. Congenital superior vena cava obstruction causing anasarca and respiratory failure in a newborn: successful transcatheter therapy. Catheter Cardiovasc Interven 2005; 65(1): 60–5.

25. Bolad I, Karanam S, Mathew D et al. Percutaneous treatment of superior vena cava obstruction following transvenous device implantation. Cathet Cardiovasc Interven 2005; 65(1): 54–9.

26. Kanzaki M, Sakuraba M, Kuwata H et al. [Stenting in obstruction of superior vena cava; clinical experience with the self-expanding endovascular prosthesis.] Kyobu Geka 2004; 57(5): 347–50; discussion 350–2.

27. Sharaf E, Waight DJ, Hijazi ZM. Simultaneous transcatheter occlusion of two atrial baffle leaks and stent implantation for SVC obstruction in a patient after Mustard repair. Cathet Cardiovasc Interven 2001; 54(1): 72–6.

28. Schneider DJ, Moore JW. Transcatheter treatment of IVC channel obstruction and baffle leak after Mustard procedure for d-transposition of the great arteries using Amplatzer ASD device and multiple stents. J Invas Cardiol 2001; 13(4): 306–9.

29. Mohsen AE, Rosenthal E, Qureshi SA, Tynan M. Stent implantation for superior vena cava occlusion after the Mustard operation. Cathet Cardiovasc Interven 2001; 52(3): 351–4.

30. El-Said HG, Ing FF, Grifka RG et al. 18-year experience with transseptal procedures through baffles, conduits, and other intra-atrial patches. Cathet Cardiovasc Interven 2000; 50(4): 434–9; discussion 440.

31. Srinathan S, McCafferty I, Wilson I. Radiological management of superior vena caval stent migration and infection. Cardiovasc Interven Radiol 2005; 28(1): 127–30.

48

Relief of right ventricular outflow tract obstruction

Neil Wilson

Relief of right ventricular outflow tract obstruction

Right ventricular outflow tract obstruction (RVOTO) can occur as an isolated congenital lesion or it can be associated with other intracardiac pathology such as ventricular septal defect (VSD) as in tetralogy of Fallot. In some patients with pulmonary atresia and VSD the pulmonary valve may be atretic and the right ventricular outflow tract well delineated. Such patients may be suitable for interventional relief of their obstruction.

As with much congenital heart disease RVOTO can exist as mild, moderate, or severe. Intervention of any sort is generally only indicated for patients with severe disease where there is concern over the long term effects of right ventricular hypertension, or when in the presence of a right to left shunt at ventricular level, pulmonary blood flow is significantly reduced and the patient is cyanosed. Interventional treatment can also be applied to patients who have undergone surgical treatment of their disease. This is seen particularly in patients with tetralogy of Fallot who have undergone reparative surgery, though the RVOTO is almost always associated with significant pulmonary regurgitation. Obstruction is also seen in chronic patients who have undergone right ventricular to pulmonary artery conduit operations of the Rastelli sort, and is acknowledged in every sort of conduit used. Obstruction may be complicated by kinking of the conduit, adhesion to the posterior aspect of the sternum, and calcification within the conduit. Calcification is a particular problem with homografts and on occasions can occur very early. Such operations are most commonly seen with repair of pulmonary atresia with VSD, complex forms of transposition of the great arteries (TGA) complicated by pulmonary stenosis and VSD, and surgical repair of truncus arteriosus. The Ross operation performed for severe aortic valve disease by necessity involves a right ventricular outflow tract conduit and this too degenerates in time and can become both stenotic and regurgitant.

Relief of the stenotic lesions in these patients is fraught with difficulty. An apparently successful result may be modified by the nature of the pathologic substrate, distal stenotic disease of the branch pulmonary arteries, calcification, infection, and/or pulmonary regurgitation. Of course in growing children, an acutely successful result will require attention as somatic growth induces recurrent stenosis; this is particularly relevant of course when stents are used.

The first documented intervention to the right ventricular outflow tract was performed by Hausdorf et al and reported in 1993.[1] They rapidly deduced that stenting was likely to be required when, having performed an acutely successful radiofrequency-assisted valvuloplasty in a patient with pulmonary atresia and VSD, severe dynamic infundibular stenosis developed, necessitating stent angioplasty to relieve the obstruction 2 weeks later. Figure 48.1 shows pre- and post-stenting of the RVOT in a baby who had undergone radiofrequency-assisted valvuloplasty for pulmonary atresia with VSD and required a stent for severe dynamic infundibular obstruction.

The futility of balloon angioplasty alone in stenosed conduits has been demonstrated by Sanatani et al,[2] where stenotic gradients were only reduced modestly and surgical conduit replacement was required in almost all of the patients reported in the study. High pressure and double balloon techniques[3] have offered good acute results, though longevity of relief in large series has not been proven. Stenting of conduits offers better results[4] and this can offer useful palliation in delaying conduit replacement surgery. In practical terms, therefore, stenting should be considered for all forms of RVOTO.

Severe muscular obstruction RVOTO is clearly unamenable to balloon angioplasty alone and stent implantation is extremely effective, as seen in Figure 48.2.

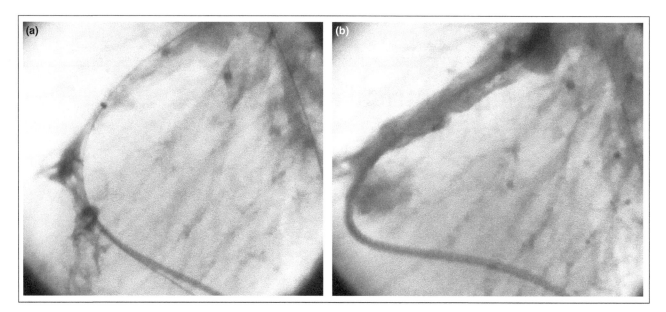

Figure 48.1
(a) Right ventricular angiogram showing severe long segment infundibular stenosis following radiofrequency-assisted valvuloplasty for pulmonary atresia with VSD. (b) Relief of RVOTO above following stent implantation.

Technique

Patients are generally selected prior to cardiac catheterization according to Table 48.1, though of course it may be impossible to predict the interventional strategy until hemodynamics and angiography are performed. Venous sheath selection should take into consideration the possible use of the diagnostic and subsequent balloon catheters. It is my usual practice to oversize the venous sheath in order to facilitate using a multi-track catheter for hemodynamic and angiographic data. Use of this catheter ensures that once a stable guidewire is in position, repeated catheter and wire replacement is not necessary. Some operators prefer to modify their own monorail type system by cutting off the end of a pigtail catheter and running it along the wire by means of the cut end hole and one of the side holes. Venous access is usually from the femoral vein, but in chronic patients thrombosis and collateralization of the iliofemoral veins may have occurred and alternative access via the right or left internal jugular vein, and exceptionally transhepatic access, may be necessary. It is recommended to have some form of arterial access for comparison of hemodynamics and beat to beat monitoring.

Right ventricular and systemic pressures should be measured simultaneously and expressed as a ratio. This is because at the end of a long procedure cardiac output may be compromised and a numerically lower right ventricular pressure may be only so because cardiac output is reduced and the systemic pressure too is reduced. It is important too to have some assessment of pulmonary regurgitation which often co-exists. This too will tend to play some part in

maintaining right ventricular pressure despite good relief of obstruction. Branch pulmonary artery anatomy is important; discrete, single, multiple, proximal, and distal stenotic lesions may maintain right ventricular hypertension when the proximal RVOTO is relieved. Branch pulmonary artery stenosis is dealt with elsewhere in this book, but it is clear that when there is co-existing significant pathology of this type it should be dealt with at the time of relief of the RVOTO. It is generally my personal practice to deal with distal lesions first, but this is a point of discussion.

Having obtained hemodynamic data with an endhole catheter of the multi-purpose type the catheter should be positioned distally in either pulmonary artery branch. It may be necessary to use a Terumo hydrophilic wire to first achieve this position.

Wire selection and positioning

A heavy duty exchange length 0.035 inch guidewire of 260 cm is then exchanged down the catheter. My personal preference is for the Amplatz range of stiff guidewires, such as the superstiff, extrastiff, or ultrastiff. These wires have a floppy end. Stability of the wire can be a potential problem as their own rigidity when under tension around the contours of the right ventricle and pulmonary arteries can induce recoil and wire position can be lost. 'Buckling' of the soft tip in the distal pulmonary artery can go some way to prevent this. Alternatively, some operators may choose to hand manufacture a bend on the stiff end of the guidewire and insert that end first. Time spent on securing a good

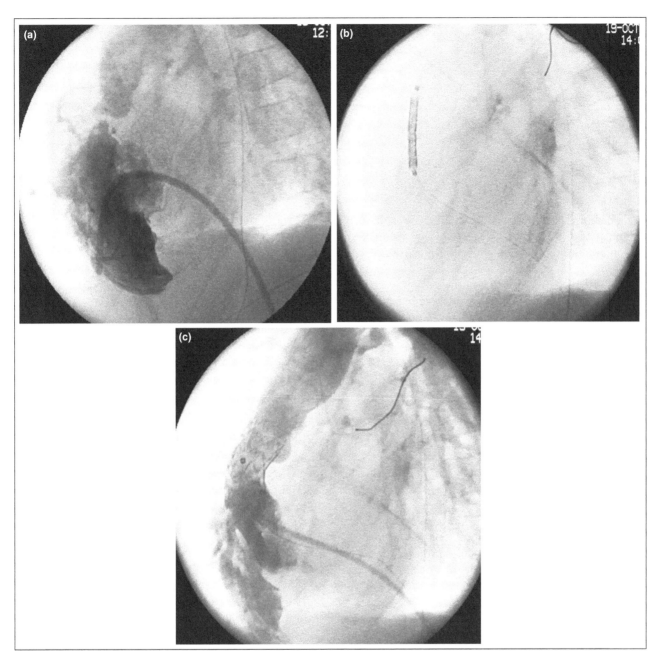

Figure 48.2
(a) Right ventricular angiogram in the lateral projection showing severe muscular RVOTO in a patient with pulmonary atresia with intact septum who had undergone surgical valvotomy as a neonate. (b) Stent in place prior to deployment. Note absence of supporting sheath in this small child. (c) Stent deployed showing complete relief of obstruction.

distal stable wire position is a worthwhile maneuver in the long run. Smaller patients will require narrower gauge wires, though support strength is still a consideration. Angiography is best performed biplane in a lateral projection and for normal sites and connections, a right anterior oblique (RAO) projection with some cranial tilt. As mentioned above, use of the multi-track catheter should be considered.

Balloon selection

The next decision is selecting the size of the balloon and stent to be used. When dealing with conduits of any sort a high pressure balloon is recommended. The Z Med balloon series has a good combination of balloon strength and shaft size. Alternatively, the BiB (NuMed) series of balloon is a

Table 48.1   *Indications for interventional relief of RVOTO*

- Symptoms: may be subjective; metabolic exercise testing helpful

- Right ventricular hypertension > 2/3 systemic level

- Right ventricular dysfunction/dyskinesis assessed by echocardiography, tissue Doppler imaging, magnetic resonance imaging

- ECG markers such as QRS duration, loss of dispersion

Table 48.2   *Arguments in favor of predilation*

- Accurately delineates the site of maximum obstruction

- Reassures compliance of the lesion if possible

- Inability to fully dilate a lesion with a stent mounted on the balloon could have disastrous consequences

- Improving compliance of a resistant lesion facilitates the next stage in the procedure, such as passage of a long, large bore sheath

- The 'denatured' balloon material allows excellent subsequent secure mounting of the stent, minimizing slippage

good choice. The Mullins balloon is exceptionally strong, though it has the drawback that if used with a stent, the balloon profile after inflation can make for considerable traction on removal. Balloon size is chosen according to the anticipated required diameter of the outflow tract. If dealing with a conduit there is clearly no need to be larger than its known diameter.

Pre-dilation of lesions in severe chronic obstruction is a debatable point. Unless using a BiB balloon which has a 'built in' pre-dilation I favor pre-dilating to 50–75% of the anticipated final balloon size. Table 48.2 outlines the advantages of pre-dilation.

Long sheath positioning

The next stage is placement of a long intracardiac sheath to a position well into either pulmonary artery along the guidewire. Sheath caliber is crucial. I choose to oversize 2–3 Fr gauges above the shaft size of the balloon catheter being used. This facilitates passage of the balloon–stent assembly through the heart without friction, minimizing the possibility of stent displacement from the balloon as it is advanced. It also allows the balloon to be removed through the long sheath after dilation. Maintaining long sheath position stabilizes wire position, facilitates passage of the multi-track catheter, and is useful back-up if a larger diameter balloon catheter is required to complete full deployment. Currently the most appropriate large bore, long sheaths are the curved Mullins series (Cook, William Cook Europe) or the Arrowflex (Arrow, Inc., Reading, PA, USA). Arrowflex sheaths are kink-resistant, though their structure of metallic wound reinforcement can lead to 'dragging' of the balloon–stent assembly as it passes through it. On the other hand, the dilator is finely tapered and runs well over the guidewire for positioning. Some operators have confidence in advancing the balloon–stent assembly through the circulation without long sheath protection, merely utilizing the short venous sheath at the groin. This technique can be successful in very small children (see Figure 48.2), and in the event of having difficulty positioning a long sheath, but it does carry a serious risk of stent dislodgement as it is advanced within

the heart. It also limits the recovery strategy in the event of complication and should not be used as a first choice technique.

Choice of stent

Currently only balloon-expandable stents are appropriate for the right ventricular outflow tract. These are of two sorts, stainless steel or platinum (Figure 48.3). Of the stainless steel series, a stent with high radial strength is recommended: either the Palmaz series (Cordis J & J Interventional Systems)[5] or the Intrastent Max LD (eV3 Plymouth, MN, USA).[6] The platinum stent (CP Stent, NuMed, Hopkinto, NY, USA)[7] is more radio-opaque and capable of large diameter dilation, and is also available covered with expanded polytetrafluoroethylene. The length of stent is chosen to cover the stenotic area, taking into consideration the effect of shortening on the initial deployment and, of course, for subsequent balloon dilation should that be necessary to keep pace with somatic growth in children. Overlong stents may be difficult to pass throught the sheath as it turns through the tricuspid valve and curves anteriorly to the outflow tract. Prior to mounting on the balloon, if the balloon has not previously been used I inflate to nominal pressure to denature the balloon material somewhat to enhance its security on the balloon. I also prefer to 'tease' open the ends of the stent as I mount it on the balloon to avoid the sharp tines of the stent puncturing the balloon. The stent is then hand crimped with a guidewire in the balloon catheter lumen to avoid crushing, which might hinder its running on the guidewire.

The balloon–stent assembly is then advanced over the wire through the long sheath as far as the main pulmonary artery, perhaps a little distal in position to that judged ideal. The sheath is then withdrawn, uncovering the stent. Angiograms are performed through the side arm of the sheath to facilitate accurate positioning. The balloon is then inflated slowly using an inflation device. One operator should be in control of the balloon catheter shaft, ready to

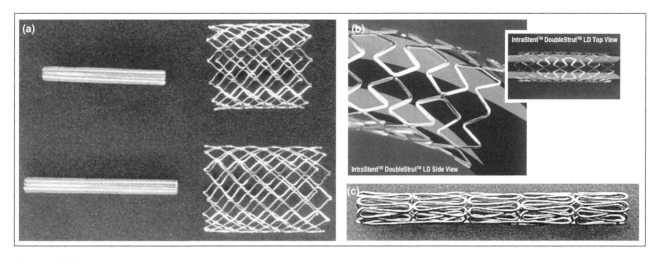

Figure 48.3

(a) Palmaz stainless steel stents. (b) Intrastent; Max series required for radial strength but offers some flexibility. (c) CP (Cheatham Platinum) stent has excellent radio-opacity and is capable of large diameter dilation.

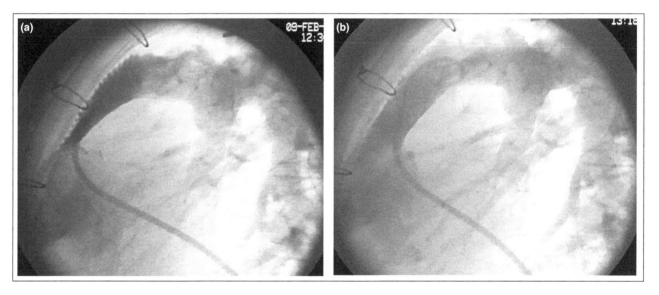

Figure 48.4

(a) Severe stenotic sternal compression in a corrugated right ventricle–pulmonary artery conduit. (b) Relief of obstruction following stent implantation.

make small adjustments of advancing or withdrawal should the balloon appear to recoil or advance away from the target. Prolonged inflation is usually not necessary, though deployment to nominal balloon pressure is almost always required to ensure proper seating of the stent. After deflating the balloon I usually wait a few seconds to ensure the balloon material has folded well. If the stent appears well applied to the lesion there is probably little need to inflate a second time,

but many operators choose to do so out of habit. After the balloon has deflated fully it is removed and hemodynamics and angiograms assessed. A second balloon can be then used if further dilation of the stent is deemed necessary.

Figure 48.4 shows relief of a right ventricle to pulmonary artery conduit which has been compressed by the posterior aspect of the sternum. Balloon angioplasty alone is ineffective in such cases. Stent implantation offers impressive relief.

Potential problems and complications

Difficulty positioning a long sheath can be experienced on two accounts. Firstly the large bore sheath may not run over even the stiffest of support guidewires and secondly, as the sheath is positioned cardiac output is compromised and systemic blood pressure falls. In the first instance consider changing to a more flexible, less stiff guidewire. The logic for this is that sometimes the wire tension presses so forcefully on the margin of the stenotic lesion that the sheath cannot advance between the lesion wall and the wire. Alternatively consider a different venous approach, say from the right internal jugular vein. In the second instance of loss of cardiac output this is usually as a consequence of the tricuspid valve being splinted open by the sheath. Again a less stiff wire may help, as might a volume infusion. Another tactic to overcome either of these issues is to 'front load' the balloon stent assembly through the long sheath, effectively using the tip of the balloon as a dilator. This can be performed starting outside the body or alternatively the sheath can be positioned say in the high inferior vena cava, the balloon–stent assembly advanced to the tip of the sheath and then the two advanced together into position, taking care not to allow the balloon–stent to protrude too far out of the end of the sheath.

Stent displacement on the balloon during advancement to the field of interest can be minimized by following the methods above to ensure good adherence of the stent by inflating the balloon prior to mounting to slightly denature the balloon fabric. Inflating the balloon a very small amount can also be used to ensure fixation of the stent and improve stability. 'Glueing' of the stent with a small amount of viscous contrast is anecdotally favored by some operators.

Displacement or embolization

This can also occur before or after balloon dilation. Providing the wire position is not lost it may be possible to secure the stent back on the balloon by advancing the balloon, partially inflating, and advancing or withdrawing to position appropriately. After stent deployment balloon removal can occasionally dislodge it. To avoid this it is recommended to keep the long sheath advanced as the balloon is first inflated than deflated as the sheath is advanced over it.[8] Displacement or embolization once inflated is a more difficult prospect and, unless the stent can be recaptured by a slightly larger balloon and manipulated into position, referral for surgical retrieval is probably prudent.

Stent compression/fracture

In the presence of pulmonary artery stenosis which maintains high right ventricular pressure it is possible that a RVOT stent may be compressed and subsequently fractured, resulting in recurrence of obstruction. Fracture has been reported with every known type of balloon-expandable stent. In most instances the fracture *per se* is not harmful as the stent struts are secured within the wall of the outflow tract. Fracture or compression can be treated by implanting a second or third stent within the existing one. Figure 48.5 demonstrates stent compression and fracture.

Homograft fracture

Calcified homografts probably undergo minor fractures quite frequently during balloon angioplasty. Major fractures can lead to disruption and dehiscence of the conduit, leading to severe hemorrhage and death. Though major fracture can be unpredictable it is appropriate to consider staged pre-dilation in patients with extensive homograft calcification, and to have a covered balloon-expandable stent such as the covered CP stent as a possible rescue strategy.[7]

Coronary artery compression

Anomalous and aberrant courses of the coronary arteries are not unusual in many of the patients undergoing angioplasty procedures to the right ventricular outflow tract. In such patients stent angioplasty rarely can lead to temporary or permanent occlusion of the coronary arteries. This is a particular hazard in patients who have undergone Rastelli type operations for complex forms of transposition of the great arteries. It is prudent therefore in such patients to delineate coronary artery anatomy relative to the RVOT, either by magnetic resonance imaging or angiography. If there is ongoing concern then a pre-dilation strategy with particular attention to signs of ischemia on the ECG is recommended.

Conclusions

Stenting offers good relief of right ventricular outflow tract obstruction in the native or conduit setting. Potential risks and complications can be kept to a minimum by meticulous technique and experience. Almost all of these patients will have chronic ongoing disease and in this setting stenting must be considered palliative, though this aim is admirable when surgical conduit replacement can be deferred.[9]

Of course the legacy of stenting in this anatomic position is that, for many patients, stenotic pathology is reduced at the expense of worsening regurgitation. It is most fitting therefore that such patients may be eminently suitable for relief of their pulmonary regurgitation by interventional implantation of a pulmonary valve mounted on a balloon-expandable stent.[10] This technique is presented in detail elsewhere in this book.

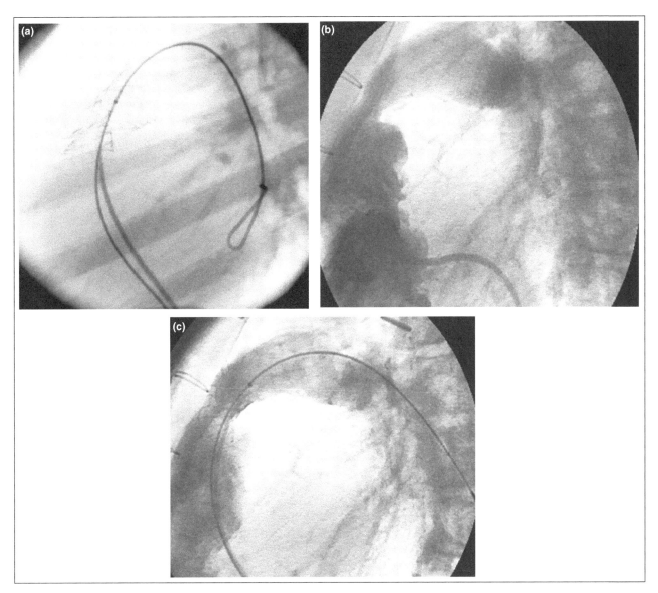

Figure 48.5
(a) Stent fracture. (b) Stent compression causing recurrent RVOTO. (c) Relief of RVOTO due to stent compression with a second stent implanted within the first.

References

1. Hausdorf G, Schulze-Neick I, Lange PE. Radiofrequency assisted construction of the right ventricular outflow tract in muscular pulmonary atresia with ventricular septal defect. Br Heart J 1993: 69; 343–6.

2. Sanatani S, Potts JE, Human DH et al. Balloon angioplasty of right ventricular outflow tract conduits. Pediatr Cardiol 2001; 22: 228–32.

3. Sreeram N, Hutter J, Silove E. Sustained high pressure double balloon angioplasty of calcified conduits. Heart 1999; 81: 162–5.

4. Ovaert CJ, Caldarone CA, McCrindle BW et al. Endovascular stent implantation of the management of postoperative right ventricular outflow tract obstruction: clinical efficacy. Thorac Cardiovasc Surg 1999; 118: 886–93.

5. O'Laughlin MP, Slack MC, Grifka RG et al. Implantation and intermediate term follow up of stents in congenital heart disease. Circulation 1993; 88: 605–14.

6. Rutledge JM, Mullins CE, Nihill MR et al. Initial experience with intratherapeutics Intrastent Doublestrut LD in patients with congenital heart defects. Cathet Cardiovasc Interven 2002; 56: 541–8.

7. Ewert P, Schubert S, Peters B et al. The CP stent for the treatment of aortic coarctation, stenosis of pulmonary arteretis and caval veins and Fontan anastomosis in children and adults. Heart 2005; 91: 948–53.

8. Recto MR, Ing FF, Grifka RG et al. A technique to prevent newly implanted stent displacement during subsequent catheter and sheath manipulation. Cathet Cardiovasc Interven 2000; 49: 297–300.

9. Sugiyama H, Williams W, Benson LN. Implantation of endovascular stents for the obstructive right ventricular outflow tract. Heart 2005; 91: 1058.

10. Khambadkone S, Coats L, Taylor A et al. Percutaneous pulmonary valve implantation in humans: results in 59 consecutive patients. Circulation 2005; 112: 1189–97.

49

Pulmonary artery stenosis

Larry Latson

Anatomy and pathophysiology

Stenotic lesions of the pulmonary arterial tree have been estimated to occur in 2–3% of patients with congenital heart disease.[1] They are most common in conotruncal abnormalities such as tetralogy of Fallot and pulmonary atresia with VSD, but have been seen in almost all forms of congenital heart disease (CHD). Stenoses may be discrete or associated with long segment hypoplasia, and may be congenital or secondary to a surgical procedure. Post-surgical stenosis is most commonly due to scarring, especially at the site of a shunt, at the ends of a patch arterioplasty, or at the anastomotic sites of unifocalized vessels. Torsion, stretching, or compression of a pulmonary artery may also occur after procedures such as the arterial switch or Norwood operations. Rarely, stenosis can be caused by mediastinal inflammatory disorders (radiation or fibrosing mediastinitis) or extrinsic compression from neoplasm.

The pulmonary artery system allows for parallel flow to both lungs and to all lung segments. Thus isolated stenosis of one pulmonary artery branch reduces flow to the affected downstream area, but may have little effect on right ventricular pressure. In most cases, however, there are multiple affected pulmonary arteries and right ventricular pressure becomes elevated. The pathophysiologic effects of pulmonary artery stenosis can be secondary to reduced segmental pulmonary flow (dyspnea, poor lung growth), or to right ventricular hypertension (right heart failure, arrhythmia, sudden death), or both.

Clinical symptoms, indications for treatment, and alternatives

Indications for treatment and symptoms of pulmonary artery branch stenosis may vary with age and associated cardiovascular defects. Congenitally stenotic lesions may improve with age, and even severe diffuse pulmonary artery stenosis unassociated with other congenital cardiovascular abnormalities rarely causes symptoms in young children.[2] We generally do not recommend treatment at less than 5 years of age in such asymptomatic patients. Patients with associated CHD, however, especially if they require repair with a Fontan type circulation, may not tolerate even relatively mild degrees of pulmonary artery stenosis. These patients may need early aggressive therapy. Older patients with otherwise normal circulation and severe pulmonary artery stenosis affecting only one lung may have symptoms due to the ventilation/perfusion mismatch (primarily dyspnea on exertion), and the potential growth of the affected lung may be reduced. In the absence of right ventricular hypertension, a large perfusion abnormality may warrant a low risk intervention, but the degree of acceptable risk must be tempered with the generally good outlook without treatment.

Older patients with otherwise normal circulation and severe bilateral proximal stenoses or multiple areas of distal stenosis may have normally distributed perfusion, but severely elevated main pulmonary artery and right ventricular pressures. The right ventricular hypertension may cause symptoms similar to those in patients with primary pulmonary hypertension, including limited ability to increase cardiac output with exercise, and a significant risk for sudden death.[3] Treatment is generally indicated in such patients if right ventricular pressure is more than 75% systemic and in some patients with lower pressures if they have significant symptoms.

History of the procedure

Balloon angioplasty of stenotic pulmonary arteries is one of the earliest transcatheter interventions performed for pediatric and congenital heart disease. Dr Lock reported on the results of balloon dilation in an experimental lamb model in 1981.[4] The first 'large' (seven patients) human experience with balloon angioplasty was reported from

Boston Children's Hospital in 1983.[5] Since then, there have been numerous articles on transcatheter treatment of various forms of pulmonary artery stenosis. Significant advances in technique included the use of high-pressure balloons, stents, and cutting balloons.

Pre-catheter imaging/assessment

Pre-catheterization assessment is essential in patients being considered for catheter treatment of pulmonary artery stenosis. The primary effects of pulmonary artery stenosis are maldistribution of blood flow to the lung parenchyma and/or elevation of right ventricular systolic pressure. Regional pulmonary blood flow is best assessed with a radionuclide quantitative perfusion scan.[6] A concurrent ventilation scan may be helpful if there is significant pulmonary parenchymal pathology or hypoplasia of a lung. A perfusion scan is strongly recommended prior to catheterization in all patients with planned pulmonary artery dilation in order to target regions of the pulmonary vasculature that are most severely affected as the primary targets. Pressure gradients across stenotic vascular lesions are the easiest parameters to measure in the cath lab, but the goal of therapy is to increase flow to underperfused regions of the lung. The perfusion scan can be readily repeated after the catheterization procedure to assess immediate and long term results.

Right ventricular pressure and function can often be conveniently evaluated by echocardiography. Right ventricular pressure can be estimated by the velocity of a tricuspid insufficiency jet if present. Proximal stenotic lesions in the pulmonary arteries may be detectable by echocardiography, but distal lesions will not be visible. CT or MRI can give excellent visualization of the peripheral pulmonary artery anatomy and MRI can quantitate regional flow in some patients.[7] Non-standard imaging planes and careful analysis are necessary to make accurate assessment of multiple stenotic vessels. Pre-cath imaging and flow studies allow the catheterization to target the most important areas in patients with multiple lesions.

Anesthesia

The choice of sedation vs general anesthesia is usually not critical. Relatively isolated lesions in older patients can often be treated conveniently with sedation alone. The younger the patient and the larger the number of lesions likely to need treatment, the more likely we are to recommend general anesthesia. Many procedures requiring treatment of multiple lesions can take several hours. Catheter manipulations may be difficult in young patients. Patients with systemic or near

systemic pressure may be in danger of acute events such as pulmonary artery rupture or abrupt decreases in cardiac output if a tricuspid or pulmonary valve is held open by the catheter. Having the patient under general anesthesia in these situations is definitely an advantage. Assessments of acute success during the catheterization procedure are generally made by angiographic measurements, pre- and post-dilation pressure gradients, and changes in right ventricular to systemic pressure ratios. These values are not dramatically affected by the use of general anesthesia.

Catheterization procedure

For most cases with pulmonary artery stenosis requiring treatment, we recommend placement of two venous sheaths and an arterial monitoring line. Arterial monitoring is optional for simple low risk procedures, but is important for high risk patients requiring prolonged procedures.

One venous catheter is used for dilation and/or stent placement in the stenotic region. The second venous catheter is used as a convenient way to perform angiograms immediately after an intervention or as a good reference during balloon dilation and stent placement. In situations where 'kissing balloons' are needed, the second sheath is utilized for placement of the second balloon. The presence of a second venous catheter is also extremely helpful in patients who suffer catastrophic complications such as vessel disruption. The second catheter provides a way to deliver drugs or blood, and to perform angiograms without the danger of losing the wire position of the original dilating catheter. We generally estimate the largest balloon size that will likely be needed and place a sheath adequate to accommodate such a balloon for the primary sheath. The secondary sheath size is chosen to be large enough for the desired angiographic catheter, or for the second balloon if simultaneous balloon inflations are anticipated.

As a routine, we perform a complete right heart catheterization to be certain that there are no unexpected shunts and to obtain accurate baseline pressure measurements in the right atrium and right ventricle. The primary catheter is advanced selectively to the desired lung. We do not perform an angiogram in the main pulmonary artery if the site of stenosis has been determined to be more peripheral by previous angiography or non-invasive evaluation. Angiographic assessment is best done with the most selective catheter position possible. We prefer to always use biplane angiography. Poorly selected angiograms that result in filling of vessels in both the left and right lungs make the lateral view difficult or impossible to accurately interpret. Non-ionic contrast is recommended since the angiographic dye load in patients requiring multiple dilations can be high. For angiograms in the central branch pulmonary arteries, we prefer to use an angiographic catheter. For more

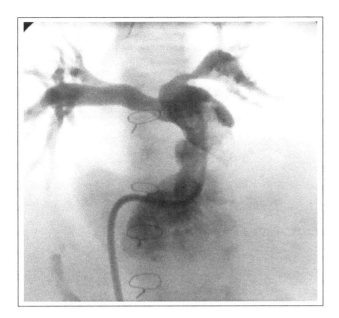

Figure 49.1
Main pulmonary arteriogram in a patient with bilateral proximal pulmonary artery stenosis. The frontal imaging system is angulated 35° cranially and slightly leftward. The length of the right pulmonary artery is well visualized. The origin of the left pulmonary artery is well seen, but this angulation results in foreshortening of the mid-portion of the vessel.

peripheral and smaller vessels, it is often advantageous to perform the angiographic injections with a catheter that has both end holes and a side hole, such as a Goodale–Lubin or other multi-purpose type catheter.

The best view of the central pulmonary arteries from a main pulmonary artery angiogram is usually with the frontal imaging system in steep cranial angulation (30+°) (Figure 49.1). The right pulmonary artery courses relatively horizontally across the right thorax and straight antero-posterior (AP) or slight right anterior oblique (RAO) angulation of the frontal radiographic imaging system, combined with a lateral projection of the lateral imaging system, provides excellent visualization (Figure 49.2). The left pulmonary artery courses leftward in a relatively steep angle from anterior to posterior. Left anterior oblique (LAO) and possibly slight caudal angulation of the frontal imaging system is usually best to evaluate the length of the major portions of the left pulmonary artery. A straight lateral view provides excellent delineation of the branches that course from anterior to posterior. Different angulations of the image intensifiers may be needed for specific portions of either the right or left pulmonary artery. At least one of the views should be varied to attempt to image the longest length of the affected vessel. If a Touhy–Borst valve is placed on the end of the catheter, a guidewire can be advanced past the area of stenosis and the angiogram can be performed with the guidewire in place and the catheter tip immediately proximal to the stenotic lesion.

Selected cannulation of the desired stenotic vessels may be challenging because of the sometimes tortuous course through the right ventricle, right ventricular outflow tract, and into sharply angulated branch vessels. Flow directed balloon catheters may tend to go to areas of high flow rather than through stenotic lesions. Catheters with excellent torque control and a relatively tight angle at the tip (such as a right coronary artery shape) may be helpful in directing the guidewire in the appropriate direction. We have also found a combination of multi-purpose guide catheter through which a hydrophilic sharply angled catheter (such as a 4 Fr Terumo angled glide catheter) may be especially helpful. The guide catheter can be shortened by cutting the proximal end. A side arm sheath (1 Fr size smaller than the guide catheter) can be cut near its hub and carefully advanced onto the cut end of the guide catheter to provide a hemostasis valve and a port for pressure monitoring or dye injection. The guide catheter provides support for the initial direction in the major branch. The sharply angled hydrophilic inner catheter can then be advanced and rotated in any direction to point to the desired branch. A hydrophilic guidewire such as a Terumo glide wire can then be advanced through the stenotic vessel and the hydrophilic catheter will often follow this type of wire through even tight stenoses.

It is absolutely essential to have excellent wire support for placement of a dilating balloon or stents. If a flexible hydrophilic wire is used to guide a small catheter across the stenotic area, the wire should generally be replaced with a stiffer wire once the initial catheter is adequately positioned. The time and effort to place a stiff wire in an excellent position definitely provide an advantage when attempting to place relatively large or stiff dilation catheters through the area of stenosis.

Stenoses may be treated by simple balloon angioplasty, cutting balloon angioplasty, or placement of a stent. Simple balloon angioplasty or cutting balloon angioplasty is preferable in young patients in whom there is an expectation of continued growth.[8] Restenosis may occur in as few as 12% of vessels when a good initial result is obtained in a small child. Placement of a stent in such patients will mandate the need for later dilation of the stent whereas successful balloon angioplasty often results in continued growth of the affected area. Balloon dilation of pulmonary artery stenoses generally requires a relatively high pressure balloon for best results.[9] For tight distal lesions less than 3 mm in diameter, we often use large, high pressure coronary balloon angioplasty catheters. The initial balloon diameter generally needs to be 3–3.5 times the diameter of the stenoses to be effective.[10] We feel that care must be taken, however, that the balloon is not larger than 1.5 times the normal vessel diameter immediately adjacent to the stenosis. Use of larger balloons extending into the distal 'normal' portions of the vessel greatly increases the risk of rupture or aneurysms in our experience. For larger vessels, we prefer to use high pressure balloons that are

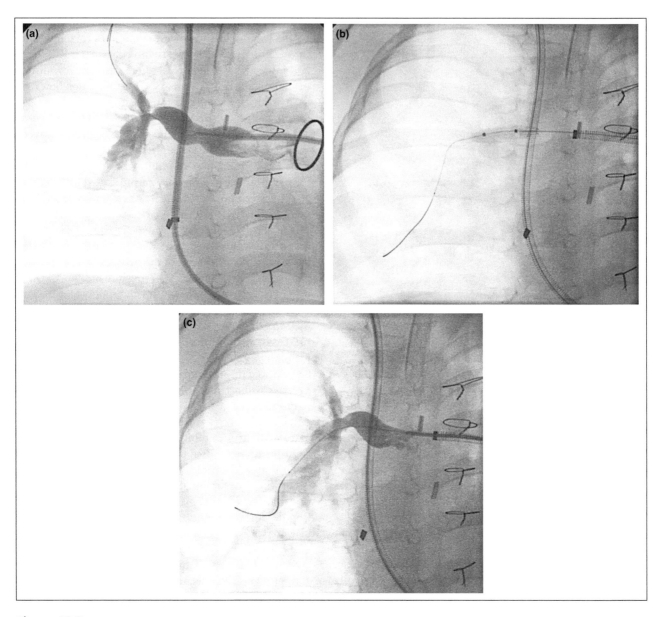

Figure 49.2

(a) Severe stenosis at the anastomosis of a central pericardial roll anastomosed to the right pulmonary artery hilum in a patient with originally discontinuous pulmonary arteries. (b) Cutting balloon inflated in the area of stenosis. Note that the three blades that are arranged along the length of the balloon are not readily visible. (c) Final result after dilation with a cutting balloon and then a slightly larger high pressure angioplasty balloon. The patient improved clinically after the procedure.

relatively flexible and that have a relatively short 'shoulder'. One example is the Zmed balloon from NuMed.

For each stenotic lesion, the guidewire is advanced into a stable position with the stiff portion of the guidewire extended past the area of stenosis to provide adequate support. The dilating balloon is advanced over the guidewire and positioned. A road map image from a prior angiogram is extremely helpful in accurate positioning. If available, a separate angiographic catheter can be used to confirm that the balloon and guidewire have not shifted the original position of the stenosis. It is also important to ensure that the tip of the balloon is not protruding into a small side branch. We are aware of cases in which pulmonary artery ruptures were caused by the tip unknowingly lodged in a very small adjacent distal vessel. When positioning is confirmed, the balloon is inflated relatively slowly. Because there are multiple parallel pathways in the pulmonary circulation, blocking one branch seldom results in severe hemodynamic instability. If there appears to be a resistant waist in the balloon that is less than half of the diameter of the remainder of the balloon, we would recommend against full inflation under high pressure initially. Such a tight waist that is subsequently eliminated under high pressure is more often associated with vascular complications. The next size smaller balloon can be used initially to assess the results, or a smaller cutting balloon may be utilized. If the waist in the balloon is larger than 50% of the balloon diameter, we generally inflate the balloon to the balloon burst pressure. Pressures are monitored with an inflation device and the burst pressure is not exceeded by more than 10%. Rupture of a balloon in a tight vascular stenosis is more likely to lead to vascular complications, and the balloon may be difficult to retrieve if it bursts in a transverse direction. The maximal pressure is maintained for 30–60 seconds if the patient is hemodynamically stable. The balloon is then deflated and withdrawn, and an angiogram is performed to assess the results. Proximal and distal pressures can be measured with the catheter maintained over the guidewire using a Tuohy–Borst type of side arm adaptor on the end of the catheter. For small vessels, the catheter may be nearly as large as the vascular opening and pressure gradients may not be accurate. The primary assessment of the result in small vessels (less than 5 mm) is therefore the angiographic appearance. An increase of 50% in diameter is generally considered a reasonable marker of success.

If simple high pressure balloon angioplasty is unsuccessful, or has been unsuccessful in the past, we would proceed to the use of the cutting balloon (Boston Scientific). This balloon has three or four microtome blades fastened along the length of the balloon. The balloon is specially designed to fold over the blades during deflation. With inflation, the blades protrude approximately 10 thousandths of an inch above the surface the balloon. These blades will create three or four equally spaced micro-incisions that ideally extend through the thickened intima and into the media of the vessel. These equally spaced weakened areas should then be the areas of expansion during angioplasty. Without these incisions, vessels may expand in only the single weakest area around the circumference. We and others have found the cutting balloons to be efficacious for lesions that have not responded to simple balloon angioplasty.[11,12] The recommended cutting balloon diameter is generally slightly less than the diameter recommended for a simple angioplasty balloon and should not exceed 10% larger than the diameter of the adjacent normal vessel. The diameter and lengths of the cutting balloon are currently somewhat limited and they are applicable primarily to smaller vessels. The blades along the balloons make them more difficult to maneuver along tortuous courses. We recommend delivering the cutting balloons through a long transseptal sheath or a guide catheter in order to minimize the possibility of damage from the blades on the balloon as the balloon traverses the tricuspid and pulmonary valves. Cutting balloons should be inflated and deflated slowly to allow for proper conformational changes in the specially configured balloon. Extreme care must be taken with withdrawal of these cutting balloons into the sheath or guide catheter to ensure that the microtome blades are not inappropriately caught on the edge of the sheath or catheter and avulsed from the balloon. These blades are extremely difficult or impossible to visualize fluoroscopically (Figure 49.2) and have the potential for significant damage if they embolize distally.

If the desired effect cannot be achieved with angioplasty (with or without cutting balloon) alone, then placement of a stent in the stenotic vessel is the next option. In patients past puberty in whom surgical intervention in the region of the stenosis is not anticipated in the near future, we will use stenting as the primary treatment for larger vessels that are not immediately adjacent to important branches. For any given balloon diameter, stenting is definitely more effective than angioplasty alone because it prevents all, or nearly all, vessel elastic recoil. Stents generally result in better stenosis relief with less risk than the alternative of using a significantly oversized balloon.[13] The primary consideration against the use of stents in all stenotic lesions is that stents will not grow. If stents are placed in younger children, it is absolutely essential that the stent type utilized can, in the future, be expanded to the full expected diameter of an adult sized vessel. Proximal main branch pulmonary arteries in adults generally grow to 16–20 mm and may be significantly larger in some patients. Primary lobar branch pulmonary arteries typically reach 5–10 mm in diameter, but may be larger in some patients. Placement of a stent that is incapable of expansion to more than 10–12 mm in a proximal branch pulmonary artery will result in eventual stenosis that can only be relieved with surgical removal or incision through the implanted stent.

Because of the prolific branching of the pulmonary vasculature, placement of a distal stent will often result in 'jailing' of the orifice of a side branch or protrusion of the stent at an angle that may make repeat crossing of the stent extremely difficult or impossible. In general, we prefer to use the shortest possible stent that can be dilated to the largest anticipated eventual diameter of the normal vessel. We do not recommend the use of self-expanding stents. Such stents cannot be expanded beyond their nominal diameter, and use of oversized self-expanding stents results in continual expansion pressure on the vessel wall that seems to encourage neointimal hyperplasia. We prefer balloon-expandable stents that have the highest radial strength. Pre-mounted stents (such as the Genesis stent) are advantageous because a long delivery sheath is not required. However, maintaining an inventory of pre-mounted stent systems of every possible balloon diameter and stent length is very costly. We often therefore use stents that are manually crimped onto an appropriate balloon and delivered through a long sheath. The sheath extends through the tricuspid and pulmonary valves in order to be certain that the stents do not become entangled or embedded in the valves or right ventricular outflow tract as the balloon traverses these regions.

The balloon size for stent implantation is chosen to equal or very slightly exceed the diameter of the normal vessel adjacent to the stenosis. Accurate placement of the balloon and stent is absolutely essential and far more important than positioning a balloon for simple angioplasty. Image intensifiers should be angled to provide the best view of the length of the vessel in which the stent will be implanted. Viewing the stent at an angle (end on) greatly reduces the accuracy of positioning. A second catheter may be extremely useful to perform small injections of contrast medium to confirm accurate placement. Alternatively, contrast may be injected through the long sheath once the balloon and stent have been extended past the tip of the sheath. Stents should be deployed with the catheter over a stiff guidewire to minimize the movement of the system during inflation. When deploying stents in a large high flow vessel, delivering the stent on a BIB balloon (NuMed, Inc.) may allow for more precise placement (Figure 49.3). In some instances, placement of the stent will result in the end of the stent encroaching on, or covering, the orifice of an adjacent important branch vessel. In this situation, it may be best to deploy stents in the two vessels simultaneously. This 'kissing balloon' technique results in a 'double barrel' opening into the adjacent pulmonary artery branches. In order to perform this type of intervention, it is necessary to have adequate personnel to hold both catheters in position while two other people inflate the balloons simultaneously.

Once stents have been deployed, extreme care must be used in removing the balloon catheter. It is often helpful to advance the long sheath over the balloon if the deflated balloon seems to be catching on the stent. Inadvertent embolization of a stent caused by careless withdrawal of the balloon is a most unfortunate event.

Pitfalls and complications

The major immediate complication of balloon angioplasty is vascular damage or even disruption. Luminal irregularities are seen in nearly all successful angioplasties, especially if evaluated by intravascular ultrasound.[14] Experimental studies have suggested that angioplasty is unlikely to be successful unless there is disruption of the intima and into the media.[4] Disruption of the inner layers of the vessel, however, may result in the formation of vascular flaps that can cause severe stenosis or occlusions. These flaps are indicated by a curtain within the vessel lumen angiographically after dilation. As long as the guidewire has not been removed, the dilating balloon can be re-advanced past the flap, then partially inflated under low pressure and withdrawn to attempt to 'tack' the disrupted inner layer back into position. The balloon can be maintained with low pressure inflation for at least 3 to 5 minutes and a repeat angiogram can be performed to see if the curtain reforms. If the intimal flap persists, placement of a stent may be necessary.

Extension of the vascular disruption past the media may result in extreme thinning of the remaining circumference of the vessel with only the adventitial layer containing the disruption. An aneurysm is frequently seen in this circumstance. These aneurysms may remain stable but definitely require follow-up evaluation by repeat catheterization or CT/MRI.[15] Some aneurysms have significantly expanded over days to months. These aneurysms may rupture catastrophically.[16] Any aneurysm seen immediately after angioplasty should be re-evaluated after 5 to 30 minutes to be certain that the aneurysm is not enlarging (Figure 49.4). Significantly enlarging aneurysms require close follow-up. If an aneurysm is enlarging rapidly or if there is disruption of a pulmonary artery seen with pulmonary imaging, the balloon catheter should be immediately re-inflated at or slightly proximal to the region of previous stenosis. Tamponading the affected vessel will reduce the chance of an urgent catastrophe. If the pressure proximal to the disruption is relatively low, coagulation parameters can be quickly normalized and the balloon can be deflated after 15–30 minutes with angiographic re-assessment. If there is continued expansion of the aneurysmal area or continued bleeding, the vessel may need to be permanently occluded with a device such as a Gianturco coil or an Amplatzer vascular plug. If a covered stent is available, this may be an alternative treatment, but placement may be difficult under emergency circumstances.

The major complication of stent placement is stent migration. Aneurysms or vascular disruptions are also possible, but should be less likely than with angioplasty alone if appropriate (smaller) balloons are utilized. The possibility of stent migration can be minimized by ensuring that the stent delivery balloon is adequate in size to result in apposition of the stent to the vessel wall over as much of its length as possible. The stent should be at least 50% larger than the stenotic area in most cases. Accurate measurements are absolutely essential. We have found that the use of a metallic sphere with an exactly known diameter as a reference for calibrating the image measurements is the most accurate method. The sphere must be positioned in the isocenter of both radiographic planes when the reference image is obtained. Changing the angles of the imaging system thereafter will have no effect on the calibration factor. However, changing the height of the table or the image intensifier will change the degree of magnification and recalibration must be performed. If a stent migrates, it is essential that the guidewire position be maintained. As long as the stent does not slip off the guidewire, it may be possible to reposition it by partially inflating a balloon in the stent and then either retracting or advancing the stent to a favorable location. In most instances, a reasonable alternative position for the stent can be found and the stent can be further dilated to maintain the new position. More sophisticated stent retrieval techniques are beyond the scope of this paper.

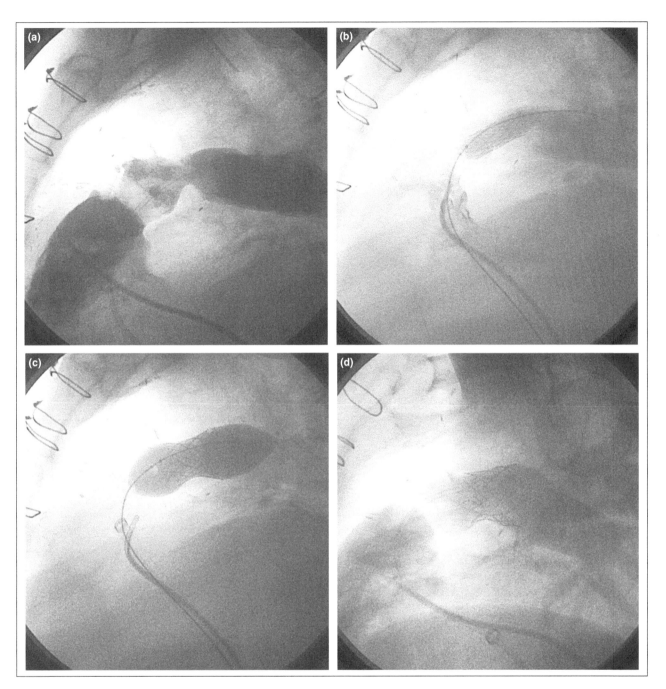

Figure 49.3
(a) Lateral view of severe supravalve main pulmonary stenosis after arterial switch procedure. (b) First stage of stent deployment using the BIB balloon. The inner balloon has been inflated to its maximal diameter and the stent has a uniform diameter that is small enough to allow slight repositioning before full deployment. (c) The outer balloon of the BIB (Balloon in Balloon, Numed Inc., Hopkinton, New York, USA) catheter has been inflated to its maximal pressure. This step must be accomplished expeditiously since the main pulmonary artery is completely occluded by the balloon at this point. (d) The final stent location is excellent with significant improvement in right ventricular pressure and no compromise of the pulmonary valve.

Post-procedure protocol

Following pulmonary artery dilation or stent deployment, most patients will be observed overnight. If stenosis relief has been successful, there will be increased flow into the affected lung segments. A reperfusion type of injury, with flash edema in portions of the lung, may occur if the pulmonary artery pressure is elevated and the stenosis has been very effectively relieved.[17] In rare instances, the degree of edema may be sufficient to lead to hemoptysis or even the

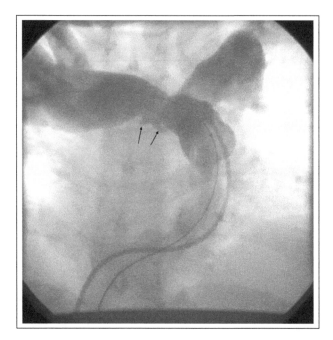

Figure 49.4
Small irregular aneurysm (arrows) at the origin of the right pulmonary artery after balloon angioplasty. In this patient, the area was unchanged 10 minutes later and also, by CT scan, one month later.

need for transient mechanical ventilation. The effects of dilation of proximal areas of stenosis can often be seen echocardiographically. A decrease in Doppler peak systolic velocity and normalization of the waveform on spectral Doppler indicates a good outcome. The effects of right ventricular pressure and size can be estimated. The best method to assess the effect on flow to the affected region is a quantitative radionuclide pulmonary perfusion scan. We generally prefer to wait for approximately one month to perform this scan after the procedure. This time frame allows for remodeling of the vasculature and resolution of any areas of mild edema that may affect the regional flow. Echocardiography and an occasional radionuclide perfusion scan may be sufficient for the follow-up of simple, proximal stenotic lesions. CT or MRI or repeat angiography may be necessary for evaluation of more distal lesions. In most cases with more than one stenotic area, and certainly if a stent is implanted, a follow-up cardiac catheterization is often needed months to years after the procedure. Timing depends upon such factors as the residual right ventricular pressure, symptoms, and results of non-invasive studies.

Catheter techniques to improve areas of stenosis in the pulmonary artery system have greatly improved outcomes over surgical management alone. Incorporation of the catheter techniques into the management plan of difficult patients has expanded surgical options for treatment of many forms of complex congenital cardiovascular malformations.

References

1. Trivedi KR, Benson LN. Interventional strategies in the management of peripheral pulmonary artery stenosis. J Interven Cardiol 2003; 16(2): 171–88.
2. Kim YM, Yoo SJ, Choi JY et al. Natural course of supravalvar aortic stenosis and peripheral pulmonary arterial stenosis in Williams' syndrome. Cardiol Young 1999; 9(1): 37–41.
3. Kreutzer J, Landzberg MJ, Preminger TJ et al. Isolated peripheral pulmonary artery stenoses in the adult. Circulation 1996; 93(7): 1417–23.
4. Lock JE, Niemi T, Einzig S et al. Transvenous angioplasty of experimental branch pulmonary artery stenosis in newborn lambs. Circulation 1981; 64(5): 886–93.
5. Lock JE, Castaneda-Zuniga WR, Fuhrman BP, Bass JL. Balloon dilation angioplasty of hypoplastic and stenotic pulmonary arteries. Circulation 1983; 67(5): 962–7.
6. Sabiniewicz R, Romanowicz G, Bandurski T. Lung perfusion scintigraphy in the diagnosis of peripheral pulmonary stenosis in patients after repair of Fallot tetralogy. Nucl Med Rev Cent East Eur 2002; 5(1): 11–13.
7. Roman KS, Kellenberger CJ, Farooq S et al. Comparative imaging of differential pulmonary blood flow in patients with congenital heart disease: magnetic resonance imaging versus lung perfusion scintigraphy. Pediatr Radiol 2005; 35(3): 295–301.
8. Mori Y, Nakanishi T, Niki T et al. Growth of stenotic lesions after balloon angioplasty for pulmonary artery stenosis after arterial switch operation. J Cardiol 2003; 91(6): 693–8.
9. Gentles TL, Lock JE, Perry SB. High pressure balloon angioplasty for branch pulmonary artery stenosis: early experience. J Am Coll Cardiol 1993; 22(3): 867–72.
10. Kan JS, Marvin WJ Jr, Bass JL et al. Balloon angioplasty–branch pulmonary artery stenosis: results from the valvuloplasty and angioplasty of congenital anomalies registry. Am J Cardiol 1990; 65(11): 798–801.
11. Rhodes JF, Lane GK, Mesia CI et al. Cutting balloon angioplasty for children with small-vessel pulmonary artery stenoses. Cathet Cardiovasc Interven 2002; 55(1): 73–7.
12. Bergersen LJ, Perry SB, Lock JE. Effect of cutting balloon angioplasty on resistant pulmonary artery stenosis. Am J Cardiol 2003; 91(2): 185–9.
13. Bacha EA, Kreutzer J. Comprehensive management of branch pulmonary artery stenosis. J Interven Cardiol 2001; 14(3): 367–75.
14. Nakanishi T, Tobita K, Sasaki M et al. Intravascular ultrasound imaging before and after balloon angioplasty for pulmonary artery stenosis. Cathet Cardiovasc Interven 1999; 46(1): 68–78.
15. Simmons PL, Scavetta KL, McLeary MS, Kuhn MA. Pulmonary artery pseudoaneurysm after percutaneous transluminal angioplasty in a pediatric patient. Pediatr Radiol 1997; 27(9): 760–2.
16. Zeevi B, Berant M, Blieden LC. Late death from aneurysm rupture following balloon angioplasty for branch pulmonary artery stenosis. Cathet Cardiovasc Diagn 1996; 39(3): 284–6.
17. Rothman A, Perry SB, Keane JF, Lock JE. Early results and follow-up of balloon angioplasty for branch pulmonary artery stenoses. J Am Coll Cardiol 1990; 15(5): 1109–17.

50

Pulmonary vein stenoses

Lee Benson

Introduction

Individual pulmonary vein stenosis, hypoplasia, or atresia is a rare congenital cardiac lesion, which may cause pulmonary hypertension. Both stenosis and atresia can occur in the same patient, and one or more veins can be involved. The obstruction may be localized to the veno-atrial junction, or may extend into the lung parenchyma for some distance. It may occur in isolation or in combination with other cardiac lesions (e.g., scimitar syndrome) (Figure 50.1) or due to compression from the left atrium and descending aorta, or from an extracardiac Fontan conduit (right-sided venous compression).[1,2] It may evolve with time and affect additional pulmonary veins.

For the interventionalist, the more common presentation will be after surgery for total anomalous pulmonary venous connection,[3–5] or after ablation techniques to address atrial fibrillation.[6–9]

In the infant, despite improved surgical repair, there continues to be a significant incidence of relentless pulmonary vein stenosis,[3–5,10] particularly common in the setting of infracardiac and mixed drainage. There have been a number of reports, primarily with short term follow-up, of the impact of balloon dilation alone or in combination with endovascular stent implantation with mixed results. Although the majority of reports document acute reduction in flow obstruction, longer term follow-up has generally found restenosis, in-stent stenosis, or progression of the disease process.[11–19] These observations contrast with the effect of stent implantation in a swine model with essentially normal pulmonary vein histology.[20] This may be due to the intrinsically abnormal histopathology noted in the congenital lesion,[21] where there is significantly increased thickness of the media of the arteries and veins, the worst examples being in those infants presenting with obstruction.[22]

This poor longer term outcome applies to acquired pulmonary vein stenosis after attempted radiofrequency ablation as well,[6,8] despite initial early enthusiasm in short term follow-up.[7,9] It appears that final stent diameter is critical, with smaller (<5 mm) implants developing in-stent restenosis sooner.

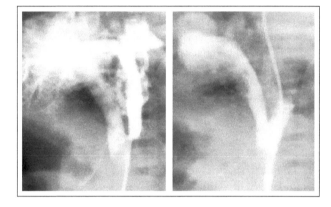

Figure 50.1
Left panel, from an angiogram of a child with the scimitar syndrome taken in the left lateral projection showing the obstructed connection to the inferior caval vein. A 3.5 mm bare metal coronary stent was implanted (right panel) for short term palliation, to avoid surgery in this 2.5 kg infant with respiratory distress syndrome and an obstructed anomalous right pulmonary vein to the inferior caval vein.

Whether adjunctive therapies (brachytherapy, sonotherapy) have a place in the growing child is a matter for future study. The concept of recurrent interventions to manage restenosis is not appealing.[3,4,6] The application of drug-eluting stents, however, may result in a renewed interest in this form of percutaneous therapy, but presently, studies are lacking to support human application.

One short term application of stent management of pulmonary vein stenosis is in the pre-operative patient with an obstructed vein, particularly if the child is not a good surgical candidate, in whom short term palliation can be achieved[23,24] (Figure 50.2).

Indications

The limited success in effective long term relief of pulmonary vein stenting restricts the application of this

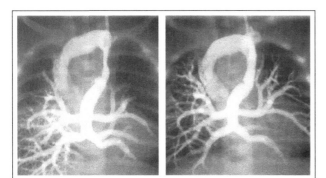

Figure 50.2
This 3 kg infant had obstructed supracardiac total anomalous venous return, complicating an unbalanced atrioventricular septal defect and right isomerism. The anatomic vertical vein obstruction was due to the left pulmonary artery anteriorly, duct or ductal ligamentum medially, and the left bronchus posteriorly. A 3 mm coronary stent was placed from the left internal jugular vein, as a bridge to a bidirectional cavopulmonary anastomosis. The angiograms shown were obtained in the frontal projection, although the left lateral was valuable for device positioning as well.

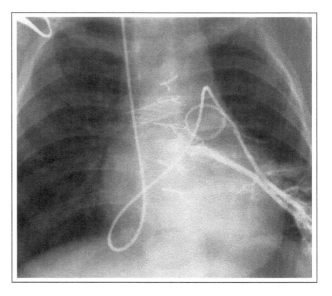

Figure 50.3
A frontal projection of a left pulmonary artery wedge injection demonstrating long segment left lower pulmonary vein stenosis, in a previously stented vein (in-stent stenosis).

technique to specific situations. If there is only one affected vein, and right ventricular pressure is not elevated, then intervention may not be indicated because of the potential complications of the interventional approach and the known outcomes.

Congenital lesions

- The infant with obstructed total or partial anomalous pulmonary venous return before surgical repair as short term palliation (Figures 50.1 and 50.2).

Acquired lesions

- The child after attempted repair of obstructed post-operative pulmonary vein stenosis, in the setting of anomalous venous return.[3–5] In this situation, a suture-line discrete stenosis may be present which might respond to angioplasty. If the lesion is not discrete, but extends into the hilar pulmonary veins, then endovascular stents can be considered, but outcomes are generally poor (Figure 50.3). The decision to place a stent must be weighed against the eventual need for treatment of in-stent stenosis, and after consideration of the absolute diameter that the implant can be dilated, as the child grows.
- Mediastinal fibrosis.
- After attempted ablation of atrial fibrillation. In this setting, the results are mixed, early studies reflecting acute

improvement, but most studies demonstrating the need for repeat catheter intervention to maintain stent patency.

Imaging

- A variety of imaging modalities can be used to perform surveillance for the development of pulmonary vein stenosis or confirm its presence, if the clinical situation demands. Transthoracic echocardiography with Doppler flow examination of pulmonary vein flow should be performed as the initial imaging modality. The practice in our unit, for infants after total anomalous pulmonary vein repair, is to perform an early post-operative echocardiogram between 2 and 3 months after discharge. Early studies are performed if the suspicion is raised in the immediate post-repair period, or clinical symptoms suggest obstruction.
- Other non-invasive imaging studies of value include magnetic resonance (MR) volume-rendering imaging, MR angiography, and spiral computed tomographic (CT) studies. As radiation exposure is an issue, MR imaging is preferred despite the need for general anesthesia to perform the study in infants (Figure 50.4). Although a previous report[25] has suggested that MRI is superior to transesophageal echocardiography, there are few data comparing MRI with spiral CT scans.
- Angiography with a balloon wedge injection is the definitive diagnostic modality and will define the extent of the lesion, and catheterization is recommended even if the

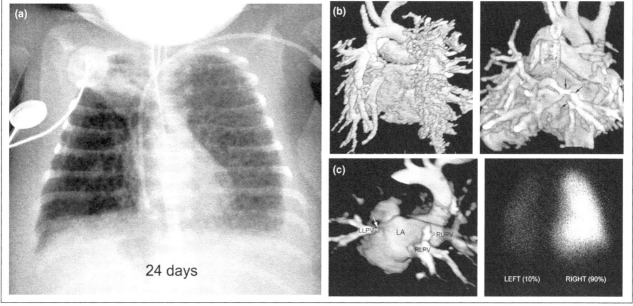

Figure 50.4

(a) Typical appearance of the chest X-ray (frontal projection) shortly after surgical repair in an infant with anomalous pulmonary venous return and persistent pulmonary vein obstruction. Note the hyperinflation and reticulated pattern of venous hypertension in the right lung. (b) A volume rendered reconstruction of the venous confluence showing right pulmonary vein stenosis in the left pane, and stenosis of the confluence (all veins – arrows in the right pane). (c) Left pane, a computed tomographic angiogram shows the reconstructed pulmonary venous confluence and left lower pulmonary vein (LLPV) stenosis. LA, left atrium; RUPV, RLPV, right upper and lower pulmonary vein. In the right panel, a perfusion scan after surgery in an infant with acquired pulmonary vein stenosis, defining little flow into the right lung.

vessel is thought to be occluded by other techniques. Initial scout views can be obtained with pulmonary artery wedge injections (catheterization procedure, below). Generally, this is performed in the frontal and left-lateral projections, but if the target lesion is known, then appropriate angulations can be performed. For right pulmonary veins, generally the frontal view is adequate, whilst for left-sided veins, either the hepatoclavicular of long axis oblique view will suffice, with a left-lateral (Figure 50.5). Although non-invasive imaging, such as a spiral CT scan, is accurate in defining mild to severe degrees of stenosis, vessels deemed occluded by these methods have been found to be patent by use of the balloon wedge angiogram technique. This is perhaps related to the dye being forced through the collapsed and stenotic vessel, with otherwise undetectable flow under normal conditions.[8]

Catheterization procedure

The goals of the procedure should be well defined beforehand. A right heart study should be performed, with selective pulmonary artery wedge injections to define the overall anatomy. Entry to the left atrium will be required, and selective pulmonary vein cannulation. Whether no intervention, balloon angioplasty alone, or stent implantation is performed will depend on the anatomy so imaged, and the management goals.

Preparation and access

The procedure should be performed under general endotracheal anesthesia. The access must be from the femoral vein(s), if there is an intact atrial septum, when a transseptal puncture must be performed. The internal jugular vein can be used if no other access is available, and if there is an atrial defect. Cannulation of the right-sided veins may be difficult from the neck. Systemic and left heart pressures should be monitored with a retrograde femoral artery catheter. The patients should be given intravenous heparin sulfate (our dose: 150 IU/kg, maximum 5000 IU). Activated clotting times (ACTs) should be monitored throughout the procedure with the goal to maintain an ACT of > 250 seconds.

Hemodynamics and angiography

Right heart hemodynamic data can be obtained with a balloon wedge catheter (6 or 7 Fr). This catheter can be used

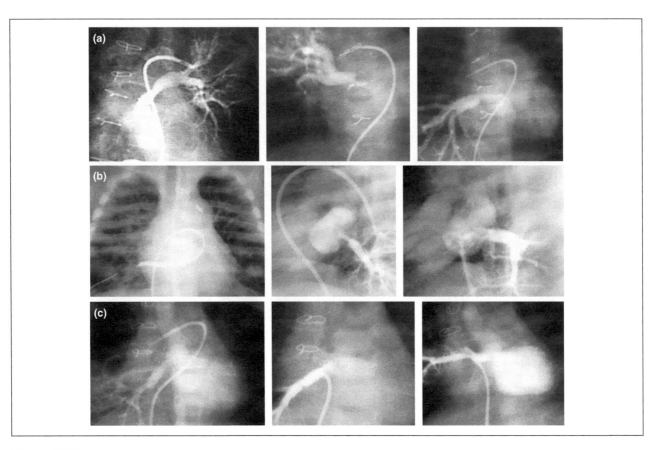

Figure 50.5
(a) Left pane, a right pulmonary artery wedge injection in a long axis oblique view, defines mild narrowing of the left upper vein as it enters the left atrium. Middle pane, in the frontal projection shows the right upper vein, and in the right pane, the right lower pulmonary vein, which are stenotic as they enter the atrium, in these infants after anomalous vein surgery. (b) Left pane, the course of a catheter to cannulate the right lower pulmonary vein is shown, while in the middle and right panes, the left-lateral view of a left lower pulmonary vein lesion before (middle) and after stent angioplasty. (c) Left pane, multiple stents are seen in this infant after anomalous vein surgery, in the left lower, and right lower and upper veins, from a right pulmonary artery wedge injection. The frontal detector was adjusted to profile the right lower lobe vein stent, to avoid foreshortening. In the middle pane, a selective injection shows evidence of restenosis within and distal to the implanted stent. The right pane shows a selective injection into the right upper vein, in which in-stent restenosis is evident.

to perform both measurements of the pulmonary artery wedge pressures and a wedge angiogram for mapping the individual pulmonary vein flow and to determine whether any segments were completely occluded (Figure 50.5). Axially angulated angiography will be required, depending on the vein under evaluation. Generally, the right-sided veins are best imaged in the frontal and left-lateral views, while the left-sided veins are profiled in the four-chamber and left-lateral views. The wedge injections can be used to improve the angulations for subsequent selective injections. The technique for obtaining a wedge angiogram is as follows:

1. Cannulate the segmental branch feeding the venous segment of interest.
2. Connect the catheter to a 20 ml syringe with 10 ml of contrast; prior to wedging the catheter tip withdraw

10 ml of the patient's blood, and by holding the syringe upright, the contrast and blood will layer, with the contrast lower than the blood.
3. Wedge the catheter and, by hand, inject the 20 ml of fluid. The contrast will enter the capillary–venous circulation, and the injected blood will force the contrast into the pulmonary vein, avoiding overlap of arterial and venous phases.

Pulmonary vein cannulation

The left atrium is then entered by a transseptal technique with a 6 or 7 Fr long sheath, depending upon the diameter of the subsequent balloon or stent to be used for the intervention. Entry into the left-sided veins follows a gentle curve from the inferior caval vein, through the atrial puncture. Lesions in the right-sided veins are more difficult to address, particularly in the smallest of patients, especially if the right middle or lower vein requires cannulation. To cannulate this vessel, a cobra-shaped catheter or one that is shaped as a hockey stick can be deflected off the lateral atrial wall to allow a direct position into the right lower pulmonary vein (Figure 50.5b). For left-sided veins, a right coronary artery catheter with a 2 or a 2.5 curve, or a cobra-shaped catheter (4 or 5 Fr), can be used to probe the individual vessels, with or without the assistance of a floppy-tipped wire (e.g. 0.035 inch glidewire, Terumo, or V-18, Boston Scientific). This catheter or a 5 Fr angled glide catheter (Medi-tech, Boston Scientific) can be used to measure the mean pressure gradient across the target lesion, angiographically study individual pulmonary venous anatomy, and position an exchange wire into the distal pulmonary vein.

A different protocol is used to engage the right lower pulmonary vein. To cannulate this vessel, we use a 7 Fr modified (length) hockey stick coronary guide catheter (Medtronic/AVE) within the left atrium, deflected off the lateral wall to allow a direct position toward the right lower pulmonary vein. This catheter is then used to guide the V-18 wire and a 5 Fr angled glide catheter as described above.

Preparation for the intervention

The diameter and length of the obstructive lesion and the distal pulmonary vein should be measured digitally, using the catheter diameter for magnification correction. Other techniques such as marker catheters can also be employed.

Intervention

Angioplasty

An angioplasty balloon, chosen not to exceed the diameter of the stenotic lesion by a factor of 3 to 4 or the distal vessel by a factor of 2, can be initially chosen, with standard angioplasty performed in each lesion. Stent implantation can be considered if there is elastic recoil of the lesion, in the absence of a fixed lesion, or a flap occurs, or when there is in-stent restenosis noted in follow-up. A variety of stents are available. In small infants, coronary stents which can be placed through a 4 Fr guide catheter and dilated to 5 or 6 mm are generally used. These stents, whilst giving early relief of the obstruction, tend to restenose, and their effectiveness is limited by the child's growth. In the older patient and adult, a larger stent (e.g., Genesis, Cordis), can be used, which can be dilated to 10 mm in diameter. If a fixed lesion is present (i.e., persistence of a waist at high inflation pressures (>8 atm)), cutting balloon angioplasty can be considered (Boston Scientific).[26] In general, the lesions should be dilated or stented to the same diameter as the distal, normal vessel.

Post-intervention assessment

After balloon angioplasty or stenting, a mean pressure gradient across the lesion should be measured. Angiography should be performed to measure the diameter of the residual lesion and assess the degree of vessel injury.

Follow-up studies are recommended due to the high rate of restenosis. Echocardiography appears to be the best initial modality for follow-up of the patient, with flow determination in the affected vein, and measurement of the right ventricular pressures. CT and MR imaging may not be useful due to the metal artifact, if the vein is stented. Repeat catheterization at 8 months to 1 year as a routine may be considered.

Interoperative placement

In the very small infant, and those children who have difficult venous access, intra-operative placement has been performed.[14–16] However, these procedures were performed at a time when the balloons and stents available were stiff, and it was difficult to maneuver tight turns, and they are probably not needed with the modern technology.

Summary and outcomes

In both acquired and congenital forms of pulmonary vein stenosis, the lesion has been uniformly frustrating to treat for cardiac surgeons and interventional cardiologists, with restenosis being a common occurrence.[3–5,11,12] Various surgical approaches have been attempted, with variable results, depending on the technique used, the anatomy, and the timing of surgery, although recent experience with a suture-less technique is promising.[27,28] In children, balloon angioplasty has been uniformly unsuccessful,[11,12] and endovascular stenting has met with little clinical success.[14–16,29–31] On the other hand, stent placement in the pulmonary veins after extrinsic compression in adults has yielded some clinical success.[18] In the setting of acquired stenosis after attempted radiofrequency ablation for atrial fibrillation, the situation may be different, as the application of energy near the orifice of the pulmonary veins results in the formation of thrombus, necrotic myocardium, and proliferation of elastic lamina and intimal proliferation.[32] This may provide a substrate for angioplasty or stent placement different from other acquired or congenital vein lesions and hence transcatheter therapy could potentially be successful. However, recent long-term follow-up studies have demonstrated restenosis and the need for frequent re-intervention.[6] Children and adults with this lesion require lifetime follow-up and potentially multiple procedures to prevent the loss of lung segments.

References

1. O'Donnell CP, Lock JE, Powell AJ, Perry SB. Compression of pulmonary veins between the left atrium and the descending aorta. Am J Cardiol 2003; 91(2): 248–51.
2. Freedom RM, Yoo SJ, Mikailian H, Williams W (eds). The Natural and Modified History of Congenital Heart Disease. New York: Blackwell Publishing, 2004; 466.
3. Caldarone CA, Najm HK, Kadletz M et al. Relentless pulmonary vein stenosis after repair of total anomalous pulmonary venous drainage. Ann Thorac Surg 1998; 66(5): 1514–20.
4. Hyde JA, Stumper O, Barth MJ et al. Total anomalous pulmonary venous connection: outcome of surgical correction and management of recurrent venous obstruction. Eur J Cardiothorac Surg 1999; 15(6): 735–40; discussion 740–1.
5. Michielon G, Di Donato RM, Pasquini L et al. Total anomalous pulmonary venous connection: long-term appraisal with evolving technical solutions. Eur J Cardiothorac Surg 2002; 22(2): 184–91.
6. Packer DL, Keelan P, Munger TM et al. Clinical presentation, investigation, and management of pulmonary vein stenosis complicating ablation for atrial fibrillation. Circulation 2005; 111(5): 546–54.
7. Purerfellner H, Aichinger J, Martinek M et al. Incidence, management, and outcome in significant pulmonary vein stenosis complicating ablation for atrial fibrillation. Am J Cardiol 2004; 93(11): 1428–31, A10.
8. Qureshi AM, Prieto LR, Latson LA et al. Transcatheter angioplasty for acquired pulmonary vein stenosis after radiofrequency ablation. Circulation 2003; 108(11): 1336–42. Epub 2003.
9. Vance MS, Bernstein R, Ross BA. Successful stent treatment of pulmonary vein stenosis following atrial fibrillation radiofrequency ablation. J Invas Cardiol 2002; 14(7): 414–16.
10. Ricci M, Elliott M, Cohen GA et al. Management of pulmonary venous obstruction after correction of TAPVC: risk factors for adverse outcome. Eur J Cardiothorac Surg 2003; 24(1): 28–36; discussion 36.
11. Driscoll DJ, Hesslein PS, Mullins CE. Congenital stenosis of individual pulmonary veins: clinical spectrum and unsuccessful treatment by transvenous balloon dilation. Am J Cardiol 1982; 49(7): 1767–72.
12. Lock JE, Bass JL, Castaneda-Zuniga W et al. Dilation angioplasty of congenital or operative narrowings of venous channels. Circulation 1984; 70(3): 457–64.
13. Tomita H, Watanabe K, Yazaki S et al. Stent implantation and subsequent dilatation for pulmonary vein stenosis in pediatric patients: maximizing effectiveness. Circ J 2003; 67(3): 187–90.
14. Coles JG, Yemets I, Najm HK et al. Experience with repair of congenital heart defects using adjunctive endovascular devices. J Thorac Cardiovasc Surg 1995; 110(5): 1513–19; discussion 1519–20.
15. Ungerleider RM, Johnston TA, O'Laughlin MP et al. Intraoperative stents to rehabilitate severely stenotic pulmonary vessels. Ann Thorac Surg 2001; 71(2): 476–81.
16. Mendelsohn AM, Bove EL, Lupinetti FM et al. Intraoperative and percutaneous stenting of congenital pulmonary artery and vein stenosis. Circulation 1993; 88(5 Pt 2): II210–17.
17. McMahon CJ, Mullins CE, El Said HG. Intrastent sonotherapy in pulmonary vein restenosis: a new treatment for a recalcitrant problem. Heart 2003; 89(2): E6.
18. Doyle TP, Loyd JE, Robbins IM. Percutaneous pulmonary artery and vein stenting: a novel treatment for mediastinal fibrosis. Am J Resp Crit Care Med 2001; 164(4): 657–60.
19. Dieter RS, Nelson B, Wolff MR et al. Transseptal stent treatment of anastomotic stricture after repair of partial anomalous pulmonary venous return. J Endovasc Ther 2003; 10(4): 838–42.
20. Hosking M, Redmond M, Allen L et al. Responses of systemic and pulmonary veins to the presence of an intravascular stent in a swine model. Cathet Cardiovasc Diagn 1995; 36(1): 90–6; discussion 97.
21. Haworth SA, Reid L. Structural study of pulmonary circulation and of heart in total anomalous pulmonary venous return in early infancy. Br Heart J 1977; 39: 80–92.
22. Yamaki S, Tsunemoto M, Shimada M et al. Quantitative analysis of pulmonary vascular disease in total anomalous pulmonary venous connection in sixty infants. J Thorac Cardiovasc Surg 1992; 104(3): 728–35.
23. Michel-Behnke I, Luedemann M, Hagel KJ, Schranz D. Serial stent implantation to relieve in-stent stenosis in obstructed total anomalous pulmonary venous return. Pediatr Cardiol 2002; 23(2): 221–3.
24. Coulson JD, Bullaboy CA. Concentric placement of stents to relieve an obstructed anomalous pulmonary venous connection. Cathet Cardiovasc Diagn 1997; 42(2): 201–4.
25. Yang M, Akbari H, Reddy GP et al. Identification of pulmonary vein stenosis after radiofrequency ablation for atrial fibrillation using MRI. J Comput Assist Tomogr 2001; 25: 34–5.
26. Sugiyama H, Veldtman GR, Norgard G et al. Bladed balloon angioplasty for peripheral pulmonary artery stenosis. Cathet Cardiovasc Interven 2004; 62(1): 71–7.
27. Najm HK, Caldarone CA, Smallhorn J, Coles JG. A sutureless technique for the relief of pulmonary vein stenosis with the use of in situ pericardium. J Thorac Cardiovasc Surg 1998; 115(2): 468–70.
28. Lacour-Gayet F, Rey C, Planche C. [Pulmonary vein stenosis. Description of a sutureless surgical procedure using the pericardium in situ.] Arch Mal Coeur Vaiss 1996; 89(5): 633–6.
29. Wax DF, Rocchini AP. Transcatheter management of venous stenosis. Pediatr Cardiol 1998; 19: 59–65.
30. O'Laughlin MP, Perry SB, Lock JE, Mullins CE. Use of endovascular stents in congenital heart disease. Circulation 1991; 83: 1923–39.
31. Cullen S, Ho SY, Shore D et al. Congenital stenosis of pulmonary veins failure to modify natural history by intraoperative placement of stents. Cardiol Young 1994; 4: 395–8.
32. Taylor GW, Kay GN, Zheng X et al. Pathological effects of extensive radiofrequency energy applications in the pulmonary veins in dogs. Circulation 2000; 101: 1736–42.

51

Discrete subaortic stenosis

José Suárez de Lezo, Manuel Pan, José Segura,
Miguel Romero, and Djordje Pavlovic

Under the term discrete subaortic stenosis (DSS) lies a spectrum of disease related to fixed and localized subaortic structures. As differentiated from idiopathic hypertrophic subaortic stenosis, three types of discrete subaortic stenosis can be distinguished:[1–3] fibromuscular collar type, the tunnel type, and the thin membranous type. However, the most common clinical presentation (85%) is that of the thin membranous type.[2] This chapter will focus on this form of the disease. The entity is surprisingly complex and the pathogenesis, natural history, and treatment of the disease remain unclear.

Although DSS has been classically considered a congenital malformation there are many patients who acquire the disease later in life without any former evidence of predisposing substrate. Indeed, although more frequently in youth, DSS may be diagnosed at any age. In addition, progression in hemodynamic severity after diagnosis may or may not develop, and we do not know yet why, when, and how it may happen. Certain observations on the follow-up of patients have shown another possible evolution of the disease, from a thin membrane to a more advanced muscular type. So, as postulated by Somerville over 25 years ago,[4] the pathologic basis seems to reside in the myocardium which could generate, by unknown mechanisms, a wide spectrum of abnormal hypertrophic responses in the left ventricular outflow tract.

The 'mildest' end of the spectrum (and the most frequent one) would be the development of a thin (1–2 mm) crescent or circumferential fibrous diaphragm traversing the anterior portion of the left ventricular outflow tract and causing a fixed subaortic obstruction. The continuous high pressure subaortic jet may damage the aortic cusps and some degree of aortic regurgitation is frequently associated. The degree of hemodynamic severity may vary from mild to severe, and may influence the rate of possible evolving complications such as the new appearance or progression of aortic regurgitation, infectious endocarditis, or extended muscular obstruction. For all these reasons, a thin DSS is considered a potentially progressive disease and all diagnosed patients should be followed up indefinitely, no matter what treatment decision we take. At present, there is no curative treatment for this disease.

Surgery and balloon dilation are only palliative procedures. Both reduce the pressure gradient to a similar degree but do not eliminate the underlying mechanism for potential disease progression.

Surgery

Surgical resection or enucleation of the membrane is an effective and safe treatment in reducing the left ventricular to aortic gradient. Indications for operation have included a pressure gradient > 50 mmHg, electrocardiographic signs of strain, or symptoms such as dyspnea, angina, or syncope.[5,6] However, the progressive nature of the disease led others[2–4,7–9] to recommend surgical treatment in patients with mild subaortic obstruction. Precise recommendations for an operation based on gradient level are not yet possible. The postoperative gradient in some reported series[2,9] is higher than the initial gradient in the treated groups with mild subaortic obstruction.[3,7] Thus, discussion still persists on when and how to operate on patients with thin DSS.[10,11] Although the pressure relief after surgical treatment persists in most patients, several reports[2,7–9,12] have shown increases in the residual gradient at late post-operative catheterization. Aortic regurgitation can be arrested but not reversed by surgical resection.[3,4] Some authors[9,13] have noted that aortic regurgitation may develop even after surgical treatment. This late complication is more frequent in patients with a high preoperative pressure gradient and seems also related to a longer time since operation. Thus, over time, a large proportion of surgically treated patients may become candidates for additional surgical procedures because of residual or recurrent stenosis or progressive deterioration of aortic valve function.

Balloon dilation

Balloon tearing of the subaortic thin membrane is also an effective and safe method for reducing subaortic obstruction.

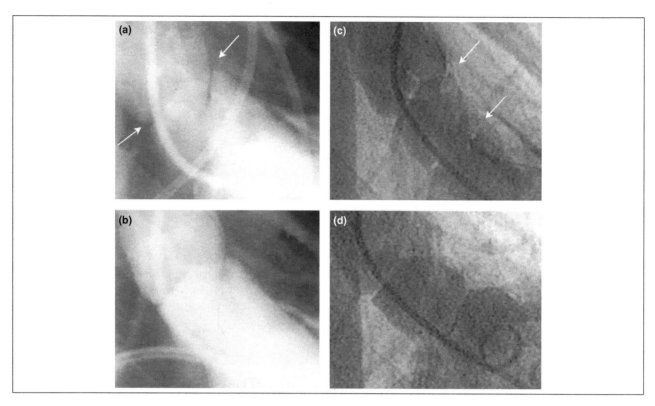

Figure 51.1
Serial left ventricular outflow angiograms (30° right anterior oblique projection) in a patient with DSS treated with balloon dilation in 1990 who developed a new distant membrane in 2002. A second balloon dilation was performed. Arrows show the aortic valve and membrane levels. (a) Before first treatment, (b) after first treatment, (c) before second treatment, (d) after second treatment.

This treatment was first described by our group in 1985.[14,15] Since then, several studies have confirmed the persistent pressure relief achieved after balloon dilation.[16–26] After this treatment, the fixed subaortic structure becomes widely mobile and fluttering in accordance with blood flow, suggesting membrane rupture as the mechanism of relief. However, only a few long term follow-up studies are available.[19,20,21,27] Following a 17-year follow-up study in 67 treated patients,[28] initial results are better in those patients with higher annulus size and in those with a membrane more distant from the aortic valve. Recurrence may appear in 17% of patients and may be secondary to restenosis (regrowth of fibrous tissue) in 14% of patients and to progression of disease in 3%. This progression may lead to extended muscular disease or to the development of a new distant membrane. Figure 51.1 shows an example of this rare (to the best of our knowledge, undescribed) late evolution after treatment. Restenosis is more frequent in patients treated by balloon dilation under the age of 13 years, and very rare when treated after puberty. The echocardiographic and angiographic features of the membrane following restenosis reproduce those observed at the first attempted dilation. In fact, mobility of the membrane could never be observed when restenosis was detected. Redilation can also be attempted

safely when needed and it is used to bring about benefits in the degree of pressure relief similar to those observed after the first dilation.[21] Figure 51.2 is a graphic representation of the gradient evolution in recurrent and non-recurrent groups of patients. The persistent pressure relief obtained in most patients may account for the favorable evolution observed in the degree of aortic regurgitation. Immediately after treatment and at follow-up, mild aortic regurgitation may not change or even disappear. Thus, balloon dilation does not seem to unfavorably affect valve competence.[21,28]

Our strategy

If we acknowledge that gradient reduction somehow prevents further complications, the percutaneous technique appears to be an attractive alternative to surgery as a first-choice treatment. The potential savings in patient discomfort are significant. Once pressure gradient relief is obtained, continued follow-up is mandatory. If recurrence develops, balloon dilation can be repeated successfully in most patients. With this strategy, surgery for a thin membrane may be delayed or even avoided.

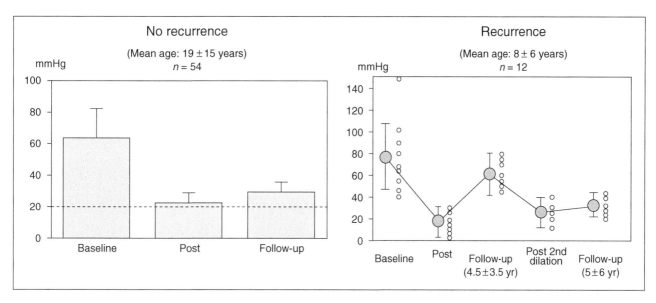

Figure 51.2
Graphic representation of gradient evolution in recurrent and non-recurrent groups of patients.

Patient selection

This is probably the most important point. The selection of patients for this treatment should be carefully analyzed by the team and meticulous non-invasive and invasive studies carried out in all candidates. The age seems an important factor. The ideal candidates for balloon dilation would be adolescents and young patients, with or without symptoms, with a thin membrane causing a significant subaortic gradient (> 50 mmHg). Younger patients with severe gradients and favorable anatomy may also be considered for a palliative procedure, whether having associated malformations or not,[23,24] but a recurrence rate of around 15% should be assumed. Adult patients with severe obstruction and favorable anatomy are also candidates. Patients of any age having a thin membrane with a mild gradient (< 50 mmHg), should be closely followed up. If progression in severity is detected they also become candidates for balloon dilation.

Previous echocardiographic study

Very clear images and measurements are necessary. If they may be obtained transthoracically we do not perform a transesophagic echocardiogram (TEE). However, we frequently need TEE, mainly in young and adult patients. The left ventricular outflow tract should be carefully inspected. The membrane causing significant obstruction must be a thin diaphragm (1–2 mm) from base to orifice. The relation to other structures like the aortic or mitral apparatus should be well established. We reject those patients having a thin membrane with a fibromuscular base in the outflow tract. These forms are almost collar types and we do not recommend

dilation because of poor results.[16,29] The most important data measurements are the following:

- subaortic Doppler gradient
- aortic annulus size
- aortic root size
- thickness of the membrane
- mean distance from the membrane to the aortic valve
- left ventricular dimensions
- diastolic left ventricular wall thickness (septum and posterior wall)
- degree of aortic valve incompetence, if any
- possible associated anomalies.

Procedure

Although the procedure can be performed without anesthesia in the young and in adults, we strongly recommend mild anesthesia in children and adolescents, at least at the critical point of balloon dilation. Complete quietness and absolute control of the patient are mandatory at that moment.

Hemodynamic and angiographic study before treatment

Three femoral punctures are performed, one venous and two arterial. We normally use the right femoral artery for the therapeutic approach and we use the left groin for monitoring and measurements. So, initially we insert a 7 Fr introducer in the right femoral artery, a 5 Fr in the left femoral artery, and a 6–7 Fr in the left femoral vein.

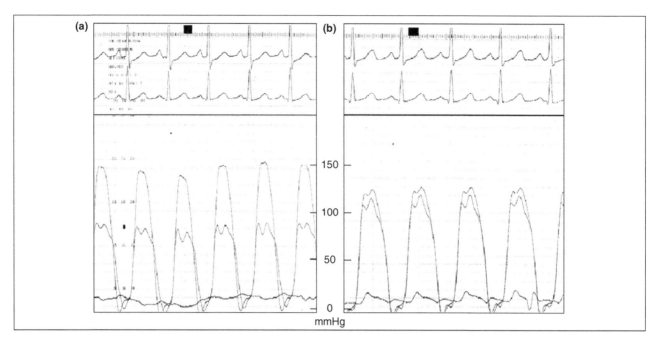

Figure 51.3
Simultaneous pressure recordings of both left ventricular chambers before (a) and after (b) balloon dilation.

Complete right and left cardiac catheterization is then performed. Simultaneous pressure measurements are obtained at all levels, especially with both arterial catheters inside the left ventricle, where the subvalvular chamber must be identified (Figure 51.3a), and then a pullback recording is performed. The baseline gradient is so obtained. Then, two left ventricular angiograms are performed, the first in the 30° right anterior oblique (RAO) projection and the second in the axial left anterior oblique (LAO) view, 25° cranial, 45° LAO. Full contrast opacification of the cavity should be obtained and careful inspection of the angiograms is needed and will be crucial for the final decision. An aortic root angiogram will be then performed in the LAO or lateral projection for evaluation of aortic valve competence. Final angiographic measurements of the aortic root and annulus, membrane thickness, and valve to membrane distance are then obtained. Selection of therapeutic materials will be based upon these angiographic measurements.

Therapeutic phase

The therapeutic target will be the rupture of the fibrous membrane without producing any damage on the valve apparatus. Selection of the appropriate material for that purpose will be the crucial point. The technique has evolved since its first description and a significant improvement in balloon dimensions and sizes makes it easier to achieve the objective. We need to quickly fully inflate a balloon catheter, of a size 1–2 mm bigger than the aortic annulus,

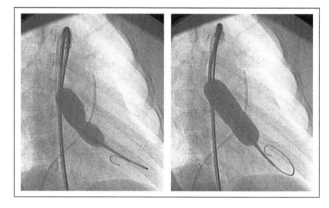

Figure 51.4
Balloon dilation of DSS in a patient. Note how the notch in the balloon disappears at full inflation.

in the left ventricular outflow tract. So, we recommend a balloon diameter 1–2 mm bigger than the angiographic annulus diameter with a balloon length of 40 to 60 mm. If the balloon remains stable during inflation, despite continuous heart beatings, and a notch in the balloon disappears at full inflation, this means that the membrane has been torn (Figure 51.4). The procedure is then most probably finished and no further inflations may be needed. However, to keep the balloon stable during inflation with potent left ventricular contractions trying to eject the inflating balloon may become a problem. The physiopathology of sudden left

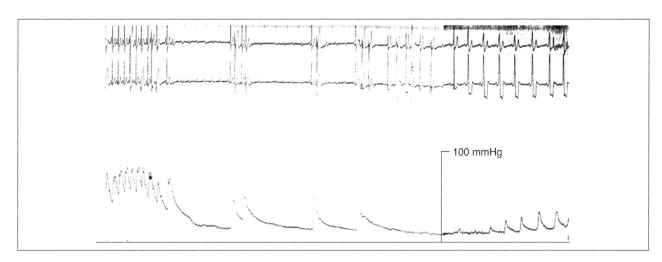

100 mmHg

Figure 51.5
Low speed aortic pressure recording during intrapulmonary infusion of adenosine. A transient AV block is obtained during which fast balloon inflation should be performed.

ventricular occlusion during balloon valvuloplasty has been studied by our group.[30,31] Surprisingly, transient aortic occlusion is well tolerated by the heart, even beating in sinus rhythm, but deep transient hemodynamic changes do occur. These changes create conditions of transient acute and complete heart failure that generate abrupt homeostatic responses detected soon after balloon inflation.[31] Recovery is always easy after balloon deflation, but extreme attention is required at this point. Transient left bundle branch block is not an infrequent finding after balloon inflation. We recommend the continuous monitoring and recording of several ECG leads and the pulmonary and aortic pressures during the balloon inflation–deflation period.

At present, we use two methods to facilitate balloon stability during inflation. One is to administer 6–12 mg of adenosine through the pulmonary catheter with the balloon catheter in place, in order to obtain a transient cardiac arrest or block while a stable full balloon inflation in the outflow tract can be easily obtained (Figure 51.5). The second, and even more efficacious, is to pace at a high rate (180 to 220 beats per minute) through an electrode with the tip properly touching the right ventricular wall. This condition always generates a transient, very low cardiac output during which the balloon can be fully expanded without much difficulty. Poor contractions at 200 beats per minute allow for a stable balloon catheter in the outflow tract during full inflation.

But let us start from the beginning. Once percutaneous treatment has been agreed by the team, full intravenous heparinization (2 mg/kg) is administered, the venous catheter is placed in the pulmonary artery for monitoring, and the 5 Fr arterial catheter will be located initially in the descending aorta for monitoring, but it may be frequently used for intermediate gradient evaluations. Then we need to

prepare the right groin for therapy. After oversizing slightly the puncture site we introduce a 0.35 inch guidewire in the descending aorta, through which we introduce a 10 Fr Perclose Tristar system, extract the threads, and leave them carefully prepared for final puncture site suture, once the procedure is finished. All these measures require continuous groin compression by an assistant to avoid bleeding. Through the remaining guidewire, which has been previously advanced to the ascending aorta, a 9 Fr to 14 Fr valved cannula with a curved tip to adapt to the aortic arch is advanced as far as the ascending aorta. We recommend the Cook cannula with a radio-opaque mark at the tip. The cannula will allow for fast interchange if needed, without causing bleeding, and will also help to fix the balloon in the outflow tract during inflation. The size of the cannula depends on the French size of the selected balloon. We must be sure that the balloon catheter is able to cross easily through the cannula. We recommend using a cannula at least 2 Fr sizes larger than that of the selected balloon catheter. Once the cannula tip is advanced to the ascending aorta, 2 to 3 cm over the aortic valve, a 7 Fr pigtail catheter is introduced and advanced through the cannula to the left ventricular cavity. At this point we always use a 30° RAO projection. The tip of the catheter is carefully located stable at the apex, without provoking premature beats. Then, a new 0.38 inch guidewire with a pre-shaped loop in the distal part, for adapting itself to the left ventricular cavity, is introduced through the pigtail catheter and carefully interchanged to allow such a looped wire delineating the left ventricular endocardial surface. The balloon catheter is now advanced through the guide and cannula to reach the left ventricular outflow tract within the marks of the balloon, with the looped wire permanently in place. At this point, the tip of the cannula is advanced close to the proximal part of the balloon to counter balloon ejection during inflation. At this point we advise repeating negative pressure on the balloon and then injecting a little contrast material to localize the notch of the membrane just in the middle of the balloon. Aortic pressure is monitored during high speed right ventricular pacing. Once a pacing rate sufficiently rapid to produce a low cardiac output is attained the balloon is inflated whilst fixing the position of the balloon catheter and sheath. Full balloon inflation with disappearance of the waist is observed. The balloon is deflated and retrieved through the sheath, maintaining the guidewire position with which we replace the 7 Fr pigtail catheter which is positioned in the left ventricle. The procedure can be repeated as many times as necessary if the balloon is not stable; we do not advise repeat balloon dilation once the notch has disappeared at full inflation.

Hemodynamic and angiographic study immediately after treatment

Simultaneous and pullback measurements are taken followed by angiography. We have not seen any degree of mitral regurgitation after treatment, though this could occur if the balloon is inadvertently inflated within the chords of the mitral valve.[32] To avoid this possibility we recommend entering the left ventricle with an angulated pigtail catheter in the RAO projection and advancing the tip to the apex before introducing the pre-shaped guidewire. The final aortogram will evaluate the changes in the degree of aortic regurgitation. In our experience, we have not seen any significant change after balloon dilation of DSS and previous mild degrees of aortic insufficiency may even disappear, once subaortic obstruction is relieved.

Groin management

Complications of the puncture site may create problems. Significant disproportion between the balloon size and that of the femoral artery is not infrequent. If the balloon is introduced directly, without a sheath, the femoral artery may be damaged, producing bleeding, hematoma, pseudoaneurysms, or ischemic complications. Thus a hemostatic sheath decreases bleeding during the procedure, facilitates interchanges, helps to fix the balloon during inflation, and seems to cause less damage to the femoral artery. Use of an arterial puncture closure device such as the Perclose system may significantly reduce femoral artery complications.

Step-by-step procedure

- Take three femoral puncture sites: two arterial and one venous.

- Make a complete hemodynamic and angiographic study.
- Make careful angiographic measurements.
- Select the balloon catheter. We use a balloon diameter 1–2 mm larger than the annulus size.
- Insert the Perclose Tristar system at the arterial puncture site, extract the threads, and leave them carefully prepared for final puncture site suture. A guidewire is maintained in the aorta.
- Using this guidewire, introduce an appropriate sized cannula and advance its tip to 1–2 cm above the aortic valve. Now, introduce a pigtail catheter in the left ventricle and exchange it with a pre-shaped long guidewire that will be looped in the cavity, remaining stable without provoking ectopic beats.
- Advance the balloon catheter over the guidewire to the left ventricular outflow tract. Adopt a 30° RAO projection. At this point, repeat vacuum to the balloon and infiltrate a small amount of contrast medium to localize the notch of the membrane in the middle of the balloon.
- Select a method to reduce left ventricular contractility, thereby improving the stability of the balloon catheter during inflation. If using adenosine, inject 6–12 mg through the catheter located in the pulmonary artery, wait for transient arrest or AV block and inflate the balloon rapidly. If using right ventricular pacing, advance a bipolar pacing electrode to the apex of the right ventricle and pace at a rate which ensures low cardiac output. Then perform rapid balloon inflation. Filmation (X-ray image acquisition during balloon inflation) of the balloon inflation will identify disappearance of the waist. Pacing is then discontinued for hemodynamic recovery.
- Replace the balloon catheter with a pigtail catheter and advance it to the left ventricle. Simultaneous pressure recordings of the left ventricle and aorta will document the hemodynamic result.
- Angiography may be repeated.
- The sheath is removed utilizing the hemostasis sutures of the Perclose device.

Pre-discharge echocardiographic study

We always perform a pre-discharge echocardiographic evaluation that will be crucial for comparison at follow-up. Besides repeat measurements in identical conditions to those obtained before treatment, we need to focus on the remaining membrane at the left ventricular outflow tract. When the tearing of the fibrous diaphragm has been successful, a mobile structure may be observed in the left ventricular outflow tract. The residual Doppler gradient should be measured and aortic valve competence evaluated. Both parameters will be of value for future follow-up studies.

References

1. Edwards JE. Pathology of left ventricular outflow tract obstruction. Circulation 1965; 31: 586–99.
2. Newfeld EA, Muster AJ, Paul MH et al. Discrete subvalvular aortic stenosis in childhood. Study of 51 patients. Am J Cardiol 1976; 38: 53–61.
3. Hardesty RL, Griffith BP, Mathews RA et al. Discrete subvalvular aortic stenosis. An evaluation of operative therapy. J Thorac Cardiovasc Surg 1977; 74: 352–61.
4. Somerville J, Stone S, Ross D. Fate of patients with fixed subaortic stenosis after surgical removal. Br Heart J 1980; 43: 629–47.
5. Hoeffel JC, Gengler L, Henry M, Pernot C. Angiocardiography in congenital subvalvular aortic stenosis: prognosis and operative indications. Ann Thorac Surg 1977; 23: 122–8.
6. Cain T, Campbell D, Paton B, Clarke D. Operation for discrete subvalvular aortic stenosis. J Thorac Cardiovasc Surg 1984; 87: 366–70.
7. Shem-Tov A, Schneeweiss A, Motro M, Neufeld HN. Clinical presentation and natural history of mild discrete subaortic stenosis. Follow-up of 1 to 17 years. Circulation 1982; 66: 509–12.
8. Katz NM, Buckley MJ, Liberthson RR. Discrete membranous subaortic stenosis. Report of 31 patients, review of the literature, and delineation of management. Circulation 1977; 56: 1034–8.
9. Brown J, Stevens L, Lynch L et al. Surgery for discrete subvalvular aortic stenosis: actuarial survival, hemodynamic results, and acquired aortic regurgitation. Ann Thorac Surg 1985; 40: 151–5.
10. de Vries AG, Hess J, Witsenburg M et al. Management of fixed subaortic stenosis: a retrospective study of 57 cases. J Am Coll Cardiol 1992; 19: 1013–17.
11. Oliver M, Gonzalez A, Gallego P et al. Discrete subaortic stenosis in adults: increased prevalence and slow rate of progression of the obstruction and aortic regurgitation. J Am Coll Cardiol 2001; 38: 835–42.
12. Kirklin JW, Barratt-Boyes BG. Congenital aortic stenosis. In: Kirklin JW, Barratt-Boyes BG, eds. Cardiac Surgery. New York: Wiley, 1986: 972–1007.
13. Bjorn-Hansen LS, Lund O, Nielsen TT et al. Aortic regurgitation after surgical relief of subvalvular membranous stenosis. A long-term follow-up study. Scand J Thorac Cardiovasc Surg 1988; 22: 275–80.
14. Suárez de Lezo J, Pan M, Herrera N et al. Left ventricular decompression through a transluminal approach in congenital aortic stenosis. Rev Esp Cardiol 1985; 38: 400–7.
15. Suárez de Lezo J, Pan M, Sancho M et al. Percutaneous transluminal balloon dilatation for discrete subaortic stenosis. Am J Cardiol 1986; 58: 619–21.
16. Lababidi Z, Weinhaus L, Stoeckle H Jr, Walls JT. Transluminal balloon dilatation for discrete subaortic stenosis. Am J Cardiol 1987; 59: 423–5.
17. Feldman T, Chiu YC, Carroll JD. Catheter balloon dilatation for discrete subaortic stenosis in the adult. Am J Cardiol 1987; 60: 403–5.
18. Arora R, Goel PK, Lochan R et al. Percutaneous transluminal balloon dilatation in discrete subaortic stenosis. Am Heart J 1988; 116: 1091–2.
19. Rao PS, Wilson AD, Chopra PS. Balloon dilatation for discrete subaortic stenosis: immediate and intermediate-term results. J Invasive Cardiol 1990; 2: 65–71.
20. Sharma S, Bhagwat AR, Loya YS. Transluminal balloon dilatation for discrete subaortic stenosis in adults and children: early and intermediate results. J Interven Cardiol 1991; 4: 105–9.
21. Suárez de Lezo J, Pan M, Medina A et al. Immediate and follow-up results of transluminal balloon dilation for discrete subaortic stenosis. J Am Coll Cardiol 1991; 18: 1309–15.
22. Shrivastava S, Dev V, Bahl VK, Saxena A. Echocardiographic determinants of outcome after percutaneous transluminal balloon dilatation of discrete subaortic stenosis. Am Heart J 1991; 122: 1323–6.
23. Ascuitto RJ, Ross-Ascuitto NT, Pickoff AS, Fox LS. Percutaneous balloon dilatation of discrete subaortic stenosis as a palliative procedure to promote recovery of left ventricular contractile function. Pediatr Cardiol 1993; 14: 122–3.
23. Gupta KG, Loya YS, Sharma S. Discrete subaortic stenosis: a study of 20 cases. Ind Heart J 1994; 46: 157–60.
24. Moskowitz WB, Schieken RM. Balloon dilation of discrete subaortic stenosis associated with other cardiac defects in children. J Invas Cardiol 1999; 11: 116–20.
25. Rao PS. Balloon angioplasty of fixed subaortic stenosis. J Invas Cardiol 1999; 11: 197–9.
26. Richartz BM, Figulla HR, Ferrari M et al. Percutaneous balloon dilatation of discrete subaortic stenosis. Z Kardiol 2002; 91: 581–3.
27. Suárez de Lezo J, Medina A, Pan M et al. Balloon valvuloplasty/angioplasty: The Spanish experience. In: Rao S, ed. Transcatheter Therapy in Pediatric Cardiology. New York: John Wiley & Sons, Inc, 1993: 471–92.
28. Suárez de Lezo J, Segura J, Medina A et al. Long-term results of percutaneous balloon dilatation for isolated discrete subaortic stenosis. A 17-year study. Circulation 2002; 106: 451.
29. Bahl VK, Radhakrishnan S, Shrivastava S. Balloon dilation of subaortic stenosis due to a thick fibrous shelf. Int J Cardiol 1988; 18: 259–60.
30. Suárez de Lezo J, Pan M, Romero M et al. Physiopathology of transient ventricular occlusion during balloon valvuloplasty for pulmonic or aortic stenosis. Am J Cardiol 1988; 61: 436–40.
31. Suárez de Lezo J, Montilla P, Pan M et al. Abrupt homeostatic responses to transient intracardiac occlusion during balloon valvuloplasty. Am J Cardiol 1989; 64: 491–7.
32. Frutos A, Sobrino N, Gallego P et al. Papillary muscle rupture during subaortic membrane balloon dilatation. Rev Esp Cardiol 1996; 49: 146–8.

52

Supravalvar aortic stenosis

José Suárez de Lezo, Manuel Pan, Miguel Romero,
José Segura, and Djordje Pavlovic

Supravalvar aortic stenosis (SAS) is a complex syndrome, which has a wide range of clinical and morphologic expression. Congenital SAS may be localized (most common) or diffuse obstruction of the ascending aorta, starting immediately above the aortic valve. It affects both sexes equally and the presentation may vary from infancy to adulthood. Frequently, it is associated with the Williams syndrome,[1] an autosomal dominant genetic disorder characterized by infantile hypercalcemia, unusual 'elfin' facies, mental retardation, mild growth deficiency, and cardiovascular disease. These patients may have associated cardiac anomalies, such as peripheral pulmonary artery stenosis, coarctation of the aorta, involvement of the supra-aortic ostial trunks, and mitral valve prolapse. However, SAS can also present as an isolated form or in familial forms of the disease without the Williams syndrome. The stenosis may vary from a localized supravalvar diaphragm to a diffusely hypoplastic ascending aorta. Because of the inability of the dysplastic aortic wall to grow adequately, its natural history shows a progression of the gradient across the aortic arch in many patients, and poor prognosis in those with severe obstruction.[2,3] From a pathophysiologic point of view, the SAS produces a left ventricular obstruction commencing above the aortic sinuses. This creates a high pressure chamber between the aortic valve and the origin of the stenosis. Besides the strain on the left ventricle, this high pressure chamber may affect competence of the aortic valve and alter coronary artery perfusion. The high coronary artery perfusion pressure may promote the development of coronary artery disease. Cardiac symptoms are common in neonates who frequently require early surgery. After 1 year of age, progression in the severity of SAS is common, whilst the severity of associated pulmonary arterial stenosis tends to improve, and only rarely alters prognosis.[2,4] Compared with an age-matched normal population, the risk of sudden death is much higher in patients with Williams syndrome.[5] Thus, life-long follow-up is necessary in all patients, even after treatment, because of the significant associated risks in a progressive disease.

Familial penetration of the disorder should always be assessed by echocardiographic screening.

Surgery

The first surgical repair was performed in 1956 by Kirklin at the Mayo Clinic.[6] Since then, different techniques of surgical aortoplasty have been developed with favorable results. Surgical correction has changed the prognosis and the long-term follow-up studies[3,7–11] show persistent relief in most patients. However, restenosis may occur and re-operation may be needed, especially in hypoplastic forms.[8] Although the localized forms may be treated successfully with patch aortoplasty, some patients with the diffuse type may require either an apical–aortic conduit or extensive endarterectomy with patch aortoplasty.[11] Thus the anatomy may influence the complexity of repair and the prognosis. In a large series of operated patients followed for a prolonged period between 1956 and 1992, the presence of associated aortic valve disease strongly correlated with late death and the need for re-operation.[7] In another large series of patients,[11] early post-operative mortality was 1% and the overall mean pressure gradient after surgery was reduced to 21 mmHg, whilst the late mortality was 2%. Thus, after almost 50 years' experience, the treatment of SAS is well established surgically, with very good initial and late results in experienced teams.

Stent treatment

Percutaneous treatment of SAS may become an attractive alternative to surgery in some patients. Although balloon dilation might be a palliative procedure in diaphragmatic forms, it fails to relieve diffuse or hypoplastic stenosis.[12,13] Based on the previous experience in long segment hypoplasia with aortic coarctation, in 1996 we reported the first two

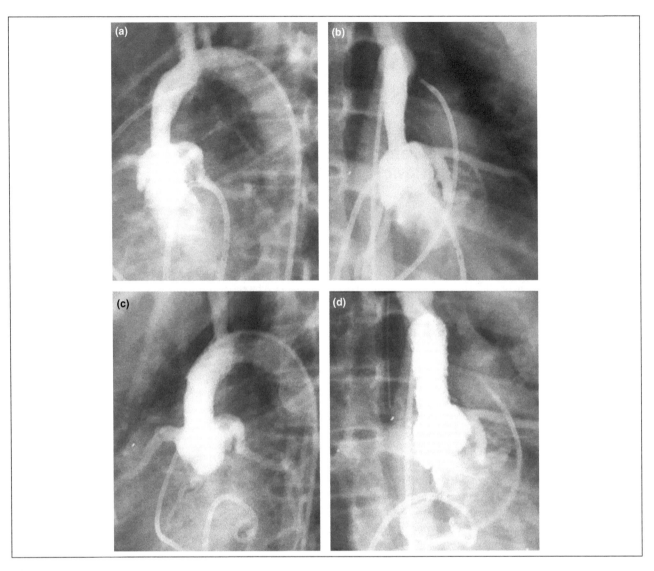

Figure 52.1
Aortograms before (a and b) and after (c and d) stent treatment; (a) and (c) are 60° LAO views; (b) and (d) are 30° RAO projections.

attempts of stent treatment for severe SAS.[14] Two sisters, aged 10 and 19 years, who had severe (peak gradient 97 and 113 mmHg, respectively), diffuse and symptomatic SAS, were successfully treated by tailored stent treatment. The younger needed a 40 mm long Palmaz stent, that was expanded to 12 mm, and the older one needed two overlapping stents, which were expanded to 15 mm diameter. After treatment, significant relief of the gradient and lumen enlargement were obtained in both patients, without altering valve competence. Figure 52.1 shows the initial angiographic result in the older patient.

After a follow-up of 10 years, both patients are alive and free of symptoms. However, both patients needed further percutaneous interventions. The younger patient showed a mild and gradual increase in the Doppler gradient over the following 5 years and, at the age of 15 years, underwent a

hemodynamic evaluation. The single implanted stent did not have any significant neointimal growth, but there was a residual gradient of 43 mmHg due to growth of the patient. Therefore the stent was re-expanded to 15 mm diameter and the residual gradient improved to 12 mmHg. The aortic valve also remained competent after this intervention. The residual Doppler gradient is currently 23 mmHg. The older patient also underwent a repeat hemodynamic evaluation 5 years after the initial intervention, because of a significant increase in the Doppler gradient. Angiography showed mild restenosis due to neointimal proliferation and some recoil of the proximal stent (Figure 52.2a). In addition, an ostial stenosis of the left common carotid artery was noted, which was not significant at the first study. A new in-stent stent, 50 mm in length, was successfully implanted and expanded to 18 mm diameter (Figure 52.2b). After this, the gradient

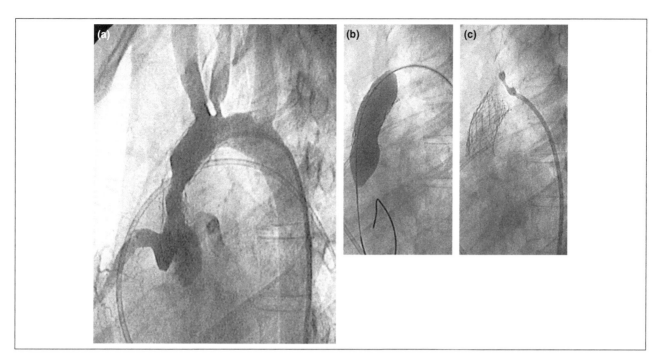

Figure 52.2
Five-year angiographic follow-up of patient from Figure 52.1 (a) Baseline 60° LAO view, showing stent recoil and neointimal proliferation. (b) A new stent is implanted inside the previous stent. (c) Stent implantation at the origin of the left carotid artery.

across the ascending aorta disappeared completely and the aortic valve remained competent. The ostial carotid artery stenosis was also treated with a short 4 mm diameter stent (Figure 52.2c). The final angiogram is shown in Figure 52.3. At present, pressure relief and valve competence persist in both patients. Finally, a third patient, aged 7 years with severe SAS, has also been treated successfully with a stent and has been described recently.[15] However, this patient developed a severe complication during treatment, which was resolved percutaneously. The leaflets of the aortic valve became trapped and held open between the expanded stent and the aortic wall, resulting in severe aortic regurgitation. By passing a wire through an open strut of the proximal part of the stent edge and externally manipulating both sides of the captured wire, the trapped cusps of the valve were freed, which was followed by an immediate and sustained recovery of the valve function. The gradient was completely abolished and the patient recovered well. After 3 years of follow-up, the pressure relief and aortic valve competence have persisted.

Thus, percutaneous experience is still too limited and cannot be recommended. Whilst stent treatment is feasible and effective in relieving severe SAS, at present, there may be an unacceptably high rate of complication of the aortic valve. New developments and materials may help in the future to reduce this complication. In addition, the technique described to release the trapped aortic leaflets may become reproducible and rapidly accomplished, if this complication occurs.

Tailored stent treatment for SAS

This technique, together with the complication mentioned above, has been described and discussed in detail.[14–16] Many current surgical treatments have evolved with time and experience. The surgeons have had to deal with expected or unexpected complications, which may appear during innovative surgical procedures, and have had to learn to treat or to avoid the complications. Interventional pediatric cardiologists may have to evolve similarly. In the near future, stent treatment for selected forms of SAS may become an alternative treatment to surgical correction. In the meantime, our experience is described below.

Patient selection

The possible candidates for an interventional treatment are children over 6 years of age, adolescents, and young adults presenting with severe SAS, with or without associated Williams syndrome. The selection of patients will need careful analysis by the team and detailed non-invasive and invasive studies will be required in all candidates. This includes evaluation of possible associated anomalies, a clearly imaged anatomy of the SAS and other adjacent structures and accurate measurements of the target obstruction. The procedure needs a tailored design,[14] so all non-invasive accurate measurements are extremely important.

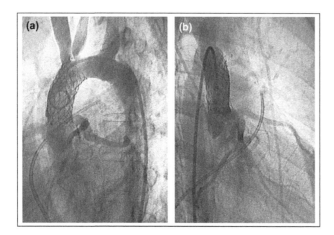

Figure 52.3
Final aortograms (a: LAO view; b: RAO projection), obtained in patient from Figures 52.1 and 52.2, after restenting. Aortic stent reconstruction can be observed.

Previous echocardiographic study

If adequate quality images are obtained by transthoracic echocardiography (TTE), there may not be a need to perform TEE. However, a TEE study is preferable in adolescents and adult patients. The presence of a patent foramen ovale should be looked for. The left ventricular outflow tract and the aortic root should be carefully inspected and the supravalvular stenosis identified. The aortic valve function should also be assessed. The most important measurements are the following: supravalvar Doppler gradient, aortic annulus size, minimal lumen diameter, length of the stenosis, the left ventricular dimensions, diastolic left ventricular wall thickness (septal and posterior wall), degree of aortic valve regurgitation, if any, and possible associated anomalies.

Procedure

The procedure should be performed under general anesthesia and TEE monitoring during the procedure, at least at the time of deployment. The patient should be kept still (if sedated).

Hemodynamic and angiographic study before treatment

One femoral venous and two femoral arterial punctures are performed. If the foramen ovale is patent, then one arterial and two venous punctures are needed, because one of the venous catheters could pass through the foramen to the left heart. Normally the right femoral artery is used for the stent implantation and the left femoral artery is used for monitoring and measurements. Initially a 7 Fr introducer sheath is inserted in the right femoral artery, a 5 Fr in the left femoral artery, and a 6–7 Fr in the left femoral vein. Complete right

and left cardiac catheterization is performed. Simultaneous pressure measurements are obtained at all levels, especially at the outflow tract. Figure 52.4a shows an example of a pullback recording before treatment. Two left ventricular angiograms are performed, the first in the 30° RAO projection and the second in the axial LAO projection, with 25° cranial, 45° LAO angulation. Two baseline aortograms are also recommended, one at 60° LAO and the other one at 30° RAO views. Accurate angiographic measurements of the diameters of the aortic root/annulus, minimal lumen diameter, lesion length, transverse aortic arch, the isthmus, and the descending aorta are obtained. Selection of balloons and stents will be based upon these angiographic measurements.

Therapeutic phase

The patient is fully heparinized with a 2 mg/kg dose of heparin. The aim is to stent the SAS without damage to the aortic valve. The proximal edge of the stent should accommodate the sinuses of Valsalva, without covering the coronary artery ostia. The recommended angiographic view during treatment is 60° LAO. In this view, the distance between the take-off of both the coronary arteries and the innominate artery origin has to be carefully measured to decide on the final length of the stent. The target stent diameter is to reach the size of the descending thoracic aorta. Selection of the appropriate equipment is based on the angiographic measurements. This diameter may be needed to be redilated at late follow-up (Figure 52.3). At present, the Cheatham-Platinum (CP) stent is used. Although the Palmaz stent has a wide range of expansion and shortening and has been successfully used, the CP stent has some advantages at the time of deployment. When implanted with a BIB balloon (balloon in balloon), initial expansion with the inner balloon may allow for repositioning of the stent before final expansion. In addition, the CP stent provides a wider range of lengths and expansion diameters, which may favor a tailored stent-covering design.

After slightly dilating the femoral puncture site, a 0.035 inch guidewire is introduced in the descending aorta, over which a 10 Fr Perclose Tristar system is passed; the threads are extracted and are left *in situ* until the procedure is finished. All these measures require continuous groin compression by an assistant to avoid bleeding. Over the guidewire, previously positioned in the ascending aorta, a 9 Fr to 14 Fr valved sheath with a curved tip (such as a Mullins sheath) is advanced to the aortic arch. The latter is recommended as it has a radio-opaque marker at the tip. Such a long sheath allows fast exchange of catheters or guidewires, if needed, without bleeding. The size of the sheath depends on the French size of the selected stent after it has been mounted on the balloon. At least 2 Fr sizes larger than the sheath recommended for the introduction of the selected balloon catheter is recommended. The other 5 Fr arterial catheter is used for repeated angiograms during

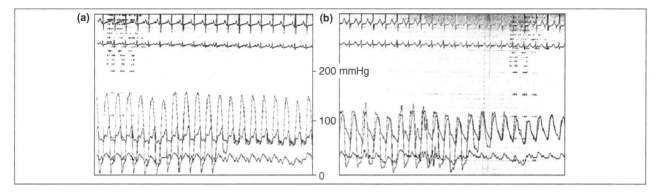

Figure 52.4
Simultaneous pressure recordings during pullback from the left ventricular cavity to the descending aorta before (a) and after treatment (b). The supravalvar gradient completely disappeared.

deployment. Once the stent is crimped onto the balloon catheter, a pre-shaped exchange length guidewire is advanced through a 7 Fr pigtail catheter and stabilized in the left ventricle. The mounted stent is advanced over the guidewire through the sheath to the target SAS. Special care has to be taken in positioning the mounted stent at exactly the desired site before inflation. To minimize the movement during systole, some maneuvers may be needed. These include (1) pharmacologic induction of transient cardiac arrest, or AV block, with intrapulmonary infusion of adenosine at a dose of 6–12 mg or (2) rapid right ventricular pacing during deployment. Simultaneous angiography during transient arrest or low cardiac output helps to opacify the whole left ventricular outflow tract, which may also help to expand the stent at the correct site.

Immediately after deployment, hemodynamic evaluation is needed. With a catheter in the left ventricle and another one at the aortic arch, changes in the gradient can be measured. Acute aortic regurgitation may be indicated by dramatic hemodynamic changes and this needs to be confirmed by angiography and TEE. If, despite all measures to avoid this complication, aortic leaflets have been trapped by the stent, rapid action is required. The surgical team should be alerted, whilst attempts are made to release the trapped cusps. Through the sheath, a Judkins right coronary catheter is advanced to the aortic root and the tip is turned towards the proximal open struts. A 0.014 inch floppy coronary guidewire is introduced through the catheter and advanced to cross the open struts. The guidewire is then directed upwards towards the aortic arch. Also through the sheath, a gooseneck snare is introduced to snare the tip of the coronary wire. Once the wire is snared, controlled traction of both ends of the wire is performed under fluoroscopic and transesophageal ultrasound guidance. With such a maneuver, the proximal part of the stent may be pulled to free the aortic valve leaflets and resolve the complication with immediate recovery of aortic valve function. If successful, a rapid hemodynamic recovery will be immediately observed and normal movements of the leaflets evidenced by TEE.[15]

Hemodynamic and angiographic study immediately after treatment

Complete hemodynamic and angiographic assessment needs to be performed after the stent has been deployed. Simultaneous pressure measurements should be repeated recording the final pullback gradient (Figure 52.4b). Finally, LAO and RAO views of the left ventricular angiograms and aortograms should be performed. Aortic valve competence, possible covering of coronary ostia, and aortic stent position should be evaluated.

Groin management

Complications of the puncture site may create problems. The size of the sheath should be large enough to allow for easy passage of the stent to the target stenosis and adequate balloon fixation during stent deployment. Both groins need to be carefully managed. The final suturing of the artery puncture hole with the Perclose system may contribute to decreasing groin complications, such as hemorrhage.

Important steps

- Three femoral puncture sites: two arterial and one venous or two venous and one arterial if there is a patent foramen ovale.
- A complete hemodynamic and angiographic study.
- Accurate detailed angiographic measurements.
- Decide on the type of stent, stent length, and degree of predicted shortening of the stent with expansion at the required expansion diameters. Aim to cover the stenosis with the stent and expand to the size of the thoracic descending aorta.

- Insert the Perclose Tristar system at the arterial puncture site, extract the threads, and leave them carefully prepared for the final puncture site repair. A guidewire is maintained in the aorta during this.
- Over this guidewire, introduce the appropriate sheath and advance it to the aortic arch.
- Through the sheath, introduce a pigtail catheter into the left ventricle and replace by a pre-shaped long guidewire looped in the cavity, which remains stable without provoking premature beats.
- Mount and crimp the stent onto the balloon. Advance the mounted stent over the guidewire and through the sheath to the target stenosis. Use a 60° LAO projection for monitoring the position of the stent.
- Select a method to decrease left ventricular contractions to avoid movement of the balloon catheter during deployment.
- If using adenosine, inject 6–12 mg through the catheter located in the pulmonary artery, wait for transient arrest or AV block and then make a rapid deployment. Angiographic monitoring at this time is crucial. An angiographic catheter in the left ventricle through a patent foramen ovale may be useful or another 5 Fr pigtail catheter that will be rapidly retrieved before deployment.
- If using rapid right ventricular pacing, advance an electrode to the apex of the right ventricle and test capture. Pace at fast frequency (180–240 beats per minute) to produce a low cardiac output and reduced aortic pressure. An angiography is performed and the stent is deployed rapidly. After deployment, pacing is stopped to allow for hemodynamic recovery.
- Exchange the balloon catheter with a 7 Fr pigtail catheter and advance it to the left ventricle. Simultaneous pressure recording and an angiogram are performed to determine whether a complication has occurred. If further expansion of the stent is needed, bigger balloons will be inflated at the stented segment.
- Final pressure recordings and angiograms are performed.
- Remove the sheath and repair the puncture site with Perclose.

Pre-discharge echocardiographic study

A pre-discharge echocardiographic evaluation is important for comparison during the follow-up period. Besides repeat measurements in identical conditions to those obtained before treatment, the whole left ventricular outflow tract should be fully imaged. The residual Doppler gradient should be obtained and aortic valve competence evaluated. All parameters are of value for future follow-up studies.

References

1. Williams JPC, Barrat-Boyes BG, Lowe JB. Supravalvular aortic stenosis. Circulation 1961; 24: 1311.
2. Wren C, Oslizlok P, Bull C. Natural history of supravalvular aortic stenosis and pulmonary artery stenosis. J Am Coll Cardiol 1990; 15: 1625–30.
3. Wessel A, Pankau R, Kececioglu D et al. Three decades of follow-up of aortic and pulmonary vascular lesions in the Williams–Beuren syndrome. Am J Med Genet 1994; 52: 297–301.
4. Eronen M, Peippo M, Hiippala A et al. Cardiovascular manifestations in 75 patients with Williams syndrome. J Med Genet 2002; 39: 554–8.
5. Wessel A, Gravenhorst V, Buchhorn R et al. Risk of sudden death in the Williams–Beuren syndrome. Am J Med Genet 2004; 127: 234–7.
6. McGoon DC, Mankin HT, Vlad P, Kirklin JW. The surgical treatment of supravalvular aortic stenosis. J Thorac Cardiovasc Surg 1961; 41: 125.
7. Van Son JAM, Danielson GK, Puga FJ et al. Supravalvular aortic stenosis. Long-term results of surgical treatment. J Thorac Cardiovasc Surg 1994; 107: 103–15.
8. Delius RE, Steinberg JB, L'Ecuyer T et al. Long-term follow-up of extended aortoplasty for supravalvular aortic stenosis. J Thorac Cardiovasc Surg 1995; 109: 155–63.
9. Hazekamp MG, Kappetein AP, Schoof PH et al. Brom's three-patch technique for repair of supravalvular aortic stenosis. J Thorac Cardiovasc Surg 1999; 118: 252–8.
10. Stamm C, Kreutzer C, Zurakowski D et al. Forty-one years of surgical experience with congenital supravalvular aortic stenosis. J Thorac Cardiovasc Surg 1999; 118: 874–85.
11. Brown JW, Ruzmetov M, Vijay P, Turrentine MW. Surgical repair of congenital supravalvular aortic stenosis in children. Eur J Cardiothorac Surg 2002; 21: 50–6.
12. Tyagi S, Arora R, Kaul UA, Khalilullah M. Percutaneous transluminal balloon dilatation in supravalvular aortic stenosis. Am Heart J 1989; 118: 1041–4.
13. Pinto RJ, Loya Y, Bhagwat A, Sharma S. Balloon dilatation of supravalvular aortic stenosis: a report of two cases. Int J Cardiol 1994; 46: 179–81.
14. Suárez de Lezo J, Pan M, Romero M et al. Tailored stent treatment for severe supravalvular aortic stentosis. Am J Cardiol 1996; 78: 1081–3.
15. Suárez de Lezo J, Pan M, Medina A et al. Acute aortic insufficiency complicating stent treatment of supravalvular aortic stenosis: successful release of trapped leaflets by wiring the stent. Cathet Cardiovasc Interven 2004; 61: 537–41.
16. Mullins CE. Not quite ready for prime time. Editorial comment. Cathet Cardiovasc Interven 2004; 61: 542.

53

Stenting in aortic coarctation and transverse arch/isthmus hypoplasia

Shakeel A Qureshi

Introduction

Stent implantation in aortic coarctation is increasingly used to treat patients who would previously have been treated by balloon angioplasty or surgery. Balloon dilation in native aortic coarctation and recoarctation has been controversial since its introduction in 1982.[1] Histologic and intravascular ultrasound studies[2–6] have demonstrated that the mechanism of angioplasty involves tearing of the intima and media. Deficient elastic and muscular lamella have been noted in ballooned sections of aorta at the time of surgery.[7] Although some of the intimal and medial tears may heal, there is concern that some may progress to aneurysms. Cystic medial necrosis may exist in the coarctation segment, suggesting that the aortic wall may be weak at the point of the stenosis.[8] A relatively high incidence of aneurysm formation of 2–20% has been reported.[9–13]

Stenting of aortic coarctation was first performed in 1991.[13] Stents tack intimal flaps to the aortic wall after tearing of the intima and media, allowing healing to occur without dissection.[14] They further reinforce the weakened areas within the aortic wall which may later predispose to formation of a pseudoaneurysm. Where intimal tears occur, the stent provides a surface for formation of neointima over the tear. Furthermore, intimal and medial damage may not occur to the same extent following stenting compared with balloon dilation, as overdilation of the aorta is avoided during stent implantation.

Initially stent implantation was used only for cases where surgery and balloon angioplasty had failed.[15] However, as experience has increased, stenting is gradually becoming the treatment of choice in aortic coarctation. This is especially the case when coarctation coexists with hypoplasia of the aortic isthmus or transverse arch, when balloon dilation tends to have a high failure rate. This and other morphologic variations such as a tortuous coarctation, long segment coarctation, or mild discrete coarctation may all be considered suitable for stenting. In other cases in whom the anatomy is more straightforward, stenting may reduce the gradient at the coarctation site more effectively than balloon dilation. In the adult patients, stenting is gradually being considered as the treatment of choice in any variant of aortic coarctation. At the other end of the scale, in children less than 10 years of age, it is preferable to avoid stenting, as several redilations may be required until the child is fully grown and there remain questions about the feasibility of redilation.

Equipment

Palmaz (Cordis Johnson & Johnson), Intratherapeutics Doublestrut (EV3), or Cheatham-Platinum (CP) (NuMed) stents have been used the most in clinical practice Figure 53.1a–e. These are balloon-expandable and so need to be mounted on the appropriate balloon diameter. A selection of balloons such as the Powerflex (Cordis Johnson & Johnson), BIB (NuMed), or Cristal (Merck) need to be kept in stock in catheter laboratories. On occasions higher pressure balloons such as Mullins balloons may be needed. A range of sizes of covered stents such as CP stents also needs to be stocked for emergency cases, as there may be the rare complication of dissection and even aortic rupture. Occasionally self-expanding stents may have some role to play but these have a limited use in pediatric cardiology practice. They have the disadvantage of lower radial strength. The choice of a stent depends on the experience and the preferences of the operator and the local cost considerations.

Technique

The procedure is performed under general anesthesia as it is painful for the patient when the balloon is inflated to deploy the stent. Access is obtained in the femoral artery as well as

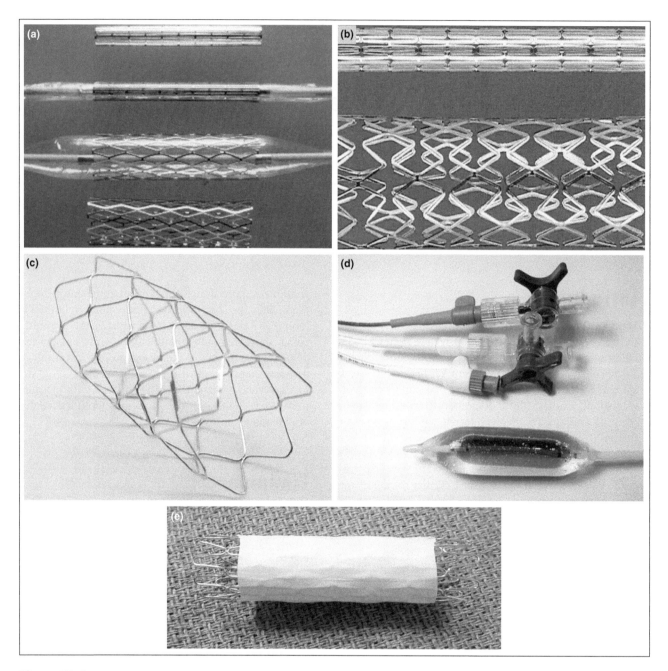

Figure 53.1
(a) Palmaz stent unexpanded, then mounted on a balloon, inflated, and then finally fully expanded. (b) Intrastent doublestrut stent unexpanded and fully expanded. (c) Expanded CP stent. (d) A BIB (balloon-in-balloon) system, which requires two inflation devices to inflate the balloons separately. (e) A covered CP stent (with expanded polytetrafluoroethylene covering).

the femoral vein. The venous access is required for the insertion and the use of a temporary pacemaker during stent implantation. This is of importance in adults with a high stroke volume, such as when aortic regurgitation is present. Rapid right ventricular pacing reduces the cardiac output in a controlled manner during the deployment of the stent, facilitating its precise positioning. In the presence of a very tight, nearly atretic, or even atretic aortic segment,

access may be needed in the right radial or brachial artery, so that a catheter can be passed from above into the descending aorta. If there is a pinhole present, the coarctation segment can be crossed from above. Rarely, carotid arterial access by a surgical arteriotomy may be required for access to the descending aorta. A Perclose (Abbott Vascular) suture is usually inserted after local angiography of the femoral arteries. This helps to produce hemostasis at the end of the procedure and may prevent complications such as hemorrhage from the arterial puncture site. This is a major advance in the methods of hemostasis. Either a single suture or occasionally two sutures are used to repair femoral arteries, in which up to 14 Fr sheaths have been inserted for the stent deployment. They have to be inserted prior to the introduction of the larger sheath.

Heparin at a dose of 50 to 100 IU/kg is given after access is obtained to maintain the activated clotting time >200–220 s during the procedure.

A 5 or 6 Fr endhole catheter is passed through the aortic coarctation and positioned in the ascending aorta. With a tight or tortuous coarctation, it is preferable to use a straight tip guidewire to cross the coarctation from below and this is followed by the catheter being passed over the wire. An Amplatz stiff exchange guidewire of 0.035 inch caliber is exchanged for the previous guidewire and, over this, a Multitrack catheter (NuMed). This catheter has a monorail system and is passed to measure withdrawal gradients across the coarctation, without losing the wire position. Angiography can be performed with this catheter, which has a 1 cm marker, allowing accurate calibration and the exact measurements of the aorta. Alternatively, a pigtail catheter with 1 cm radio-opaque markers is used for angiography. Angiography is performed in the left lateral and either shallow left anterior oblique (LAO) or right anterior oblique (RAO) views (if biplane facilities are available). The diameters of the distal transverse arch (just proximal to the origin of the left subclavian artery), the aortic isthmus (just distal to the origin of the left subclavian artery), the site of coarctation, and the descending aorta above the diaphragm are measured using catheter magnification or the calibration markers on the catheters. The diameter of the aorta at maximum systolic expansion is measured and is used to select the appropriate diameter balloon.

The length of the chosen stent is based on the distance between the left subclavian artery (or the left common carotid if the subclavian artery has been used at previous surgery or if the subclavian artery is intimately related to the site of coarctation) to about 15 mm beyond the site of the coarctation. The maximum balloon diameter on which the stent is mounted is based on either the transverse or the distal arch diameter, whichever is the greater, and on occasions 1–2 mm greater.

The types of stents in use for this procedure include the Palmaz 2910 (29 mm long, nominal diameter 3.4 mm, dilates to 8–12 mm), 4014 (4 cm long, nominal diameter 4.6 mm, dilates to 14–25 mm) and 5014 (5 cm long, nominal diameter 4.6 mm, dilates to 14–25 mm), the various sizes of the Intratherapeutics doublestrut stents and the CP stents available in 22, 28, 34, 39, and 45 mm. The latter stents have a slightly higher profile and are more rigid with higher radial strength than other stents and so are preferable in adult patients and those with aortic recoarctation after previous surgery.

A long Mullins sheath (length 75 cm) is passed over a 0.035 inch stiff exchange length guidewire positioned in the ascending aorta for stent delivery. As an alternative, the guidewire may be positioned in either the innominate artery or the left subclavian artery. The sheath size ranges between 10 and 14 Fr for bare stents or covered stents, and is generally 2–3 Fr larger than that required for the introduction of the balloon catheter alone. The stent is manually crimped on to the selected balloon tightly enough to ensure that it does not slip off the balloon during insertion through the tight diaphragm of the sheath. To avoid the stent from slipping off the balloon, a small piece of sufficient length of a similar size short sheath is cut to cover the stent and this covering is used to pass the stent/balloon assembly through the diaphragm of the sheath. The various steps of the technique are shown in Figure 53.2a–f. Angiography is performed through the side-arm of the sheath to check the position of the stent across the site of coarctation prior to inflation of the balloon. In the past, adenosine was used to produce transient asystole during balloon inflation, but more recently, rapid right ventricular pacing has been used with good effect. The rate of pacing varies between 180 and 240 beats per minute. The exact rate can be determined at the outset by monitoring the pressure in the ascending aorta whilst pacing the heart at different rates. The rate for pacing which reduces the blood pressure in the ascending aorta to less than 50 mmHg is used.

The stent/balloon assembly is advanced through the long sheath and positioned across the site of the coarctation. Optimal positioning is confirmed by small hand injections of contrast through the side-arm of the Mullins sheath or alternatively by hand injections through a second catheter placed in the descending aorta. Whilst maintaining the balloon catheter and wire in position, the Mullins sheath is withdrawn to expose the stent/balloon assembly in position at the site of the coarctation. Rapid right ventricular pacing is initiated and almost simultaneously the balloon is inflated with an inflation device so that pressures up to the balloon burst pressure can be delivered. The final part of stent expansion may sometimes occur slowly with sustained pressure. Once the stent is deployed, pacing is stopped and the balloon is deflated. Further dilation with a larger balloon is performed in some cases until satisfactory relief of the stenotic waist is attained. If a BIB balloon is used, then two inflation devices are needed. As soon as rapid pacing is started, one operator inflates the inner balloon and the other operator the outer balloon. The inner balloon is inflated first, followed by the outer balloon, and a similar sequence is followed for deflation.

Although a bare stent can be expanded to the diameter of the normal vessel either side of the coarctation, in a tight coarctation, either an undersized balloon is chosen or the balloon is not fully expanded to the normal vessel diameter, to reduce the likelihood of aortic wall damage and dissection. The stent is expanded to approximately 60–80% of the diameter of the descending aorta at the diaphragm at

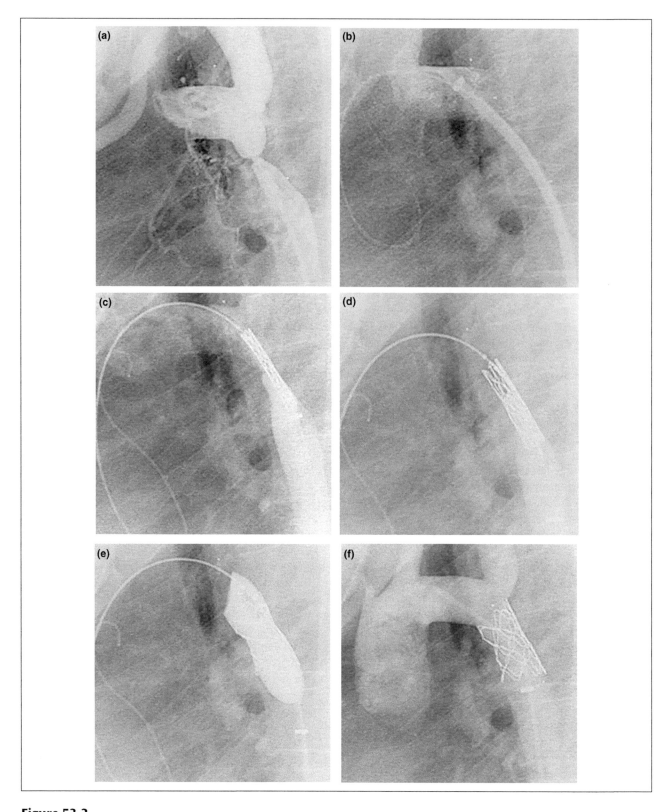

Figure 53.2

(a) A discrete aortic coarctation just beyond the left subclavian artery with mild distal isthmic hypoplasia. (b) The guidewire is positioned in the ascending aorta and the Mullins sheath is placed in the transverse aortic arch. (c) The stent/balloon assembly is positioned at the site of coarctation and the Mullins sheath is withdrawn to expose the stent. (d) The inner balloon-in-balloon (BIB) balloon is inflated and an angiogram performed to check for the satisfactory position of the stent. (e) The outer BIB balloon is inflated to deploy the stent fully. A mild residual waist is kept on the balloon on occasions, cespecially if a tight coarctation is present, to reduce the possibility of a dissection. (f) An angiogram after stent implantation showing good position of the stent and excellent relief of coarctation.

implantation. Flaring of the ends of the stent to achieve contact with the aortic wall at all points is not performed.

After deflation, the balloon is withdrawn carefully so as not to dislodge the stent. The gradient across the stent is remeasured, by recording simultaneous pressures from the angiographic catheter passed over the wire to above the stent and the long sheath placed below the stent. An aortogram is repeated to exclude dissection or aneurysm formation.

After removal of the sheath, hemostasis is achieved with the Perclose suture. After the procedure, subcutaneous low molecular weight heparin is administered for 24 hours. Antibiotics (flucloxacillin and gentamycin or cefuroxime) are given at the beginning of the procedure and continued for 24 hours. Aspirin is administered to all the patients the evening prior to the procedure at a dose of 3–5 mg/kg, and continued for up to 6 months.

Follow up is arranged for 4 weeks, 6 months, and 1 year after the procedure and spiral CT scanning is performed 4–6 weeks after the procedure to exclude aneurysm formation, dissection, and stent thrombosis. Recatheterization is performed only if there is clinical recoarctation, continuing hypertension, or CT evidence of aneurysm formation. Elective recatheterization is performed after 6 to 12 months to carry out stent redilation when there is residual stenosis as a result of the stent having been intentionally underinflated initially.

Disadvantages of stenting

Relatively large 10–14 Fr Mullins delivery sheaths are used to deliver the stent/balloon assembly across the coarctation. Whilst there may be a higher risk of femoral artery occlusion with stenting than with balloon angioplasty, this has not been a problem in adult patients.[16,17] If it was crucial to avoid a larger sheath and the coarctation was tight enough, then the stent could initially be deployed using an 8 or 10 mm Powerflex balloon or another lower profile balloon (introduced through an 8 or 9 Fr sheath) and then expanded to the final size with a larger balloon, thereby minimizing sheath size and trauma to the femoral artery.[18] A possible disadvantage with unknown consequences may be the introduction of a non-compliant and non-pulsatile section in the aorta at the stent site and its possible effects on the systolic blood pressure on exercise in the future.[19]

Complications of stenting

Complications of the stenting procedure include femoral artery disruption or thrombosis, stent migration at implantation, delayed stent migration, acute aortic rupture, paradoxic hypertension, thrombotic occlusion of the stent (described in stenting of the abdominal aorta), and endocarditis.[20–26]

Most of these complications can be dealt with by medical treatment or catheter techniques. Stent thrombosis can be

treated with local thrombolysis. Stent migration is best dealt with by implanting and dilating the stent in an alternative safe location. If a dissection occurs, this can be managed conservatively if small or by implanting a bare or a covered stent, if large. The occurrence of an aneurysm can also be treated similarly (Figure 53.3a–c). Rarely if aortic rupture occurs, then the availability of a covered stent, which can be rapidly inserted percutaneously, can save the day and avoid the need for emergency surgery. Paradoxic hypertension can be treated by aggressive medical treatment.

Measures of success

In the adult population, the initial gradient across the coarctation may not reflect its severity as there may be extensive collateral vessels decompressing the aorta proximal to the stenosis. Resolution of hypertension cannot necessarily be used as a measure of efficacy because the incidence of hypertension may be masked by antihypertensive treatment. Some adult patients without residual stenosis at the coarctation site will continue to be hypertensive.[27–30] However, their blood pressure control may become easier after stenting. Stenting appears to be effective in reducing resting blood pressure to normal levels in the majority of children and adults.[26–31] There is no information on how stenting affects exercise tolerance or how well the stented coarctation segment responds to the increased cardiac output in pregnancy.

Staged dilation

Aortic rupture, although rare, is well documented after balloon angioplasty.[32,33] The risk of pseudoaneurysm formation after balloon angioplasty may be associated with overdilation.[34] Although stenting avoids overdilation, there may still be insufficient vascular tissue to stretch to a normal aortic diameter when the coarctation is tight. There is, therefore, a risk of rupture and aneurysm formation when a severely stenotic coarctation is stretched to the diameter of the adjacent vessel. Staged dilation, in which stents are expanded to a diameter less than the adjacent aorta and redilated a few months later, may overcome the possible risks of disruption. A controlled injury is allowed time to heal and the arterial wall to remodel before full expansion is attempted. However, even with this approach, aneurysm formation may not be avoidable.

Aneurysm formation after stenting

The incidence of aneurysms following stenting is low. It is possible that medial injury from compression by the stent

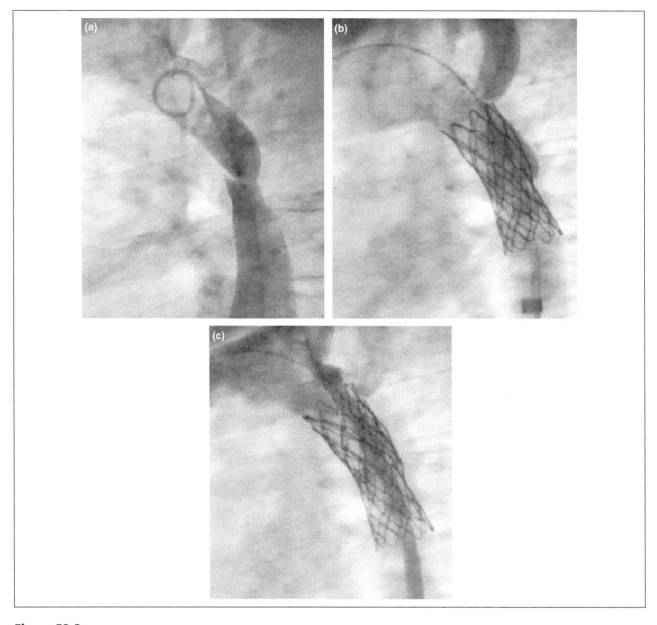

Figure 53.3
(a) An unusual native aortic coarctation with a small duct ampulla and moderate distal arch/isthmic hypoplasia. (b) After implantation of a Cheatham-Platinum (CP) stent, there is evidence of a small aneurysm posteriorly related to upper edge of the stent. (c) Angiogram after implantation of an overlapping covered CP stent showing exclusion of the small aneurysm.

struts or intimal and medial tears at the time of stent implantation creates a substrate for late aneurysm formation. Several reports describe sporadic cases of aneurysm formation.[23,26,31,34] Pre-dilation may be a risk factor for subsequent aneurysm formation. If aneurysm occurs after redilation of a previously implanted stent, this can easily be treated now with a covered stent, as can any aneurysms (Figure 53.4).

Allowance for growth/redilation

If stents are implanted in smaller patients, somatic growth of the patient will require redilation and so it is best to avoid stenting in infants and smaller children. In this age group, stenting should be reserved for exceptional clinical

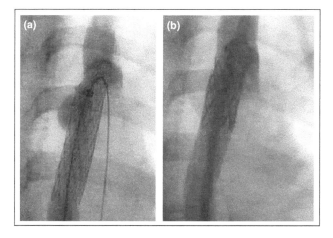

Figure 53.4
(a) An angiogram showing an aneurysm after redilation of a previously implanted Palmaz stent. (b) This was treated by implantation of an overlapping covered CP stent.

indications rather than routine use because excellent surgical results can be obtained with extended arch repair.

Covered stents

Covered stents could ultimately replace uncovered stents, especially in the treatment of aortic coarctation in adults. Although covered stents should prevent formation of aneurysms, there is some concern that they may occlude aortic side branches to the spinal cord and therefore carry a risk of paraplegia. However, the arterial supply to the spinal cord usually originates below the aortic isthmus in the region of T9–T12 vertebrae and so, in the usual location of aortic coarctation, there should not be any incidence of paraplegia. Indeed this was the case in two recent small series after stent-graft insertion.[35,36] However, a larger series reported a 3.6% paraplegia rate after stent-grafting,[37] suggesting that there is a small but significant risk. This is supported by data from surgical series in which the risk of paraplegia from surgery has been reported to be under 1% for procedures at the upper end of the aorta, but over 10% for procedures in the mid-portion of the aorta just above the diaphragm.[38] Nevertheless, stent grafts have now established an important role in the treatment of thoracic aortic aneurysms.[39]

Covered stents have been used recently to treat aortic coarctation.[40] They are being used predominantly in adults, but rarely they may need to be used in children also.[41] The recent introduction of the CP stent is an example of an expanded polytetraflouroethylene (ePTFE) covered stent in the early phase of clinical trials and is now becoming an important part of the stock of catheter laboratories (Figure 53.1e).[42–44] It may be indicated in adults with very tight aortic coarctation, in atretic or subatretic coarctation,

in complex tortuous coarctation, with hypoplasia of the isthmus, or when there is an aneurysm, either native or after previous balloon dilation or surgery, or after redilation of a previously implanted stent, or rarely when there is a native coarctation associated with a patent arterial duct in an adolescent or an adult (Figures 53.3 and 53.4).[42–45]

Covered stents can be implanted using the same technique as described above for the bare stents. A Mullins sheath of 1–2 Fr larger than that needed for implantation of a bare stent is used. A short covering sheath is important to allow introduction of the covered stent through the diaphragm of the Mullins sheath, otherwise the covering may be stripped off from the stent if it is introduced without a protective covering. Experience with stent grafts for thoracic aortic aneurysms suggests that the origin of the left subclavian artery (although best avoided) can be covered with a covered stent to treat coarctation without any ill effects.[39,42] However, it is important to avoid covering the origins of the left common carotid artery.

Stenting for transverse aortic arch/isthmic hypoplasia

Whilst the commonest indication for stenting is discrete aortic coarctation, there are some patients in whom there is a residual gradient because of an associated transverse arch or isthmic hypoplasia. Indeed it has been shown that the aortic arch anatomy (in particular transverse and distal arch hypoplasia) plays an important role in a less than optimal result such as risk of recoarctation or residual coarctation.[24,46,47] There may also be occasional patients in whom the coarctation is diffuse and located in the transverse arch (Figure 53.5). These are difficult patients to treat. The surgical treatment option for transverse arch hypoplasia is to perform an extended arch repair, which frequently requires cardiopulmonary bypass and is not risk free. Thus if such lesions can be treated in the adult patients with non-surgical means, such as by using a stent, then clearly there are benefits for the patient.

The technique of stent implantation is similar to that described above for conventional implantation of a stent in aortic coarctation. An ascending angiogram is performed in the left lateral and either LAO or RAO projection with the aim of defining the arch anatomy as well as the origins of the innominate, the left common carotid, and the left subclavian arteries. Accurate measurements of the aortic arch at different locations are crucial in the decision making. The largest diameter of the aortic arch (usually just beyond the left carotid artery or between the innominate artery and the left common carotid artery) is taken as a guide for the selection of the stent and the balloon. The distance between the origins of these vessels is also measured and this helps in the selection of an appropriate length stent. The balloon

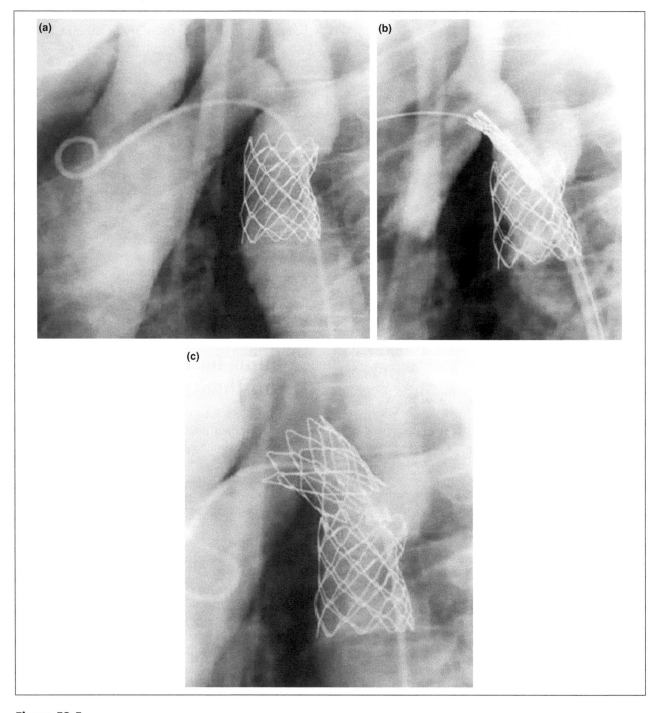

Figure 53.5
(a) Angiogram of an unusual native aortic coarctation. The usual typical coarctation site has been treated with a bare CP stent just distal to the origin of the left subclavian artery. There is additional severe transverse arch hypoplasia between the origins of the left common carotid and left subclavian arteries with a tortuous aorta. (b) A further bare CP stent is positioned in the transverse aortic arch.
(c) Angiogram after full inflation of the bare CP stent showing a good result. The residual gradient was abolished.

needs to be 1–2 mm larger than the largest diameter of the aortic arch and the stent needs to be about 3–5 mm longer than the distance between the origins of the vessels where the aorta is to be stented. The size of the Mullins sheath is determined by the diameter and the type of the balloon on which the stent is to be mounted. The sheath should be 2 Fr larger than that needed to introduce the balloon alone in order to allow the stent to pass through it when mounted on

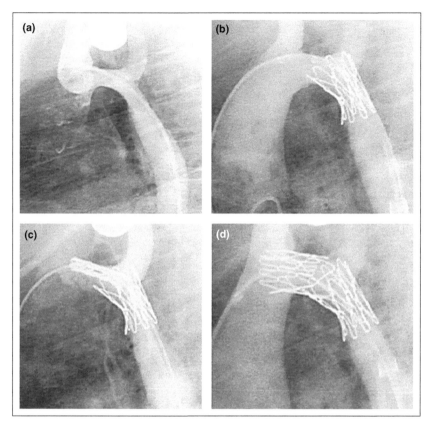

Figure 53.6
(a) Angiogram of a post-surgical aortic recoarctation combined with transverse arch hypoplasia (between the left common carotid artery and the innominate artery). (b) A bare CP stent has been implanted across the recoarctation site. (c) A further CP stent positioned in the transverse aortic arch. (d) After inflation of the stent, an angiogram shows a good result. A few millimeters of the stent protrude into the origin of the left common carotid artery.

the same balloon. Rapid right ventricular pacing is essential during the placement of the stent, as it is possible to displace the stent/balloon assembly distally during inflation of the balloon because of a relatively large stroke volume in an adult patient.

The stiff Amplatz exchange length guidewire is positioned in the ascending aorta. Once the Mullins sheath is in place across the hypoplastic arch, the stent/balloon assembly is passed through this (using a short covering sheath during passage through the diaphragm of the Mullins sheath) until it is at the tip of the sheath. Frequent angiograms are performed through the side-arm of the Mullins sheath to check for accurate positioning of the stent. In case of hypoplasia of the arch between the left common carotid artery and the left subclavian artery (the most frequently encountered lesion), the stent is positioned such that only about 2–3 mm of the stent are protruding across the origin of the left carotid artery. On balloon inflation, the stent will tend to shorten and so will be clear of the origin of the carotid artery. Stent struts covering the origin of the left subclavian artery are not of concern (Figure 53.6a–d). The Mullins sheath is withdrawn whilst keeping the stent/balloon assembly in position so as to expose the stent. After accurate positioning has been checked, rapid right ventricular pacing is initiated and the balloon is inflated rapidly to a pressure recommended by the manufacturer so as to deploy the stent. After full inflation is

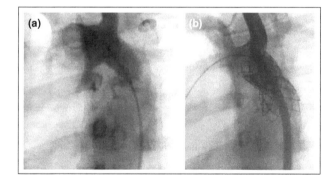

Figure 53.7
(a) Angiogram showing arch hypoplasia distal to the left common carotid artery – treated with a covered CP stent. (b) The diameter of the stent matches the aorta proximal to the left common carotid artery.

achieved, pacing is terminated and gradually the balloon is deflated and gently withdrawn back into the Mullins sheath. An angiogram is repeated, either through the Mullins sheath or through a pigtail catheter advanced over the guidewire into the ascending aorta. The pigtail catheter is withdrawn over the guidewire and an endhole multi-purpose catheter advanced over the wire in order to remove the guidewire from the ascending aorta and then to measure the pressure gradient across the stented vessel. If a covered stent is used, then it can be inflated to its full size without too much concern about dissection (Figure 53.7).

Conclusions

Stents are an important advance in the treatment of aortic coarctation. Their use should be limited to children more than 10 years old and adults. Whilst stents can be used to treat localized aortic coarctation, they are indicated in adolescents and adults with long segment coarctation, or when there is associated hypoplasia of the isthmus or transverse arch, or in a tortuous aortic coarctation, in recoarctation after previous balloon or surgery, or when an aneurysm has developed after previous treatment. With any form of treatment for aortic coarctation, a small incidence of aneurysm formation is inevitable. However, most of these complications can be treated with covered stents, which may in due course become the treatment of choice in adolescents and adults.

References

1. Singer MI, Rowen M, Dorsey TJ. Transluminal aortic balloon angioplasty for coarctation of the aorta in the newborn. Am Heart J 1982; 103: 131–2.
2. Ho SY, Somerville J, Yip WC et al. Transluminal balloon dilation of resected coarcted segments of thoracic aorta: histological study and clinical implications. Int J Cardiol 1988; 19: 99–105.
3. Lock JE, Castaneda-Zuniga WR, Bass JL et al. Balloon dilatation of excised aortic coarctations. Radiology 1982; 143: 689–91.
4. Ino T, Kishiro M, Okubo M et al. Dilatation mechanism of balloon angioplasty in children: assessment by angiography and intravascular ultrasound. Cardiovasc Interven Radiol 1998; 21: 102–8.
5. Rothman A, Ricou F, Weintraub RG et al. Intraluminal ultrasound imaging through a balloon dilation catheter in an animal model of coarctation of the aorta. Circulation 1992; 85: 2291–5.
6. Sohn S, Rothman A, Shiota T et al. Acute and follow-up intravascular ultrasound findings after balloon dilation of coarctation of the aorta. Circulation 1994; 90: 340–7.
7. Brandt Bd, Marvin WJ Jr, Rose EF et al. Surgical treatment of coarctation of the aorta after balloon angioplasty. J Thorac Cardiovasc Surg 1987; 94: 715–19.
8. Isner JM, Donaldson RF, Fulton D et al. Cystic medial necrosis in coarctation of the aorta: a potential factor contributing to adverse consequences observed after percutaneous balloon angioplasty of coarctation sites. Circulation 1987; 75: 689–95.
9. De Lezo JS, Sancho M, Pan M et al. Angiographic follow-up after balloon angioplasty for coarctation of the aorta. J Am Coll Cardiol 1989; 13: 689–95.
10. Shaddy RE, Boucek MM, Sturtevant JE et al. Comparison of angioplasty and surgery for unoperated coarctation of the aorta [see comments]. Circulation 1993; 87: 793–9.
11. Rao PS, Galal O, Smith PA et al. Five- to nine-year follow-up results of balloon angioplasty of native aortic coarctation in infants and children. J Am Coll Cardiol 1996; 27: 462–70.
12. Fletcher SE, Nihill MR, Grifka RG et al. Balloon angioplasty of native coarctation of the aorta: midterm follow-up and prognostic factors. J Am Coll Cardiol 1995; 25: 730–4.
13. O'Laughlin MP, Perry SB, Lock JE et al. Use of endovascular stents in congenital heart disease. Circulation 1991; 83: 1923–39.
14. Trent MS, Parsonnet V, Shoenfeld R et al. A balloon-expandable intravascular stent for obliterating experimental aortic dissection. J Vasc Surg 1990; 11: 707–17.
15. Rosenthal E, Qureshi SA, Tynan M. Stent implantation for aortic recoarctation. Am Heart J 1995; 129: 1220–1.
16. Lee HY, Reddy SC, Rao PS. Evaluation of superficial femoral artery compromise and limb growth retardation after transfemoral artery balloon dilatations. Circulation 1997; 95: 974–80.
17. Burrows PE, Benson LN, Babyn P et al. Magnetic resonance imaging of the iliofemoral arteries after balloon dilation angioplasty of aortic arch obstructions in children. Circulation 1994; 90: 915–20.
18. Bjarnason H, Hunter DW, Ferral H et al. Placement of the Palmaz stent with use of an 8-F introducer sheath and Olbert balloons. J Vasc Interven Radiol 1993; 4: 435–9.
19. Xu J, Shiota T, Omoto R et al. Intravascular ultrasound assessment of regional aortic wall stiffness, distensibility, and compliance in patients with coarctation of the aorta. Am Heart J 1997; 134: 93–8.
20. Suarez de Lezo J, Pan M, Romero M et al. Balloon-expandable stent repair of severe coarctation of aorta. Am Heart J 1995; 129: 1002–8.
21. Magee AG, Brzezinska-Rajszys G, Qureshi SA et al. Stent implantation for aortic coarctation and recoarctation. Heart 1999; 82: 600–6.
22. Thanopoulos BD, Hadjinikolaou L, Konstadopoulou GN et al. Stent treatment for coarctation of the aorta: intermediate term follow up and technical considerations. Heart 2000; 84: 65–70.
23. Marshall AC, Perry SB, Keane JF et al. Early results and medium-term follow-up of stent implantation for mild residual or recurrent aortic coarctation. Am Heart J 2000; 139: 1054–60.
24. Pihkala J, Pedra CA, Nykanen D et al. Implantation of endovascular stents for hypoplasia of the transverse aortic arch. Cardiol Young 2000; 10: 3–7.
25. Brzezinska-Rajszys G, Qureshi SA, Ksiazyk J et al. Middle aortic syndrome treated by stent implantation. Heart 1999; 81: 166–70.
26. Suarez de Lezo J, Pan M, Romero M et al. Immediate and follow-up findings after stent treatment for severe coarctation of aorta. Am J Cardiol 1999; 83: 400–6.
27. Kaemmerer H, Oelert F, Bahlmann J et al. Arterial hypertension in adults after surgical treatment of aortic coarctation. Thorac Cardiovasc Surg 1998; 46: 121–5.
28. Gunthard J, Buser PT, Miettunen R et al. Effects of morphologic restenosis, defined by MRI after coarctation repair, on blood pressure and arm–leg and Doppler gradients. Angiology 1996; 47: 1073–80.
29. Guenthard J, Zumsteg U, Wyler F. Arm–leg pressure gradients on late follow-up after coarctation repair. Possible causes and implications. Eur Heart J 1996; 17: 1572–5.
30. Gardiner HM, Celermajer DS, Sorensen KE et al. Arterial reactivity is significantly impaired in normotensive young adults after successful repair of aortic coarctation in childhood. Circulation 1994; 89: 1745–50.
31. Bulbul ZR, Bruckheimer E, Love JC et al. Implantation of balloon-expandable stents for coarctation of the aorta: implantation data and short-term results. Cathet Cardiovasc Diagn 1996; 39: 36–42.
32. Balaji S, Oommen R, Rees PG. Fatal aortic rupture during balloon dilatation of recoarctation. Br Heart J 1991; 65: 100–1.
33. Rao PS. Aortic rupture after balloon angioplasty of aortic coarctation. Am Heart J 1993; 125: 1205–6.
34. Fletcher SE, Cheatham JP, Froeming S. Aortic aneurysm following primary balloon angioplasty and secondary endovascular stent placement in the treatment of native coarctation of the aorta. Cathet Cardiovasc Diagn 1998; 44: 40–4.
35. Kato N, Dake MD, Miller DC et al. Traumatic thoracic aortic aneurysm: treatment with endovascular stent-grafts. Radiology 1997; 205: 657–62.
36. Rousseau H, Soula P, Perreault P et al. Delayed treatment of traumatic rupture of the thoracic aorta with endoluminal covered stent. Circulation 1999; 99: 498–504.
37. Mitchell RS, Miller DC, Dake MD. Stent-graft repair of thoracic aortic aneurysms. Semin Vasc Surg 1997; 10: 257–71.

38. Connolly JE. Hume Memorial lecture. Prevention of spinal cord complications in aortic surgery. Am J Surg 1998; 176: 92–101.

39. Taylor PR, Gaines PA, McGuinness CL et al. Thoracic aortic stent grafts-early experience from two centers using commercially available devices. Eur J Vasc Endovasc Surg 2001; 22: 70–6.

40. Gunn J, Cleveland T, Gaines P. Covered stent to treat co-existent coarctation and aneurysm of the aorta in a young man. Heart 1999; 82: 351.

41. Khan MS, Moore JW. Treatment of abdominal aortic pseudoaneurysm with covered stents in a paediatric patient. Cathet Cardiovasc Interven 2000; 50: 445–8.

42. Qureshi SA, Zubrzycka M, Brzezinska-Rajszys G et al. Use of covered Cheatham-Platinum stents in aortic coarctation and recoarctation. Cardiol Young 2004; 14: 50–4.

43. Ewert P, Abdul-Khalid H, Peters B et al. Transcatheter therapy of long extreme subatretic aortic coarctations with covered stents. Cathet Cardiovasc Interven 2004; 63: 236–9.

44. Forbes T, Matisoff D, Dysart J et al. Treatment of coexisting coarctation and aneurysm of the aorta with covered stent in a pediatric patient. Pediatr Cardiol 2003; 24: 289–91.

45. Sadiq M, Malick NH, Qureshi SA. Simultaneous treatment of native coarctation of the aorta combined with patent ductus arteriosus using a covered stent. Cathet Cardiovasc Interven 2003; 59: 387–90.

46. Kaine SF, Smith EO, Mott AR et al. Quantitative echocardiographic analysis of the aortic arch predicts outcome of balloon angioplasty of native coarctation of the aorta. Circulation 1996; 94: 1056–62.

47. Walhout RJ, Lekkerkerker JC, Ernst SM et al. Angioplasty for coarctation in different aged patients. Am Heart J 2002; 144: 180–6.

54

Middle aortic syndrome

Grazyna Brzezinska-Rajszys and Shakeel A Qureshi

Middle aortic syndrome (MAS) (abdominal coarctation, mid-aortic dysplastic syndrome), first described in 1963,[1] is an uncommon cause of arterial hypertension in children and young adults. It is characterized by segmental narrowing of the distal thoracic and/or abdominal aorta (Figure 54.1).[2–7] It accounts for 0.5–2% of cases of coarctation of the aorta. Stenosis of the aorta may be associated with stenoses of aortic side branches, mostly renal and visceral arteries (Figure 54.2).

The exact etiology of MAS remains unknown, but most often it is acquired, caused by non-specific inflammatory arteritis, or Takayasu's disease, fibromuscular dysplasia, retroperitoneal fibrosis, radiation-induced arterial fibrosis, or congenital (developmental anomaly in the fusion and maturation of the paired embryonic dorsal aortas). MAS is reported in association with neurofibromatosis, Alagille syndrome, and the Williams syndrome.[2,3,5,7–12]

Stenosis of the aorta causes upper limb hypertension. Additionally, reduction of perfusion to one or both kidneys causes severe renovascular hypertension. MAS is considered to be life-threatening as a result of the complications associated with severe hypertension. The prognosis in untreated patients is poor, with death usually occurring in the fourth decade.

Whatever the etiology of MAS, assuming that active aortic inflammation has been medically treated and is in a burnt-out state, patients with aortic narrowing, who have clinical symptoms such as severe arterial hypertension, lower extremity claudication, or mesenteric ischemia will need revascularization.[2–4,13]

Depending on the experience of the units and the anatomic forms of MAS, several management strategies are used in different centers. Surgery is widely accepted especially in older patients and in complex MAS associated with renal and visceral arterial stenosis.[2,3,6,7,10,14–17] The type of surgery may involve thoracoabdominal to infrarenal aortic bypass with renal artery re-implantation, splenorenal bypass, aortorenal bypass, and autotransplantation. In children, surgical bypass using conduits is difficult and complicated and the tube graft may need to be replaced at a later date.[5,7,11]

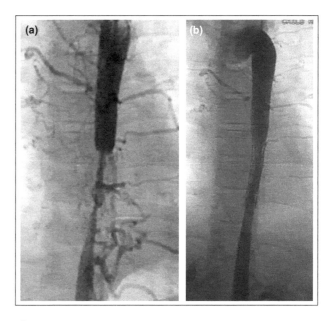

Figure 54.1
Middle aortic syndrome, narrowing of the distal thoracic aorta before (a) and after (b) stent implantation.

Experience over the last decade has shown that MAS can be treated with percutaneous techniques, such as balloon angioplasty or stent implantation, depending on the anatomy and age of the patient.[11,18]

The mechanism of relief of narrowing after balloon dilatation is similar to that of dilatation of coarctation and intimal tears may be seen on intravascular ultrasound.[18] Percutaneous transluminal balloon angioplasty is reported to be effective in relieving short segment stenosis (<3 cm) of the aorta due to aortic arteritis in children,[13,19,20] but the results may be unpredictable and unsatisfactory in other forms of MAS. Stent implantation for long segment lesions or after unsuccessful angioplasty of the aorta, in which there may be incomplete relief of stenosis or dissection, is associated with good early and immediate results (Figure 54.3).

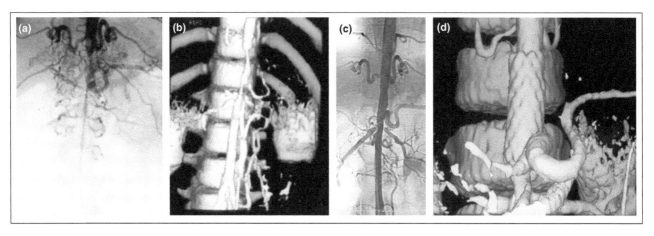

Figure 54.2
Middle aortic syndrome, narrowing of the abdominal aorta associated with stenoses of renal and visceral arteries. Angiography (a) and computed tomography angiography (3D reconstruction) (b) before treatment. Angiography (c) and computed tomography angiography (3D reconstruction) (d) after stent implantation into the aorta.

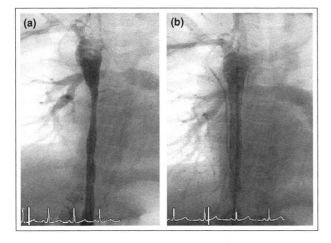

Figure 54.3
Ventricular septal defect with pulmonary atresia after two Blalock–Taussig shunts with severe long segment stenosis of the thoracic aorta. Aortography one year after two balloon angioplasties (a). Aortography after implantation of two stents into the aorta (b).

Indeed, in some centers it may be the primary therapy of MAS.[19,21–24] As the risk of dissection, aneurysm, and rupture of the aorta exists with this type of treatment, covered stents for bailout purposes should be available. In some patients covered stents may be used as primary therapy. In carefully selected cases of severe aortic narrowing in very small children, cutting balloons have been used (J Cheatham, personal communication).

In complex forms of MAS, for example those associated with renal artery stenosis, dilation of the aorta should be combined with treatment of renal artery stenosis. In patients with discrete renal artery stenosis, balloon angioplasty of the stenotic renal arteries is highly effective, but in diffuse stenosis, renal autotransplantation may be associated with better results (Figure 54.4).[13,25] Besides the good immediate results of treatment, progression of the arterial occlusive process may occur afterwards, therefore careful follow-up of patients with MAS is mandatory.[10,11,26]

Pre-intervention imaging

The site and type of obstruction of aorta and additional arterial stenosis can be shown in detail by magnetic resonance imaging (MRI), computed tomography (CT), or aortography. MRI and CT can accurately illustrate the site and extent of the obstruction of the aorta, and involvement of its branches and collaterals. Analysis of MRI or CT angiography may reduce the need for angiography in the planning of the required treatment. Breath-hold gadolinium-enhanced MRI and contrast-enhanced CT angiography can demonstrate thickening of the arterial wall with crescents and indistinct outlines typical for the acute phase of arteritis, which may be important for the timing of interventions.[27,28]

Modern spiral and multi-detector CT, which can be used for rapid imaging of large scan volumes using thin section collimation, allows for the evaluation of the arterial system without anesthesia, even in small children (Figure 54.5).

Ultrasonography can demonstrate vascular stenoses in accessible areas, and their location may help in diagnosing MAS, but ultrasonography is mostly important for the follow-up assessment of the results of interventions.

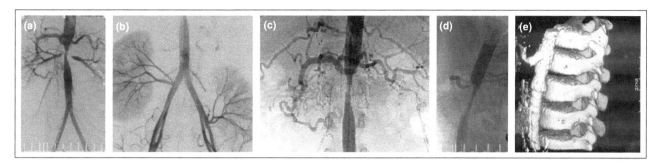

Figure 54.4
Middle aortic syndrome, narrowing of abdominal aorta and diffuse stenosis of both renal arteries; angiography before treatment (a). Angiography after renal autotransplantation. Both renal arteries transplanted to iliac arteries (b). Severe stenosis of abdominal aorta (c) and celiac artery (d). Computed tomography angiography 3 years after stent implantation into the aorta and celiac artery (e).

Technique of interventional therapy (balloon angioplasty and stent implantation in the aorta)

Dilation of the aorta should be performed under routine or general anesthesia, depending on the experience of the center and the age of the patient. The standard access for dilation of MAS is by femoral arterial percutaneous puncture. In small children, surgical cut-down on to the iliac artery or carotid artery may be needed. In complex MAS, femoral artery access is also used for dilatation of the renal and celiac arteries. The brachial artery approach may be helpful in some cases. The vascular access depends on the anatomy of the stenosed vessels and should facilitate the intervention.

Heparin is administered intravenously, at a dose of 100 IU/kg; a maximum of 5000 units is given and repeated as needed to maintain the activated clotted times (ACTs) above 200 seconds during the procedure.

The pre-interventional diagnostic procedure consists of obtaining hemodynamic and angiographic data. From the femoral arterial approach, a multi-purpose catheter is used to cross the stenosis in the aorta with the help of a guidewire, which is put in a stable position across the stenosis and located in the ascending or thoracic aorta, depending on the location of the narrowing. A J-curve guidewire may be helpful to avoid entering the collateral arteries. An angiographic catheter, such as a pigtail, multi-purpose, or multi-track, is introduced over the wire into the aorta above the stenosis. The advantage of using the multi-track catheter is that the guidewire position can be maintained whilst repeated pullback measurements and angiography are performed. Hemodynamic measurements are recorded with the aortic pressures in the ascending and descending aorta and the gradient is obtained. Aortography in the antero-posterior and lateral projections and, in complex

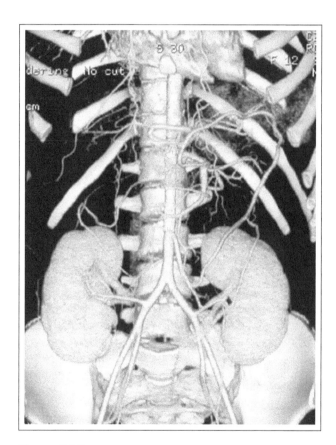

Figure 54.5
Computed tomography (3D reconstruction). Middle aortic syndrome after renal autotransplantation and stent implantation into the aorta.

cases, in the LAO or RAO projections is performed using any of the previously mentioned angiographic catheters. The projection is variable and depends on the anatomy.

Measurements of the anatomic details are performed using the antero-posterior and lateral projection. The measurements, which are needed to determine the size of the balloon, should be accurate as errors may lead to complications. The measurements include the minimum diameter of the stenotic aorta and the diameter above and below the stenosis. In cases in which there are co-existing additional stenoses of the aortic branches (e.g., renal or celiac arteries), measurements on these vessels, with the minimum diameter of the stenosis and the diameter of the normal vessel, should be performed. The stiff exchange length guidewire (such as an Amplatz wire) is positioned across the stenosis with the soft J-curve in the ascending or in the thoracic aorta, depending on the anatomy.

Balloon angioplasty of MAS

Balloon angioplasty of MAS is based on the same rules as balloon angioplasty of coarctation of the aorta. Low pressure balloon catheters (such as Tyshak balloons) may be effective in discrete stenosis and in the younger children, but high pressure balloons are usually more effective. The balloon diameter should not exceed the diameter of the aorta above the stenosis and also should not exceed 3 times the diameter of the stenosis. The guidewire lumen of the balloon catheter is flushed and air is also removed from the balloon with a syringe by creating a vacuum. Over the wire, the angiography catheter is exchanged for the balloon catheter. The correct sized sheath, according to the recommendation of the balloon catheter manufacturer, should be introduced into the artery. The side-port of the sheath can be connected to the pressure monitoring system for immediate assessment of the hemodynamic result. A balloon catheter is placed at the level of the stenosis. The balloon is inflated with diluted contrast material (25% contrast + 75% saline). An inflation device is useful to control and monitor the balloon pressure, but manual inflation can be performed in low pressure balloons. This choice depends on the experience of the individual operator. Appearance of a waist on the balloon indicates the site of stenosis. The balloon is inflated until the waist disappears. The balloon is kept inflated for approximately 10–30 seconds, after which the balloon is deflated as quickly as possible. Additional balloon inflation may be required if the balloon slips during inflation or if the waist has not been completely abolished. Occasionally, rapid right ventricular pacing may be useful for stabilization of the balloon position during inflation, in particular in older patients. After dilation, the contrast material is removed from the balloon and the balloon catheter is withdrawn through the sheath. Continuous negative pressure applied on the balloon lumen should diminish its profile and allow for easy withdrawal. The wire position should be maintained and a Multitrack catheter is inserted over the wire into the aorta above the area of dilation. It is important to avoid manipulation of the tip of the catheter or guidewire in the dilated area, and avoid losing guidewire position or trying to recross the recently dilated lesion.

Final aortography, in the same projection as prior to balloon dilation, is performed to check the anatomic result

of dilation and the diameter of the stenosis. The hemodynamic measurements, with pressures in the aorta, using a pullback method, are performed as well. A reduction of the pressure gradient below 10 mmHg secondary to an increase in the diameter of the aorta at the level of the stenosis constitutes a good result of the angioplasty.

Stent implantation in MAS

In patients with suboptimal reduction of the gradient, those with long segment stenosis of the aorta, or those accepted for primary stent implantation into the aorta, the technique of implantation is very similar to that used in typical coarctation of the aorta. After the diagnostic part of procedure, consisting of hemodynamic and angiographic data acquisition, an appropriate balloon catheter and stent are selected. The balloon diameter should be similar to the diameter of the aorta above the stenosis. A long segment narrowing of the aorta may mimic serial vessel obstructions. Low pressure balloon inflation may show a beady appearance with multiple waists due to the multiple stenoses. These waists can be a marker for precise placement of a stent. The length of the balloon should be similar to the length of the stent, and certainly not shorter than the stent. The balloon-in-balloon (BIB) catheter is preferable for stent implantation in the aorta, but other types of high pressure balloons can also be used.

Pre-mounted or manually mounted stents can be used. Nowadays, stents used in this situation include the Palmaz, Palmaz Genesis, or the Cheatham-Platinum stents. In some situations, self-expanding stents are also used. The choice of stent depends on the technical properties of the stent and, in particular, the need for the stent to be dilatable to the diameter of the adult aorta.

The guidewire lumen of the balloon catheter is flushed and the air removed from the balloon with a syringe by creating a vacuum. The BIB catheter preparation is similar, but the air should be removed from both balloons with syringes by creating a vacuum, after which both balloon hubs are connected to the inflation devices. The appropriate stent is mounted on the balloon in a position related to the markers on the balloon catheters. If there is any uncertainty, the position of the stent on the balloon should be checked under fluoroscopy prior to the final crimping. The stent is crimped manually onto the balloon. An appropriate diameter and length sheath with a radio-opaque marker at its tip (such as the Mullins sheath) is placed in the aorta. The sheath should be at least 1–2 Fr sizes larger than that recommended for the introduction of the balloon catheter. This depends on the type of stent being used. The sheath and its dilator are flushed with saline and introduced over the guidewire and the sheath is placed across the stenosis with the marker above the stenosis.

For insertion of the stent/balloon assembly into the long sheath, a small piece of tubing of appropriate French size is prepared to cover the stent/balloon assembly. This will prevent the stent from slipping off the balloon during its introduction through the diaphragm of the long sheath. The tubing may be the cut piece of a short sheath or the plastic or metal tube included in the stent package. The stent/balloon assembly is advanced through the sheath under fluoroscopic guidance and placed across the stenosis. Special care should be taken to maintain the guidewire position throughout the procedure. The long sheath is withdrawn to completely uncover the stent/balloon assembly. The accurate positioning of the stent is checked with hand injections of contrast through the side-port of the sheath.

The balloon is inflated with diluted contrast (25% contrast + 75% saline). When using the BIB balloon, initially inflation of the inner balloon is performed with the inflation device to reach the pressure recommended by the manufacturer. After inflation, the stopcock connected to the inner balloon should be closed and aortography is performed through the long sheath or through a second catheter, if inserted, to check the position of the stent. If needed, the position of the stent can be adjusted at this stage. The outer balloon is then inflated with the inflation device also to reach the pressure recommended by the manufacturer. Full inflation of the balloon should be maintained for approximately 10–30 seconds. The stent position should be checked under fluoroscopy during the balloon inflation. The inner balloon is deflated first followed by the outer balloon. With continuous negative pressure applied on both balloons, the balloon catheter is carefully withdrawn under fluoroscopy. Occasionally it is helpful to advance the sheath over the balloon whilst taking care not to push the stent upwards. A Multitrack catheter is inserted over the exchange wire into the aorta above the dilated area and aortography is repeated in the same projection as prior to stent implantation to check the anatomic result of dilation and measure the diameter of the stent.

Finally, the post-procedure pressures in the aorta are recorded by the pull-back method. A reduction of pressure gradient below 10 mmHg secondary to the increased diameter of the stented aorta at the level of stenosis is considered a good result of the procedure. After balloon angioplasty or stent implantation, aspirin at a dose of 3–5 mg/kg is given daily for 3–6 months and antihypertensive treatment is maintained or started.

Spiral CT or MRI assessment should be performed, preferably before discharge if there have been any complications during the procedure, or one year later if the procedure was uncomplicated. In complex forms of MAS with stenosis of the aorta co-existing with stenosis of the renal and other branches of the abdominal aorta, interventional dilation should be considered. In discrete forms of renal artery stenosis, balloon angioplasty usually produces good results. In long segment renal artery stenosis, balloon angioplasty may be ineffective and the risks of damage to the artery wall, spasm, dissection,

and rupture are higher. In such cases, surgery should be considered. Celiac trunk stenosis or mesenteric artery stenosis can be treated with balloon angioplasty but, in some cases, stent implantation should be considered. In some variants, immediate implantation of stents into the aorta and its branches may be needed. In cases of aorta narrowing in the region of the renal orifices, balloon angioplasty of renal arteries should be the first step in the procedure followed by stent implantation in the aorta. It should be stressed that balloon angioplasty of renal arteries, especially their orifice, may be the origin of a dissection of the aorta. Balloon angioplasty of the aorta with guidewires positioned in the renal arteries to protect their flow after tear of the aortic intima has been reported.

Complications

The main complications of balloon angioplasty of MAS relate to aortic wall damage. A small aortic dissection should be treated with additional prolonged balloon inflation maintained for approximately 1–2 minutes or even longer. If repeat spiral CT or MRI scans show progress of the dissection, implantation of a bare or covered stent should be performed. A large dissection should be treated with a bare or covered stent implanted during the same procedure.[19]

A small aneurysm should be followed with repeat spiral CT or MRI scans. If necessary, when the diameter of the aneurysm increases or when there is a spiral aneurysm, implantation of a bare or covered stent should be performed. A large or increasing aneurysm should be treated immediately with implantation of a covered stent.

Aortic rupture is an indication for emergency surgery or implantation of a single or multiple covered stents.[29] Another complication is damage to the femoral artery, which should be treated with thrombolysis or surgical repair.

The main complications of stent implantation into the aorta in MAS are mostly related to stent migration and malposition, even though these are rare. Implantation of the migrated stent below or above the stenosis, depending on the anatomy, allows for completion of the procedure. Migration of the stent to the ascending aorta has been reported and may be more difficult to treat. An expanded stent can be retrieved percutaneously, but this is very difficult and requires a combination of snares, tip-deflectors, forceps, and large sheaths. In some situations, surgery is recommended. Aortic wall complications are sporadic during stent implantation in MAS. In such situations, treatment is the same as discussed earlier. During the follow-up period, restenosis of the stent may occur due to neointimal hyperplasia or growth of the patient. This can generally be treated successfully with balloon redilation. Stent fracture may occur rarely in patients in whom the stent is only partially expanded. If this results in stent restenosis, a further stent or a covered stent is implanted.

Conclusion

Middle aortic syndrome is an uncommon cause of arterial hypertension. In The Children Memorial Health Institute, Warsaw, 17 children (aged 3–17 years, mean age 11.6 years) with severe arterial hypertension resistant to multi-drug therapy and a diagnosis of MAS underwent interventional treatment. Sixteen had narrowing of the thoracic and/or abdominal aorta (length of stenosis 3–9 cm, minimum diameter 1.5–5 mm); one aortic atresia was below the origin of the stenosed left renal artery. Aortic narrowing was isolated in 7 patients and co-existed with renal, celiac, and mesenteric artery stenosis in 9 patients. Aortic narrowing was treated in 13 with stent implantation (8 as primary treatment, 5 after balloon angioplasty), and in 3 with balloon angioplasty. Additional interventional or surgical procedures were performed (renal arteries balloon angioplasty: 7 patients, renal artery autotransplantation: 3 patients, celiac artery balloon angioplasty: 5 patients, mesenteric balloon angioplasty: 2 patients, stent implantation to truncus coeliacus: 1 patient, heminephrectomy: 1 patient). A good hemodynamic and anatomic result of stent implantation with diminished gradient (from a mean of 43 mmHg to a mean of 11 mmHg) and an increased diameter of the aorta (from a mean of 3 mm to a mean of 9.8 mm) was achieved. In a mean of 50.4 months follow-up, 4 patients had elective stent redilation, 4 had successful redilations due to neointimal hyperplasia, 2 had second stent implantations (aneurysm formation: 1 patient, progressive aorta narrowing: 1 patient). Balloon angioplasty of the aorta was performed in a complex form of MAS or in very young patients as a primary treatment which temporarily improved the pressure control. The antihypertensive medication was continued in all patients, but the dosage was reduced with improved control of the blood pressure during follow-up. The progression of vascular changes was observed during follow-up in 4 patients (3 with neurofibromatosis). From these experiences, interventional treatment of children with MAS is effective in early and mid-term follow-up. Due to the complexity of the disease, combined interventional and surgical treatment may be necessary.

References

1. Sen PK, Kinare SG, Engineer SD et al. The middle aortic syndrome. Br Heart J 1963; 25: 610–18.
2. Graham LM, Zelenock GB, Erlandson EE et al. Abdominal aortic coarctation and segmental hypoplasia. Surgery 1979; 86: 519–29.
3. Lewis VD III, Meranze SG, McLean GK et al. The midaortic syndrome: diagnosis and treatment. Radiology 1988; 167: 111–13.
4. Poulias GE, Skoutas B, Doundoulakis E. The middle aortic dysplastic syndrome: surgical considerations with a 2 to 18 year follow-up and selective histopathology study. Eur J Vasc Surg 1990; 4: 75–82.
5. Sumboonnananda A, Robinson BL, Gedroyc WM et al. Middle aortic syndrome: clinical and radiological findings. ADIC 1992; 67: 501–5.
6. Panayiotopoulos YP, Tyrrell MR, Koffman G et al. Mid-aortic syndrome presenting in childhood. Br J Surg 1996; 83: 235–40.
7. Connolly JE, Wilson SE, Lawrence PL, Fujitani RM. Middle aortic syndrome: distal thoracic and abdominal coarctation, a disorder with multiple etiologies. J Am Coll Surg 2002; 194(6): 774–81.
8. Pagni S, Denatale RW, Boltax RS. Takayasu's arteritis: the middle aortic syndrome. Am Surg 1996; 62: 409–12.
9. Shefler AG, Chan MK, Ostman-Smith I. Middle aortic syndrome in a boy with arteriohepatic dysplasia (Alagille syndrome). Pediatr Cardiol 1997; 18: 232–4.
10. Radford DJ, Pohlner PG. The middle aortic syndrome: an important feature of Williams' syndrome. Cardiol Young 2000; 10: 597–602.
11. Criado E, Izquierdo L, Lujan S et al. Abdominal aortic coarctation, renovascular, hypertension, and neurofibromatosis. Ann Vasc Surg 2002; 16(3): 363–7.
12. Delis KT, Gloviczki P. Middle aortic syndrome: from presentation to contemporary open surgical and endovascular treatment. Perspect Vasc Surg Endovasc Ther 2005; 17: 187–203.
13. D'Souza SJ, Tsai WS, Silver MM et al. Diagnosis and management of stenotic aorto-arteriopathy in childhood. J Pediatr 1998; 132: 1016–22.
14. Stanley JC, Graham LM, Whitehouse WM et al. Developmental occlusive disease of the abdominal aorta and the splanchnic and renal arteries. Am J Surg 1981; 142: 190–6.
15. Reiher L, Sandmann W. Coarctation of the thoracoabdominal aorta. Chirurgie 1998; 69: 753–8.
16. Upchurch GR Jr, Henke PK, Eagleton MJ et al. Pediatric splanchnic arterial occlusive disease: clinical relevance and operative treatment. J Vasc Surg 2002; 35: 860–7.
17. Terramani TT, Salim A, Hood DB, Rowe VL, Weaver FA. Hypoplasia of the descending thoracic and abdominal aorta: a report of two cases and review of the literature. J Vasc Surg 2002; 36: 844–8.
18. Kashani IA, Sklansky MS, Movahed H et al. Successful balloon dilation of an abdominal coarctation of the aorta in patient with presumed Takayasu's aortitis. Cathet Cardiovasc Diagn 1996; 38: 406–9.
19. Tyagi S, Kaul UA, Arora R. Endovascular stenting for unsuccessful angioplasty of the aorta in aortoarteritis. Cardiovasc Interven Radiol 1999; 22: 452–6.
20. Tyagi S, Khan AA, Kaul UA, Arora R. Percutaneous transluminal angioplasty for stenosis of the aorta due to aortic arteritis in children. Pediatr Cardiol 1999; 20: 404–10.
21. Brzezinska-Rajszys G, Qureshi SA, Ksiazyk J et al. Middle aortic syndrome treated by stent implantation. Heart 1999; 81: 166–70.
22. Bali HK, Bhargava M, Jain AK. De novo stenting of descending thoracic aorta in Takayasu arteritis: intermediate-term follow-up results. J Invas Cardiol 2000; 12: 612–17.
23. Keith DS, Markey B, Schiedler M. Successful long-term stenting of an atypical descending aortic coarctation. J Vasc Surg 2002; 35: 166–7.
24. Sharma BK, Jain S, Bali HK. A follow-up study of balloon angioplasty and de-novo stenting in Takayasu arteritis. Int J Cardiol 2000; 75 (Suppl 1): S147–52.
25. Tyagi S, Singh B, Kaul UA. Balloon angioplasty for renovascular hypertension in Takayasu's arteritis. Am Heart J 1993; 125: 1386–93.
26. Liang P, Tan-Ong M, Hoffman GS. Takayasu's arteritis: vascular interventions and outcomes. J Rheumatol 2004; 31: 102–6.
27. Choe YH, Han BK, Koh EM. Takayasu's arteritis: assessment of disease activity with contrast-enhanced MR imaging. Am J Roentgenol 2000; 175: 505–11.
28. Yamada I, Nakagawa T, Himeno Y et al. Takayasu arteritis: diagnosis with breath-hold contrast-enhanced three-dimensional MR angiography. J Magn Reson Imaging 2000; 11: 481–7.
29. Deshmukh HL, Rathod KR, Sheth RJ, Garg A. Fatal aortic rupture complicating stent plasty in a case of aortoarteritis. Cardiovasc Interven Radiol 2003; 26: 496–8.

Section XI

Hypertrophic obstructive cardiomyopathy

55

Catheter intervention for hypertrophic obstructive cardiomyopathy

Ulrich Sigwart and Haran Burri

Introduction

About 25% of patients with hypertrophic cardiomyopathy (HCM) have left ventricular outflow obstruction under resting conditions.[1,2] Medical therapy with negative inotropic drugs may alleviate symptoms in many of these patients; however, a certain number may remain refractory to drug therapy. This subset of patients may represent 5–10% of the total population with this disease.[3] Surgical myectomy has been shown to reduce outflow gradients, and has been practiced since the 1960s. Some patients may, however, not be regarded as favorable candidates for this major intervention because of advanced age, concomitant medical conditions, or previous cardiac surgery.[4] In 1994, a catheter treatment using absolute alcohol to induce a myocardial infarction localized to the interventricular septum was introduced as an alternative to surgery. Since the first series of three patients reported in 1995,[5] there has been growing enthusiasm for this technique. During the first 5 years this technique was performed in over 800 cases,[6] the number is now several thousand.

Patient selection

In addition to stable patients, those at high risk of surgical morbidity and mortality (including patients of advanced age or with co-morbidities such as pulmonary or renal disease) may be evaluated for alcohol ablation. The criteria outlined in Table 55.1 may be used to select candidates. Septal wall thickness should be ≥ 18 mm, and the anatomy of the septal perforator branches should be adequate. It has been a subject of debate whether patients with gradients that are present only by provocation benefit from alcohol ablation. A report compared patients in New York Heart Association (NYHA) classes III and IV with gradients of > 30 mmHg at rest, to those whose gradient was only present after an extrasystolic beat, and found that the hemodynamic and functional benefits

Table 55.1 *Patient selection criteria for alcohol septal ablation*

- New York Heart Association (NYHA) or Canadian Cardiovascular Society (CCS) class III or IV despite drug therapy with a resting gradient of > 30 mmHg or ≥ 60 mmHg under stress[7] (a gradient of > 50 mmHg at rest and/or with exercise has also been proposed[8])
- NYHA or CCS class II with a resting gradient of > 50 mmHg or > 30 mmHg at rest and ≥ 100 mmHg under stress[9]
- Patients who are symptomatic after having to discontinue medication due to side-effects
- Previous but hemodynamically unsuccessful surgical myectomy or pacemaker therapy

were similar in both groups.[10] Little experience with alcohol ablation has been reported so far in patients with mid-ventricular obstruction, although this is technically feasible. Surgical myectomy is preferable to septal alcohol ablation in patients with concomitant cardiac conditions requiring surgery, such as extensive coronary artery disease or valvular disease, and morphologic changes of the mitral valve and papillary muscles responsible for gradient formation or mitral regurgitation.

Mechanisms of treatment efficacy

Alcohol ablation induces a well demarcated subaortic necrosis, corresponding to approximately 10% of the left ventricle by PET and SPECT imaging.[11–13] However, with the current technique and ethanol doses, the amount of necrosis is probably significantly less.

The left ventricular outflow tract (LVOT) gradient usually falls immediately after alcohol ablation, with a further fall in the gradient over the following months. Alcohol ablation results in an acute decrease in septal contraction, thus reducing subaortic narrowing in systole.[14–16] The long term relief in outflow obstruction is probably linked to LVOT remodeling with widening due to infarction necrosis and myocardial scar formation.[14,15] Furthermore, there appear to be geometric changes in the left ventricle, resulting in a more parallel angle between ejection flow and the mitral valve, with fewer drag forces leading to systolic anterior motion.[14]

In addition to relief of LVOT obstruction, changes in diastolic function also seem to improve long term hemodynamics resulting from alcohol ablation.[17–19] Outflow tract obstruction relief may increase coronary flow, thus decreasing ischemia which may participate in the patients' symptoms.[17] Lastly, reductions in the severity of mitral regurgitation may contribute to clinical improvement.[20]

The technique
Measurement of outflow gradient

Most operators use hemodynamic measurement of outflow gradient during the procedure, although some centers only measure the gradient non-invasively using echocardiography. A 5 Fr pigtail or multi-purpose catheter with side holes situated close to the tip can be used to measure pre-stenotic pressure. It is important to place the catheter close to the apex, particularly in cases with mid-ventricular hypertrophy. A J-wire may sometimes be useful for advancing the catheter further towards the apex. Attention should be paid to avoid entrapment in the myocardium, as this may exaggerate the gradient. Injecting a small volume of contrast via the catheter, and checking for proper clearance of the dye, can verify the absence of entrapment.

Many operators prefer to introduce the catheter retrogradely via a contralateral femoral arterial puncture, rather than perform transseptal puncture with a Brockenbrough catheter as described initially.[5] The post-stenotic pressure is measured through a 7 or 8 Fr guiding catheter (for example a short tip Judkins type that allows deep intubation of the vessel in case of need) placed in the ascending aorta. A 6 Fr catheter should not be used, as it causes excessive pressure damping with concomitant use of a balloon catheter required for alcohol injection later during the procedure. After having excluded a valvular gradient, the peak-to-peak intraventricular gradient should be measured at rest, during isoproterenol infusion, and after extrasystoles. Isoproterenol infusion may be particularly useful to unmask a gradient in sedated patients. Isoproterenol may be administered by diluting 200 μg in 50 ml of saline, injecting a bolus of not more than 1–3 ml and then carefully adding supplemental boluses until a heart rate of 100–120 beats per minute is reached.

A temporary pacing wire should be placed in the right ventricle to ensure back-up pacing in the advent of AV block. The pacing wire may also serve to measure the post-extrasystolic gradient by programmed stimulation (with coupling intervals of about 370 ms), if extrasystoles are not observed spontaneously. Beta-blockers should be discontinued due to the risk of block, and also in order to assess the underlying gradient.

Positioning and testing of the balloon catheter

A left coronary angiogram is performed (Figure 55.1a). Milking of the septal perforators supplying the hypertrophied segments is often observed and may be a good indicator identifying the target vessel. Positioning the guidewire in the septal branch may sometimes be difficult due to a steep take-off angle. Pre-shaping the guidewire with two angles through a needle as shown in Figure 55.2 (rather than a curve) may be of help. A floppy guidewire should be tried first, and pushed distally into the septal perforator to ensure stability. Stiffer guidewires (intermediate or, in rare cases, a standard wire) may be necessary to make the balloon follow over steep angles. In exceptional cases a 4 Fr catheter with a sharp angle (for example an internal mammary catheter) may be used as an inner catheter to pre-select septal branches with extremely steep take-offs for placing the 0.014 inch guidewire. However, extreme caution must be used in manipulating the catheter to avoid dissection. As a last resort, another balloon catheter may be briefly inflated just distally to the septal branch, and the 0.014 inch guidewire bounced off into the targeted vessel.

The targeted septal branch should be at least 1.5 mm in diameter. The shortest available balloon catheter (a 10 × 2 mm balloon is suitable for most cases) is then placed as proximally as possible in a stable position after intravenous administration of heparin. The balloon should be slightly oversized (usually 2–3 mm), and adapted to the dimension of the vessel. Standard angioplasty balloons may be used, although balloons dedicated to this procedure have been developed. In case of proximal branching of the septal perforator, a very short balloon (e.g., 5 mm, supplied for example by Schwager Medica, Winterthur, Switzerland) may be used. The guiding catheter may then have to be positioned more deeply, in order to provide more support for the balloon catheter and avoid recoil during injection. The balloon should be inflated with a pressure of 4–6 bar, and correct positioning verified by injecting contrast agent into the left coronary artery (Figure 55.1b), and then distally via the lumen of the balloon catheter using about 1 ml of contrast dye (Figure 55.1c). Absence of retrograde leakage and stability of balloon position (especially with shorter balloons) should be verified attentively. A very important point is to inject the contrast *forcefully* via the inflated balloon catheter when testing for stability. Furthermore, the extent of myocardium supplied by the septal branch and shunting of flow to non-targeted regions can also be analyzed, ideally using two different projections. The injection of contrast

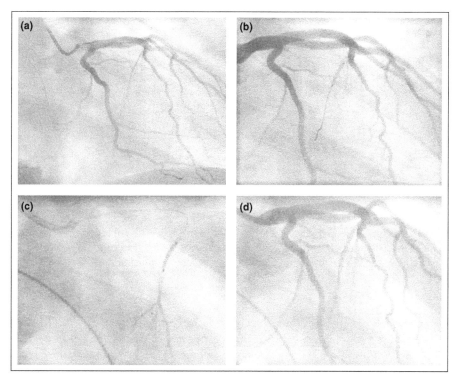

Figure 55.1
Challenging coronary anatomy for septal ablation; the target vessel resisted intubation on a previous attempt elsewhere because of the acute angle take-off just after a bend in the left anterior descending artery (LAD). This type of anatomy highlights the usefulness of the double bend of the guidewire tip (Figure 55.2). (a) Right anterior oblique 30° angiogram of the left coronary artery. (b) Balloon catheter inflated and positioned in the first septal branch over a 0.014 inch guidewire. (c) Contrast dye is injected forcefully via the balloon catheter to confirm stability and absence of retrograde leakage. (d) Angiogram after alcohol injection. Note that the first septal branch is still patent.

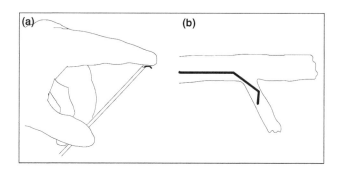

Figure 55.2
(a) Pre-shaping the 0.014 inch guidewire with two angles through a blunt needle. (b) Positioning of the guidewire in a septal branch.

agent also serves to accentuate ischemia to the territory of the septal branch. The outflow gradient should be monitored continuously to check for a drop in the resting gradient by > 30 mmHg or the post-extrasystolic gradient by > 50 mmHg within 5 minutes of balloon occlusion. If these criteria are not met (as is the case in about 20% of patients[21]), the balloon catheter may be positioned in another septal branch. Occasionally, the target vessel may originate from an intermediate or diagonal branch,[22] or from the posterior descending artery in case of a dominant right coronary artery.

Myocardial contrast echocardiography has proved to be extremely useful in targeting the desired septal branch, increasing success rates despite reduced infarct size, which in turn reduces complications.[13,22,23] Before injecting alcohol, 1–2 ml of echo contrast (for example, Sonovue®, Levovist®, Optison®, Albunex®, etc.) is injected via the inflated balloon catheter under transthoracic echography in the apical four- and five-chamber views (Figure 55.3a). This serves to ascertain whether the opacified myocardium is adjacent to the region of anterior mitral leaflet septal contact and maximal flow acceleration, and to withhold alcohol injection in case of a suboptimal irrigation pattern, such as, for example, if the right side of the interventricular septum is predominantly opacified.[24] Furthermore, this technique also helps in delineating the infarct zone and to rule out retrograde leakage or involvement of myocardium distant from the expected target region,[25] such as the ventricular free wall[13,23] or papillary muscles.[23,26] With echo contrast volumes of more than 1 ml, transcapillary passage of the contrast medium into the ventricles, more often the right than the left, is usually observed during the injection (Figure 55.3b). If echo contrast is not

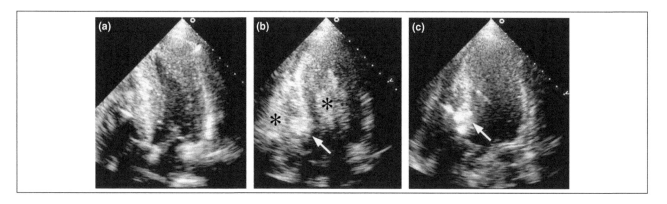

Figure 55.3
(a) Apical four-chamber echocardiogram showing the hypertrophied septum. (b) Injection of echo contrast (Levovist®) via the occluded balloon catheter positioned in the first septal perforator, with opacification of the basal septum (arrow). Note the presence of echo contrast (asterisks) within both ventricles due to transcapillary passage. (c) After alcohol injection, the area of necrosis becomes echodense (arrow).

available, echocardiography may also be performed during regular contrast dye injection in the septal perforator via the occluded balloon catheter. Contrast dye injections through the inflated balloon should not be done before echographic imaging (e.g., when testing for balloon stability), as this may opacify the myocardium and make the images difficult to interpret for subsequent injections.

Alcohol injection

Once the septal perforator is considered suitable and the balloon position stable without retrograde spilling, 0.7–3 ml of 96% alcohol may be slowly injected through the inflated balloon catheter. The volume injected will depend on the size of the vessel and the volume of the targeted myocardium. The alcohol may be either injected as a bolus, or slowly over 2 minutes. We prefer the former technique, as this may allow more efficient dissipation of the alcohol over a larger volume of myocardium (and avoid preferential streaming to a single region). However, it may be argued that slow injection may allow for longer contact of the alcohol with the myocardium (for instance by initially inducing capillary leakage which may then allow more alcohol extravasations into the interstitial tissue). The electrocardiogram should be monitored closely, and the injection aborted upon the development of atrio-ventricular block. There has been a tendency over recent years to reduce the amount of alcohol injected to a maximum of 2 ml,[11,21] which may reduce complications. The balloon should be kept inflated for at least 5 minutes (to enhance the contact of alcohol with the tissue, and to avoid reflux into the left anterior descending artery). Analgesics may be given before alcohol administration as they may reduce chest pain. Left coronary angiography should be repeated after balloon deflation in order to confirm patency of the left anterior

descending artery (Figure 55.1d). The target septal vessel may not necessarily be occluded, although flow is usually sluggish. It is not known whether this has an impact on treatment efficacy. Echocardiographically, the injection of alcohol results in a significant contrast effect, which is much stronger than currently available echo contrast agents (Figure 55.3c).

If the residual gradient after alcohol injection is > 30 mmHg at rest (after 5–10 min following the last injection of alcohol), the balloon may be positioned more proximally inside the same septal branch, or a shorter balloon used if branches of the septal perforator were occluded by the balloon inflation during the first injection. Alternatively, a second septal perforator may be targeted using the same procedure as for the first branch. Most patients will require one target perforator branch only, especially since the advent of myocardial contrast echocardiography. A residual gradient of < 30 mmHg is often acceptable, as it has been shown that a further decrease in outflow gradient due to ventricular remodeling may be observed over the following months in about 50% of patients.[23,27,28] Some operators therefore prefer a 'one vessel per session' approach, and it is still unclear whether more than a single septal perforator should be targeted initially. Occasionally, an initial increase in gradient compared to the acute result may be observed in the days following the procedure, followed by a decrease. This may be due to collateral edema caused by the infarct, which then subsides.

Post-procedural management

Vascular sheaths may be removed after normalization of coagulation parameters. We do not continue heparin at therapeutic levels after the procedure. All patients should receive aspirin (e.g. 100 mg/d) before the procedure, which is then continued for 1 month due to the risk of mural thrombosis resulting from the infarct. Creatinine kinase (CK) levels should be dosed every 4 hours in order to measure peak values. Peak rises are usually observed in the range of 750–1500 U/l. Patients should be observed in the coronary care unit for 48 hours, with removal of the temporary pacing wire at the end of this period in the absence of atrio-ventricular block. The patient may then be transferred to a telemetry unit for the remainder of the hospital stay (which is usually 1 day).

Treatment efficacy

There is growing evidence to indicate that alcohol ablation is comparable to surgical myectomy with respect to hemodynamic and functional improvement,[19,29–31] although no randomized comparative studies exist to this date. Gradient reduction can be achieved acutely in about 90% of patients.[20,22,32] In a series of 241 patients, acute reductions in mean rest gradients from 72 to 20 mmHg and mean post-extrasystolic gradients from 148 to 62 mmHg were achieved.[33]

Although very long term follow-up data are still lacking, reports indicate maintenance of clinical and hemodynamic benefits for at least a year.[20,21,32,34,35] In a series of 178 patients observed for 2–5 years,[35] gradients at baseline compared to last follow-up were 60±35 mmHg versus 7±14 mmHg ($p < 0.001$) at rest and 127±50 mmHg versus 20±28 mmHg ($p < 0.001$) with Valsalva. The outflow gradient may even decrease over time,[22,23,27,28] indicating a remodeling process. Functional class, exercise capacity, and quality of life are also significantly improved over follow-up.[20,27,32,35–37]

Repeat procedures may sometimes be required due to recurring gradients and symptoms despite initial success, as in one series proved necessary in 7 of 50 patients.[20]

Risks of the procedure

Mortality associated with the procedure is low, ranging from 0 to 4%, which is comparable to that with surgical myectomy. In the registry from the German Cardiac Society,[38] among 264 patients there was an in-hospital mortality rate of 1.2%. There are also reports of death due to stroke,[32,34] complete heart block,[32,34] dissection of the left anterior descending artery,[20] and right coronary artery thrombosis.[20] A dreaded complication is retrograde leakage of alcohol into the left anterior descending artery, which may result in a massive infarct.[37,39] However, this complication is extremely rare and avoidable, and the importance of checking for leakage before alcohol injection cannot be overemphasized.

Spontaneous ventricular fibrillation and tachycardia have been reported to occur within 48 hours of the procedure.[32,36,37]

The most frequent complication of alcohol ablation however is transient (up to 70%) or permanent (now around 10%) complete atrio-ventricular block.[22] The block is usually observed shortly after alcohol injection (but may even appear at 72 hours[40]) and is most often transient. Complete heart block may resolve within the first 12 hours of alcohol ablation, and then recur within the following week, requiring pacemaker implantation.[21] We and others[10,41] implant a pacemaker if the block persists for > 48–72 hours, although with longer observation, atrio-ventricular conduction may recover in many patients. About 1 out of 10 patients ultimately requires a pacemaker. In a recent series of 224 patients, the incidence of pacemaker implantation was 14%.[41] The German registry[38] reported implantation of a pacemaker in 9.6% of patients due to complete heart block. Baseline conduction abnormalities (especially pre-existing left bundle branch block) may increase the risk for complete heart block after ablation.[12,41,42] Other factors found to be independently predictive of pacemaker implantation are female gender, bolus injection of ethanol, and injection into more than one septal artery.[41] Use of myocardial contrast echography helps limit infarct size, and in one series reduced the need for permanent pacemaker implantation from 17 to 7%,[22] which is still higher than the reported 2% incidence with surgical myectomy.[30,43]

Right bundle branch block following the procedure may be observed in over half of the patients.[21,42,44] This is not surprising, as the right bundle is a discrete structure that is vascularized by septal branches from the left anterior coronary artery in 90% of patients, whereas the left bundle is fan-like and receives a dual blood supply from perforator branches of both the left anterior descending and posterior descending arteries. The left conduction system may nevertheless be involved, and left anterior fascicular block is reported to appear in 11% of patients.[42]

Alcohol ablation may result in loss of capture in patients implanted with a pacemaker if the ventricular lead is placed near the septum.[45] It may be prudent to increase pacing to maximal output during the first days following the procedure in these patients.

There was no evidence for the creation of an arrhythmogenic substrate by alcohol ablation as assessed by serial electrophysiologic studies before and after the procedure in a total of 78 patients in two different series,[21,32] and none of the published reports indicate an increase in incidence of ventricular arrhythmias or sudden death over follow-up.

Conclusion

Alcohol ablation is progressively replacing surgical myectomy as the first treatment of choice for drug-resistant obstructive HCM. Data indicate that procedural success is high, and comparable to that of surgery, with the advantage that it may be performed in patients in whom major surgery may be considered unsuitable. Benefits in comparison to myectomy also include shorter hospitalization, minimal pain, and avoidance of complications associated with surgery and cardiopulmonary bypass. Alcohol ablation has an important learning curve, with potentially serious complications, the most frequent of which is atrio-ventricular block requiring a pacemaker in about 10% of patients. Although these rates are declining with continuing experience and with the advent of imaging techniques such as myocardial contrast echocardiography, the procedure should only be practiced by experienced operators in appropriate centers and on carefully selected patients.

References

1. Maron BJ, Olivotto I, Spirito P et al. Epidemiology of hypertrophic cardiomyopathy-related death: revisited in a large non-referral-based patient population. Circulation 2000; 102: 858–64.
2. Maron MS, Olivotto I, Betocchi S et al. Effect of left ventricular outflow tract obstruction on clinical outcome in hypertrophic cardiomyopathy. N Engl J Med 2003; 348: 295–303.
3. Maron BJ, Bonow RO, Cannon RO 3rd et al. Hypertrophic cardiomyopathy. Interrelations of clinical manifestations, pathophysiology, and therapy (1). N Engl J Med 1987; 316: 780–9.
4. Maron BJ. Hypertrophic cardiomyopathy: a systematic review. JAMA 2002; 287: 1308–20.
5. Sigwart U. Non-surgical myocardial reduction for hypertrophic obstructive cardiomyopathy. Lancet 1995; 346: 211–14.
6. Spencer WH, III, Roberts R. Alcohol septal ablation in hypertrophic obstructive cardiomyopathy: the need for a registry. Circulation 2000; 102: 600–1.
7. Braunwald E, Seidman CE, Sigwart U. Contemporary evaluation and management of hypertrophic cardiomyopathy. Circulation 2002; 106: 1312–16.
8. Maron BJ, McKenna WJ, Danielson GK et al. American College of Cardiology/European Society of Cardiology clinical expert consensus document on hypertrophic cardiomyopathy. A report of the American College of Cardiology Foundation Task Force on Clinical Expert Consensus Documents and the European Society of Cardiology Committee for Practice Guidelines. J Am Coll Cardiol 2003; 42: 1687–713.
9. Seggewiss H. Medical therapy versus interventional therapy in hypertropic obstructive cardiomyopathy. Curr Control Trials Cardiovasc Med 2000; 1: 115–19.
10. Gietzen FH, Leuner CJ, Obergassel L et al. Role of transcoronary ablation of septal hypertrophy in patients with hypertrophic cardiomyopathy, New York Heart Association functional class III or IV, and outflow obstruction only under provocable conditions. Circulation 2002; 106: 454–9.
11. Kuhn H, Gietzen FH, Schafers M et al. Changes in the left ventricular outflow tract after transcoronary ablation of septal hypertrophy (TASH) for hypertrophic obstructive cardiomyopathy as assessed by transoesophageal echocardiography and by measuring myocardial glucose utilization and perfusion. Eur Heart J 1999; 20: 1808–17.
12. Lakkis NM, Nagueh SF, Kleiman NS et al. Echocardiography-guided ethanol septal reduction for hypertrophic obstructive cardiomyopathy. Circulation 1998; 98: 1750–5.
13. Nagueh SF, Lakkis NM, He ZX et al. Role of myocardial contrast echocardiography during nonsurgical septal reduction therapy for hypertrophic obstructive cardiomyopathy. J Am Coll Cardiol 1998; 32: 225–9.
14. Flores-Ramirez R, Lakkis NM, Middleton KJ et al. Echocardiographic insights into the mechanisms of relief of left ventricular outflow tract obstruction after nonsurgical septal reduction therapy in patients with hypertrophic obstructive cardiomyopathy. J Am Coll Cardiol 2001; 37: 208–14.
15. Henein MY, O'Sullivan CA, Ramzy IS et al. Electromechanical left ventricular behavior after nonsurgical septal reduction in patients with hypertrophic obstructive cardiomyopathy. J Am Coll Cardiol 1999; 34: 1117–22.
16. Park T-H, Lakkis NM, Middleton KJ et al. Acute effect of nonsurgical septal reduction therapy on regional left ventricular asynchrony in patients with hypertrophic obstructive cardiomyopathy. Circulation 2002; 106: 412–15.
17. Nagueh SF, Lakkis NM, Middleton KJ et al. Changes in left ventricular diastolic function 6 months after nonsurgical septal reduction therapy for hypertrophic obstructive cardiomyopathy. Circulation 1999; 99: 344–7.
18. Nagueh SF, Lakkis NM, Middleton KJ et al. Changes in left ventricular filling and left atrial function six months after nonsurgical septal reduction therapy for hypertrophic obstructive cardiomyopathy. J Am Coll Cardiol 1999; 34: 1123–8.
19. Sitges M, Shiota T, Lever HM et al. Comparison of left ventricular diastolic function in obstructive hypertrophic cardiomyopathy in patients undergoing percutaneous septal alcohol ablation versus surgical myotomy/myectomy. Am J Cardiol 2003; 91: 817–21.
20. Lakkis NM, Nagueh SF, Dunn JK et al. Nonsurgical septal reduction therapy for hypertrophic obstructive cardiomyopathy: one-year follow-up. J Am Coll Cardiol 2000; 36: 852–5.
21. Boeksteegers P, Steinbigler P, Molnar A et al. Pressure-guided nonsurgical myocardial reduction induced by small septal infarctions in hypertrophic obstructive cardiomyopathy. J Am Coll Cardiol 2001; 38: 846–53.
22. Faber L, Seggewiss H, Gleichmann U. Percutaneous transluminal septal myocardial ablation in hypertrophic obstructive cardiomyopathy: results with respect to intraprocedural myocardial contrast echocardiography. Circulation 1998; 98: 2415–21.
23. Faber L, Seggewiss H, Ziemssen P et al. Intraprocedural myocardial contrast echocardiography as a routine procedure in percutaneous transluminal septal myocardial ablation: detection of threatening myocardial necrosis distant from the septal target area. Cathet Cardiovasc Interven 1999; 47: 462–6.
24. Okayama H, Sumimoto T, Morioka N et al. Usefulness of selective myocardial contrast echocardiography in percutaneous transluminal septal myocardial ablation: a case report. Jpn Circ J 2001; 65: 842–4.
25. Faber L, Ziemssen P, Seggewiss H. Targeting percutaneous transluminal septal ablation for hypertrophic obstructive cardiomyopathy by intraprocedural echocardiographic monitoring. J Am Soc Echocardiogr 2000; 13: 1074–9.
26. Harada T, Ohtaki E, Sumiyoshi T. Papillary muscles identified by myocardial contrast echocardiography in preparation for percutaneous transluminal septal myocardial ablation. Acta Cardiol 2002; 57: 25–7.
27. Faber L, Meissner A, Ziemssen P et al. Percutaneous transluminal septal myocardial ablation for hypertrophic obstructive cardiomyopathy: long term follow up of the first series of 25 patients. Heart 2000; 83: 326–31.
28. Seggewiss H, Faber L, Meissner A et al. Improvement of acute results after percutaneous transluminal septal myocardial ablation in hypertrophic obstructive cardiomyopathy during mid-term follow-up. J Am Coll Cardiol 2000; 35: 188A.
29. Firoozi S, Elliott PM, Sharma S et al. Septal myotomy-myectomy and transcoronary septal alcohol ablation in hypertrophic obstructive cardiomyopathy. A comparison of clinical, haemodynamic and exercise outcomes. Eur Heart J 2002; 23: 1617–24.
30. Nagueh SF, Ommen SR, Lakkis NM et al. Comparison of ethanol septal reduction therapy with surgical myectomy for the treatment of

hypertrophic obstructive cardiomyopathy. J Am Coll Cardiol 2001; 38: 1701–6.

31. Qin JX, Shiota T, Lever HM et al. Outcome of patients with hypertrophic obstructive cardiomyopathy after percutaneous transluminal septal myocardial ablation and septal myectomy surgery. J Am Coll Cardiol 2001; 38: 1994–2000.

32. Gietzen FH, Leuner CJ, Raute-Kreinsen U et al. Acute and long-term results after transcoronary ablation of septal hypertrophy (TASH). Catheter interventional treatment for hypertrophic obstructive cardiomyopathy. Eur Heart J 1999; 20: 1342–54.

33. Seggewiss H, Faber L, Ziemssen P et al. Age related acute results of percutaneous septal ablation in hypertrophic obstructive cardiomyopathy. JACC 2000; 35: 188A.

34. Oomman A, Ramachandran P, Subramanyan K et al. Percutaneous transluminal septal myocardial ablation in drug-resistant hypertrophic obstructive cardiomyopathy: 18-month follow-up results. J Invas Cardiol 2001; 13: 526–30.

35. Welge D, Faber L, Werlemann B et al. Long-term outcome after percutaneous septal ablation for hypertrophic obstructive cardiomyopathy. JACC 2002; 39: 173A.

36. Kim JJ, Lee CW, Park SW et al. Improvement in exercise capacity and exercise blood pressure response after transcoronary alcohol ablation therapy of septal hypertrophy in hypertrophic cardiomyopathy. Am J Cardiol 1999; 83: 1220–3.

37. Knight C, Kurbaan AS, Seggewiss H et al. Nonsurgical septal reduction for hypertrophic obstructive cardiomyopathy: outcome in the first series of patients. Circulation 1997; 95: 2075–81.

38. Kuhn H, Seggewiss H, Gietzen FH et al. Catheter-based therapy for hypertrophic obstructive cardiomyopathy. First in-hospital outcome analysis of the German TASH Registry. Z Kardiol 2004; 93: 23–31.

39. Dimitrow PP, Dudek D, Dubeil JS. The risk of alcohol leakage into the left anterior descending coronary artery during non-surgical myocardial reduction in patients with obstructive hypertrophic cardiomyopathy. Eur Heart J 2001; 22: 437–8.

40. Kern MJ, Holmes DG, Simpson C et al. Delayed occurrence of complete heart block without warning after alcohol septal ablation for hypertrophic obstructive cardiomyopathy. Cathet Cardiovasc Interven 2002; 56: 503–7.

41. Chang SM, Nagueh SF, Spencer I et al. Complete heart block: determinants and clinical impact in patients with hypertrophic obstructive cardiomyopathy undergoing nonsurgical septal reduction therapy. J Am Coll Cardiol 2003; 42: 296–300.

42. Runquist LH, Nielsen CD, Killip D et al. Electrocardiographic findings after alcohol septal ablation therapy for obstructive hypertrophic cardiomyopathy. Am J Cardiol 2002; 90: 1020–2.

43. ten Berg JM, Suttorp MJ, Knaepen PJ et al. Hypertrophic obstructive cardiomyopathy. Initial results and long-term follow-up after Morrow septal myectomy. Circulation 1994; 90: 1781–5.

44. Kazmierczak J, Kornacewicz-Jach Z, Kisly M et al. Electrocardiographic changes after alcohol septal ablation in hypertrophic obstructive cardiomyopathy. Heart 1998; 80: 257–62.

45. Valettas N, Rho R, Beshai J et al. Alcohol septal ablation complicated by complete heart block and permanent pacemaker failure. Cathet Cardiovasc Interven 2003; 58: 189–93.

56

Hypertrophic obstructive cardiomyopathy – radiofrequency septal reduction

Joseph V De Giovanni

Pathophysiology

Hypertrophic obstructive cardiomyopathy (HOCM) is a congenital, sometimes hereditary, defect of the amino acid sequence, which can manifest itself by inappropriate hypertrophy of the myocardium, often involving the septum more than the rest of the heart to a varying degree. Histologically, the myocardial cells are abnormal with myocardial disarray and short, broad myocardial cells. Functionally, there is good systolic but impaired diastolic function due to poor myocardial relaxation. Additional hemodynamic problems include outflow tract obstruction (usually involving the left more than the right, but it could involve both sides), mitral regurgitation, and coronary artery compression due to myocardial bridging.

Symptoms

Many patients remain asymptomatic until this condition has progressed to an advanced degree, but eventually they can develop reduced exercise tolerance, chest pain, exercise-induced syncope, arrhythmias (some potentially fatal), or sudden death.

Treatment options

The condition is incurable and any treatment is directed at management of arrhythmias (anti-arrhythmic drugs, +/− pacing, +/− implantable cardiovertor defibrillator) or improvement in mechanical function to relieve symptoms (e.g., drugs such as beta-blockers, calcium channel blockers, or disopyramide, relief of right ventricular or left ventricular outflow tract by myotomy or myectomy, mitral valve replacement, or relief of myocardial bridging). Interventional procedures have been used to replace these surgical options. For instance, myocardial bridging can be overcome by placement of a coronary stent and future transcatheter techniques for mitral regurgitation may prove useful in this setting. The main advance in interventional procedures for HOCM has been to tackle the outflow tract obstruction.

Methods for relief of left ventricular outflow tract obstruction

1. Surgery: myotomy, myectomy, diathermy.
2. Interventional septal reduction:
   (a) alcohol injection in the septal branches of the left anterior descending coronary
   (b) coil embolization of septal branches
   (c) covered stent to exclude septal branches
   (d) radiofrequency directly to the ventricular septum.
3. Electrical: pacing with short AV delay.

Diagnosis and indications for treatment

Initial assessment of HOCM is carried out by echocardiographic and Doppler studies. Apart from making a diagnosis largely based on asymmetric septal hypertrophy, quantitative or semi-quantitative assessment of the left ventricular outflow gradient and mitral regurgitation can also be carried out. Obstruction within the left ventricle can be multi-level and is usually dynamic. Indications for detailed invasive evaluation and possible intervention include the presence of symptoms (e.g. shortness of breath, chest pain, dizziness or syncope on exercise) or increasing hemodynamic deterioration especially worsening outflow gradient, and mitral regurgitation. In addition, intervention is also indicated in those considered at high risk, such as those with a septal thickness of more than 2 cm, a strong family history of sudden death, or documented arrhythmias. It is unusual for symptoms to arise until the left ventricular outflow velocity is more than 4 m\s and, therefore, intervention is usually indicated when the velocity exceeds this and, more often, when it exceeds 4.5 m\s. The radiofrequency technique can be used when there is a contraindication to surgery or alcohol ablation.

History

The first and most extensively used and evaluated catheter interventional method was pioneered by Sigwart[1] and involved the selective injection of absolute alcohol into the appropriate septal branch/branches of the left coronary artery. An alternative to this is the use of radiofrequency to create lesions in the septum, which lead to muscle atrophy and hence a reduction in outflow obstruction. This latter technique, first used by De Giovanni in 1998 and presented at the Third International Workshop on Interventional Pediatric Cardiology which was held in Milan in 2001, is of particular benefit to children, whereas alcohol septal ablation is not a practical option in young patients.

The use of electrical energy to treat HOCM was first described by Armistead and Williams[2] when they recommended using diathermy to remove septal muscle that was causing obstruction during open surgery; this was suggested as an alternative to myotomy or myectomy. In 1994, Dalvi[3] proposed using radiofrequency ablation to create left bundle branch block, which was designed to create paradoxic septal motion (an effect similar to that which results from right ventricular pacing), with the expectation of gradient reduction on the left side. Our recommendation has been to apply radiofrequency energy directly to the septal bulge in the left ventricular outflow tract;[4] others have suggested applying radiofrequency to the right side of the ventricular septum and have claimed improvement in the gradient.[5] Conceptually, it is difficult to see how it could improve the left-sided obstruction as the lesions created are unlikely to be more than 6 mm and the septal thickness is usually over 2 cm. Moreover, there are no technical advantages to this over the left-sided approach.

The rest of this chapter concentrates on the technique of radiofrequency septal reduction.

Technique

Invasive assessment and radiofrequency septal reduction can be technically carried out under sedation with local anesthesia but, in children, this is usually carried out under general anesthesia as the procedure can take a long time, making it difficult for patient co-operation. It is important for the anesthetist to avoid using potent systemic vasodilators or drugs with a positive sympathomimetic action.

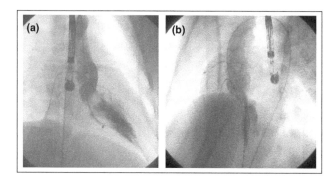

Figure 56.1
Left ventriculogram in RAO 30° (a) and LAO 60° (b) showing features of HOCM with severe outflow obstruction. Note two temporary pacing wires in the right atrium and ventricle and the TEE probe.

Cardiac catheterization is carried out with biplane fluoroscopy and facilities for intracardiac electrograms as well as disposables and a generator for delivering radiofrequency energy are crucial. These are standard equipment in institutions, where radiofrequency ablation for arrhythmias is conducted. The procedure requires several steps:

1. Transesophageal echocardiography (TEE) to obtain detailed assessment of the ventricular outflow obstruction and to correlate this with angiography. It also helps to target delivery of radiofrequency energy to the site of obstruction.
2. Hemodynamic assessment of the right and left ventricular side of the heart with specific quantitation of the right ventricular outflow and the left ventricular outflow tract gradients, usually without pharmacologic enhancement. This is accompanied by detailed biplane angiography, usually in right anterior oblique (RAO) 30° and left anterior oblique (LAO) 60° projections (Figure 56.1). Angiography will show the level, length, and the number of obstructions within the ventricle and whether this also involves the right side, although the usual and more important obstruction is often on the left side (Figure 56.2). In addition, mitral regurgitation can be assessed and selective coronary angiography is carried out to look for coronary artery compression from myocardial bridging, as this may determine whether to proceed with intervention or surgery. Although stent implantation is an option for coronary compression from myocardial bridging, this is not a recommended option in young patients, in whom surgery is preferable.[6]

Having determined the resting gradient, two temporary bipolar pacing wires are introduced through the femoral venous sheaths, which are usually 5 or 6 Fr. One of the temporary wires is placed in the right atrial appendage and one

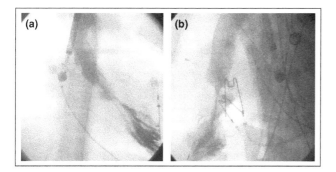

Figure 56.2
Left ventriculogram in the anterior-posterior (AP) and left anterior oblique (LAO) projections showing multiple and long segment muscular obstructions in the context of HOCM. Two surface electrode markers for the LocaLisa system are seen in (a).

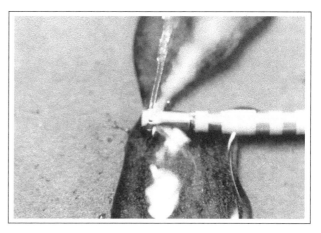

Figure 56.3
ThermoCool ablation cool tip catheter with four electrodes. The tip electrode is 4 mm and irrigation ports are seen by the production of a jet of saline.

in the apex of the right ventricle. A baseline PR interval is measured in sinus rhythm and ventricular pacing with atrial tracking is carried out, whilst measuring the gradient across the left ventricular outflow tract. The AV delay is reduced from baseline by 20 millisecond increments, whilst monitoring the change this produces to the left ventricular outflow gradient. The lowest AV delay is usually 60 ms. If the gradient is substantially reduced by altering the AV delay (arbitrarily more than 50% reduction in the gradient), this can determine how aggressively septal reduction is carried out, particularly if the muscular obstruction is in the vicinity of the HIS bundle. In other words, if the obstruction is close to the HIS bundle and there is improvement in the gradient with a short AV delay pacing, a balanced judgment would be to attempt septal reduction, even if this results in heart block which requires pacing. The temporary wire acts as a back-up should heart block occur during ablation. Radiolucent defibrillator pads are placed over the chest for remote defibrillation should this become necessary during the procedure.

If the obstruction is significant on the basis of the gradient and angiographic observations, a radiofrequency ablation catheter is introduced into the left ventricle through a femoral artery sheath, which is usually 7 Fr. Standard intracardiac electrograms can be recorded, but the alternative is to use an electro-anatomic mapping system, such as the LocaLisa navigation system. For the LocaLisa recordings, a surface reference electrode is placed on the skin of the chest and a temporary pacing lead is placed transvenously in the right ventricle; there is a specifically designed temporary screw-in lead for this purpose which can be delivered through a 5 Fr Judkins right coronary guiding catheter. An electrode plate is placed over the back, the buttock or the thigh as an earthing electrode for the radiofrequency delivery. If the LocaLisa is used, the His and the left bundle with its anterior and posterior fascicles are identified, mapped, and plotted with the radiofrequency catheter prior to

administration of energy. A note is made of the anatomic relationship between the muscular obstruction and the conducting system prior to ablation. A standard or a cool tip ablation catheter can be used. If a standard radiofrequency ablation catheter is used, a longer tip electrode, i.e. 8 mm (e.g. Celsius, Cordis), is preferable. A cool tip catheter (e.g. Thermocool by Biosense Webster or Sprinkler by Medtronic) can theoretically produce a deeper lesion of up to 6 mm compared with a 3 mm lesion using the standard ablation catheter (Figure 56.3). With cool tip catheters, fluid administration must be kept under control, especially in small children. During mapping and catheter placement, a normal saline infusion through a cool tip catheter is run at 30 ml per hour, whereas during ablation this is increased to between 300 and 600 ml per hour. It is important to reduce the flow once ablation has stopped to avoid fluid overload.

During energy application, the AV conduction is observed closely and radiofrequency application is stopped if there is evidence of heart block. The energy delivered is 60 watts and each application is for one minute, unless there are conduction problems or arrhythmias.

Radiofrequency delivery is carried out sequentially using the angiographic images of the obstruction, TEE, and electro-anatomic mapping, if this is available. Radiofrequency application is commenced distally away from the His bundle, working proximally towards the aortic valve. Prior to each application of energy, the intracardiac ECG is checked for evidence of a His bundle, signal, avoiding energy delivery if at all possible in this region. It is important to appreciate the difference between His bundle signals and one produced by a fascicle of the left bundle. Linear application of radiofrequency energy is carried out along different planes of the ventricular septum until the area of obstruction is covered, as assessed by biplane fluoroscopy,

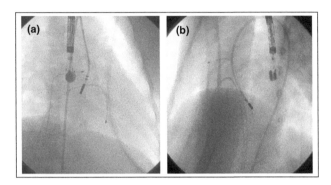

Figure 56.4
Standard 8 mm Celsius ablation catheter during radiofrequency application to the ventricular septum at the site of obstruction (a) in RAO 30° and (b) in LAO 60°. Note the direct approach to the ventricular septum with only a gentle curve.

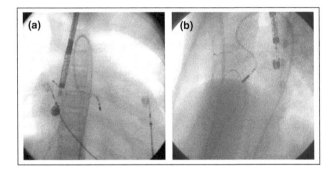

Figure 56.5
(a) Use of a Mullins sheath to adjust catheter orientation in the left ventricle combined with curvature of the catheter. (b) Celsius 8 mm standard ablation catheter in LAO. Note the more anteriorly placed tip compared with Figure 56.4a and also the more exaggerated curve at the tip.

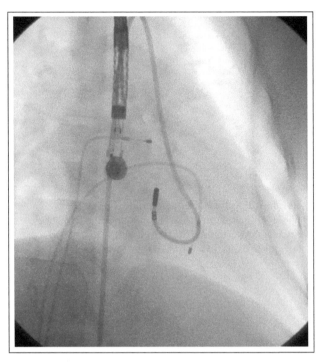

Figure 56.6
Celsius 8 mm ablation catheter curved on itself within the left ventricle and gently opened to reach the target area on the ventricular septum. This is guided by fluoroscopy and TEE.

electro-anatomic mapping, or TEE (Figure 56.4). During the application of energy, it is important to observe the impedance and temperature, bearing in mind that the temperature rise with cool tip catheters is lower than with standard catheters; this usually does not rise much above 50°C. On many occasions, the steerable ablation catheter can be directed towards the obstructing muscle simply by adjusting the curve and orientation of the catheter tip, but it is sometimes necessary to curve the catheter tip on itself within the left ventricle and then gently release the curve until it abuts against the area of interest (Figures 56.5 and 56.6). Using the LocaLisa navigation system, for anatomic mapping, helps to ensure that the treatment area covers the site of obstruction and avoids damage to the His bundle; moreover, it reduces the need for fluoroscopy (Figure 56.7). The area of muscle treated by radiofrequency becomes

more echogenic compared with the rest of the myocardium. This is a helpful observation in directing the ablation catheter towards the obstructing muscle band (Figure 56.8).

During the procedure, the patient is given heparin 100 units/kg and an activated clotting time (ACT) is checked 1–1½ hours later. We aim to keep the ACT between 250 and 300 seconds. The number of radiofrequency applications required depends on the size of the patient, the severity and the nature of the obstruction (multiple or long segment), and the appearance of echogenic changes on TEE. Usually, between 20 and 50 radiofrequency applications are required. As the radiofrequency lesions may initially lead to edema before atrophy produces regression, the gradient at the end of the procedure is meaningless; indeed, this may be higher, especially for right-sided lesions, because of the anatomy of the infundibulum. Echocardiographic assessment at the end of the procedure consists of evaluation of the septal lesions, ensuring that there is no aortic regurgitation or worsening of mitral regurgitation and excluding thrombus or pericardial effusion.

The appearance of left bundle branch block is not of concern and may indeed prove of additional benefit by encouraging paradoxic septal motion and hence an improvement in the left ventricular tract obstruction.

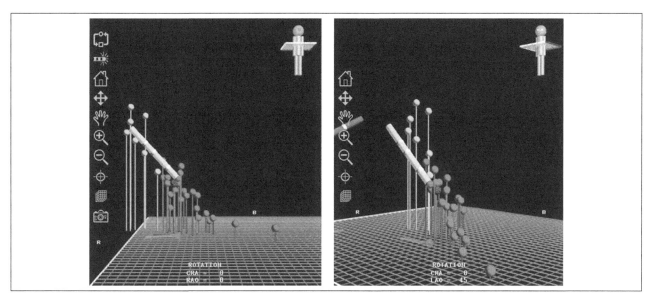

Figure 56.7
LocaLisa images with no cranial or RAO rotation in (a) but with LAO rotation of 45° in (b). The His and left bundle are shown in aquamarine and the areas where radiofrequency has been applied are shown by the red markers. The ablation catheter in aquamarine with white strips and red tip indicates the position at the time of energy application without requiring fluoroscopy. Courtesy of Professor N Sreeram. (See also color plate section.)

Post-operative observations

These include an ECG, cardiac enzymes, and an echocardiogram/Doppler; some have used three-dimensional (3D) echocardiography to assess the result following alcohol septal ablation and this could be applied to the radiofrequency technique. Aspirin in an antiplatelet dose (5 mg/kg per day) is prescribed for 6 months. If heart block results, a short course of steroids is recommended prior to considering permanent pacing.

Usually patients are kept overnight after the procedure before discharge. If radiofrequency application has been successfully delivered to the culprit area, a reduction in gradient is often seen within 2–3 days, but it may take up to 3 months for the maximum effect to be seen, until muscle atrophy occurs.

The benefits of this procedure compared with others include:

1. The technique uses a single radiofrequency catheter and standard equipment usually available in most units which carry out ablation for arrhythmias.
2. It is a more controlled tissue reduction procedure than alcohol ablation and, therefore, of particular benefit to children.
3. The procedure may be repeated if required.
4. There are minimal complications.
5. It does not preclude other forms of treatment if required.
6. It is minimally traumatic to patients.

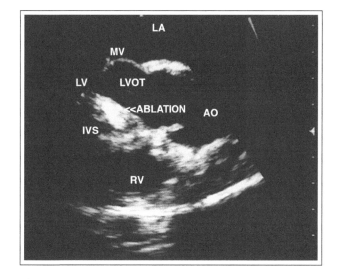

Figure 56.8
TEE long-axis view at the end of the radiofrequency procedure showing the area of ablation below the aortic valve. Note the thick ventricular septum and the increased echogenicity at the site of radiofrequency application. LA, left atrium; MV, mitral valve; IVS, interventricular septum; LVOT, left ventricular outflow tract; RV, right ventricle; AO, aorta.

7. Constant intracardiac ECG helps to reduce the risk of heart block.
8. It is cost-effective.

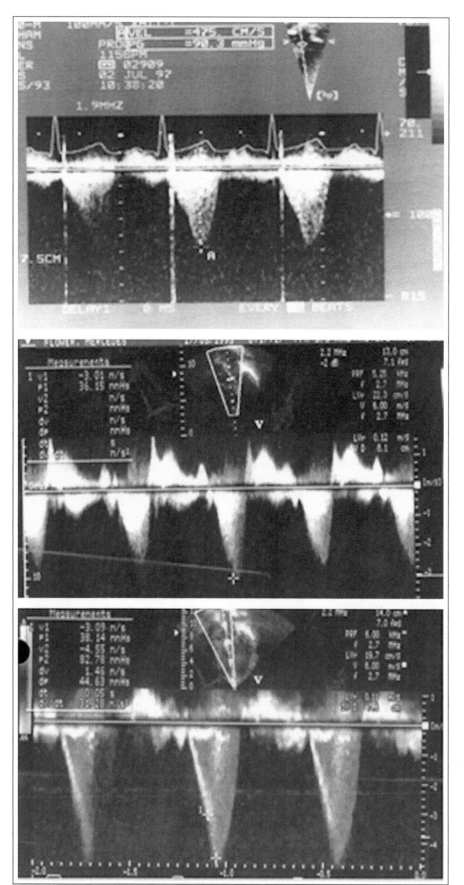

Figure 56.9
Sequential spectral Doppler of left
ventricular outflow tract. Top: in 1997,
prior to septal reduction (velocity
4.75 m/s, peak gradient 90 mmHg);
middle: in 2001, 3 years after ablation
(velocity 3.01 m/s, peak gradient
36 mmHg); and bottom: velocity of
4.55 m/s (peak gradient 83 mmHg)
7 years later.

Potential complications

Complications are uncommon but are similar to those encountered in most interventional procedures and include thromboembolic, vessel thrombosis or damage, cardiac perforation or tamponade, aortic/mitral valve damage, inadvertent entry +/– radiofrequency application within the coronary artery, heart block, and ventricular fibrillation.

Results

Since 1998, 10 procedures have been carried out on 8 patients, ranging in age from 4 to 15 years. All had left-sided septal reduction and one also had radiofrequency application to the right side of the septum because of bilateral obstruction. Two patients have required a second procedure, 1 after 5 years and another 6.5 years after the original ablation, due to gradual recurrence of the left ventricular outflow tract gradient (Figure 56.9). One patient developed transient heart block and this lasted more than 48 hours. As the patient had shown benefit with short AV pacing, it was decided to implant a permanent dual chamber pacemaker, but the heart block resolved. One patient developed two episodes of ventricular fibrillation during the procedure, one during catheter manipulation and one during application of radiofrequency energy, responding to DC shock each time. Two patients developed left bundle branch block, with no consequence other than potential enhancement of gradient relief. One patient developed a large groin hematoma, needing 2 extra days in hospital, but there was no need for active intervention.

Gradient reduction was noted in 7 out of the 8 patients. The one who showed no improvement, despite a good rise in troponin post-procedure (3.7 μg/l at the end of the procedure, reaching a peak of 11.24 after 12 hours and dropping to 6.6 after 24 hours) was referred for surgical myectomy, which is still awaited. Overall, the left ventricular outflow gradient or velocity has dropped. Cardiac enzymes rose in all patients, but were variable. This is partly due to the new nature and evolution of the technique, where initially a limited number of radiofrequency applications were carried out using a standard 4 mm tip catheter.

Role of radiofrequency

This technique is new and has been carried out in a small number of young patients, but with encouraging results. Recurrence is inevitable as the condition is progressive and this is more likely to take place in growing children. The procedure can, however, be repeated. Apart from children, adults who have a contraindication for surgery or alcohol septal ablation may also qualify, although repeated procedures may be required to remove sufficient myocardium to achieve hemodynamic or clinical improvement. Experience and better mapping have evolved the technique to a more aggressive approach with improved results. If the technique continues to show promise, less symptomatic patients may be considered for treatment on the basis of risk stratification.[7]

An extension of this technique is envisaged for muscular infundibular stenosis, such as that associated with Fallot's tetralogy, and this could form part of an interventional repair for the condition in selected patients, in whom the ventricular septal defect may be amenable to closure with a device.

References

1. Sigwart U. Non-surgical myocardial reduction for hypertrophic obstructive cardiomyopathy. Lancet 1995; 346(8969): 211–14.
2. Armistead SH, Williams BT. Hypertrophic cardiomyopathy. The use of a diathermy loop for septal resection. J Cardiovasc Surg 1984; 25(2): 185–6.
3. Dalvi B. Percutaneous radiofrequency ablation of the left bundle branch; an alternative modality of treatment for patients with hypertrophic cardiomyopathy. Med Hypoth 1994; 43(3): 141–4.
4. Emmel M, Sreeram N, De Giovanni JV, Brockmeier K. Radiofrequency catheter septal ablation for hypertrophic obstructive cardiomyopathy in childhood. Z Kardiol 2005; 94(10): 699–703.
5. Lawrenz T, Kuhn H. Endocardial radiofrequency ablation of septal hypertrophy. A new catheter-based modality of gradient reduction in hypertrophic obstructive cardiomyopathy. Z Kardiol 2004; 93(6): 493–9.
6. Downar J, Williams WG, McDonald C et al. Outcomes after 'unroofing' of a myocardial bridge in the left anterior descending coronary artery in children with hypertrophic cardiomyopathy. Pediatr Cardiol 2004; 25(4): 390–3.
7. McKenna WJ, Behr ER. Hypertrophic cardiomyopathy; management, risk stratification and prevention of sudden death. Heart 2002; 87(2): 169–76.

Section XII

Aneurysms

57

Aortic aneurysms

JP Morales and John F Reidy

Introduction

Aortic aneurysms are common degenerative conditions that affect mainly elderly people. They are three times more frequently found in men than women.[1] The overall mortality rate from aneurysm rupture is of the order of 65–85% in the abdominal aorta and even higher in the thoracic aorta.[2] Of the deaths attributed to ruptured aneurysms, about half occurred before the patient reached hospital[3] and, for those who survived the initial period, the mortality rate from emergency open surgical treatment is between 30% and 70%.[2,3]

Late aneurysm formation has been reported after surgical repair of aortic coarctation in young people, with rupture of such aneurysms being responsible for approximately 7% of all deaths. Secondary surgical repair in these patients carries a significant mortality and morbidity.[4]

Volodos et al[5] in 1988 reported the first case of endovascular treatment of a thoracic aortic aneurysm followed by Parodi et al,[6] who published the first case concerning the abdominal aorta. At that time the size and quality of devices were very limited, but now with the help of technologic advances, an increasing number of commercial devices have become available. It is estimated that since the first cases were reported, more than 25 000 patients have received an aortic stent-graft worldwide[7] and many studies have suggested that endovascular aneurysm repair offers an important new alternative to open repair of both abdominal and thoracic aneurysms, especially in older patients with significant co-morbidity.[8–11] According to the current limited experience of small series and short periods of follow-up, endoluminal repair appears to be a promising alternative to re-operations for post-surgical thoracic aneurysms associated with coarctation repair.[4,12,13]

To date, four second generation thoracic endograft devices such as Valiant (Medtronics), TX-2 (Cook), TAG (Gore), and Relay (Bolton) have mainly been used, although these manufacturers have continued to modify and improve their devices.

Symptoms

Most patients with aortic aneurysms have no symptoms attributable to the aneurysm when first diagnosed,[14] explaining why the diagnosis of aneurysm, particularly thoracic, is rarely made on physical examination. However, the only common presenting symptom is vague chest, back, flank, or abdominal pain. The pain may increase steadily as the aneurysm enlarges, or the patient may experience a sudden, sharp pain due to rapid expansion and impending rupture. Occasionally the aneurysm might compress or erode into adjacent structures, yielding diagnostic clues such as hoarseness, tracheal deviation, hemoptysis, dysphagia, hematemesis, or neurologic and musculoskeletal complaints. Superior and inferior vena cava syndrome can also occur secondary to expanding thoracic or abdominal aneurysms. Patients may present with symptoms from the abdominal aortic aneurysm. These include gastrointestinal hemorrhage from duodenal erosion, compression of the porta hepatis leading to jaundice, and a palpable pulsatile mass in the upper abdomen.[15]

Pre-procedure imaging

Endovascular aneurysm repair requires far more detailed assessment than is necessary for open surgery. This is necessary to plan the procedure and to assess length and diameter of the devices needed. Ultrasound (US) in the abdomen is used to identify aneurysms that are large enough to require treatment. Until recently computed tomography (CT) and angiography were required for the full assessment of aneurysms. CT allows the physician to measure the maximum diameter of the aneurysm and wall thickness, and to measure the diameters of the aneurysm necks and other landmarks (Figure 57.1a,b). CT allows the measurement of the diameter of the normal aorta on either side of the aneurysm, which is necessary to plan the endovascular procedure and to select an adequate size of device. More

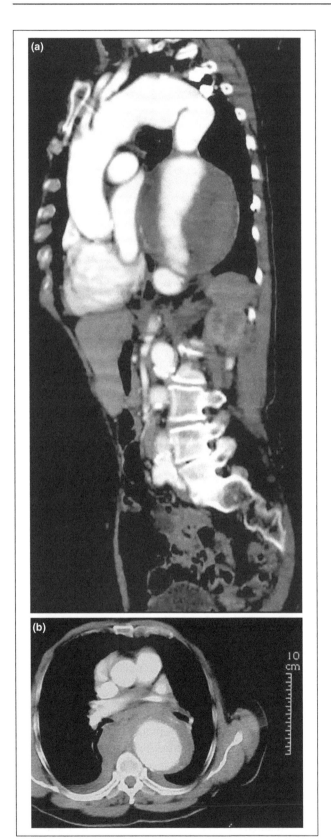

Figure 57.1
(a) Sagittal view of CT scan demonstrates a descending thoracic aortic aneurysm. (b) Axial view of CT scan demonstrates a descending thoracic aortic aneurysm with bilateral pleural effusion.

sophisticated multi-slice (MS) CT scans with three-dimensional (3D) reconstructions are extremely helpful to assess the aneurysm morphology and can accurately measure aneurysm length and dimensions, but in some cases this has not eliminated the need for an angiogram. Although MS CT scans produce excellent quality pictures, there is a concern, particularly in children, regarding the high X-ray dose, and in patients with renal pathology where contrast media is contraindicated. In these cases, magnetic resonance imaging (MRI) and magnetic resonance angiography (MRA) are used, because they do not utilize ionizing radiation and provide detailed vascular imaging without the use of iodinated contrast media. However, MRI/MRA are not currently widely used. Calibrated angiography is still used to measure aneurysm dimensions; however, with new 3D reconstruction MS CT scanners and 3D MRI/MRA, it is likely to be superseded.

Assessment

There are three areas of particular importance in endovascular stent-grafting:

Access: The currently available 24–46 mm devices can be introduced via 21–28 Fr sheaths. Diseased and tortuous iliac arteries (Figure 57.2) may prevent passage of the delivery system. Endovascular stent-grafting is contraindicated in patients with iliac artery diameter less than 8 mm, tortuosity with more than one > 90° angulation and with heavy calcification. In these cases, iliac conduit can be performed prior to the endovascular procedure.

Anchorage sites: Suitable diameters and lengths for the proximal and distal stents are normally ≥ 2 cm. It is contraindicated when the proximal neck length is less than 1.5 cm, proximal neck angulation ≥ 60°, and when a tapering neck is present.

Adequate visceral blood supply: The graft material of the stent-graft must not cover vital arteries to the intestine or kidneys.

Anesthesia

The anesthesia of choice for endovascular repair of aortic aneurysms in adults is the epidural, as it is easy to identify any neurologic and visceral complications. If the patient were to develop paraplegia, insertion of a cerebrospinal fluid (CSF) drain must be considered urgently. However, general anesthesia is the method of choice in children.

Procedure

Arterial access for the devices is usually via the right common femoral arteriotomy (CFA). Five thousand units of

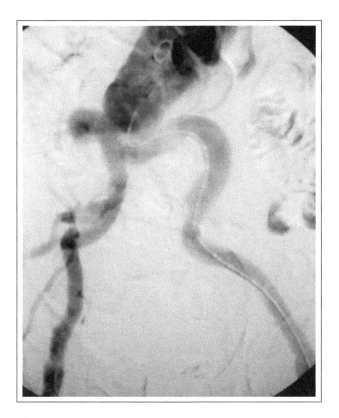

Figure 57.2
Angiography demonstrates tortuous iliac arteries.

unfractionated heparin (adult dose) and prophylactic antibiotics are given intravenously before insertion of the delivery sheath. A contralateral percutaneous femoral puncture is used for an angiographic catheter (5 Fr) as well as initial angiography to give an overview of the aneurysm. The device is inserted over an extra stiff guidewire (Lunderqvist®; Cook, Inc., Bloomington, Indiana, USA) and advanced through the aortic lumen. The device is oversized by a minimum of 10% relative to the normal aorta at the fixation sites, and deployed in the optimal position with a minimum of 2 cm of normal aorta proximal and distal to achieve a good seal. Positioning of the graft is achieved ideally under biplane fluoroscopy and digital subtraction angiography. Single plane fluoroscopy is acceptable when previous CT or MR scans have been performed to choose the right angulations. In thoracic aneurysms, the origin of the left subclavian artery is covered when necessary to achieve a good seal of the stent-graft (Figure 57.3a,b). No surgical reconstruction of the subclavian artery is routinely performed. In order to cover the origin of the left common carotid artery (LCCA) it is necessary to perform a right to left carotid–carotid bypass prior to the stenting. In infrarenal abdominal aortic aneurysms, suprarenal fixation can be used when there is a short neck. An angiogram is performed on completion of the procedure to confirm adequate placement of the stent-graft and occlusion of the aneurysm sac.

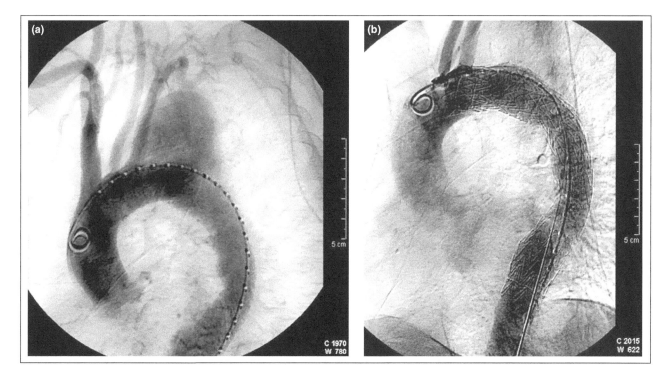

Figure 57.3
(a) Aortography demonstrates a sacular aneurysm proximal to the left subclavian artery. (b) Post-procedure aortography demonstrates successful exclusion of the aneurysm covering the left subclavian artery.

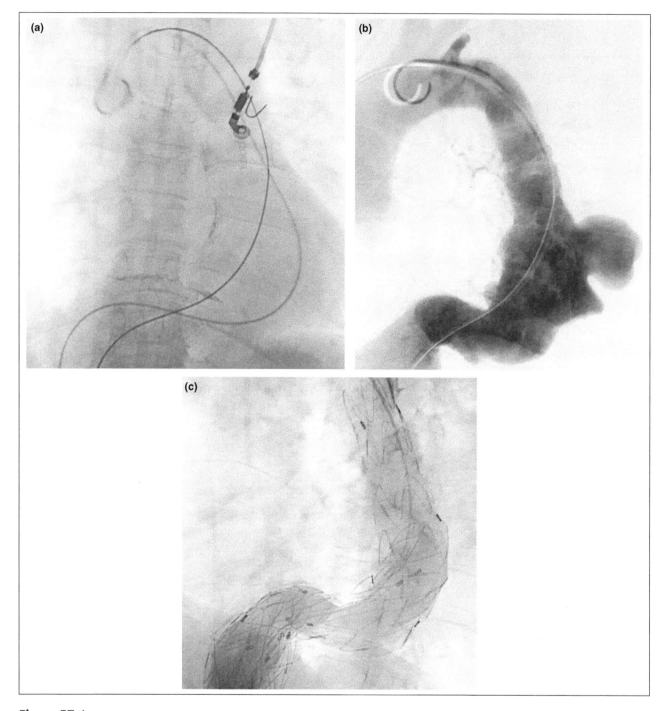

Figure 57.4
(a) Plain fluoroscopy demonstrates the pigtail catheter in the aortic arch. (b) Initial aortography performed to give an overview of the aneurysm. (c) Post-procedure aortography confirms satisfactory position and no endoleaks.

Basic steps for the endovascular procedure

1. Surgical cutdown to access CFA to allow introducer device placement.
2. A 4 or 5 Fr pigtail catheter is placed just proximal to the aneurysm from the contralateral groin (Figure 57.4a).

3. Initial angiography is performed to give an overview of the aneurysm (Figure 57.4b).
4. Insertion of the delivery system just above the proximal portion of the aneurysm.
5. Magnified angiogram to demonstrate the position of the left common carotid and left subclavian arteries (thoracic aneurysms), the position of the renal arteries

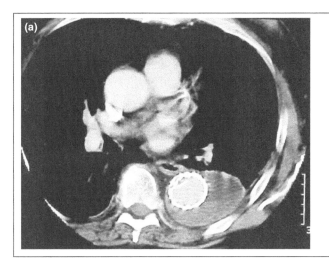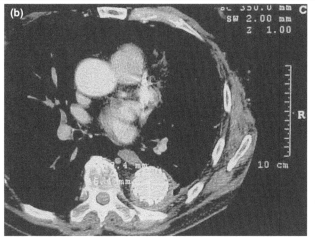

Figure 57.5
(a) Three month CT scan demonstrates stent-graft *in situ* with no endoleaks. (b) Two year CT scan demonstrates stent-graft *in situ* with no endoleaks and further aneurysm shrinkage.

(abdominal aneurysms), and location of internal iliac artery. The table is locked in position.

6. Deploy the stent-graft using continuous fluoroscopy.
7. Balloon top and bottom sides of stent, and overlapping joints where there are two or more stents.
8. Repeat angiogram to confirm satisfactory position and to check for endoleaks (Figure 57.4c).

Follow-up

As stent-grafts are a new modality treatment of aortic aneurysm, either CT or MR scans should be performed at 3 months and then yearly thereafter in order to assess aneurysm sac shrinkage (Figure 57.5a,b) as well as for detection of possible complications such as endoleaks, migration, or stent fracture.

Conclusion

We believe that with better patient selection and improvements in stent-graft design, there will be an increase in the number of aortic aneurysms suitable for endovascular repair.

References

1. MacSweeney ST, O'Meara M, Alexander C et al. High prevalence of unsuspected abdominal aortic aneurysm in patients with confirmed symptomatic peripheral or cerebral arterial disease. Br J Surg 1993; 80: 582–4.

2. Kniemeyer HW, Kessler T, Reber PU et al. Treatment of ruptured abdominal aortic aneurysm, a permanent challenge or a waste of resources? Prediction of outcome using a multi-organ-dysfunction score. Eur J Vasc Endovasc Surg 2000; 19: 190–6.

3. Wilmink TB, Quick CR, Hubbard CS, Day NE. The influence of screening on the incidence of ruptured abdominal aortic aneurysms. J Vasc Surg 1999; 30: 203–8.

4. Gawenda M, Aleksic M, Heckenkamp J et al. Endovascular repair of aneurysm after previous surgical coarctation repair. J Thorac Cardiovasc Surg 2005; 130: 1039–43.

5. Volodos NL, Karpovich IP, Shekhanin VE et al. A case of distant transfemoral endoprosthesis of the thoracic artery using a self-fixing synthetic prosthesis in traumatic aneurysm. Grudnaia Khirurgiia 1988; 6: 84–6.

6. Parodi JC, Palmaz JC, Barone HD. Transfemoral intraluminal graft implantation for abdominal aortic aneurysms. Ann Vasc Surg 1991; 5: 491–9.

7. Jacobs TS, Won J, Gravereaux EC et al. Mechanical failure of prosthetic human implants: a 10-year experience with aortic stent graft devices. J Vasc Surg 2003; 37: 16–26.

8. Biebl M, Lau LL, Hakaim AG et al. Midterm outcome of endovascular abdominal aortic aneurysm repair in octogenarians: a single institution's experience. J Vasc Surg 2004; 40: 435–42.

9. Rigberg DA, Dorafshar A, Sridhar A et al. Abdominal aortic aneursym: stent graft vs clinical pathway for direct retroperitoneal repair. Arch Surg 2004; 139: 941–6.

10. Bell RE, Taylor PR, Aukett M et al. Mid-term results for second-generation thoracic stent grafts. Br J Surg 2003; 90: 811–17.

11. Bell RE, Taylor PR, Aukett M et al. Results of urgent and emergency thoracic procedures treated by endoluminal repair. Eur J Vasc Endovasc Surg 2003; 25: 527–31.

12. von Segesser LK, Marty B, Tozzi P et al. Endovascular surgery for failed open aortic aneurysm repair. Eur J Cardiothorac Surg 2004; 26: 614–20.

13. Bell RE, Taylor PR, Aukett M et al. Endoluminal repair of aneurysms associated with coarctation. Ann Thorac Surg 2003; 75: 530–3.

14. Fann JI. Descending thoracic and thoracoabdominal aortic aneurysm. Coronary Artery Disease 2002; 13: 93–102.

15. Knaut AL, Cleveland JC. Aortic emergencies. Emerg Med Clin N Am 2003; 21: 817–45.

58

Catheter interventions in dissecting aneurysms of the aorta

Tim C Rehders, Hüseyin Ince, Stephan Kische,
Michael Petzsch, and Christoph A Nienaber

Conventional treatment of *Stanford type A* (De Bakey type I, II; Figure 58.1) dissection of the aorta consists of surgical reconstruction of the ascending aorta with complete or partial resection of the dissected aortic segment; thus in type A dissections interventional endovascular strategies have no clinical application except to relieve critical malperfusion to various organs prior to surgery of the ascending aorta by distal fenestration in cases of thoracoabdominal extension (De Bakey type I) and peripheral ischemic complications. Conversely, placement of stent-grafts aims at remodeling of the descending thoracic aorta, typically in Stanford type B (deBakey type III; Figure 58.1) by sealing one (or multiple) proximal entry tears with a Dacron-covered stent, thus initiating thrombosis of the false lumen.[1–4] In addition, reconstruction of a collapsed true lumen might result in re-establishment of flow in side branches (Figure 58.2). Various scenarios of malperfusion syndrome are amenable to endovascular management. These include static or dynamic (by invagination of the intima) collapse of the true aortic lumen (so called 'pseudo-coarctation', Figure 58.3), static or dynamic occlusion of one or more vital side branches (Figure 58.4), or enlarging false aneurysm due to patent proximal entry tear.

Although deficit of the peripheral pulses can be acutely reversed with surgical repair of the dissected thoracic aorta in approximately 90%, patients with mesenteric or renal ischemia do not fare well. Mortality of patients with associated renal ischemia is 50 to 70% and increases to as high as 87% when mesenteric ischemia is present.[5–7] Surgical mortality rates in patients with acute peripheral vascular ischemic complications are similar to those with mesenteric ischemia, approaching in-hospital mortality rates of 89%.[8–11] Operative mortality of surgical fenestration of the dissection varies from 21 to 61%. This has encouraged percutaneous interventional management by endovascular balloon fenestration of a dissecting aortic membrane to treat mesenteric ischemia, a concept discussed as a niche indication in such complicated cases of malperfusion.[10–12]

The interventional management of *Stanford type B* (De Bakey type III; Figure 58.1) dissection and the use of stent-grafts evolved slowly in anticipation of the risk of paraplegia resulting from spinal artery occlusion, which may occur in up to 18% of cases after open surgery.[11,12] With further technical improvements, a large series of cases has now been successfully treated in various specialized centers by placement of endovascular stent-grafts covering the entry tears in the descending aorta as well as in the aortic arch. Recent studies have demonstrated that closure of proximal entry tears is essential to reconstruct the aortic wall and to reduce the total aortic diameter. Closure of entry tears promotes decompression of the false lumen, formation of thrombus in the false lumen (Figure 58.5), and remodeling of the entire aorta.[2,3,12] In the near future, combined surgical and interventional procedures, even for proximal dissection, are likely to evolve.[13–15]

Current indications for fenestration and endovascular aortic repair

The exact role of percutaneous fenestration and stent-grafting in the treatment of *aortic dissection* is not fully established yet. There appears to be a role for interventional management in several aspects of the treatment. These include treatment of static or dynamic obstruction of aortic branch arteries, overcoming static obstruction of a branch by placing endovascular stents in the ostium of the compromized side branch, and treating dynamic obstruction with stents in the aortic true lumen with or without additional fenestration with a balloon or stenting of a side branch. In classic aortic dissection, successful fenestration leaves the pressure in the true lumen unchanged.[16] Sometimes bare stents deployed from the true lumen into side branches are

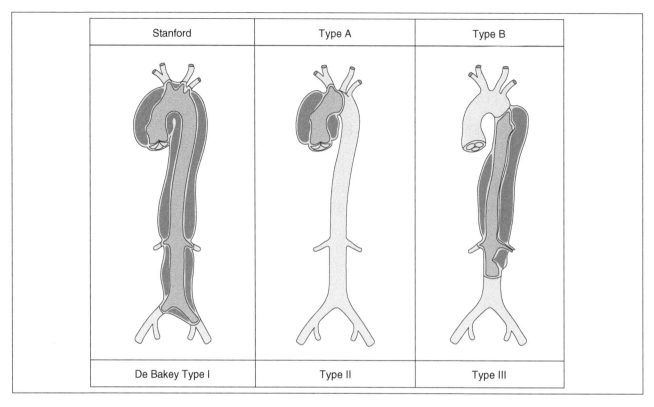

Stanford	Type A	Type B
De Bakey Type I	Type II	Type III

Figure 58.1

For aortic dissection two classification systems predominate: the DeBakey and the Stanford. Descriptive definitions:

Stanford type A: all dissections involving the ascending aorta, regardless of the site of origin

Stanford type B: all dissections *not* involving the ascending aorta

De Bakey type I: originates in the ascending aorta, propagates at least to the aortic arch and often beyond it distally

De Bakey type II: originates in and is confined to the ascending aorta

De Bakey type III: originates in the descending aorta and extends distally down the aorta or, rarely, retrograde into the aortic arch and ascending aorta.

useful to buttress the flap in a stable position.[17] In chronic dissection, in which fenestration of a fibrosed dissecting membrane may result in the collapse of the connection between the true and false lumen, a stent may be necessary to keep the fenestration open. A rare use of fenestration is to create a re-entry tear for the dead-end false lumen back into the true lumen with the aim of preventing thrombosis of the false lumen and compromise of branches fed exclusively from the false lumen or jointly from the false and true lumen. This concept, however, lacks clinical proof of its efficacy. Conversely, fenestration may increase the long-term risk of aortic rupture, because a large re-entry tear promotes flow in the false lumen and provides the basis for aneurysmal expansion of the false lumen. There is also a risk of peripheral embolism from a patent but partly thrombosed false lumen.[17,18]

The most effective method to exclude an enlarging and aneurysmally dilated false lumen is to seal the proximal entry tears with a customized stent-graft; the absence of a distal re-entry tear is desirable for optimal results but not a prerequisite. Adjunctive treatment by fenestration and/or ostial bare stents may help to establish blood flow to the compromised aortic branches. Compression of the true aortic lumen cranial to the main abdominal branches with distal malperfusion (so called pseudo-coarctation) may also be corrected by stent-grafts that enlarge the compressed true lumen and improve distal aortic blood flow.[2,3,10,12] Decompression and shrinking of the false lumen is the most beneficial result to be gained, ideally followed by complete thrombosis of the false lumen and remodeling of the entire dissected aorta (Figure 58.6), and on rare occasions, even in retrograde type A dissection.[14] As in previously accepted indications for surgical intervention in type B dissection, scenarios such as intractable pain with descending aortic dissection, rapidly expanding diameter of the false lumen, extra-aortic blood collection as a sign of imminent rupture, or distal malperfusion syndrome are accepted indications for emergency placement of stent-grafts.[15,17–19] Moreover, late onset of complications such as malperfusion of vital side branches of the aorta may justify endovascular

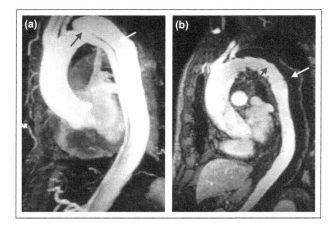

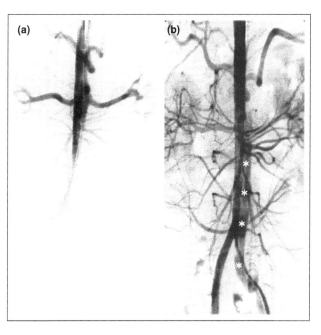

Figure 58.2
Magnetic resonance angiograms obtained before and after placement of a stent-graft. (a) Three-dimensional, maximum-intensity projection after injection of gadolinium-diethylenetriamine pentaacetic acid (DTPA). There is a dual, open-lumen type B dissection; the entry to the perfused false lumen (black arrow) is located in the distal arch directly adjacent to the left subclavian artery. The white arrow indicates the false lumen. (b) Three months after successful placement of a TALENT™ stent-graft (Dacron covered) directly onto the entry of the false lumen. The entry is completely sealed by the stent-graft and the false lumen in the thoracic and abdominal aorta is thrombosed (white arrow). The left subclavian artery is widely patent and the true lumen (black arrow) has widened as evidence of aortic remodeling.

Figure 58.3
Digital subtraction angiography in thoraco-abdominal type B dissection. (a) Dynamic obstruction of the true lumen distally to the renal arteries causing malperfusion of the mesentery and both lower extremities. (b) At follow-up (3 months after stent-graft placement in the proximal descending aorta) the true lumen has widened as a consequence of aortic remodeling and the patient is asymptomatic. However, the false lumen (white stars) in the abdominal aorta is not completely thrombosed.

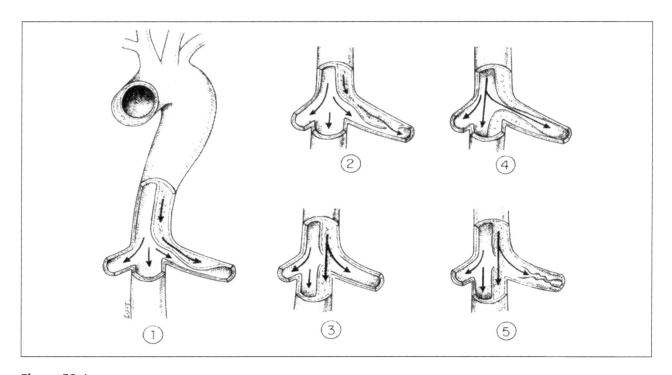

Figure 58.4
Possible variants of static or dynamic occlusion of aortic side branches in aortic dissection.

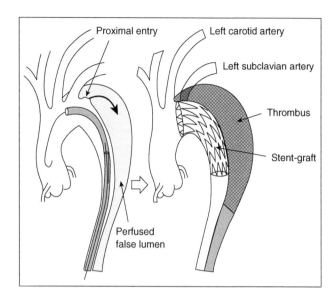

Figure 58.5
Concept of interventional reconstruction of the dissected aorta with sealing of the proximal entries, depressurization of the false lumen, and initiation of false lumen thrombosis.

stent-grafting of an occlusive lamella (or fenestration) to improve flow in the distal true lumen as a first option. Only after an unsuccessful attempt may surgery be employed, considering that surgical repair has failed to prove its superiority over interventional treatment even in uncomplicated cases; in complicated cases the concept of endoluminal treatment is currently replacing open surgery in advanced aortic centers.[1–3,17–20] A summary of treatment options is listed in Table 58.1.

Technique of aortic stent-graft placement

Aortic stent-grafts are primarily used to treat compression of the supplying true lumen cranial to major aortic branches and to increase distal blood flow. Moreover, proximal communications should be sealed to decompress the false lumen, to direct flow into the true lumen, and to induce thrombosis in the false lumen with fibrotic transformation and subsequent remodeling of the aortic wall. Placement of a stent-graft across the origin of the celiac, superior mesenteric, and renal arteries is strongly discouraged.

Based on the measurements obtained during aortic angiography, transesophageal echocardiography, computed tomography, magnetic resonance imaging, or intravascular ultrasound, customized stent-grafts (Figure 58.7) should be used in covering up to 20 cm (and sometimes even more) of the dissected aorta and the major tear(s). The procedure is best performed in the catheterization and imaging laboratory using digital angiography and under general anesthesia. The femoral artery is the commonest site of vascular access and can usually accommodate a 24 French stent-graft system.

Using the Seldinger technique a 260 cm stiff guidewire is placed through a pigtail catheter, which has been navigated with a soft wire ensuring its placement in the true lumen under both fluoroscopic and transesophageal ultrasound guidance. In complex cases with multiple re-entries in the abdominal aorta, the 'embracing-technique' with the use of two pigtail catheters is useful (Figure 58.8). A pigtail catheter which has been positioned in the true aortic lumen via the left brachial artery picks up the femoral pigtail catheter in the true lumen of the abdominal aorta and pulls it up into the aortic arch. This procedure ensures definitive correct positioning of the stiff guidewire in the true lumen, which is essential for the correct deployment of the stent-graft. By carefully advancing over the stiff guidewire the stent-graft is delivered, with the blood pressure briefly lowered to 50–60 mmHg by infusing sodium nitroprusside to prevent migration of the stent-graft.[21] After deployment, a short inflation of a latex balloon may be used to improve apposition of the stent struts to the aortic wall, but only if proximal sealing of thoracic communications is incomplete.

Both Doppler ultrasound and contrast fluoroscopy are instrumental in assessing the immediate result or in initiating adjunctive maneuvers. For thoracic aortic aneurysms or ulcers, the navigation of wires and instruments is markedly easier, but meticulous imaging using ultrasound and fluoroscopy simultaneously is equally important. A frequent anatomic consideration is the close vicinity of the origin of the left subclavian artery (LSA) and the primary tear in type B dissections. For this reason, complete covering of the ostium of the LSA has to be accepted at times to perform endovascular aortic repair in this aortic pathology and is unavoidable. According to observational evidence, prophylactic surgical maneuvers are not essential for safety reasons, but may be relegated to an elective measure after an endovascular aortic intervention when intolerable signs or symptoms of limb ischemia occur.[22] However, prior to intentional covering of the LSA, careful attention has to be paid to potential supra-aortic variants (e.g. the presence of a lusorian artery, a non-intact vertebro-basilar system, or vertebral arteries, which originate directly from the aortic arch; Figure 58.9) and pathologies during pre-interventional imaging and vascular staging.

Interventional therapy in an elective setting

With both bare stents in side branches and sometimes fenestrating maneuvers, compromised flow can be restored in more than 90% (range 92–100%) of vessels obstructed

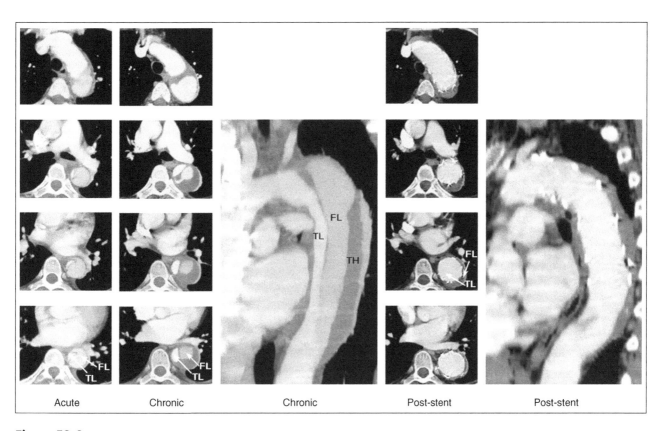

| Acute | Chronic | Chronic | Post-stent | Post-stent |

Figure 58.6

Type B aortic dissection in a 48-year-old man; note the dynamic obstruction of the true lumen (TL) in the acute phase. After stent-graft placement across the proximal thoracic entry, the entire true lumen of the thoracic aorta is reconstructed with time, with complete 'healing' of the dissected aortic wall and shrinking of the completely thrombosed false lumen (FL).TH, thrombus.

Table 58.1 *Considerations for surgical, medical, and interventional therapy in aortic pathologies*

Surgery

- Treatment of choice in acute type A dissection
- Acute type B dissection complicated by the following

  ▸ retrograde extension into the ascending aorta
  ▸ dissection in Marfan's syndrome
  ▸ rupture or impending rupture (historically classic indication)
  ▸ progression with compromise of vital organs

Medical therapy

- Treatment of choice in uncomplicated type B dissection
- Stable, isolated arch dissection
- Stable type B dissection (chronic, ≥ 2 weeks of onset)

Interventional therapy

- Stent-grafts to seal entry to false lumen of aortic dissection and to enlarge compressed true lumen

  ▸ unstable type B dissection
  ▸ malperfusion syndrome (proximal aortic stent-graft and/or distal fenestration/stenting of branch arteries)
  ▸ stable type B dissection (under study)

- Stent-grafts to exclude thoracic aortic aneurysm (≥ 5.5 cm)
- Stent-grafts to cover perforating aortic ulcers (especially deep, progressive ulcers)
- Stent-grafts to reconstruct the thoracic aorta after traumatic injury
- Stent-grafts as an emergency treatment of evolving or imminent aortic rupture

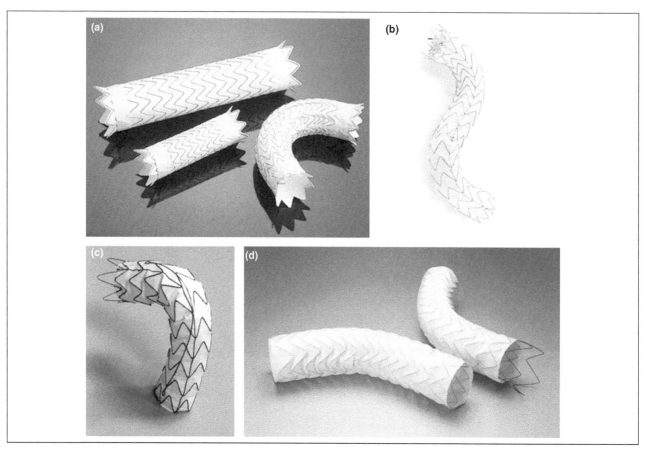

Figure 58.7
A selection of thoracic stent-grafts currently available in Europe: (a) TAG by GORE, Flagstaff, Arizona, USA; (b) Valiant by Medtronic AVE, Minneapolis, Minnesota, USA; (c) Relay Thoracic Stent-Graft by Bolton Medical Inc., Sunrise, Florida, USA; (d) EndoFit by LeMaitre Vascular, Phoenix, Arizona, USA.

from the aortic dissection. The average 30-day mortality rate is 10% (range 0–25%) and additional surgical revascularization is rarely needed.[23] Most patients remain asymptomatic over a mean follow-up time of approximately one year. Fatalities related to the interventional procedure may occur as a result of irreversible ischemic complications, progression of the dissection, or complications of additional reconstructive surgical procedures on the thoracic aorta.[1–3,17,20] Potential problems may arise from unpredictable hemodynamic alterations in the true and false lumens after fenestration and stenting of side branches. These alterations can result in loss of previously well perfused arteries, or in loss of initially salvaged side branches.

Recent reports suggest that percutaneous placement of stent-grafts in the dissected aorta is safer and produces better results than surgery for type B dissection. Paraplegia may occur after use of multiple stent-grafts, but still appears to be a rare phenomenon, especially when the stented segment does not exceed 16 cm. However, paraplegia in particular remains the most dreadful potential complication of stent-graft placement as for surgical repair of type B dissection. At

present, the exact mechanism is not completely understood; however, occlusion of numerous critical intercostal arteries (Adamkiewicz artery) by stent-grafts is commonly believed to determine an increased risk of paraplegia.[24] In particular, simultaneous abdominal and thoracic aortic repair with loss of lumbar and intercostal arteries appears to pose an increased risk of spinal cord damage caused by insufficient collateral circulation.[25] Eggebrecht and co-workers showed that the overall risk of neurologic complications with stent-grafting ranges between 2.9 and 3.4%.[26] The 1% risk of paraplegia appears to be remarkably low, considering that contemporary studies have suggested the risk of paraplegia after surgical repair of the descending thoracic aorta to be between 7 and 26%.[27] Successful treatment of stent-graft induced paralysis with cerebrospinal drainage has been previously reported.[28,29] Results of short term follow-up are excellent with a one-year survival rate of >90%; tears can be re-adapted and aortic diameters generally decrease with complete thrombosis of the false lumen. This suggests that stent placement may facilitate healing of the dissection, sometimes of the entire aorta, including abdominal segments

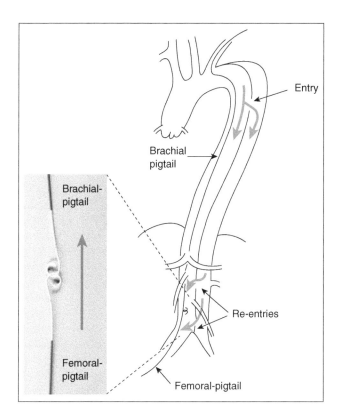

Figure 58.8
'Embracing pigtails' technique to ensure navigation of the guidewire in the true lumen before stent-graft placement.

(Figure 58.6). However, late reperfusion of the false lumen has been observed occasionally, underlining the need for stringent follow-up imaging. In some patients, follow-up imaging has revealed tears that had initially been overlooked, but required additional stents.

Interventional therapy in an emergency setting

Inclusion criteria for endovascular treatment of acute type B aortic dissection have been reported by Shimono et al.[30] In our opinion, the following criteria should apply when an emergency placement of a stent-graft is considered:

1. Identification of at least one patent primary entry tear in the descending thoracic aorta.
2. Major entry tear located in the descending aorta proximal to the 10th thoracic vertebra.
3. Absence of severe dilatation (>38 mm in diameter) and/or severe atherosclerotic alterations in the landing zone for stent-grafting.
4. Exclusion of severe aortic regurgitation.
5. Exclusion of coronary artery or aortic arch branch ischemia.

6. Femoral and iliac arteries of sufficient size and quality (absence of kinking or significant stenosis) to permit passage of at least a 22 French stent graft delivery system (vessel diameter ≥7.5 mm).

Few cases of emergency placement of stent-grafts have been described so far. We have recently reported a series of 11 patients treated by emergency endovascular aortic repair of dissection and compared these with historic-matched control patients subjected to conventional therapy. All the patients had acute type B aortic dissection complicated by loss of blood into the periaortic space. All procedures were performed successfully with no evidence of periprocedural morbidity, abolishing the leakage, and ensuring satisfactory reconstruction of the dissected aorta; at a mean follow-up of 15±6 months, no deaths were seen in the stent-graft group, whereas four patients had died with conventional treatment. Also, as previously seen in elective endovascular procedures, emergency stent-grafting of aortic dissection was not associated with excessive peripheral or neurologic complications.[18]

Nevertheless, whilst patients who suffer from post-surgery aortic dissection and who receive stent grafting seem to show better outcome than those in whom a second surgical intervention is attempted, endovascular repair in impending rupture or para-aortic leakage has not yet proved to be always effective.[30]

Conclusions

Current advances with stent-graft thoracic intervention must be viewed as exciting new developments that offer hope to many patients with type B dissection. Technical strategies and devices continue to evolve and it is likely that these techniques will soon become first-line therapy for most patients presenting with anatomically suitable thoracic and thoraco-abdominal aortic lesions.

Considering both the aging patient population in Western societies with prolonged survival despite hypertension and the better diagnostic strategies available to more patients, the cardiovascular community faces an increasing incidence of acute and chronic aortic problems such as dissection, aneurysm, intramural hematoma, ulcerations, and traumatic lesions that desperately need to be stratified using both early biomarkers of a dissecting process and functional imaging of the aortic wall. At this pivotal point in time, an elevated level of awareness in clinical cardiology and the availability of modern imaging technology should trigger the interest in diagnosing and treating the complex of acute aortic syndromes similar to previous efforts in acute coronary syndromes. Cardiologists should improve diagnostic pathways and vascular staging in acute and chronic aortic diseases, form regional referral networks and allocation systems, and utilize uniform follow-up programs. Moreover, precise

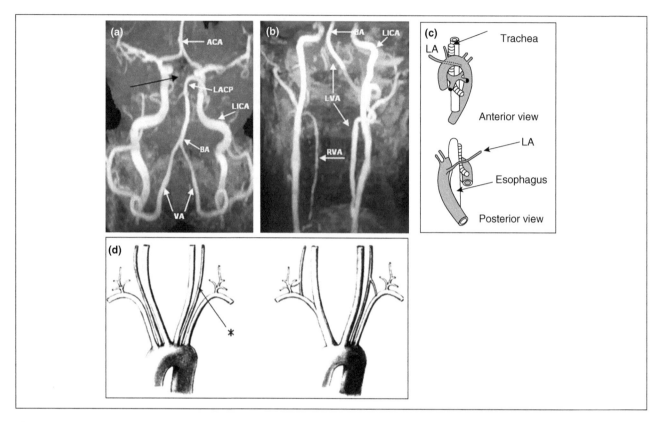

Figure 58.9

(a) Three-dimensional reconstruction of contrast-enhanced MRA in a patient with a regular vertebral-basilar system but incomplete circle of Willis. The right arteria cerebri posterior is probably aplastic (black arrow), since the left arteria cerebri posterior (LACP) has almost the same caliber as the basilar artery (BA). Nevertheless, in this patient intentional LSA occlusion during stent-graft implantation was performed since MRA documented an intact vertebral-basilar system. (b) The arterial anatomy in a patient with an incomplete vertebral-basilar system. The proximal segment of the right vertebral artery (RVA) is hypoplastic compared to the left vertebral artery (LVA). In addition the right vertebral artery does not join the basilar artery. In this case primary bypass surgery would be urgently necessary before stent-induced occlusion of the left subclavian artery. (c) The pattern of a lusorian artery. The aberrant right subclavian artery (LA) originates distally to the left subclavian artery and usually runs dorsal to the esophagus. (d) Variants of vertebral arteries originating directly from the aortic arch. The left diagram shows the variant without a connection (*) to the left subclavian artery. ACA, arteria cerebri anterior; LICA, left internal carotid artery; VA, vertebral arteries.

definitions of pathology using clear semantics should be integrated into prospective registries of aortic diseases by a multi-disciplinary team of physicians in an attempt to validate previous retrospective observations and to make the best use of evolving diagnostic and endovascular treatment strategies. Finally, cardiologists are in need of credible prognostic models that can support decisions for individual patient care independent of investigators, at different times, and in worldwide locations.

Acknowledgment

We are indebted to Mrs Knoop and Mrs Heine for their professional support in preparing the manuscript and the artwork.

References

1. Ince H, Nienaber CA. The concept of interventional therapy in acute aortic syndrome. J Card Surg 2002; 17: 135–42.
2. Nienaber CA, Fattori R, Lund G et al. Nonsurgical reconstruction of thoracic aortic dissection by stent-graft placement. N Engl J Med 1999; 340: 1539–45.
3. Dake MD, Kato N, Mitchell RS et al. Endovascular stent-graft placement for the treatment of acute aortic dissection. N Engl J Med 1999; 340: 1546–52.
4. Walkers PJ, Miller DC. Aneurysmal and ischemic complications of type B (type III) aortic dissections. Semin Vasc Surg 1992; 5: 198–214.
5. Bossone E, Rampoldi V, Nienaber CA et al. Usefulness of pulse deficit to predict in-hospital complications and mortality in patients with acute type A aortic dissection. Am J Cardiol 2002; 89: 851–5.
6. Cambria RP, Brewster DC, Gertler J et al. Vascular complications associated with spontaneous aortic dissection. J Vasc Surg 1988; 7: 199–209.

7. Laas J, Heinemann M, Schaefers HJ et al. Management of thoracoabdominal malperfusion in aortic dissection. Circulation 1991; 84: 20–4.

8. Miller DC. The continuing dilemma concerning medical versus surgical management of patients with acute type B dissections. Semin Thorac Cardiovasc Surg 1993; 5: 33–46.

9. Miller DC, Mitchell RS, Oyer PE et al. Independent determinants of operative mortality for patients with aortic dissections. Circulation 1984; 70: 153–164.

10. Elefteriades JA, Hartleroad J, Gusberg RJ et al. Long-term experience with descending aortic dissection: the complication-specific approach. Ann Thorac Surg 1992; 53: 11–20.

11. Walker PJ, Dake MD, Mitchell RS et al. The use of endovascular techniques for the treatment of complications of aortic dissection. J Vasc Surg 1993; 18: 1042–51.

12. Fann JI, Sarris GE, Mitchell RS et al. Treatment of patients with aortic dissection presenting with peripheral vascular complications. Ann Surg 1990; 212: 705–13.

13. Yano H, Ishimaru S, Kawaguchi S et al. Endovascular stent-grafting of the descending thoracic aorta after arch repair in acute type A dissection. Ann Thorac Surg 2002; 73: 288–91.

14. Kato N, Shimono T, Hirano T et al. Transluminal placement of endovascular stent-grafts for the treatment of type A aortic dissection with an entry tear in the descending thoracic aorta. J Vasc Surg 2001; 34: 1023–8.

15. Iannelli G, Piscione F, Di Tommaso L et al. Thoracic aortic emergencies: impact of endovascular surgery. Ann Thorac Surg 2004; 77: 591–6.

16. Saito S, Arai H, Kim K et al. Percutaneous fenestration of dissecting intima with a transseptal needle. A new therapeutic technique for visceral ischemia complicating acute aortic dissection. Cathet Cardiovasc Diagn 1992; 26: 130–5.

17. Nienaber CA, Ince H, Petzsch M et al. Endovascular treatment of thoracic aortic dissection and its variants. Acta Chir Belg 2002; 102: 292–8.

18. Nienaber CA, Ince H, Weber F et al. Emergency stent-graft placement in thoracic aortic dissection and evolving rupture. J Card Surg 2003; 18: 464–70.

19. Beregi JP, Haulon S, Otal P et al. Endovascular treatment of acute complications associated with aortic dissection: midterm results from a multicenter study. J Endovasc Ther 2003; 10: 486–93.

20. Bortone AS, Schena S, D'Agostino D et al. Immediate versus delayed endovascular treatment of post-traumatic aortic pseudoaneurysms and type B dissections: retrospective analysis and premises to the upcoming European trial. Circulation 2002; 106: 234–40.

21. v Knobelsdorff G, Hoppner RM, Tonner PH et al. Induced arterial hypotension for interventional thoracic aortic stent-graft placement: impact on intracranial haemodynamics and cognitive function. Eur J Anaesthesiol 2003; 20: 134–40.

22. Rehders TC, Petzsch M, Ince H et al. Intentional occlusion of the left subclavian artery during endovascular stent-graft implantation in the thoracic aorta: risk and relevance. J Endovasc Ther 2004; 11: 659–66.

23. Slonim SM, Nyman U, Semba CP et al. Aortic dissection: percutaneous management of ischemic complications with endovascular stents and balloon fenestration. J Vasc Surg 1996; 23: 241–51.

24. Fattori R, Napoli G, Lovato L et al. Descending thoracic aortic diseases: stent-graft repair. Radiology 2003; 229: 176–83.

25. Mitchell RS, Miller DC, Dake MD et al. Thoracic aortic aneurysm repair with an endovascular stent-graft: the 'first' generation. Ann Thorac Surg 1999; 67: 1971–4.

26. Eggebrecht H, Nienaber CA, Neuhauser M et al. Endovascular stent-graft placement in aortic dissection: a meta-analysis. Eur Heart J 2006; 27: 489–98.

27. Umana JP, Miller DC, Mitchell RS. What is the best treatment for patients with acute type B aortic dissections – medical, surgical, or endovascular stent-grafting? Ann Thorac Surg 2002; 74: S1840–3.

28. Tiesenhausen K, Amann W, Koch G et al. Cerebrospinal fluid drainage to reverse paraplegia after endovascular thoracic aortic aneurysm repair. J Endovasc Ther 2000; 7: 132–5.

29. Ortiz-Gomez JR, Gonzalez-Solis FJ, Fernandez-Alonso L et al. Reversal of acute paraplegia with cerebrospinal fluid drainage after endovascular thoracic aortic aneurysm repair. Anesthesiology 2001; 95: 1288–9.

30. Shimono T, Kato N, Yasuda F et al. Transluminal stent-graft placement for the treatments of acute onset and chronic aortic dissections. Circulation 2002; 106: 241–7.

Section XIII

Hybrid procedures

59

A hybrid strategy for the initial management of hypoplastic left heart syndrome: technical considerations

Mark Galantowicz and John P Cheatham

Introduction

A collaborative interaction between pediatric cardiothoracic surgeons and interventional cardiologists, coupled with new technology, has enabled the development of new hybrid treatment strategies for patients with congenital heart disease. The goal of hybrid therapies is to reduce the accumulated insults of necessary interventions over the lifetime of a child with complex congenital heart disease, thereby improving their quantity and quality of life. The short and long term outcomes for children with hypoplastic left heart syndrome (HLHS) using traditional staged open heart procedures remain suboptimal. Further improvement using these traditional strategies may not be possible given the nature of the disease, the physiology established, and the accumulated insults. A recent report from the Congenital Heart Surgeon's Society, from 1994 to 2000 involving 29 institutions, demonstrated only a 54% survival after 5 years using conventional palliative techniques for HLHS.[1] In addition, only 28% of patients underwent Fontan completion with another 20% as potential candidates. This report again identifies the period around the Stage 1 Norwood operation as the greatest risk for mortality and morbidity.

Our hybrid strategy for the initial management of HLHS involves an innovative combination of surgical and transcatheter techniques creating a stable physiology to palliate the neonate until a comprehensive procedure can be performed at 6 months of age. This new hybrid palliation controls pulmonary blood flow, provides reliable systemic cardiac output through the PDA, and creates unobstructed flow from the left atrium all performed without cardiopulmonary bypass. We review the technical aspects of this hybrid procedure from a surgeon's and an interventional cardiologist's perspective. Emphasis is placed on highlighting the lessons learned from our experience,[2] so that the significant learning curve may be shortened or avoided by other teams embarking on this hybrid approach.

Pre-operative management

The goal of the pre-operative management of newborns with HLHS is to balance the systemic, pulmonary, and coronary circulations. There are many strategies to accomplish this goal. Our typical patient is supported with prostaglandin to maintain a patent ductus arteriosus (PDA), is extubated on room air, receives oral digoxin and lasix, and is beginning enteral feeding. If they manifest pulmonary overcirculation, a nitrogen hood is placed over the head to create a subambient inspired oxygen content. During this period of time an echocardiogram is performed to establish the anatomy, to assure an unrestrictive atrial septum, and to rule out retrograde, transverse aortic arch stenosis. A general neonatal survey is performed including a head and abdominal ultrasound. Parental counseling of the nature of HLHS and treatment options is ongoing.

Contraindications to a Hybrid Stage 1 procedure

All forms of hypoplastic left heart syndrome, including aortic atresia/mitral atresia, have been successfully palliated with a hybrid approach. However, there was one death secondary to an unusual anatomic variant which we now consider a contraindication to the Hybrid Stage 1 procedure. This child had an undetected, congenital stenosis of the retrograde orifice of the transverse arch which was established at autopsy (Figure 59.1). When the PDA stent was deployed it created critical occlusion of retrograde flow into the transverse arch, thereby creating fatal coronary and cerebral ischemia leading to death within hours. Typically, children with HLHS, even aortic atresia/mitral atresia with a diminutive ascending aorta, have an adequate size transverse aortic arch that opens even further at the ductal connection.

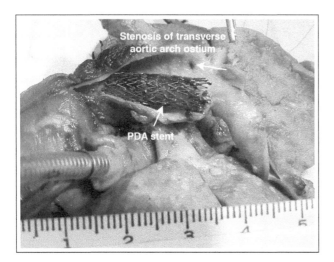

Figure 59.1
This autopsy photograph illustrates the congenital, critical stenosis of the transverse aortic arch. (Reproduced from Hill, Galantowicz and Cheatham[3])

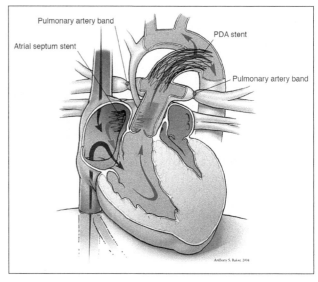

Figure 59.2
The Hybrid Stage I palliation. Note pulmonary artery (PA) bands on the left and right PAs, proximal to the upper lobe branches. Stents span the length of the PDA and atrial septum (if necessary). (Reproduced from Hill, Galantowicz and Cheatham[3]) (See also color plate section.)

This area of connection can be imaged effectively with echocardiography. If there is a small retrograde orifice, or signs of flow acceleration consistent with stenosis, the child is at risk of the stent distorting this orifice, further creating critical or fatal limitation to retrograde perfusion of the heart or brain. We have detected this type of stenosis in two subsequent patients who went on to have a successful, traditional Norwood Stage 1 procedure. Currently we have no other contraindications to a hybrid approach including patient size or degree of prematurity.

Hybrid Stage 1: evolution of a novel technique

The evolution of the new initial palliation for HLHS has occurred over the past 4 and a half years with modifications based on clinical experiences and outcomes. The goals of the initial palliation include (1) unobstructed systemic output through the PDA, (2) balanced pulmonary and systemic blood flows, and (3) an unobstructed atrial septal defect (Figure 59.2) This is currently accomplished by placing bilateral pulmonary artery bands and a PDA stent via a median sternotomy as one hybrid procedure in a specially designed Hybrid Suite (Figure 59.3), followed by a balloon atrial septostomy several days later prior to discharge. However, this procedure was and can be performed in a traditional operating room or cath lab as sequential procedures or combined in either venue. If a combined hybrid approach is desired in the operating room a portable, digital C-arm in the lateral position can give adequate angiographic guidance for the PDA stent deployment or in the cath lab the

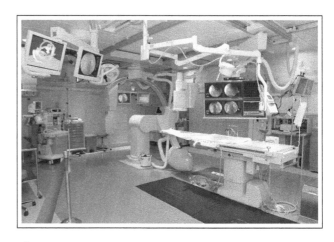

Figure 59.3
A photograph of the specially designed Hybrid Suite at the Heart Center, Columbus Children's Hospital.

surgeon needs to adapt to the limitations of a cath lab bed for patient positioning and visualization.

Several lessons learned during this experience have led to our current approach. First, placing the bands before the stent is important. The PDA stent does not change the patient's hemodynamics or add any stability over an open PDA secondary to prostaglandin. However, adequately placed branch pulmonary artery bands will improve the hemodynamics by balancing the circulation, improving systemic perfusion which helps stabilize the patient for any subsequent procedures. Moreover, with the PDA stent in place the left pulmonary artery is harder to isolate for banding and the stent is at greater risk for distortion or perforation while trying to get around the left pulmonary artery.

Second, any transcatheter wire course through the HLHS heart can lead to hemodynamic compromise secondary to acute tricuspid and pulmonary valve insufficiency from wire distortion. This can lead to end organ damage or rarely valve damage. Therefore we now avoid any wire course through the heart by placing a sheath directly into the main pulmonary artery above the pulmonary valve, through which the PDA stent can be deployed without crossing any valves.

Finally, creating an unrestrictive, durable atrial septal communication in the HLHS heart is more difficult than a standard balloon septostomy for other anomalies. This has to do with the size and location of the defect, the size of the left atrium, and the stability of the patient. We have varied the timing of the procedure, utilized other techniques including static balloon dilatation with and without cutting balloons, and have even placed atrial septal stents. No technique yielded a reliable, reproducible result until our current approach.

Hybrid Stage 1: current technique

The typical neonate comes to the hybrid suite extubated, on prostaglandin as the only intravenous medication. The goal of the anesthetic management is to extubate the child at the end of the procedure. Appropriate venous and arterial access is established. The surgical team starts with a median sternotomy and creation of a pericardial well to expose the heart. From a standard 3.5 mm Gore-Tex (WL Gore & Associates, Flagstaff, AZ, USA) tube graft an approximately 1 mm wide ring is cut to serve as the pulmonary artery band material. The ring is opened and passed around the right and left pulmonary artery (RPA and LPA). On the right exposure is straightforward and the band is positioned on the RPA between the ascending aorta and superior vena cava proximal to the right upper pulmonary artery take-off. Exposure on the left is much more difficult. It is easier to visualize and maneuver a clamp around the LPA with the surgeon standing on the patient's left side. Stay stitches pull the main PA–PDA junction rightward, exposing the take-off of the left pulmonary artery. A small gauze can help push the left atrial appendage out of its usual position on top of the LPA. Using sharp dissection the veil of tissue between the LPA and PDA is cleared, allowing a right angle clamp to be passed around the origin of the LPA to position the band. The bands are then tightened by reclosing the band with a 5-0 horizontal mattress suture. An additional stitch is placed through the band and tacked to the local adventitia to resist band migration. The tightness of the band is an

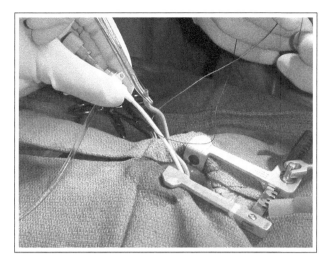

Figure 59.4
This photograph demonstrates the sheath and dilator being secured in the pulmonary artery with a snare in order to facilitate atraumatic delivery of the PDA stent through a limited, median sternotomy, off cardiopulmonary bypass.

intraoperative decision based on the child's size, pulmonary artery size, systemic blood pressure and saturation response to tightening. However, experience has shown that bands closed to approximately 3.3 mm (slightly smaller than the original diameter of the shunt) will adequately balance the circulations and protect the pulmonary bed, while not becoming too tight with resultant cyanosis as the child grows to around 5.5 kg at 6 months of age when the Comprehensive Stage 2 procedure is performed.

After the bands are placed, a 6 Fr introducer and sheath with side-arm is pre-shaped to simulate the course of the PDA and descending aorta. A silk suture is placed around the distal sheath approximately 2 mm from the tip to serve as an external marker for the surgeon as to how far to insert the sheath. This is important in order to avoid the sheath being inserted too far into the pulmonary artery, hindering deployment of the stent to cover the entire length of the PDA. The introducer is then pulled back into the sheath exposing approximately 5 mm beyond the tip of the sheath. A pursestring in the main pulmonary artery just above the sinotubular junction is placed and the sheath and dilator advanced through a small incision. After the sheath is advanced to the external suture, the dilator is removed and the snare tightened (Figure 59.4). The side-arm of the sheath is then flushed to clear any remaining air or blood.

Next, the surgeon stabilizes the sheath by holding gentle finger pressure around the distal end while moving forward toward the patient's head. The lateral fluoroscopic camera is then moved into place for angiography and PDA stent placement (Figure 59.5). A V-18 Control Wire (Boston Scientific Corp., Miami, FL) is pre-shaped and passed through the sheath, into the PDA, and down the descending aorta. A

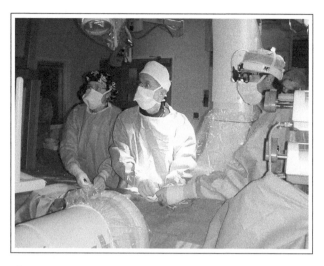

Figure 59.5
The Hybrid team is seen here preparing to deliver the PDA stent in the Hybrid Suite. The surgeon has moved around the lateral camera to hold the sheath in place, while the interventional cardiology team places a guidewire through the sheath, into the PDA, and down the aorta. An angiogram will be performed through the side-arm of the sheath to demonstrate the PDA anatomy.

small hand injection of contrast through the side-arm of the sheath nicely defines the PDA, left pulmonary artery, descending aorta, and retrograde aortic flow. The PDA length and diameter are measured at the distal, middle, and proximal ends, and the appropriate stent is chosen. We prefer to perform the angiogram after the guidewire is in position,

simulating any distortion that will be present during stent delivery.

In our early experience, there were very few appropriate size pre-mounted stents available in the United States. Therefore, we used self-expandable biliary stents which were available in diameters from 6 to 10 mm, but in lengths of only 20 mm, 30 mm, etc. We chose 20 mm long stents from 7 to 9 mm in diameter, attempting to cover the entire length of the PDA from the junction with the LPA to the aorta distal to the left subclavian artery, where the typical coarctation shelf was located. This necessitated extending the bare stent across the orifice of the transverse aortic arch in most patients, which allows retrograde flow to the coronary arteries. The self-expandable nitinol stents used were the Smart® or Precise® (Johnson and Johnson, Cordis Division, Miami, FL), Protégé™ GPS™ (eV3 Inc., St Paul, MN), or the Zilver® 518 (Cook, Inc., Bloomington, IL). All have slightly different delivery systems and characteristics, but the deployment required a slow, controlled pulling of the outer catheter to allow the nitinol stent to self-expand (Figure 59.6). Unfortunately, there were three technical problems:

1. The stents tended to 'jump' out of the delivery catheter due to the relative short length. In addition, there was little ability to control or reposition the stent during deployment, although the Protégé™ delivery system did allow the partially deployed stent to be pulled back before final deployment.
2. The position of the delivery sheath would sometimes interfere with the stent opening at the PDA–LPA junction.
3. The action of pulling back on the outer catheter tended to drag the delivery sheath with it, forcing the surgeon

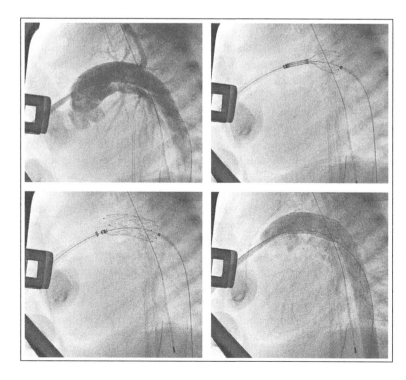

Figure 59.6
In this series of angiograms performed through the side-arm of the sheath using the lateral camera, the PDA is nicely demonstrated, along with the banded LPA, as well as the retrograde aortic flow. The Protégé™ self-expandable stent is deployed by slowly pulling the outer catheter back, allowing the nitinol stent to expand. A follow-up angiogram demonstrates the stent to be completely covering the entire PDA.

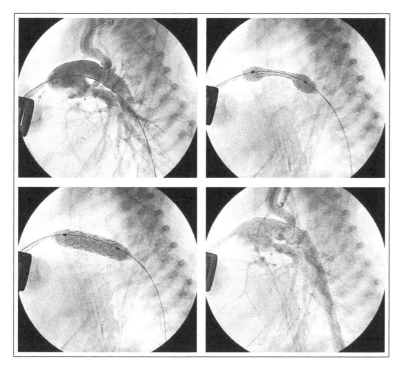

Figure 59.7
The balloon-expandable, pre-mounted Genesis stent is shown here being deployed to cover the entire PDA. Note the stent crossing the origin of the aortic arch with retrograde flow filling the atretic ascending aorta and coronary arteries.

to counteract this force by pushing forward on the sheath in order to avoid dislodgement of the sheath, making the precise deployment more difficult.

After the pre-mounted Palmaz® Genesis stents (Johnson & Johnson, Cordis Division, Miami, FL) became available in the United States, we began to use this balloon-expandable stainless steel stent with lengths of 12, 15, 18, and 24 mm and diameters from 4 to 8 mm. We found these stents easier and more familiar to deploy, with more precise placement and a greater choice of stent lengths (Figure 59.7). In addition, the surgeon did not have to exert force on the delivery sheath. However, either the self-expandable or balloon-expandable stents may be used successfully and should be left to the interventionalist's discretion.

After the stent is deployed, the delivery catheter or balloon is removed and a final angiogram is performed. Although we now typically also remove the guidewire before the angiogram is performed, it can be left in place until enough experience is gained by the Hybrid team. If necessary, a second stent can be deployed coaxially to cover the entire PDA. However, we have found this to be relatively uncommon (< 10%) with increasing experience and the variable stent lengths now available. In newborns > 2.5 kg, a 24 mm long stent premounted on an 8 mm Slalom balloon was used in over 90% of our patients. The smallest diameter of deployed stent was 7 mm and the largest 9 mm.

Once the stent position is confirmed to completely cover the ductus the sheath is removed and the pursestring tied. After hemostasis is assured the pericardium, sternum, and skin are closed. Typically there is no need for inotropic support, the prostaglandin is stopped, and the child is extubated prior to transport to the cardiac intensive care unit.

A baseline echocardiogram is performed on the first post-operative day. Observation for 24–48 hours in the Cardiac ICU is typical, during which time oral feeding is started as well as digoxin, lasix, and aspirin therapy. Once reliable caloric intake is established and the child is a day or two away from being discharged home they return to the cath lab for a balloon atrial septostomy.

While it is tempting to perform transcatheter creation of a larger ASD at the time of the hybrid procedure, there are several caveats. Some surgeons will choose to perform PA banding in the conventional operating room, followed by PDA stent placement in the cath lab. Performing balloon atrial septostomy at the same time seems like a natural choice. However, creation of an adequate ASD that will last long enough until the Comprehensive Stage 2 repair is performed can be problematic. The left atrium in the newborn with HLHS is extremely small. The latex Miller–Edwards balloon atrial septostomy catheter and the 2 ml (13.5 mm) NuMED balloon atrial septostomy catheter (NuMED, Inc., Hopkinton, NY) will not 'fit' in the small left atrium. Therefore, as a compromise, the 1 ml (9.5 mm) NuMED catheter was used. However, the ASD typically becomes too restrictive within 2–3 months and creates a scenario of either repeat balloon atrial septostomy or early Comprehensive Stage 2 repair. We also attempted static balloon atrial septoplasty with and without Cutting Balloon™ (Boston Scientific Corp., Murrieta, CA) septoplasty as an alternative in these newborns. However, an ASD large enough to last until 6 months was rare. Therefore, we changed to our current

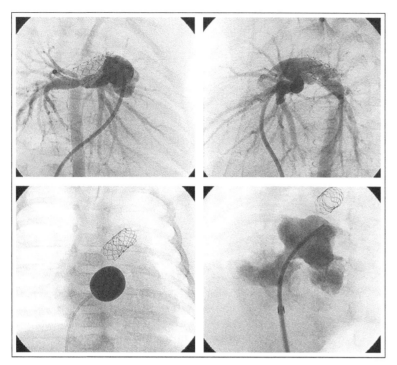

Figure 59.8
The day prior to discharge, the neonate returns to the Hybrid Suite for a short hemodynamic study, angiography, and balloon atrial septostomy. The right pulmonary artery band is best shown in the RAO projection, while the left pulmonary artery band and PDA stent are seen in the LAO view. A 2 ml (13.5 mm) NuMED balloon atrial septostomy catheter is used to create an ASD that will remain unrestrictive until the comprehensive Stage II repair at 6 months.

protocol and elected to defer balloon atrial septostomy until the day before the patient was to be discharged or after discharge when the mean Doppler gradient was > 5–8 mmHg. At this time, the 2 ml NuMED balloon atrial septostomy can be used (Figure 59.8). The left atrium is large enough to accommodate the 2 ml (13.5 mm) balloon at this time. In our experience, this creates an unrestrictive ASD that lasts until the Comprehensive Stage 2 repair can be performed at 6 months in over 90% of patients. Usually the atrial tissue around the defect is thin enough to allow safe and successful creation of an adequate ASD. This anatomic characteristic should be remembered when considering stent therapy.

While it is tempting to stent all patients with HLHS to ensure unrestricted atrial flow for a length of time until Comprehensive Stage 2 repair is performed, there are reasons to be cautious. Typically, and as mentioned earlier, the atrial septum is thin adjacent to the fossa ovalis defect, while the septum inferiorly near the atrioventricular valves is quite thick. The secure placement of a stent relies on the adjacent thickness of the septum, as well as the length of stent able to be used. Stent embolization is more likely in this scenario with the thin septum primum being pushed downward during balloon expansion of the stent, only to recoil with deflation and guidewire removal, thus 'pushing' the stent from the LA to the RA. Therefore, our prejudice is to only implant stents in the atrial septum when there is a severely restrictive ASD or intact atrial septum as a newborn. This is an urgent or emergent situation that must be addressed shortly after birth and before the PA bands or PDA stent is placed. We prefer to perform this procedure in the Hybrid Suite using transvenous access from the right femoral vein and echo guidance during radiofrequency perforation of the septum

using the Nykanen catheter (Baylis Medical Company, Montreal, Canada). This is much easier and safer than attempting transseptal puncture in these critically ill newborns with a small 'flat' left atrium. A premounted Genesis Palmaz Stent is then delivered over the 0.018 inch guidewire and expanded. Typically a 12 mm long stent pre-mounted on an 8 mm balloon is used (Figure 59.9). We have also used a Cutting Balloon™ after successful RF perforation followed by static balloon septoplasty, but now feel stent therapy is the best choice (Figure 59.10). Regardless, be cautious of stenting the atrial septum as a 'routine' procedure and reserve it for specific indications. After the child is discharged home close interstage monitoring is critical.

Interstage monitoring

Close interstage monitoring has been the key to minimizing interstage mortality, as well as perioperative complications at the Comprehensive Stage 2 procedure. After discharge home, the infants are followed closely with a minimum of every other week cardiology assessment. Echocardiography is used liberally to monitor for obstruction through the PDA stent, retrograde into the transverse aortic arch, at the atrial septum or decreased right ventricular function or increased tricuspid regurgitation as another indicator of obstruction. Any evidence of obstruction or decreased ventricular function leads to a catheterization to diagnose and treat the level of obstruction. In addition we routinely perform a surveillance cardiac catheterization at 6–8 weeks post-Hybrid Stage 1. A commitment to aggressive re-intervention in the cath lab to relieve obstruction, whether emergently or at the time

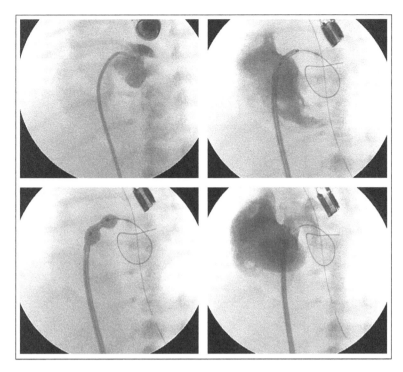

Figure 59.9
A 12 mm long pre-mounted Genesis stent on an 8 mm diameter Slalom balloon is delivered through a 6 Fr long sheath over a 0.018 inch guidewire. TEE is used to help guide placement of the interatrial stent. Follow-up angiography demonstrates a widely patent ASD and small decompressed LA.

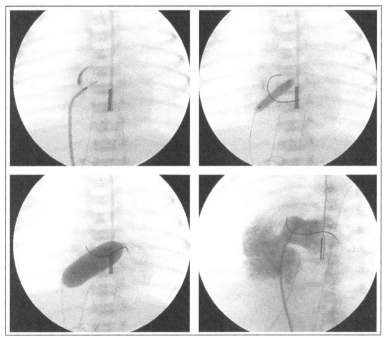

Figure 59.10
Radiofrequency perforation of the intact atrial septum using the Nykanen RF catheter with an intracardiac echocardiography (ICE) probe placed transesophageal is shown here. A 4 mm diameter Cutting Balloon is expanded, followed by a 10 mm static balloon septoplasty, resulting in a moderate ASD.

of the surveillance catheterization, is necessary. Given the volume load on the heart after the initial palliation, any increased afterload leads to the rapid development of right ventricular dysfunction with or without tricuspid regurgitation. Early detection and treatment of obstruction of flow through the PDA stent related to coarctation to antegrade or retrograde aortic flow is mandatory. Restriction of the atrial septum may manifest as tachypnea and/or cyanosis. Maintaining ventricular function has been the key to survival through the Comprehensive Stage 2 procedure. The patients

are scheduled for their Comprehensive Stage 2 surgery at 6 months of age.

Comprehensive Stage 2

This is a formidable operation. Despite the magnitude, the resultant circulation in series rather than in parallel, outside of the neonatal period has been well tolerated. Unexpected benefits of the new initial hybrid palliation have been the growth of the native pulmonary arteries and the transverse aortic arch. Because the transverse arch/innominate artery junction has grown, the aortic cannula can be positioned into the innominate artery during arch reconstruction, thereby removing the need for circulatory arrest with its associated risks. Moreover, much of the procedure can be done with the heart beating on bypass without aortic cross-clamping, thereby minimizing the period of cardiac ischemia.

The open heart surgery consists of removal of the PDA stent and PA bands, repair of the aortic arch and pulmonary arteries (if necessary), division of the diminutive ascending aorta with re-implantation into the pulmonary root, main PA to reconstructed aorta anastomosis, atrial septectomy with removal of the atrial stent (if present), and a modified cavopulmonary anastomosis (Figure 59.11). All of these steps are familiar to a pediatric cardiothoracic surgeon with single ventricle experience, except for the removal of the PDA stent. This is the most intimidating aspect of the procedure because of the delicate nature of removing the distal part of the stent that continues into the descending thoracic aorta. Moreover, injury of the aorta at this level has very few reasonable bail-out options. Therefore widespread acceptance of the Hybrid Stage 1 procedure will be dependent on surgeons' comfort with the Comprehensive Stage 2 procedure. Hopefully, with future stent development specifically designed for this procedure, stent removal or better yet absorbable stents will make this significant technical hurdle obsolete for surgeons.

Conclusion

The goal of the Hybrid Stage 1 approach for the initial management of HLHS is to effectively palliate patients through the neonatal period with minimal morbidity and mortality, preserving ventricular function, while allowing normal growth and development, especially of the pulmonary vascular bed. Thus the patient is prepared for a comprehensive open heart procedure that yields a circulation in series rather than parallel, with expected improved hemodynamic stability resulting in reduced morbidity and mortality. This hybrid approach combining surgical and transcatheter techniques can achieve acceptable short term outcomes in patients with HLHS. Long term studies will be necessary. We are now beginning an Institutional Review Board (IRB) approved, prospective trial of this novel hybrid strategy to determine its usefulness which can lead to a multi-institutional trial. Continued collaboration between cardiothoracic surgeons, interventional cardiologists, and industry is necessary to further develop innovative hybrid management strategies for HLHS as well as other congenital heart anomalies.

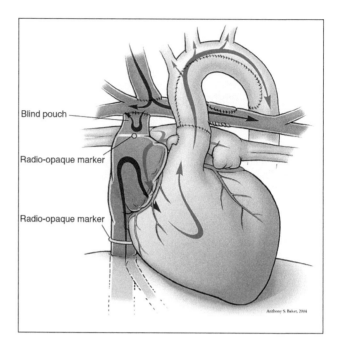

Figure 59.11
Illustration of the anatomy after the Comprehensive Stage 2 procedure. (See also color plate section.)

References

1. Ashburn DA, McCrindle BW, Tchervenkov CI et al. Outcomes after the Norwood operation in neonates with critical aortic stenosis or aortic valve atresia. J Thorac Cardiovasc Surgery 2003; 125(5): 1070–82.
2. Galantowicz M, Cheatham JP. Lessons learned from the development of a new hybrid strategy for the management of hypoplastic left heart syndrome. Pediatr Cardiol 2005; 26: 190–9.

Further reading and additional sources

1. Akinturek H, Michael-Behnke I, Valeske K et al. Stenting of the arterial duct and banding of the pulmonary arteries. Basis for combined Norwood stage 1 and 2 repair in hypoplastic left heart. Circulation 2002; 105: 1099–103.
2. Gibbs JL, Wren C, Watterson KG et al. Stenting of the arterial duct combined with banding of the pulmonary arteries and atrial septectomy or septostomy: a new approach to palliation for the hypoplastic left heart syndrome. Br Heart J 1993; 69: 551–5.
3. Hill SL, Galantowicz M, Cheatham JP. Emerging strategies in the treatment of HLHS: combined transcatheter & surgical techniques. Pediatr Cardiol Today 2003; 1(3): 1–5.
4. Hill SL, Mizelle K, Vellucci SM et al. Radiofrequency perforation and cutting balloon septoplasty of intact atrial septum in a newborn with hypoplastic left heart syndrome using transesophageal ICE probe guidance. Cathet Cardiovasc Interven 2005; 64: 214–17.

60

Alternative procedures for hypoplastic left heart syndrome as a bridge to transplantation

Ryan R Davies, Mark M Boucek, and Jonathan M Chen

Introduction

Hypoplastic left heart syndrome (HLHS) is a lethal congenital malformation of the left ventricle, aorta, and associated valves that occurs at a rate of approximately 0.23 per 1000 live births or 1500 cases per year in the United States.[1,2] Prior to 1980, HLHS was uniformly fatal, with most infants dying within one month of birth. Following the pioneering efforts of Norwood and Bailey, two treatment options are now available: staged reconstruction and cardiac transplantation.[3]

Although Norwood's procedure represented an important advance in the management of infants with HLHS, initial survival was poor, ranging only from 9% to 47% in early series.[4–6] Such results led Bailey and colleagues to advocate cardiac allotransplantation as primary therapy for infants with HLHS. However, neonatal transplantation for HLHS requires life-long immunosuppression and is associated with a waiting list mortality of 20–25% owing to a distinct shortage of donors of appropriate size. Improvements in pre-transplant survival are thus necessary before cardiac transplantation can be an epidemiologically viable therapeutic alternative for all newborns with HLHS.

Staged reconstruction: the Norwood principle

The concept of the Norwood procedure is predicated upon many of the same principles that underlie catheter-based procedures for the palliation of HLHS. The essential components of the Norwood procedure are: (1) unobstructed pulmonary venous return, (2) unobstructed systemic blood flow from the single ventricle to the systemic circulation, (3) adequate pulmonary blood flow without volume overload, and (4) unobstructed mixing at the atrial level.[7] Most commonly, this is accomplished through construction of a neo-aorta consisting of pulmonary artery and aortic tissue, closure of the patent ductus arteriosus, atrial septectomy, and creation of a modified Blalock–Taussig shunt (or Sano right ventricular to pulmonary artery (RV–PA) connection) to provide regulated pulmonary blood flow.

Stage II is performed between 4 and 6 months of age; it consists of a hemi-Fontan or bidirectional Glenn procedure, and involves removal of the systemic (or RV) pulmonary shunt and creation of a cavopulmonary shunt.[8] The Fontan procedure, which completely separates the pulmonary and systemic circulations, is typically performed between 18 months and 3 years of age.[9] Transplantation may be performed at (or between) any of these stages, often with outcomes comparable to patients transplanted for primary cardiomyopathy. However, those transplanted after a failed 'high risk' Glenn or Fontan procedure have impaired outcomes when compared with those undergoing interval transplantation in lieu of staged succession.

Outcomes

In the 25 years since the introduction of the Norwood procedure, significant changes in both surgical technique and perioperative management have resulted in improved survival to Fontan completion. However, operative mortality remains high, and is primarily related to the stage I repair.[10] Data from the early 1990s described a 1-year survival of only 36–42% in patients undergoing staged repair of HLHS. Continued improvement in techniques and experience has resulted in significant improvements over time, but overall 1-year survival remains only 70 to 85% in even the best series.[11–15]

Because HLHS includes a range of anatomic defects, from mitral or aortic stenosis through complete atresia of one or both valves with variable atrial septal anatomy, attempts at improving outcomes with staged reconstruction have focused on improved patient selection and perioperative management based on pre-operative anatomic and physiologic factors predictive of poor outcomes following repair. Such research has identified several factors that increase the risk to children undergoing the Norwood procedure. Patients with larger ascending aortic arch diameter have improved survival.[11,14,16–18] Older patients tend to have significantly

Table 60.1 *Predictors of poor outcome following stage I Norwood reconstruction*

- Low operative weight[15,18,19] or low birth weight[10]
- Atresia of one or both of the left ventricular valves[10,11]
- Pre-operative ventricular dysfunction[24]
- Moderate or severe tricuspid regurgitation[17,21]
- High pre-operative creatinine[10]
- Pre-operative acidosis[11,18]
- Highly restrictive atrial septal defect[22] or need for pre-operative septostomy[10]
- Severe pulmonary venous obstruction[23]
- Significant non-cardiac congenital conditions[23]

higher mortality rates, especially those aged > 1 month at the time of operative repair.[15,19] Patients with increased PVR are particularly prone to lethal pulmonary vascular crises.[20]

A variety of other risk factors have been identified for poor outcomes following stage I reconstruction (Table 60.1).[10,11,15,17–19,21–24] However, despite this extensive list of risk factors, an analysis of the causes of death following stage I found that most (77%) were related to largely correctable surgical technical problems associated with perfusion of the lungs, myocardium, and systemic organs,[21] thus explaining the improved survival in the most recent series. Long term survival should improve dramatically as the higher short term survival following stage I in contemporary series is translated into intermediate and long term improvements after subsequent stages.[15,25]

Cardiac transplantation for HLHS

Following the first report of cardiac transplantation in HLHS by Bailey and colleagues in 1986, transplantation has become the preferred method of surgical treatment at some institutions.[26] It offers several obvious advantages over staged reconstruction, most notably a single, definitive operative repair with return to normal circulatory physiology. The transplant procedure is performed in a fashion similar to transplants into patients with normal physiology, although the donor aorta is used to reconstruct the ascending aorta and aortic arch under deep hypothermic circulatory arrest.[27,28]

Both short and long term outcomes following transplantation have been excellent. Early post-operative survival approaches 90% in some series,[11,29] and long term survival in those surviving the first 2 years of life is excellent.[29] The main limitation, therefore, to the use of transplantation in all infants with HLHS has been the relative shortage of donor organs. In addition to an increased risk of death on the waiting list, longer waiting times result in a higher risk of removal from the list for organ failure and may result

in impaired long term survival following transplantation.[10,30–32] Furthermore, if an infant waits on the transplant list without receiving an organ and ultimately requires surgical palliation, survival following the Norwood procedure is likely to be compromised.[16,19,30]

Mechanical devices as a bridge-to-transplantation have been used extensively in adult patients and have lately been extended to select groups of pediatric patients with heart failure. Until recently, device size limited the use of ventricular assist devices to adolescents, precluding their use in the neonatal and infant population. In addition, congenital physiology may limit the application of either ventricular support or extracorporeal membrane oxygenation (ECMO). In general, patients with single-ventricle physiology have poor outcomes with ECMO support, where delivering an adequate mechanically supported systemic cardiac output without causing pulmonary volume overload makes the use of ECMO or ventricular assist devices particularly challenging.[33] Thus, although only limited data are available, prospects for an effective mechanical bridge-to-transplant technique in this population are poor.

Catheter-based interventions in HLHS

The high mortality associated with waiting for donor organ availability, as well as the surgical mortality that continues to be associated with stage I reconstruction, demonstrates that there is significant room for improvement in the early management of infants with HLHS. Several catheter-based techniques have been proposed, both as measures to increase survival prior to transplantation and – more recently – as alternatives to stage I palliation (covered in Chapter 59). Advances in interventional techniques and in pre-natal diagnostic methods have also enabled the treatment of some of the anatomic defects associated with HLHS *in utero*.

Fetal interventions
Balloon atrial septostomy

Surgical reconstruction with the Norwood procedure (and ultimately the hemi-Fontan and Fontan procedures) requires low pulmonary vascular resistance in order to enable adequate pulmonary blood flow and normal systemic pressures.[3,14,34,35] Similarly, the risk of cardiac transplantation has been directly associated with reversibility and/or a lower baseline pulmonary vascular resistance. The presence of a restrictive atrial communication in infants with HLHS results in higher left atrial pressures, which, when transmitted to the pulmonary vascular bed, may lead to pulmonary venous hypertension *in utero*.[22,36] While some infants may benefit from early postnatal atrial septostomy[37] or open atrial septectomy, the resultant pulmonary vascular changes may be only partially reversible.[22,36] In addition, balloon atrial septostomy can be technically difficult in these patients, owing to the posterior deviation of the interatrial septum and its thick integrity. Moreover, staged open septectomy with subsequent Norwood procedure (or transplantation) naturally also carries an increased risk of morbidity and mortality.

Accordingly, some investigators have proposed enlargement of the foramen ovale *in utero* in patients with HLHS who have an apparent restrictive atrial communication.[38] Marshall and colleagues recently published a report of seven fetuses with prenatally diagnosed HLHS demonstrating the feasibility of *in utero* atrial septostomy.[38] Their technique draws both on experience with neonatal atrial septostomy as well as fetal valvuloplasty and cardiocentesis. In this procedure, an introducer is advanced through the maternal abdominal wall and the uterus, then through the fetal chest wall and ultimately into the right atrium. A needle is then passed through the atrial septum and an angioplasty balloon advanced and used to perform the septostomy.

In Marshall's series, the procedure was technically successful in 6 of 7 fetuses, however one of the 6 died within 4 hours due to procedural complications (right hemothorax, small hemopericardium), potentially related to the use of a larger introducer in this patient to enable creation of a larger atrial septal defect (ASD). The size of the ASD remains one of the primary drawbacks of the technique, as an ASD of > 2 mm could only be created in 4 of the fetuses. Only two patients remained alive and well following Norwood stage I. Obviously, significant work remains both in surpassing the technologic hurdles and in demonstrating survival advantages to this technique; however, the poor outcome in patients with restrictive ASDs, with either cardiac transplantation or surgical reconstruction,[37,39] argues in favor of continued attempts to mitigate the pulmonary vascular damage occurring prior to birth.[36]

Aortic valvuloplasty

HLHS consists of a wide range of anatomic defects from complete mitral and aortic atresia without an appreciable left ventricular (LV) cavity, to those with severe aortic stenosis and a diminutive LV. Those in the latter category may in fact have had a morphologically normal LV outflow tract early in gestation, but with reduced flow consequently evolved either poor LV development or a hypoplastic outflow tract and aortic arch.[40,41] Some have suggested that the ability to identify patients with critical pre-natal aortic stenosis and perform valvuloplasty *in utero* might allow for more normal left ventricular growth with the potential to allow a post-natal two-ventricle repair with its attendant improved survival.[17,36,41] Naturally, an incomplete result with this technique still

allows for subsequent procedures. However, the creation of significant valvar insufficiency could render the staged procedure unlikely to succeed and thus render transplantation the only remaining option post-natally.

To date, several case reports have been published describing the use of pre-natal aortic valvuloplasty.[42–44] The results of these studies, comprising a total of 12 human fetal patients, were analyzed in 2000 by Kohl and colleagues.[45] As with atrial septostomy described above, fetal cardiac access is obtained via insertion of a needle through the maternal abdominal wall and uterus and then into the fetal chest and the hypoplastic ventricle. Coronary artery balloons are used to perform the valvuloplasty. Of the 12 patients, 3 required emergency C-sections for either sustained bradycardia or chorioamnionitis. Four fetuses (25%) died within 24 hours of the procedure either from bleeding, sustained bradycardia, or in one case at open operative valvotomy following emergency delivery. Only one patient with a technically successful valvuloplasty survived long term.[45] Despite the need for multiple subsequent valvuloplasties in the post-natal period, by 4 years of age, this patient had near normal cardiac contractility and ejection fraction.[42] Further advances in the equipment, techniques, and, most importantly, in patient selection are necessary before the wider adoption of pre-natal intervention to treat critical aortic stenosis. Furthermore, fetoscopic or open procedures may have higher success rates than ultrasound-guided direct cardiac punctures.[45] However, the anecdotal results in this patient population combined with the growing understanding of flow-dependent cardiac chamber growth *in utero* suggests that prenatal intervention could potentially have a role in the treatment of patients along the spectrum of HLHS.

Neonatal interventions

Pre-operative preparation of patients with HLHS for either surgical palliation or for transplantation requires optimization of the balance between systemic and pulmonary circulations, maintenance of ductal patency, adequate restriction of pulmonary blood flow, and creation of unobstructed atrial mixing. Several non-interventional therapies have been used to achieve this goal: maintenance of ductal patency via prostaglandin-E1 (PGE1) infusion as well as adjustment of the ratio of systemic to pulmonary vascular resistances using inspired hypoxic air, nitrogen, carbon dioxide, or the use of inotropes and vasodilators.[46–48] Although these treatments may be successful, in some patients, pharmacologic and inhalational techniques may not provide adequate resuscitation. Accordingly, several investigators have developed mechanical techniques for improving systemic blood flow and limiting pulmonary flow, including balloon atrial septostomy (described previously), mechanical stenting of the ductus arteriosus and pulmonary artery banding.

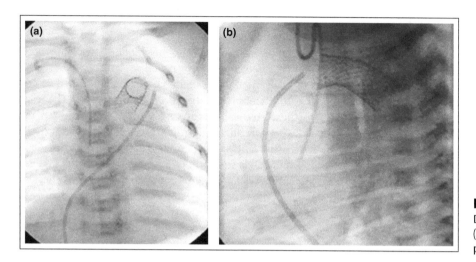

Figure 60.1
Ductal stent deployed in
(a) postero-anterior and (b) lateral
projections.

Stenting of the ductus arteriosus

Successful stenting as a palliative procedure in anticipation of transplantation was first reported by Ruiz and colleagues at Loma Linda in 1993.[49] Four of the five infants reported in the series were successfully bridged to transplantation. Access was first obtained with a 6 Fr sheath through which a 5 Fr Berman catheter was introduced and advanced through the main pulmonary artery into the ductus. A 7 Fr sheath was then introduced and a 2.5 mm by 2 cm pre-mounted Palmaz–Schatz balloon-expandable stent placed. The sheath was retracted, the balloon (5 Fr Medi-Tech PE-MT balloon) inflated, and the stent deployed. In this technique, the authors note that particular care must be taken to prevent protrusion of the device into either the pulmonary artery or isthmus of the descending aorta, and while stent migration is unlikely, it did occur in the one patient who died. Additionally, balloon inflation naturally compromises cardiac output during stent expansion. Later studies by Gibbs and colleagues in the UK were less favorable, owing partially to progressive endothelialization of the stent and procedural morbidities.[50]

Subsequent technologic advances have allowed for the use of self-expanding nitinol stents, which may be delivered through smaller sheaths (5 or 6 Fr) and whose delivery does not impair cardiac output (Figure 60.1). A more recent review of the 4-year experience at Denver Children's Hospital demonstrated 40 patients to have been successfully stented.[51] The mean age of the patients was 1.6 ± 1.2 months, with a mean weight of 3.8 ± 0.9 kg (the smallest weighing 2.1 kg). Stent deployment was performed with sedation and under fluoroscopic guidance. A 4 Fr Berman catheter was placed and the ductal size and diameter measured using biplane angiography. The lateral projection was the most useful during positioning of the stent delivery sheath. Biplane imaging was helpful in infants with a distal, inferior insertion of the aortic end of the ductus arteriosus. A stent was then chosen at least 2 mm larger than the minimal ductal diameter and 1 mm

larger than the maximum ductal diameter, and deployed through a 6 or 7 Fr sheath; ideally, the stent was opened in the aortic ampulla of the ductus and the distal aspect of the stent was allowed to flare into both the aortic isthmus and descending aorta. In the lateral projection the distal end of the stent was at the anterior border of the spinal bodies.

Angiography was also useful to demonstrate ductal anatomy. Approximately 70% of infants with HLHS were found to have favorable ductal anatomy which would allow the distal end of the stent to be placed in the aortic ampulla and avoid placement into the descending aorta. About 25% of infants with HLHS had transitional ductal anatomy which could require stent placement beyond the aortic ampulla into the descending aorta. In 5% of infants the ductal anatomy was felt to be unsuitable for stenting.

Of interest, heparinization to an activated clotting time (ACT) > 200 seconds was employed, as were six doses of 1 mg/kg of dipyridamole therapy and two doses of 0.5 mg/kg enoxaparin post-procedurally, as well as 5–10 mg/kg of acetylsalicylic acid daily until stent removal.

There were no deaths in this series related to the ductal procedure, with a mean follow-up of 65 ± 65 days; however, there was one late death possibly related to stenting at 3 months (during re-admission for coarctation angioplasty). Only one patient was deemed unstentable, owing to a short ductus measuring less than 10 mm, and a posterior ductal ridge. In 6 patients, two stents were required for complete coverage of ductal tissue (the mean length of the ductus in these patients was 22.4 mm, the mean length for the entire population was 16.3 ± 4.4 mm). One patient required a second stent due to stent migration. The mean ductal diameter of the entire population was 6.6 ± 1.2 mm. Procedural complications included bradycardia (3), hypotension (4), respiratory arrest (1), and transient heart block (1). Of note, morbidity was siginificantly higher among patients with either type 2 or 3 ductal anatomy (ductal orientation ≤ 10° leftward from the vertical plane),[51] suggesting that certain anatomic variants may be better managed with earlier

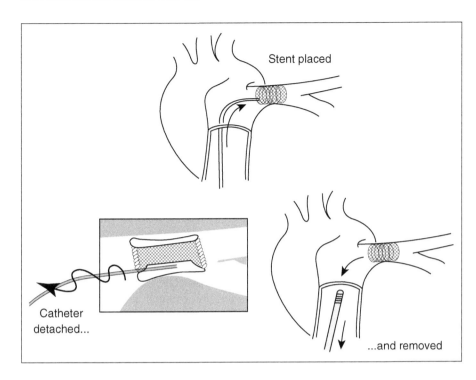

Figure 60.2
Schematic of percutaneous pulmonary band placement and deployment.

surgical palliation or transplantation. Two patients developed coarctation adjacent to the distal stent, one of whom underwent successful balloon angioplasty, the other of whom died pre-procedurally.

Longer term follow-up has been reported in 20 patients undergoing combined ductal stenting and pulmonary artery banding by Michel-Behnke and colleagues.[52] In their series, two patients died during the stent insertion or PA banding. Two patients received heart transplantation (57 and 331 days following stenting), although two also died awaiting transplantation at similar time periods (58 and 193 days).[52] Ten patients had undergone a combined stage I and II Norwood surgical repair with only 10% mortality in these patients. Perhaps most encouragingly, two patients with multiple left heart obstructive lesions (one with HLHS, the other with interrupted aortic arch and hypoplastic aortic valve annulus) were successfully palliated with ductus arteriosus (DA) stenting and PA banding, enabling eventual biventricular repair with its attendant improved long term prognosis.[17,53]

Pulmonary artery banding

Several investigators have recently promoted the concept of a hybrid first stage procedure (ductal stenting, open pulmonary artery banding) as an alternative to the Norwood procedure for HLHS (discussed in Chapter 59).[52] These same strategies to allow for ductal patency but limited pulmonary blood flow may also be adopted as a means to 'bridge' such patients to transplantation. In fact, the banding

of the pulmonary arteries has been a strategy employed in older infants with HLHS who have experienced prolonged severe pulmonary overcirculation, but who may not yet have developed fixed pulmonary hypertension.[54]

Mitchell and colleagues[54] performed open bilateral pulmonary artery banding with 2 mm PTFE bands. These were placed on the branch pulmonary arteries and secured to reduce pulmonary arterial pressure to 50% of systemic. The distal pulmonary arterial pressures were measured with 3 Fr catheters advanced into the distal pulmonary arteries, the right directly, and the left via a pursestring suture on the pulmonary trunk. Subsequently, intravascular branch pulmonary artery flow limiting devices delivered via femoral venous techniques were employed. The flow limiting devices are constructed of nitinol mesh and sized to fit securely in the proximal right and left pulmonary arteries. The device has a fixed internal lumen which reduces the effective orifice, reducing distal pressure and flow in a predictable fashion (Figure 60.2).

The order in which the ductal stent and pulmonary banding procedures are done varies. Some have suggested performing a one time procedure in the neonatal period (Figure 60.3).[52] Others have supported a staged procedure, unless the child is to undergo balloon atrial septostomy. These authors have suggested that waiting for pulmonary banding until 3–4 months of age can allow for good distal pulmonary artery growth prior to band procedures, and does not appear to impact upon pulmonary vasoreactivity.[54] Children in their study demonstrated a mean interval from PDA stent to band placement of 76±52 days. With the use of internal bands the mean age of banding decreased and procedures were performed in the first several weeks of life.

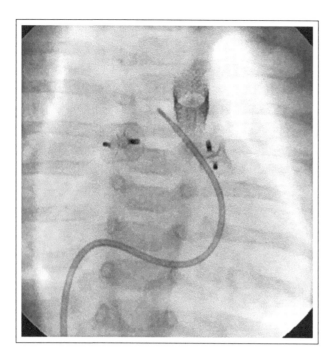

Figure 60.3
Ductal stent and pulmonary bands placed in a patient with HLHS.

As experience develops with internal bands one would anticipate routine use during interventional catheterization by 2 weeks of age. Internal bands may also provide an option for patients who were diagnosed late or were unsuitable for early palliative surgery before one month of age.

Transplantation

Orthotopic heart transplantation for HLHS following any of the prior interventional palliative procedures must be performed under deep hypothermic circulatory arrest (usually limited to the aortic arch reconstruction). In PA band patients, often the bands are removed and the branch pulmonary arteries snared to prevent run-off. Alternatively, the ductus can be clamped or snared if a self-expanding stent has been placed in the ductus. These stents do not crush and will re-expand if the clamp needs to be removed. The internal bands are then removed from the branch pulmonary arteries by separating the devices from the intimal surface of the artery. After circulatory arrest, the ductal stent is removed by dividing the ductus (and stent) at its mid-point. The remaining stent in the aorta is carefully removed during the arch reconstruction; all residual ductal tissue within the descending aorta must be excised (often requiring removal of the isthmus and anastomosis of the posterior wall of the aorta from the distal descending aorta to the underside of the left subclavian artery). The branch pulmonary arteries should be dilated (5–7 mm Hegar dilators) prior to pulmonary arterial anastomosis. Any residual stenosis should be addressed by patch arterioplasty at the time of transplantation.

For those with internal pulmonary arterial flow limiters, the stent and ductus are clamped in their mid-point after bypass is initiated. The stent in the ductus must be removed first, the internal flow limiting devices extracted through the divided pulmonary trunk and again dilators passed to confirm the patency and integrity of the branch pulmonary arteries.

In all cases, it is essential to assure that the donor procurement team retrieve all of the donor aortic arch and branch pulmonary arterial vessels so that arch reconstruction can be completed with donor aorta and that, in the event that pulmonary artery reconstruction must occur, donor pulmonary artery tissue may be used for onlay patch angioplasty. Of note, in the cases reported by Mitchell et al using internal bands, none required pulmonary artery reconstruction or repair after band removal. Furthermore, none of these patients developed late branch pulmonary artery stenosis, and 1 year after transplant, follow-up catheterizations documented appropriate pulmonary arterial growth.[54]

Norwood or cardiac transplant, which for whom?

Several recent studies have attempted to establish whether the Norwood procedure or primary transplantation affords the greatest survival to infants with HLHS. The rapidity with which (1) percutaneous strategies for interval palliation as well as (2) technical advances in the management of Norwood patients have evolved has rendered the results of these earlier decision analyses somewhat difficult to interpret in the current era. Importantly, however, while a recent transplant multi-center analysis demonstrated a 25% waiting list mortality for infants with HLHS, the post-transplant survival of this subgroup did not differ from those patients with other pre-transplant diagnoses.[55] Five-year survival from listing through transplantation in this series was 54% for infants with HLHS, a finding comparable to the long term survival after the Norwood procedure in recent reports.[56]

Jenkins et al reported the results of a comparison study between infants undergoing staged palliation or transplantation for HLHS.[29] Here, with 118 patients intended for staged surgery, and 124 intended for transplantation, transplantation resulted in greater survival rates at 1 and 5 years (61% and 55%) when compared with staged surgery (42% and 38%). A later comparison study evaluated a decision analysis involving six strategies: staged surgery, transplantation, stage I surgery as an interim to transplantation, and listing for transplant for 1, 2, or 3 months before performing surgery if a donor were unavailable.[10] In this study, it was suggested that the optimal strategy for individual centers should be guided by their center's historical donor organ availability and stage 1 surgical mortality, since optimal outcome necessarily involves a balance of these risks. In

Table 60.2	*Loma Linda pre-operative scoring system*
Variable	Points
Ventricular function	
poor	0
marginal	1
good	2
Tricuspid regurgitation	
severe	0
moderate	1
mild or less	2
Ascending arch size (mm)	
<3	0
≥3	2
ASD characteristics	
restrictive	0
non-restrictive	1
Blood type	
A, B, AB	0
O	1
Age at surgery (days)	
>21	0
14–21	1
<14	2

Total score <7 points is a recommendation to proceed to surgical palliation, stage I (Norwood procedure); ≤7 points is a recommendation to list for transplantation.
ASD, atrial septal defect.
Adapted from Checchia PA, Larsen R, Sehra R et al.[13] Copyright 2004, with permission from the Society of Thoracic Surgeons.

centers where <10% of patients receive an organ within 3 months of birth, and where stage I operative mortality is <20%, staged surgery appears to offer the higher survival.[10] In contrast, where organ donation rates exceed 30% in 3 months, optimal treatment would include waiting 1 month on the transplant list followed by stage I surgery if an organ fails to become available.[10] Their analysis suggested that performing stage I surgery before listing, or performing it after a 2- or 3-month wait on the transplant list were rarely optimal choices.

In order to more accurately delineate optimal treatment in individual patients (versus treatment preferences in programs overall), the group from Loma Linda has developed a scoring system to predict those patients with higher mortality risk after stage I repair. Their scoring system used several factors known to increase the risk of surgical palliation (Table 60.2); patients with scores greater than 7 were selected for early surgical palliation, while transplant was used in those with lower scores. Following the implementation of this system (as well as modifications in the perioperative care of all patients with HLHS), they reported significant increases in post-operative survival with the

Norwood procedure (48 hour survival 88% versus 40% and 1 year survival 50% versus 10%) while transplant outcomes remained unchanged.[13] These reports suggest that the survival of patients following staged reconstruction can be significantly improved through an appropriate treatment algorithm tailored both to the program performing the repairs and to the individual patient.

Summary

The optimal treatment of neonates with HLHS is a process in evolution. The rapid growth and development of hybrid procedures as an alternative to the Norwood procedure as first stage palliation has also promoted several strategies for catheter based palliation of neonates as a 'bridge' to heart transplantation. A medical program involving maintenance of ductal patency with either PGE1 or ductal stenting, and a limiting of pulmonary blood flow with nitrogen or allowance of a mildly restrictive atrial septum, has even allowed for home discharge in some series, with a reduction in waiting list mortality to 15%.[48] In parallel with these advances are those of the recent Sano modification of the Norwood procedure, which has reportedly improved first-stage survival to as high as 90%.[57,58] Only with continued re-evaluation in light of further evolution of these processes will the optimal treatment strategy for neonates with HLHS become evident.

References

1. Fixler DE, Pastor P, Sigman E, Eifler CW. Ethnicity and socioeconomic status: impact on the diagnosis of congenital heart disease. J Am Coll Cardiol 1993; 21(7): 1722–6.
2. Fyler DC. Report of the New England Regional Infant Cardiac Program. Pediatrics 1980; 65(2 Pt 2): 375–461.
3. Norwood WI, Lang P, Hansen DD. Physiologic repair of aortic atresia–hypoplastic left heart syndrome. N Engl J Med 1983; 308(1): 23–6.
4. Lang P, Norwood WI. Hemodynamic assessment after palliative surgery for hypoplastic left heart syndrome. Circulation 1983; 68(1): 104–8.
5. Meliones JN, Snider AR, Bove EL et al. Longitudinal results after first-stage palliation for hypoplastic left heart syndrome. Circulation 1990; 82(5 Suppl): IV151–6.
6. Sade RM, Crawford FA Jr, Fyfe DA. Symposium on hypoplastic left heart syndrome. J Thorac Cardiovasc Surg 1986; 91(6): 937–9.
7. Norwood WI, Kirklin JK, Sanders SP. Hypoplastic left heart syndrome: experience with palliative surgery. Am J Cardiol 1980; 45(1): 87–91.
8. Pridjian AK, Mendelsohn AM, Lupinetti FM et al. Usefulness of the bidirectional Glenn procedure as staged reconstruction for the functional single ventricle. Am J Cardiol 1993; 71(11): 959–62.
9. Bove EL, Ohye RG, Devaney EJ. Hypoplastic left heart syndrome: conventional surgical management. Semin Thorac Cardiovasc Surg Pediatr Card Surg Ann 2004; 7: 3–10.
10. Jenkins PC, Flanagan MF, Sargent JD et al. A comparison of treatment strategies for hypoplastic left heart syndrome using decision analysis. J Am Coll Cardiol 2001; 38(4): 1181–7.

11. Bando K, Turrentine MW, Sun K et al. Surgical management of hypoplastic left heart syndrome. Ann Thorac Surg 1996; 62(1): 70–6; discussion 76–7.

12. Bu'Lock FA, Stumper O, Jagtap R et al. Surgery for infants with a hypoplastic systemic ventricle and severe outflow obstruction: early results with a modified Norwood procedure. Br Heart J 1995; 73(5): 456–61.

13. Checchia PA, Larsen R, Sehra R et al. Effect of a selection and postoperative care protocol on survival of infants with hypoplastic left heart syndrome. Ann Thorac Surg 2004; 77(2): 477–83; discussion 483.

14. Bove EL. Current status of staged reconstruction for hypoplastic left heart syndrome. Pediatr Cardiol 1998; 19(4): 308–15.

15. Mahle WT, Spray TL, Wernovsky G et al. Survival after reconstructive surgery for hypoplastic left heart syndrome: a 15-year experience from a single institution. Circulation 2000; 102(19 Suppl 3): III136–41.

16. Jonas RA, Hansen DD, Cook N, Wessel D. Anatomic subtype and survival after reconstructive operation for hypoplastic left heart syndrome. J Thorac Cardiovasc Surg 1994; 107(4): 1121–7; discussion 1127–8.

17. Lofland GK, McCrindle BW, Williams WG et al. Critical aortic stenosis in the neonate: a multi-institutional study of management, outcomes, and risk factors. Congenital Heart Surgeons Society. J Thorac Cardiovasc Surg 2001; 121(1): 10–27.

18. Forbess JM, Cook N, Roth SJ et al. Ten-year institutional experience with palliative surgery for hypoplastic left heart syndrome. Risk factors related to stage I mortality. Circulation 1995; 92(9 Suppl): II262–6.

19. Iannettoni MD, Bove EL, Mosca RS et al. Improving results with first-stage palliation for hypoplastic left heart syndrome. J Thorac Cardiovasc Surg 1994; 107(3): 934–40.

20. Duncan BW, Rosenthal GL, Jones TK, Lupinetti FM. First-stage palliation of complex univentricular cardiac anomalies in older infants. Ann Thorac Surg 2001; 72(6): 2077–80.

21. Bartram U, Grunenfelder J, Van Praagh R. Causes of death after the modified Norwood procedure: a study of 122 postmortem cases. Ann Thorac Surg 1997; 64(6): 1795–802.

22. Graziano JN, Heidelberger KP, Ensing GJ et al. The influence of a restrictive atrial septal defect on pulmonary vascular morphology in patients with hypoplastic left heart syndrome. Pediatr Cardiol 2002; 23(2): 146–51.

23. Bove EL, Lloyd TR. Staged reconstruction for hypoplastic left heart syndrome. Contemporary results. Ann Surg 1996; 224(3): 387–94; discussion 394–5.

24. Andrews R, Tulloh R, Sharland G et al. Outcome of staged reconstructive surgery for hypoplastic left heart syndrome following antenatal diagnosis. Arch Dis Child 2001; 85(6): 474–7.

25. Chang RK, Chen AY, Klitzner TS. Clinical management of infants with hypoplastic left heart syndrome in the United States, 1988–1997. Pediatrics 2002; 110(2 Pt 1): 292–8.

26. Bailey LL, Nehlsen-Cannarella SL, Doroshow RW et al. Cardiac allotransplantation in newborns as therapy for hypoplastic left heart syndrome. N Engl J Med 1986; 315(15): 949–51.

27. Vricella LA, Razzouk AJ, del Rio M et al. Heart transplantation for hypoplastic left heart syndrome: modified technique for reducing circulatory arrest time. J Heart Lung Transplant 1998; 17(12): 1167–71.

28. Bailey L, Concepcion W, Shattuck H, Huang L. Method of heart transplantation for treatment of hypoplastic left heart syndrome. J Thorac Cardiovasc Surg 1986; 92(1): 1–5.

29. Jenkins PC, Flanagan MF, Jenkins KJ et al. Survival analysis and risk factors for mortality in transplantation and staged surgery for hypoplastic left heart syndrome. J Am Coll Cardiol 2000; 36(4): 1178–85.

30. Razzouk AJ, Chinnock RE, Gundry SR et al. Transplantation as a primary treatment for hypoplastic left heart syndrome: intermediate-term results. Ann Thorac Surg 1996; 62(1): 1–7; discussion 8.

31. Chiavarelli M, Gundry SR, Razzouk AJ, Bailey LL. Cardiac transplantation for infants with hypoplastic left-heart syndrome. JAMA 1993; 270(24): 2944–7.

32. Tweddell JS, Canter CE, Bridges ND et al. Predictors of operative mortality and morbidity after infant heart transplantation. Ann Thorac Surg 1994; 58(4): 972–7.

33. Morris MC, Ittenbach RF, Godinez RI et al. Risk factors for mortality in 137 pediatric cardiac intensive care unit patients managed with extracorporeal membrane oxygenation. Crit Care Med 2004; 32(4): 1061–9.

34. Jonas RA, Lang P, Hansen D et al. First-stage palliation of hypoplastic left heart syndrome. The importance of coarctation and shunt size. J Thorac Cardiovasc Surg 1986; 92(1): 6–13.

35. Norwood WI, Jacobs ML. Fontan's procedure in two stages. Am J Surg 1993; 166(5): 548–51.

36. Goldberg CS, Gomez CA. Hypoplastic left heart syndrome: new developments and current controversies. Semin Neonatol 2003; 8(6): 461–8.

37. Rychik J, Rome JJ, Collins MH et al. The hypoplastic left heart syndrome with intact atrial septum: atrial morphology, pulmonary vascular histopathology and outcome. J Am Coll Cardiol 1999; 34(2): 554–60.

38. Marshall AC, van der Velde ME, Tworetzky W et al. Creation of an atrial septal defect in utero for fetuses with hypoplastic left heart syndrome and intact or highly restrictive atrial septum. Circulation 2004; 110(3): 253–8.

39. Canter C, Naftel D, Caldwell R et al. Survival and risk factors for death after cardiac transplantation in infants. A multi-institutional study. The Pediatric Heart Transplant Study. Circulation 1997; 96(1): 227–31.

40. Allan LD, Sharland G, Tynan MJ. The natural history of the hypoplastic left heart syndrome. Int J Cardiol 1989; 25(3): 341–3.

41. Hornberger LK, Sanders SP, Rein AJ et al. Left heart obstructive lesions and left ventricular growth in the midtrimester fetus. A longitudinal study. Circulation 1995; 92(6): 1531–8.

42. Maxwell D, Allan L, Tynan MJ. Balloon dilatation of the aortic valve in the fetus: a report of two cases. Br Heart J 1991; 65(5): 256–8.

43. Allan LD, Maxwell DJ, Carminati M, Tynan MJ. Survival after fetal aortic balloon valvoplasty. Ultrasound Obstet Gynecol 1995; 5(2): 90–1.

44. Lopes LM, Cha SC, Kajita LJ et al. Balloon dilatation of the aortic valve in the fetus. A case report. Fetal Diagn Ther 1996; 11(4): 296–300.

45. Kohl T, Sharland G, Allan LD et al. World experience of percutaneous ultrasound-guided balloon valvuloplasty in human fetuses with severe aortic valve obstruction. Am J Cardiol 2000; 85(10): 1230–3.

46. Mora GA, Pizarro C, Jacobs ML, Norwood WI. Experimental model of single ventricle. Influence of carbon dioxide on pulmonary vascular dynamics. Circulation 1994; 90(5 Pt 2): II43–6.

47. Tweddell JS, Hoffman GM, Fedderly RT et al. Phenoxybenzamine improves systemic oxygen delivery after the Norwood procedure. Ann Thorac Surg 1999; 67(1): 161–7; discussion 167–8.

48. Bourke KD, Sondheimer HM, Ivy DD et al. Improved pretransplant management of infants with hypoplastic left heart syndrome enables discharge to home while waiting for transplantation. Pediatr Cardiol 2003; 24(6): 538–43.

49. Ruiz CE, Gamra H, Zhang HP et al. Brief report: stenting of the ductus arteriosus as a bridge to cardiac transplantation in infants with the hypoplastic left-heart syndrome. N Engl J Med 1993; 328(22): 1605–8.

50. Gibbs JL, Uzun O, Blackburn ME et al. Fate of the stented arterial duct. Circulation 1999; 99(20): 2621–5.

51. Boucek MM, Mashburn C, Kunz E, Chan KC. Ductal anatomy: a determinant of successful stenting in hypoplastic left heart syndrome. Pediatr Cardiol 2005; 26(2): 200–5.

52. Michel-Behnke I, Akintuerk H, Marquardt I et al. Stenting of the ductus arteriosus and banding of the pulmonary arteries: basis for various surgical strategies in newborns with multiple left heart obstructive lesions. Heart (Br Card Soc) 2003; 89(6): 645–50.

53. de Leval MR. Surgical management of the neonate with congenital heart disease. Br Heart J 1986; 55(1): 1–3.

54. Mitchell MB, Campbell DN, Boucek MM et al. Mechanical limitation of pulmonary blood flow facilitates heart transplantation in older infants with hypoplastic left heart syndrome. Eur J Cardio-Thorac Surg 2003; 23(5): 735–42.

55. Chrisant MR, Naftel DC, Drummond-Webb J et al. Fate of infants with hypoplastic left heart syndrome listed for cardiac transplantation: a multicenter study. J Heart Lung Transplant 2005; 24(5): 576–82.

56. Ashburn DA, McCrindle BW, Tchervenkov CI et al. Outcomes after the Norwood operation in neonates with critical aortic stenosis or aortic valve atresia. J Thorac Cardiovasc Surg 2003; 125(5): 1070–82.

57. Sano S, Ishino K, Kawada M, Honjo O. Right ventricle-pulmonary artery shunt in first-stage palliation of hypoplastic left heart syndrome. Semin Thorac Cardiovasc Surg Pediatr Card Surg Annu 2004; 7: 22–31.

58. Sano S, Ishino K, Kado H et al. Outcome of right ventricle-to-pulmonary artery shunt in first-stage palliation of hypoplastic left heart syndrome: a multi-institutional study. Ann Thorac Surg 2004; 78(6): 1951–7.

61

Intraoperative VSD device closure

Zahid Amin

Introduction

Currently, surgery and transcatheter techniques are employed for closure of ventricular septal defects (VSDs). With surgery, almost all perimembranous and most muscular VSDs can be closed, regardless of the patient's size or weight. Muscular VSDs, however, have been a challenge to the surgeons because of their location and right ventricular trabeculations, and because the defects cannot be effectively closed through the right atrium, necessitating right or left ventriculotomy which is fraught with its own complications.[1] Amongst the muscular VSDs, the apical and anterior muscular VSDs are difficult to visualize intra-operatively and, hence, closure is either incomplete or not possible.[1,2] Surgical closure may be prolonged and this in turn increases the cardiopulmonary bypass (CPB) time, and its associated complications.[3] On the other hand, transcatheter techniques are being employed with increasing frequency to close muscular and perimembranous VSDs.[4] These techniques, with several advantages when compared to surgery, have limitations primarily because of patients' weight and size. If the patient has concomitant cardiac defects, the defect may be closed in the operating room for obvious reasons.

Pre- and intra-operative device closure of VSDs was first introduced in 1991;[5–7] after the patient was placed on CPB, a Clamshell (NMT Medical, Boston, MA) device was used to close complicated muscular VSDs under direct visualization. This procedure was, however, inadequate because visualization of the VSD was difficult as the heart was flaccid. The Clamshell is a non-centering device, delivered through a large and stiff delivery sheath; the residual defect rate was high and, hence, the results were less than optimal.[6]

After the introduction of the Amplatzer (AGA Medical, Golden Valley, MN) Septal Occluder device, we directed our attention to design a muscular VSD device specifically for closure of muscular VSDs.[8] During our initial experiments in the dog model, we created a muscular VSD (with a 10 mm sharp punch device) through the right ventriculotomy, under epicardial echocardiographic guidance. These procedures were performed while the heart was beating, through the free wall of the right ventricle, without CPB. After creation of the defect, we let the animal recuperate from the procedure and about 3 weeks later closed the defect with the Amplatzer muscular VSD device, using the transcatheter approach. At the time of creation of the defect, intraoperative echocardiography was utilized during the procedure to measure the defect and to specify its location. After successfully closing the defect using the *percutaneous* approach,[8] we decided to close the muscular VSD immediately after creation in the operating room. Utilizing epicardial echocardiography, we were able to close several defects immediately after creation while the heart was beating.[9] The closure was performed by introducing the delivery sheath through the free wall of the right ventricle. We named this the *perventricular* technique, as opposed to the percutaneous technique.[9] Later we reported successful application of the technique in humans[10–12] and extended its application to perimembranous VSDs.[13]

In this chapter I will describe the evolution of the perventricular approach and its use for closure of muscular VSDs and perimembranous VSDs, and its potential for deployment of the pulmonary valve with self-expanding and balloon-expandable stents.

Methods

Patient population

As the use of the perventricular technique increases, we believe that there will be some changes in the patient population in whom this technique can be used. At the current time, we recommend this procedure in patients who, first and foremost, are not good candidates for the transcatheter procedure in the cardiac catheterization laboratory. The indications for perventricular closure are low weight, issues with vascular access, inability or failed attempt to close the defect in the catheterization laboratory for any reason, concomitant lesions that require a visit to the operating room, and patients who have had pulmonary artery banding in the past for VSD and require debanding of the pulmonary artery in addition to closure of the defect. In addition, the use may increase in the Third World countries as the overall cost of the procedure will be low because of no CPB, shorter hospital stay, and the patient's ability to resume daily activities in a relatively short period of time, etc.

The devices

Amplatzer muscular and perimembranous VSD devices were used for the perventricular approach. These devices have distinct advantages over the other currently available devices. They are circular in shape, hence no hooks or pointed corners; they are self-expandable, hence maneuvering to ensure disk formation is not required; they are easily retrievable, hence no extensive maneuvers are needed to withdraw them back into the delivery sheath, if needed; they can be delivered through a relatively small sheath size when compared to other devices, hence a minimal chance of traumatizing the ventricle during the perventricular closure; and they are self-centering, hence encroachment of the atrioventricular and semi-lunar valves is less likely. The device size corresponds to the connecting waist. The above mentioned attributes of the devices make them ideal for this approach.

Muscular VSD occluder

The Amplatzer muscular VSD occluder is made of 0.005 inch wires that are woven to form two disks. The disks are connected to each other via a connecting waist. It is the size of the waist that tells us the size of the device. The disks are 8 mm larger than the waist. The waist is 7 mm in length to accommodate the thickness of the muscular ventricular septum. The available sizes range from 4 mm to 18 mm in 2 mm increments. For defects that are larger than 18 mm, a post-infarction muscular VSD device can be used. This device is similar to the muscular VSD occluder in design, except that the waist is 10 mm in length and the disks are 10 mm larger than the waist. A Dacron mesh is sewn inside the nitinol wire mesh to enhance closure rate. A female screw is welded in the middle of one disk (a would-be right ventricular disk) for attachment to the delivery sheath.

Membranous VSD occluder

The membranous VSD device is also made from 0.005 inch nitinol wire, but has a completely different design. The waist of the device tells us the size of the device but the disks are uneven in size and eccentric in design. The right ventricular disk is 4 mm larger than the waist and the left ventricular disk is 6 mm larger than the waist. However, the left ventricular disk is only 0.5 mm larger than the waist on one side and 5.5 mm larger on the opposite side. The unique device design ensures that there will be no aortic valve encroachment after the device is deployed. In order to have optimal left disk position, it is important to have a delivery mechanism that will ensure proper device position. Hence, the delivery sheath for the membranous VSD device is different from the muscular VSD device. In addition to the regular delivery cable, there is a pusher catheter that latches on to the device so that the left disk orientation after it is deployed in the left ventricle keeps the smaller edge of the disk toward the aortic valve.

The delivery sheath

For the perventricular approach, the delivery sheath does not need to be 60 or 80 cm in length. A short sheath would suffice, as the part of the delivery sheath which has to be inside the ventricles may not be more than 5 cm in length (it depends upon the size of the ventricles). Although a long sheath can be used, it does make the procedure cumbersome and device deployment a bit more difficult. A short sheath has been used successfully, and a sheath designed specifically for perventricular closure is being developed by AGA Medical Corporation.

For perventricular delivery of the perimembranous VSD, the pusher catheter is not needed as the sheath can be rotated clockwise or anticlockwise if the left disk orientation is incorrect.

The procedure

The key to a successful procedure is collaboration between the surgeon and the interventionalist. The procedure is performed in the operating room with or without the availability of fluoroscopy. Ideally, transesophageal echocardiography (TEE) is used, but in smaller patients where use of the TEE probe is not possible because of small patient size or other anatomic issues, epicardial echocardiography can be utilized. In addition, an intracardiac echocardiographic probe can be used in the smaller population, as it can be accommodated by small babies. However, it is not recommended for use with TEE at the current time.

The septum is carefully scanned from apex to the base of the heart, and from anterior to posterior. Particular vigilance should be given to trouble spots such as the apical and the anterior septum. The defect is measured in two views during ventricular diastole (or the largest diameter of the defect is measured), in order to select the appropriate sized device. Usually a device that is 2 mm larger than the defect is chosen for a muscular VSD, and a device that is equal to or 1 mm larger than the defect in the perimembranous VSD.

After the patient is draped and prepped in sterile fashion, a median sternotomy is performed. In the first few cases,

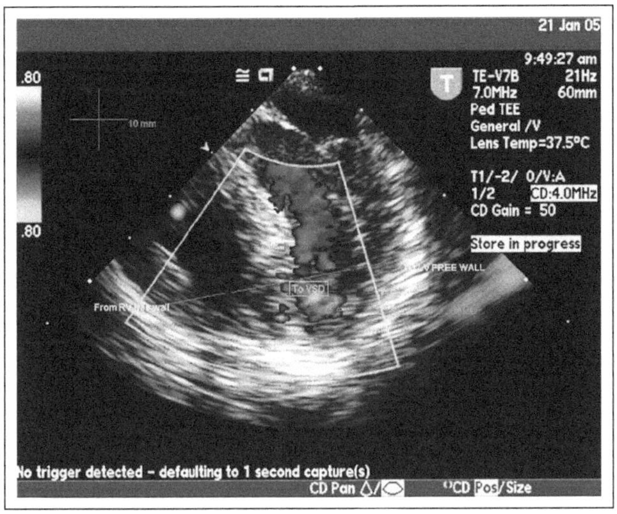

Figure 61.1
Echocardiographic still frame from a patient with a muscular VSD. It is crucial to measure the distance from the free wall of the right ventricle to the VSD, and, from the free wall of the right ventricle to the free wall of the left ventricle. (See also color plate section.)

we recommend that a complete median sternotomy be performed; a mini-sternotomy can be performed in the subsequent procedures as the learning curve is steep. After the sternum is divided, the pericardium is opened longitudinally and a pericardial cradle made. Depending upon the location of the muscular VSD, a pursestring suture is placed (opposite to the defect) on the free wall of the right ventricle. If the defect is apical, it is of paramount importance not to place the pursestring suture close to the apex (*vide infra*). In order to be as close to the defect as possible, a gentle pressure on the right ventricular free wall and echocardiographic assistance is helpful in locating an optimal spot for placement of the pursestring suture. Once the pursestring suture is placed on the free wall of the right ventricle, the distance from the right ventricular free wall to the middle of the defect is measured. Subsequent to that, the maximum distance from the free wall to the left ventricular free wall (with a straight line passing through the middle of the VSD) is measured (Figure 61.1). This distance is important because it helps in determining how deep the delivery sheath can be advanced without injuring the left ventricular free wall. Usually the dilator of the sheath is 3–4 cm longer than the sheath, if the distance from right ventricular free wall to the left ventricular free wall is 4 cm, it is clear that as soon as the dilator is introduced through the right ventricle, the sheath has to be advanced over the dilator, without advancing the dilator further, otherwise left ventricular free wall injury or perforation can occur.

An angio-catheter is advanced through the pursestring over the right ventricle, and once it is in the lumen of the right ventricle, the needle is removed. Under TEE guidance, a glide wire (Figure 61.2a) is advanced and directed toward the VSD. The angio-catheter is ideally held by the surgeon as their knowledge of the location of the VSD in the operating room is helpful in directing the catheter toward the VSD. Once the glide wire crosses the defect, it is maneuvered and advanced through the aortic valve or toward the left ventricle (Figure 61.2a). The angio-catheter is removed and an appropriate sized dilator (1 Fr larger than the delivery sheath chosen to place the device) is advanced to predilate the right ventricle muscle. The dilator is removed and the delivery sheath is advanced over the wire (Figure 61.2b). The dilator is removed after ensuring that the sheath is in the left ventricle or ascending aorta. The sheath is allowed to back bleed and is flushed. Gently pull the sheath back if spontaneous back bleeding does not occur when the dilator is removed. Flush the sheath with saline. The flushing of the sheath will clear blood from the sheath and also help you accurately locate the sheath tip (saline contrast echocardiography). The Amplatzer device is then advanced through the sheath to the tip of the sheath (Figure 61.2c). The whole system is pulled back, if the tip is in the ascending aorta (for a perimembranous VSD, the tip should be in the ascending aorta), the left disk is deployed by both pulling on the delivery sheath and advancing the cable (Figure 61.2d). Once the left disk is completely deployed, the whole system is pulled toward the ventricular septum and, while the delivery cable is kept stable in one location, the delivery sheath is pulled to deploy the waist and the right disk (Figure 61.2e, f). Gentle repositioning of the sheath is necessary to avoid pulling the left disk into the defect. If the device appears stable, after gentle pull–push maneuvers, it is released by anticlockwise rotation of the delivery cable. The procedure can be repeated if there are multiple defects. The sheath and the cable are removed and the pursestring suture tightened to achieve hemostasis. The chest is closed in the routine fashion.

If the defect is apical (*vide supra*), we recommend not placing the pursestring suture adjacent to the defect. The deployment of the right ventricular disk is difficult because, as the sheath is withdrawn, the disk may protrude out of the right ventricle free wall. In this situation place the pursestring suture away from the RV apex and make a loop with the delivery sheath as if the device was being deployed from the internal jugular vein. Deploy the waist and part of the RV disk into the left ventricle, pull the sheath and the cable to approximate the left disk to the LV side of the ventricular septum, and deploy the right disk very slowly while advancing the cable and retracting the sheath. If the device protrudes out of the RV free wall, advance the delivery sheath over the device and reposition the right disk.

There are subtle but distinct differences between muscular and membranous device deployment. For a muscular VSD, the waist can be deployed in the left ventricle cavity before pulling the whole system toward the septum. For a perimembranous VSD (Figure 61.3a–g) the left disk should

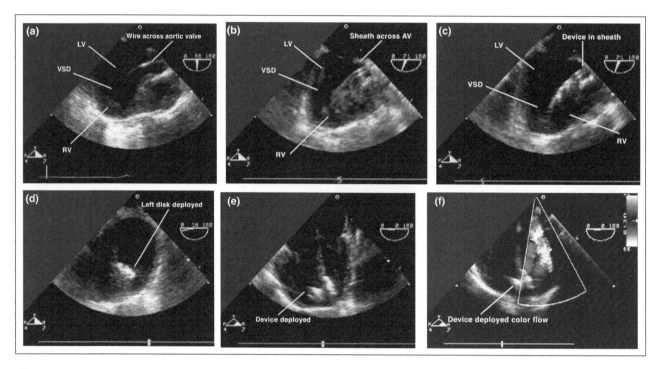

Figure 61.2
(a)–(f) Echocardiographic still frames of muscular VSD closure. See text for detail. LV, left ventricle; RV, right ventricle; VSD, ventricular septal defect. (61.2 (f), see also color plate section.)

approximate the septum before the waist is deployed, as the waist is much shorter than the muscular VSD device.

Results

The use of the perventricular technique for closure of muscular VSDs has been widespread, with estimated procedures exceeding 80. The majority of these procedures were performed in patients who were high risk candidates for conventional surgery and transcatheter closure. In our personal experience of 40 procedures that were performed in the US and several other countries, the results have been excellent. The technical success of the procedure was 100%. In one patient the device had to be removed because of significant residual shunt. One patient developed complete heart block. This patient had high inlet VSD with significant failure to thrive. The initial procedure was attempted in the cardiac catheterization laboratory where heart block was noted when the wire advanced across the defect. Later, the procedure was performed in the operating room. The patient developed heart block several hours after the procedure, requiring a permanent pacemaker. Device embolization was encountered in one patient. This patient had pulmonary

artery banding for multiple VSDs. The patient had suprasystemic right ventricular pressures intra-operatively. The larger defect was closed successfully with the perventricular technique. The patient was then placed on CPB to repair the banded pulmonary artery. Unfortunately, the banded area repair required several runs of bypass with inadequate relief of the stenosis. It was unclear when the device embolized to the left ventricle.

Perimembranous VSD

There have been a total of four patients with perimembranous VSD in whom perventricular closure was attempted. Three had successful closure and in one patient the device closure was not attempted. Minor left ventricle free wall injury was encountered in one patient. This patient had significant and chronic lung disease. The patient was born at 26 weeks estimated gestational age and at the time of the procedure was only 2 kg. TEE was not possible and the patient had a very large conal branch on the surface of the right ventricular outflow tract. We were not able to find an optimal place for pursestring suture and device closure was not attempted. The patient underwent patch repair of the VSD.

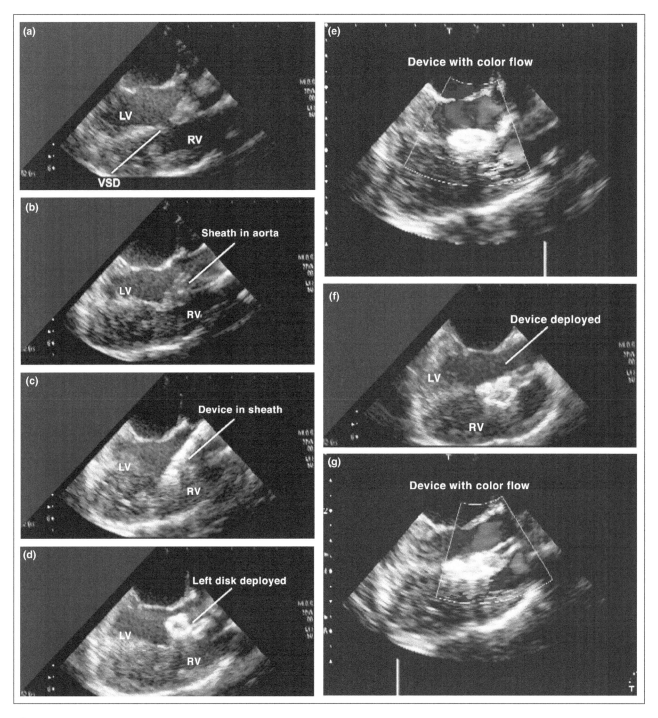

Figure 61.3

Echocardiographic still frames from a patient who underwent device closure of a perimembranous VSD. (a) The perimembranous VSD in the modified four-chamber view. (b) The delivery sheath is across the defect and the delivery sheath. (c) The device in the delivery sheath. (d) The left disk has been deployed below the aortic valve. (e) The right disk has been deployed. (f) and (g) Color flow evaluation after device deployment. LV, left ventricle; RV, right ventricle; VSD, ventricular septal defect. (61.3 (f) and 61.3 (g), see also color plate section.)

Robotic assisted perventricular VSD closure

The robotic system is frequently used to repair congenital and acquired cardiac defects. Its use should minimize the trauma secondary to median sternotomy or mini-sternotomy. We recently completed robotic assisted perventricular closure of perimembranous VSD in a Yucatan pig model.[14] The procedure was performed using three robotic ports, two for instruments and one for the endoscope. Transthoracic echocardiography was performed during the procedure. The procedure was attempted in 7 Yucatan pigs and was successful in 5. We believe that once smaller ports become available, the procedure can be performed in small children. We do recommend more research before conducting human trials.

Closure of post-myocardial infarction (post-MI) VSD with the perventricular technique

To date, there have been at least two patients who benefited from perventricular closure of post-MI VSD. One procedure was performed by us in the US and the second procedure in Santiago, Chile (Leopoldo Romero, personal communications). Both procedures were successful.

Perventricular placement of the pulmonary valve

Percutaneous placement of the pulmonary valve is being performed with increasing frequency. The sheath size required to place the valve is large and hence its application in smaller children is limited. We conducted experimental work in a sheep model, with a self-expandable valve.[15] We used a Cook Z-stent (Cook Inc., Bloomington, IN) and Shelhigh (Shelhigh, Newark, NJ) porcine valve for the experiment. The procedure was performed successfully through the free wall of the right ventricle using the perventricular approach. The preliminary results are encouraging.

Conclusions

The perventricular technique is a relatively new technique for closure of VSDs. It has been used successfully in several other institutions with excellent results.[12,16] The procedure can also be used with robotic assistance with positive results in the animal model. In the near future, the procedure will become useful for pulmonary valve insertion and for aortic or atrioventricular valve insertion. At the current time, the technique has only been used for VSD closure in the high risk and hemodynamically significant defects, with excellent

results. The use of the technique has and can be extended to patients with concomitant lesions to shorten total CPB time. For muscular VSDs which are difficult to close once the patient is under CPB, this technique is ideal as the defect is clearly seen by echocardiography, as the heart is beating during the procedure. The procedure decreases the risks associated with CPB, can be performed with limited sternotomy, and, in the future, we may be able to do the procedure with the assistance of a robotic system. No CPB also reduces the number of days the patient has to spend in the hospital. Since a trip to the cardiac catheterization laboratory is avoided, all potential complications of catheterization are avoided. There is no risk from radiation, contrast, and the cumbersome catheter course which may cause arrhythmias, decreased cardiac output, and hemodynamic compromise.

We believe that this technique will be used with increasing frequency in the future as collaboration between the surgeon and the cardiologists increases. Its use may increase significantly when perventricular closure of perimembranous VSDs starts, which we hope is going to be in the near future.

References

1. Serraf A, Lacour-Gayet F, Bruniaux J et al. Surgical management of isolated multiple ventricular septal defects. J Thorac Cardiovasc Surg 1992; 103: 437–43.
2. Singh AK, de Leval MR, Stark J. Left ventriculotomy for closure of muscular ventricular septal defects. Ann Surg 1997; 86: 577–80.
3. Kern FH, Hickey PR. The effects of cardiopulmonary bypass on the brain. In: Jonas RA, ed. Cardiopulmonary Bypass in the Neonates, Infants and Young Children, 1st edition. Boston: Blackwell Science, 1994: 263–78.
4. Chessa M, Carminati M, Cao Qi-Ling et al. Transcatheter closure of congenital and acquired muscular ventricular septal defects using the amplatzer device. J Invas Cardiol 2002; 14: 322–7.
5. Bridges ND, Perry SB, Goldstein SA et al. Preoperative transcatheter closure of congenital muscular ventricular septal defects. N Engl J Med 1991; 324(19): 1312–17.
6. Fishberger SB, Bridges ND, Keane JF et al. Intraoperative device closure of ventricular septal defects. Circulation 1993; 88(pt 2): 205–9.
7. Okubo M, Benson LN, Nykanen D et al. Outcomes of intraoperative device closure of muscular ventricular septal defects. Ann Thorac Surg 2001; 72: 416–23.
8. Amin Z, Gu X, Berry JM et al. A new device for closure of muscular ventricular septal defects in a canine model. Circulation 1999; 100: 320–8.
9. Amin Z, Gu X, Berry JM et al. Perventricular closure of ventricular septal defects without cardiopulmonary bypass. Ann Thorac Surg 1999; 68: 149–54.
10. Amin Z, Berry JM, Foker J et al. Intraoperative closure of muscular ventricular septal defect in a canine model and application of the technique in a baby. J Thorac Cardiovasc Surg 1998; 115: 1374–6.
11. Amin Z, Berry JM, Danford D et al. Intraoperative closure of muscular ventricular septal defects without cardiopulmonary bypass: preliminary results of the perventricular approach. Circulation 2001; 104(Suppl 17): II-710.
12. Maheshwari S, Suresh PV, Bansal M et al. Perventricular device closure of muscular ventricular septal defects on the beating heart. Ind Heart J 2004; 56: 333–5.

13. Amin Z, Danford D, Lof J et al. Intraoperative device closure of perimembranous ventricular septal defects without cardiopulmonary bypass: preliminary results with the perventricular technique. J Thorac Cardiovasc Surg 2004; 127: 234–41.

14. Amin A, Woo R, Danford D et al. Rabotically assisted perventricular closure of perimembranous ventricular septal defects: Preliminary results in Yucatan pigs. J Thorac Cardiovasc Surg 2006; 131: 427–32.

15. Amin Z. Available transcatheter pulmonary valves: Perventricular technique with the Shelhigh valve. In: Hijazi Z, BonHoeffer P, Feldman TE, Ruiz C (eds), Transcatheter Valve Repair. Abingdon, Oxford: Taylor and Francis 2006: 89–95.

16. Bacha E, Cao Q, Starr JP et al. Perventricular device closure of muscular ventricular septal defects on the beating heart: technique and results. J Thorac Cardiovasc Surg 2003; 126: 1718–23.

62

Intra-operative stent implantation

Evan M Zahn

Introduction

Since 1990, transcatheter implantation of intravascular stents has been extensively described as an effective form of therapy for a variety of acquired and congenital vascular stenoses.[1-7] Congenital lesions treated by stent placement include central and branch pulmonary artery stenosis, native and recurrent coarctation of the aorta, a variety of venous stenoses, intra- or extracardiac baffle obstructions, and conduit narrowing. More recently, stents and covered stents have been utilized as a means of creating or maintaining new vascular channels, such as transcatheter Fontan baffle placement or long term maintenance of ductal arteriosus patency.[8-12] Although the effectiveness of stent therapy is well accepted, the technical demands of implantation have at times limited the applicability of these devices, particularly in small, critically ill children. While improvements in delivery technique, balloon, stent, and sheath technology have made percutaneous stent implantation a more accomplishable procedure,[13-15] there are numerous clinical scenarios where intra-operative stent implantation may be preferable. In this chapter we will discuss the techniques utilized for intra-operative implantation of stents in the pulmonary arteries and aorta.

History

Intra-operative stent implantation was first reported in 1992.[16] This and all other subsequent reports describe stent implantation under direct visualization in the operating room with essentially no immediate post-procedural assessment. Despite the obvious pitfalls of such techniques, the results reported for intra-operative pulmonary artery stent implantation have been good, with improvements in vascular diameter (as measured in follow-up) comparable to those reported using standard percutaneous implantation.[17-19] A more limited experience with intra-operative placement of pulmonary vein stents indicates good initial results with high early restenosis rates, similar to those described with the percutaneous treatment of this lesion. Proponents of intra-operative stent implantation tout the speed and ease of implantation as important advantages of this technique.

Indications and advantages of intra-operative stent implantation

Previously described[19] indications for intra-operative stent implantation include:

1. a need for a concomitant surgical procedure
2. limited vascular access
3. small patient size
4. and as rescue therapy after failed percutaneous stent placement.

In our institution we also advocate this approach in selected patients requiring stent placement in the early post-operative period as an alternative to surgical arterioplasty.[20] One important advantage of intra-operative or hybrid stent implantation is that, regardless of patient size, a stent ultimately capable of achieving an adult diameter can nearly always be implanted. The majority of children requiring stent implantation at any age would ideally receive stents capable of being expanded to 'adult size' (e.g. 16–20 mm in diameter) as the child grows. Despite dramatic improvements in stent technology, relatively large stiff delivery systems are still required for deployment of 'adult size' stents (e.g. a large XD Genesis typically requires at least an 8 Fr delivery system). In small infants or children, particularly those with tenuous hemodynamics, the placement of these delivery systems often produces such profound hemodynamic compromise as to preclude safe completion of the procedure. Even stable infants and toddlers (< 15 kg) can present significant challenges for percutaneous implantation of adult size stents across certain lesions (e.g. tortuous left pulmonary artery stenosis in the setting of a redundant outflow tract after repair of tetralogy of Fallot). Additional technical issues which may negatively impact percutaneous stent placement include:

1. an excessively tortuous catheter course with numerous acute angles to navigate
2. pronounced delivery system movement during implantation (e.g. as a result of pulmonary insufficiency)
3. close proximity of important vascular structures to the target lesion (e.g. origin of the right pulmonary artery when attempting to stent an ostial stenosis of the left pulmonary artery).

Utilizing a hybrid technique in these instances may mean the difference between a successful result and a 'nightmare case'.

Techniques

Over the last decade we have utilized two distinct methods for hybrid stent delivery. The first technique, *videoscopic-guided stent implantation*, has been used solely for the treatment of branch pulmonary artery stenosis and, typically, is a planned procedure which takes place in the operating room. The second technique, *stent implantation via surgically provided vascular access*, has been used to treat a wide variety of lesions including branch pulmonary artery stenoses, recurrent aortic arch obstruction (after HLHS palliative surgery), and shunt occlusion/stenosis. This approach can be performed in either the catheterization laboratory, surgical suite, or a hybrid suite.

Videoscopic-guided stent implantation

In our experience all of these procedures have been performed in conjunction with other surgical procedures, most commonly right ventricular outflow reconstruction (including conduit replacement) and/or delayed ventricular septal defect (VSD) closure in the setting of pulmonary atresia and VSD. A critical component to the success of this technique is an exhaustive evaluation of the pertinent anatomy *prior* to the operative procedure. To date this has been done with pre-operative angiography, although it is likely that pre-operative MRI and/or CT angiography will replace the need for this in the near future.[21]

During the pre-operative catheterization, selective pulmonary angiography using multiple axial angulated views aimed at obtaining optimal images of the target lesion and surrounding vascular structures is performed. Since we do not routinely employ angiography during videoscopic stent placement, decisions regarding stent type/length, implantation diameter, and precise implant location are decided *prior* to surgery based upon these pre-procedural angiograms (Figure 62.1). A stent with the largest future potential diameter (i.e., an 'adult sized' stent) is chosen in most cases. An important exception occurs in neonates or small infants where implantation diameter is limited by adjacent small native vessel size *and* further future surgery will be required (e.g. conduit replacement). In these cases smaller stents, with potential diameters less than adult size, may be implanted and either removed or altered surgically at subsequent operations. The balloon diameter used for implantation is chosen to match the diameter of the nearest adjacent normal vessel (typically distal to the target lesion) regardless of the stenosis diameter. We try not to oversize stent diameter at implantation secondary to concerns regarding accelerated stenosis at transition zones when implant diameters greatly exceed adjacent vessel diameters.[22,23] Stent length is determined by obtaining the optimal length desired as measured on the pre-operative angiogram and using known foreshortened length–diameter relationships provided by the manufacturers. A stent length is selected for which the predicted foreshortened length best approximates the desired ideal length, paying careful attention to the location of side branch take-offs. We attempt to avoid crossing side-branches whenever possible.

Implantation procedures are performed with general anesthesia with the patient maintained on cardiopulmonary bypass. Timing of stent placement in relation to other portions of the operation is decided upon by the cardiac surgeon and varies according to the specific anatomy of the patient, location of the lesion(s) being treated, and the operation being performed. The interventional cardiologist and an experienced catheter laboratory technician scrub into the case and temporarily replace the surgical first assistant at the left side of the table while the cardiac surgeon remains at the right side of the table. A separate sterile 'interventional table', easily accessible to the interventional team, is set up on the left side of the table with all of the devices and equipment which would be needed for a particular case.

Since in most institutions the catheterization laboratory and operating room are in separate physical locations, duplicates of the catheterization-related inventory which could be needed are brought into the operating room, as well as a wide range of balloons and stents on either end of the predicted stent and balloon, which were calculated from the pre-operative angiograms. This saves precious minutes when an unanticipated finding occurs or equipment fails. Additionally, a second catheter laboratory technician is always present to be used as a 'runner' should more supplies be needed from the catheterization laboratory. These issues

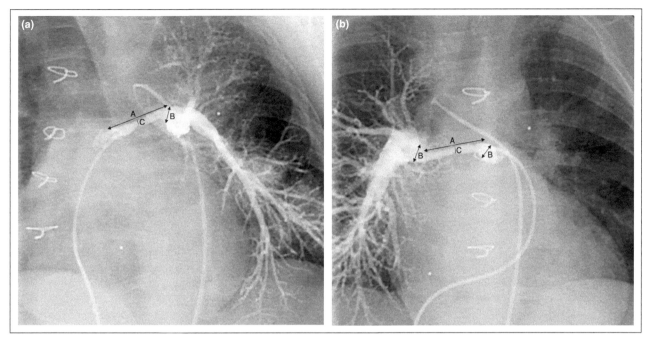

Figure 62.1
Pre-operative selective pulmonsary angiography performed in the left and right pulmonary arteries of a 6-month-old with bilateral severe branch pulmonary artery hypoplasia associated with pulmonary atresia/ventricular septal defeat (VSD), status post-neonatal right ventricular outflow reconstruction (VSD left open). Measurements used for stent/balloon selection are vessel length to be stented (A), diameter of adjacent 'normal vessel' (B), and narrowest stenosis diameter (C).

can be minimized or eliminated when these procedures are performed in a true hybrid suite.

The interventional table typically holds a heparinized bowl of saline, a small curved surgical clamp, a 0.035 inch Wholey Hi-torque floppy guidewire (Mallinckrodt, St Louis, MO), a digitized pressure manometer, and the pre-determined stent and balloon. Prior to implantation the target vessel is examined externally and internally with a digital videoscope (Image 1 digital camera, Karl Storz Endoscopy, Culver City, CA), operated by the cardiac surgeon. Use of this imaging technique limits the amount of dissection required around the target vessel, thereby minimizing trauma to surrounding structures (e.g. phrenic nerve), shortening operative time, and preserving supporting tissue as the target vessel is forced to expand under the tension of the stent and balloon. The videoscopic images are compared with the pre-procedural angiograms which are available for viewing in the operating room through a digital network (Siemens ACOM NET, Erlangen, Germany) and the location of side branch take-offs and target vessel length are confirmed or altered accordingly. Based on these observations the surgeon and interventional cardiologist make a final decision regarding implantation diameter and the length of vessel to be covered by the stent.

The interventional cardiologist and technician then prepare the stent for delivery on the interventional table. The delivery balloon lumen is flushed with saline and the

balloon inflated and deflated using a manometer syringe filled with saline (there is no need for contrast media with this method). We find that refolding the balloon improves stent adherence to the lower profile delivery balloons which we prefer for this application. We prefer balloons with moderate burst pressures (8–12 atm) and low deflation profiles to minimize the possibility of stent dislodgement during balloon removal following implantation. Most commonly we employ Cordis Opta Pro and Power-flex balloons (Cordis Endovascular, Miami Lakes, FL) for this application. Balloons with larger deflation profiles (e.g. Z-Med, Numed, Hopkinton, NY) have been more difficult to remove after stent deployment and, on occasion, have resulted in intra-operative stent dislodgement requiring stent removal and replacement. We have tended *not* to utilize high pressure balloons and inflation pressures (> 14 atm) with this technique secondary to concerns about transmural vessel tear or rupture in this setting. The stent is hand crimped onto the delivery balloon in a similar fashion to percutaneous deployment. Our current preferred stent for this application is the Palmaz Genesis XD series (Cordis Endovascular, Miami Lakes, FL) with the length determined by the above described method. As discussed above, if the implantation diameter is restricted to < 6 mm (such as in a small baby or severely hypoplastic vessel and the child will require further surgery) we will use stents with smaller ultimate diameter potential (Palmaz Genesis medium

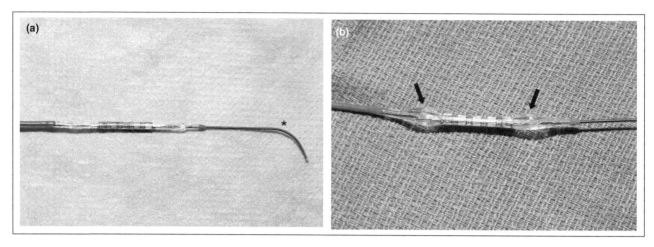

Figure 62.2
Genesis 1910B XD stent mounted on low profile balloon (Cordis Opta Pro) before (a) and after (b) slight inflation to create a 'dumbbell' (black arrows) shape on either side of the stent to secure the position on the balloon. Note the soft-tipped curved Wholey wire (*) which has been placed through the catheter lumen to assist with guiding the stent/balloon complex across the stenosis.

transhepatic biliary stent, Cordis Endovascular) secondary to concerns regarding early thrombosis and/or rapid neointimal build-up if a large stent is used in that situation. After crimping the stent onto the balloon, firm but gentle traction is placed on the stent to test for the possibility of stent slippage. This is particularly important since fluoroscopy is not used during stent deployment. Prior to deployment if the stent slips easily upon the balloon surface, the balloon is inflated slightly to form a 'dumbbell' shape, thereby further improving stent adherence (Figure 62.2). Since there is no requirement to fit the stent/balloon complex within a delivery sheath, the diameter of this partially inflated balloon is irrelevant. A slight 'hockey stick' curve is placed on the soft tip of a Wholey guidewire which is then advanced through the balloon lumen until a few centimeters extend from the balloon tip.

The entire apparatus is then moved over to the operating table with the interventional cardiologist positioned at the head of the patient, handling the front end of the stent/balloon complex, and the technician handling the manometer and back end of the balloon and wire toward the patient's feet. Access to the branch pulmonary arteries is provided by the surgeon either directly at the bifurcation (more distal lesions) or through a proximal anastomosis of a conduit whose distal anastomosis has already been completed. The balloon tip is positioned by the interventional cardiologist near the vessel orifice using a pair of forceps and the tip of the Wholey wire torqued (by the technician) to align with the course of the vessel to be stented. The wire tip is then gently advanced using the delivery forceps down the vessel lumen. If early resistance is encountered a different wire angle is tried until several centimeters of wire have been passed down into the distal vessel. With the back of the

wire held in place by the technician, the balloon-mounted stent is advanced to the target lesion by the interventional cardiologist, being careful not to damage either the stent or balloon with the forceps. Prior to deployment, positioning is checked with the videoscope (Figure 62.3). The balloon is then inflated to the manufacturer's rated burst pressure. Because it is not possible using this technique to visualize the entire length of the balloon/stent complex during the inflation, we suggest using a pressure manometer for this procedure and making sure that at a minimum the nominal pressure for complete balloon expansion is reached.

The balloon is deflated in the usual fashion and removed over the wire, which is left in place should further expansion of the stent be needed. The surgeon places gentle pressure on the proximal struts of the stent with a forceps during balloon removal to prevent accidental stent dislodgement. With the guidewire still in place, the videoscope is carefully passed down through the stented vessel to examine the result (Figure 62.3). Particular attention is paid to the appearance of any transmural tears, the degree of apposition of the stent to the vessel wall, the location and patency of any side branches in close proximity to the stent, and the integrity of any suture lines which were crossed by the stent. If further stent expansion is required due to residual stenosis or failure of complete stent apposition to the vessel wall, a second balloon with a higher inflation pressure or larger diameter can be advanced over the guidewire and inflated. For ostial lesions where a small amount of stent must protrude into the main pulmonary artery, the surgeon often will carefully flare the proximal struts by gently bending each cell with a forceps to better appose the device to the ostium of the vessel (Figure 62.4). This facilitates future catheter entry into the vessel as well as protects against stent migration. We

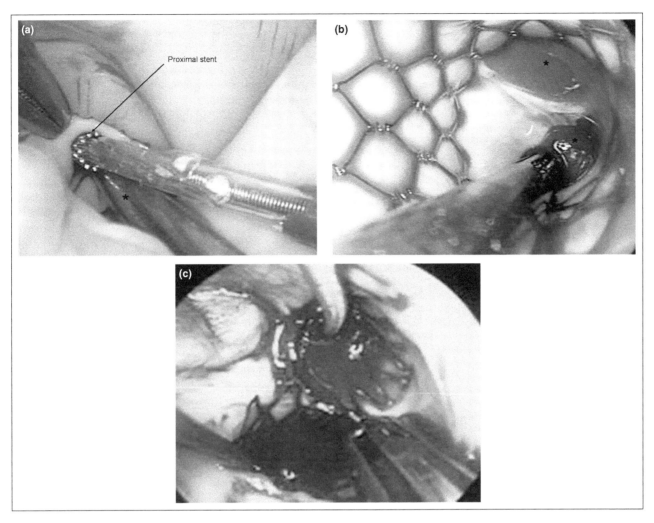

Figure 62.3
(a) Prior to inflation of the balloon the proximal stent is positioned using videoscopic guidance to cover the most proximal portion of the stenosis. The suction tip (*) is used to stabilize the pulmonary artery during positioning. (b) After stent expansion, apposition to the vessel wall and position in relation to side branch takeoff (*) are examined. (c) Final result of 'adult sized kissing stents' placed in the 6-month-old seen in Figure 62.1.

believe that cutting of the stent should be avoided as the sharp edges which result can make further balloon expansion in the catheter laboratory difficult secondary to balloon rupture. After final assessment with the videoscope, the guidewire is removed and the intervention completed.

Potential pitfalls

While this is a simple technique which offers several potential advantages over the more commonly performed percutaneous technique, this procedure places the interventional cardiology team in what is initially an unfamiliar environment using new types of equipment and eliminating such fundamental tools as angiography and fluoroscopy. Therefore, meticulous attention to detail, careful pre-procedural planning, and good co-operation with the surgical team are

all essential to a successful outcome. Because intraprocedural angiography is not used, one must be sure that the measurements made prior to the hybrid procedure are accurate. The most common causes for inaccurate vessel measurement are erroneous calibration for magnification and lack of proper profiling of a given vessel. These pitfalls must be avoided to have consistent success with hybrid stent implantation. As an example, we have experienced a case where underestimation of a pre-procedural measurement of a distal vessel diameter resulted in a late distal migration of an intra-operatively implanted stent which, in retrospect, we underexpanded. Use of a soft-tipped guidewire and avoidance of high inflation pressures are important safety measures to prevent vessel perforation, particularly from the distal tip of the balloon which is not visualized during inflation with this technique. Stents which fail to expand

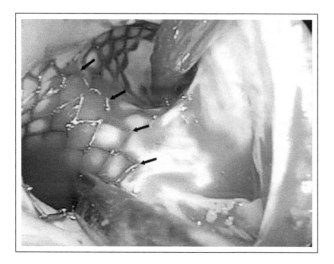

Figure 62.4
Following implantation of left (LPA) and right (RPA) proximal branch pulmonary artery stents, the proximal struts (arrows) of the RPA stent have been flared by the surgeon to facilitate future catheter passage in the RPA as well as limit the cutting effect these struts could have on future angioplasty balloons in the proximal LPA.

completely secondary to resistant stenoses can be left in place, with the intent of proceeding with high pressure balloon inflation at a later date using percutaneous techniques.

Institutional experience

Between October 1998 and September 2005 we utilized this approach to implant 33 stents into the pulmonary arteries of 27 patients. The median weight in this group was 16 kg (2.9–67 kg). There was one procedural failure in a child with previously implanted stents that were incompletely removed at another institution. The metal fragments from the partially removed stents repeatedly resulted in rupture of the implantation balloon and prevented hybrid stent placement. All other hybrid stent implant procedures were technically successful (96% success of implantation). There were no instances of excessive post-operative bleeding, suture disruption, or early stent migration. Later follow-up indicates maintenance of improved vessel diameters, minimal tissue build-up within stented vessels, and the consistent ability to further expand hybrid stents in a manner similar to stents placed percutaneously. The one instance of late stent migration was noted above and resulted in no clinical sequelae.

Stent implantation via surgically provided vascular access

A second hybrid approach to stent implantation involves the use of surgical techniques to provide a variety of access ports to place stents into otherwise difficult areas to reach within the vascular system. These procedures can be performed in either the catheterization laboratory or operating room, with or without the use of cardiopulmonary bypass. In our experience these techniques are typically utilized in two distinct groups of patients: (1) infants and neonates who are critically ill in the early post-operative period or (2) comparatively healthy outpatients presenting with unusual lesions or limited vascular access which makes conventional stent implantation impossible. The indications and advantages of this approach are similar to those noted above for videoscopic-guided stent implantation. These approaches, however, utilize fluoroscopy and angiography and allow access to a wider range of target vessels than the videoscopic hybrid technique. Using these approaches we have successfully placed stents to treat branch pulmonary artery stenoses, recurrent aortic arch obstruction, modified Blalock–Taussig, and central shunt stenosis/occlusion, and to create extracardiac Fontan fenestrations.

Cases are performed using general anesthesia with endotracheal intubation. Most cases begin with a diagnostic catheterization performed from a conventional access route (most often femoral artery or vein) if one is available. Based upon the particular lesion being treated and the patient's individual anatomy, the best access route for stent placement is chosen. The cardiac surgical team then enters the case and the appropriately sized introducer sheath (based upon the predicted balloon and stent which will be utilized) is placed under direct vision through an incision into the chosen access location. Vessels utilized for this purpose have included carotid artery, innominate vein, ascending aorta, and right ventricular outflow tract. Utilization of various vascular access routes is discussed in Chapter 2 and we will therefore confine our discussion in this section to the techniques used for stent implantation via surgically provided access through the open chest in a beating heart.

Pulmonary artery stent implantation via the right ventricular outflow tract

Significant residual branch pulmonary artery stenosis may result in unfavorable hemodynamics in the early post-operative period and negatively influence outcome.[24,25] It is our institutional bias that aggressive treatment of these types of stenoses is warranted and may significantly improve outcome in terms of hospital morbidity, mortality, and the long term fate of the right ventricle. Re-operation in this setting incurs more trauma, is technically difficult, and has limited success. Balloon angioplasty may be effective in the early post-operative period, however, its inherent unreliability coupled with the requirement to oversize balloons in order to achieve an effective result make it an unattractive option in critically ill post-operative patients. Stent implantation with

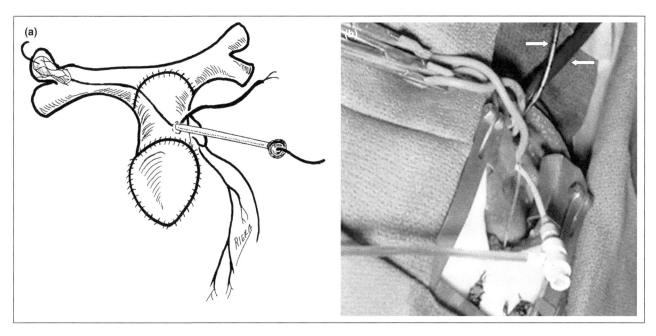

Figure 62.5
Diagrammatic representation (a) and digital photo (b) of sheath placement via an incision into a right ventricle–pulmonary artery homograft conduit of a patient with severe early pulmonary artery stenosis after complete repair of pulmonary atresia and ventricular septal defect. Note the arterial and venous cannulas (white arrows) required to perform this intervention on cardiopulmonary support.

its more predictable result can be hampered by the technical issues of implantation discussed previously. These issues may be compounded when the goal is to put in a stent capable of achieving adult diameter. We have found that implantation directly via the right ventricular outflow tract greatly facilitates stent placement in this group of patients.

Implantation technique   All of our experience with this procedure is in patients in the early post-operative period who arrive in the catheterization laboratory with their sternum open. Typically a diagnostic catheterization using femoral venous access is performed to delineate the hemodynamics and the post-operative anatomy. The surgical team then scrubs into the case and places a pursestring suture in the proximal right ventricular outflow tract. An arteriotomy is made with an 11 blade and a standard sheath and dilator are directly inserted through the arteriotomy (Figure 62.5). The dilator is removed and, after confirming proper position with fluoroscopy, the pursestring suture is tightened around the sheath to secure position. Care must be taken to ensure that enough distance exists between the tip of the sheath and the area to be stented so that the delivery balloon can be fully expanded without constraint from the sheath. Repeat angiography is performed through the side-arm of the sheath using non-diluted contrast media injected by hand (Figure 62.6). This injection is then used as a roadmap for performing stent implantation. A soft-tipped guide wire (typically a 0.035 inch Wholey or

Glide wire, Terumo Medical Corporation, Summerset, NJ) is then advanced across the stenosis with or without the assistance of a catheter as needed. The wire tip is positioned as far distally into a lower lobe branch as possible. This wire can then be exchanged for a slightly stiffer wire (0.035 inch Rosen guidewire, Boston Scientific Corporation, Natick, MA) to be used for stent positioning if needed. An appropriately sized stent is then chosen and hand-crimped upon a delivery balloon in the usual fashion. We always attempt to implant stents with 'adult size potential' whenever possible. Using this technique, sheath size is never a limiting factor. A delivery balloon diameter equal to the adjacent normal vessel diameter is chosen and overexpansion of the stent is avoided.

The stent/balloon complex is then advanced through the sheath, over the guidewire, and across the stenosis. It is often not necessary to 'protect' the stent/balloon complex with the sheath since the distance traveled is typically short and the catheter course straight. Serial angiography through the side-arm of the delivery sheath aids with precision of stent placement prior to deployment. The balloon is then inflated using a pressure manometer and the stent deployed. Angiography through the side-arm of the sheath is used to assess the adequacy of the result and, if deemed satisfactory, the delivery balloon is removed over the guidewire. A final angiogram is performed, the guidewire removed, and the surgical team then re-enters the case, removes the sheath, and repairs the arteriotomy. Minimal

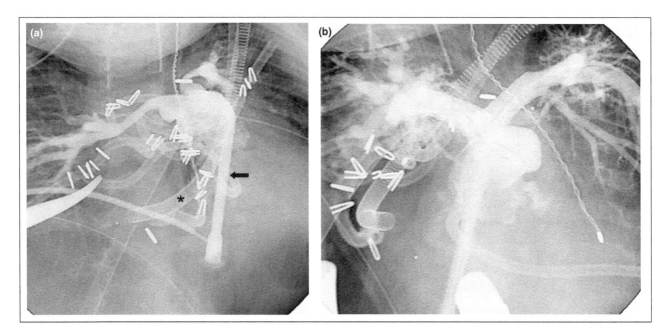

Figure 62.6

(a) Pulmonary angiogram performed through the side-arm of a sheath (arrow) in the right ventricular outflow tract in a 6.2 kg, 9-month-old following complete repair of pulmonary atresia using a homograft conduit. Note the severe hypoplasia of the branch pulmonary arteries as well as the presence of bypass cannulas (*) as this child required mechanical cardiopulmonary support for this procedure. (b) Repeat angiogram following placement of adult sized Genesis stents into both branch pulmonary arteries.

hemodynamics, including pressure measurements, are performed in these cases.

Advantages

Typically these children are young, small, and hemodynamically unstable with open chests. They may require mechanical cardiopulmonary support. In these instances we have found that the use of the right ventricular outflow tract for stent placement offers numerous important advantages, including freedom from sheath size constraints, simplification of the catheter course making passage of the rigid stents much simpler, and avoidance of tension upon the tricuspid valve and right ventricle. This results in the ability to implant larger stents more precisely in a shorter time with more stable patient hemodynamics during the case. It also ensures in-room surgical back-up should an untoward event occur.

Results

Between 1999 and 2004, 9 patients underwent placement of 10 pulmonary artery stents using this technique. The patients were generally small (median weight 6.2 kg) and all were critically ill, requiring mechanical ventilation and inotropic support, and on mechanical cardiopulmonary support in several cases. There were no procedural

complications or deaths. All stent placements were considered successful as judged by standard criteria as well as clinical improvement. In follow-up, all stents placed in this fashion have been amenable to further balloon expansion via conventional access routes and there have been no instances of late complications.

Aortic stent implantation via the right ascending aorta

Survival after stage 1 palliative surgery for hypoplastic left heart syndrome (HLHS) has improved remarkably over the past decade, however recurrent or residual aortic arch obstruction continues to be a common and serious problem.[26–28] Typically, aortic obstruction occurs in the area of the distal anastomosis of the aortic gusset with the thoracic aorta. In addition to upper body hypertension, aortic obstruction in this setting may result in a number of other undesirable physiologic effects including pulmonary overcirculation resulting in ventricular volume overload, systemic atrioventricular valve insufficiency, and diminished cardiac output. This constellation of hemodynamic abnormalities may be poorly tolerated by an already overburdened systemic right ventricle. Surgical revision of the distal aortic arch reconstruction is difficult and may not completely relieve the obstruction. Balloon angioplasty does not

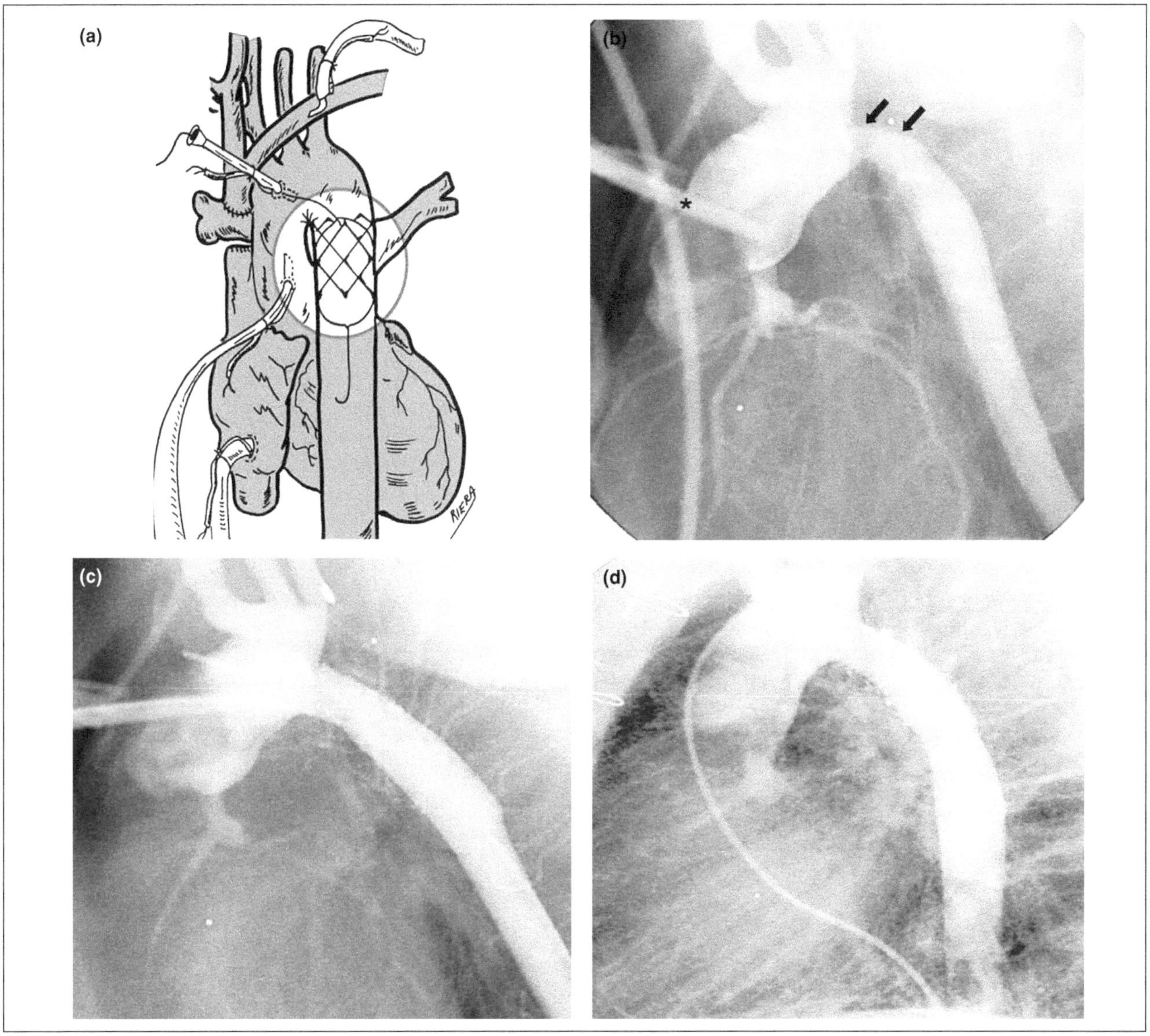

Figure 62.7

Hybrid stent implantation for treatment of resistant aortic re-obstruction after hypoplastic left heart palliation. Diagrammatic representation (a) demonstrating the location used for sheath placement in the distal ascending aorta. Aortogram (b) performed through the side-arm of the sheath (*) placed in the neo-ascending aorta demonstrating recurrent/residual distal aortic arch/isthmus hypolasia (black arrows). Follow-up aortogram (c) after hybrid stent implantation with a large Genesis stent showing improvement in hypoplastic aortic segment. Follow-up aortogram (d) performed following balloon expansion of the hybrid stent 3 years after implantation.

always provide long term relief and may carry an increased risk compared with simple recurrent coarctation angioplasty. In infants who have persistent aortic obstruction despite aortic angioplasty, we have utilized a hybrid approach to place adult sized stents into the aorta at the time of their cavo-pulmonary anastomosis.

Technique

These procedures are typically performed in the operating room using a portable digital C-arm for imaging, although we have performed one case in the catheterization laboratory. After dissecting out the neo-aortic root, but prior to placing the patient on bypass, the surgeon places a pursestring suture in the ascending neo-aorta. Via a small incision, a standard vascular sheath large enough to accommodate the stent/balloon complex is placed a short distance into the aorta (Figure 62.7). It is important that the access site leaves enough room for the sheath to be pulled back proximally enough as to not interfere with balloon inflation. After removing the dilator and de-airing the sheath an angiogram is performed by hand injection through the side-arm of the sheath using 20–30° of left anterior oblique (LAO) angulation. This image is stored to be used as a roadmap. Stent length and implantation diameter are chosen prior to the intervention based upon the pre-operative angiograms. Implant diameter is chosen to match the aortic diameter at the level of the diaphragm. Only stents with the potential to achieve adult diameter are used for this application. Currently we prefer the large Genesis XD stents in as short a length as possible due to the small size of these children (typically between 3 and 6 months of age). The stent is mounted and hand-crimped on a delivery balloon in the usual fashion employed for transcutaneous deployments. Using the initial angiogram as a roadmap, a 0.035 inch Wholey wire with a curved tip is advanced directly through the sheath, across the stenosis, and down into the descending aorta. Once again, due to the simplicity of the 'catheter course' a catheter is not needed. The balloon-mounted stent is advanced through the sheath over the guidewire until it straddles the stenosis. Because of the short, straight wire path we have not found it necessary to advance the sheath across the stenosis prior to or during passage of the stent. Once the stent is in position, serial angiography is used to confirm precise positioning and then the stent is deployed by manometer-guided balloon inflation. After removal of the balloon one final angiogram is performed and then the sheath and guidewire are removed by the surgeon and the small aortic incision closed. The remainder of the operation is then completed.

Advantages

This is a very simple technique that allows an adult sized stent to be placed into the aorta of a young infant when balloon angioplasty has not adequately alleviated recurrent aortic obstruction. It is far less traumatic than attempted repeat surgical repair and offers the possibility of a lifetime 'cure' with repeated stent expansion as the patient grows.

Results

To date we have performed this procedure in 8 children with successful stent implantation in all. There were no procedural complications. In follow-up all stents have been successfully redilated when needed, although the maximum follow-up to date is short. In the single case where a Double Strut LD stent (ev3, Plymouth, MN) was implanted we observed significant stent distortion when redilation was performed, prompting surgical removal of the stent at the time of the Fontan operation. We no longer use this device for this application. While we have seen no other evidence of stent failure in follow-up, unfortunately several of the patients who have undergone this procedure have had persistent poor ventricular function. This may represent the cumulative negative effects of early

continued arch obstruction after stage I palliation for hypoplastic left heart syndrome.

Conclusion

Most patients with structural heart disease can undergo successful stent implantation into a wide variety of vascular and intracardiac locations using standard percutaneous techniques. A select group which includes small children and neonates, hemodynamically unstable children, and those with poor vascular access may greatly benefit from the hybrid techniques described in this chapter. With experience these procedures are relatively simple to perform, require a minimal amount of inventory, and appear to provide excellent results. Careful consideration of the long term medical and surgical management of these patients as well as excellent communication between the interventional cardiologist and cardiac surgeon are mandatory for ultimate success.

References

1. Palmaz JC, Garcia OJ, Schatz RA et al. Placement of balloon-expandable intraluminal stents in iliac arteries: first 171 procedures. Radiology 1990; 174: 969–75.
2. O'Laughlin MP, Perry SB, Lock JE, Mullins CE. Use of endovascular stents in congenital heart disease. Circulation 1991; 83: 1923–39.
3. Moore JW, Kirby WC, Lovett EJ, O'Neill JT. Use of an intravascular endoprosthesis (stent) to establish and maintain short-term patency of the ductus arteriosus in newborn lambs. Cardiovasc Interven Radiol 1991; 14: 299–301.
4. Beekman RH, Muller DW, Reynolds PI et al. Balloon-expandable stent treatment of experimental coarctation of the aorta: early hemodynamic and pathological evaluation. J Interven Cardiol 1993; 6: 113–23.
5. Hosking MCK, Benson LN, Kakanishi T et al. Intravascular stent prosthesis for right ventricular outflow obstruction. J Am Coll Cardiol 1992; 20: 373–80.
6. O'Laughlin MP, Slack MC, Grifka RG et al. Implantation and intermediate-term follow-up of stents in congenital heart disease. Circulation 1993; 88: 605–14.
7. Benson LN, Nykanen D, Freedom RM. Endovascular stents in pediatric cardiovascular medicine. J Interven Cardiol 1995; 8: 767–75.
8. Akintuerk H, Michel-Behnke I, Valeske K et al. Stenting of the arterial duct and banding of the pulmonary arteries: basis for combined Norwood stage I and II repair in hypoplastic left heart. Circulation 2002; 105: 1099–103.
9. Boucek MM, Mashburn C, Chan KC. Catheter-based interventional palliation for hypoplastic left heart syndrome. Semin Thorac Cardiovasc Surg Pediatr Card Surg Ann 2005; 72–7.
10. Galantowicz M, Cheatham JP. Fontan completion without surgery. Semin Thorac Cardiovasc Surg Pediatr Card Surg Ann 2004; 7: 48–55.
11. Michel-Behnke I, Akintuerk H, Thul J et al. Stent implantation in the ductus arteriosus for pulmonary blood supply in congenital heart disease. Cathet Cardiovasc Interven 2004; 61(2): 242–52.
12. Alwi M, Choo KK, Latiff HA et al. Initial results and medium-term follow-up of stent implantation of patent ductus arteriosus in

duct-dependent pulmonary circulation. J Am Coll Cardiol 2004; 44(2): 438–45.

13. McMahon CJ, El Said HG, Vincent JA et al. Refinements in the implantation of pulmonary arterial stents: impact on morbidity and mortality of the procedure over the last two decades. Cardiol Young 2002; 12(5): 445–52.

14. Pass RH, Hsu DT, Garabedian CP et al. Endovascular stent implantation in the pulmonary arteries of infants and children without the use of a long vascular sheath. Cathet Cardiovasc Interven 2002; 55: 505–9.

15. Qureshi SA, Sivasankaran S. Role of stents in congenital heart disease. Expert Rev Cardiovasc Ther 2005; 3: 261–9.

16. Houde C, Zahn EM, Benson LN et al. Intraoperative placement of endovascular stents (letter). J Thorac Cardiovasc Surg 1992; 104: 530–2.

17. Mendelsohn AM, Bove EL, Lupinetti FM et al. Intraoperative and percutaneous stenting of congenital pulmonary artery and vein stenosis. Circulation 1993; 88(5 Pt 2): II210–17.

18. Bokenkamp R, Blom NA, De WD et al. Intraoperative stenting of pulmonary arteries. Eur J Cardiothorac Surg 2005; 27: 544–7.

19. Ungerleider RM, Johnston TA, O'Laughlin MP et al. Intraoperative stents to rehabilitate severely stenotic pulmonary vessels. Ann Thorac Surg 2001; 71: 476–81.

20. Zahn EM, Dobrolet NC, Nykanen DG et al. Interventional catheterization performed in the early postoperative period after congenital heart surgery in children. J Am Coll Cardiol 2004; 43: 1264–9.

21. Lardo AC. Real-time magnetic resonance imaging: diagnostic and interventional applications. Pediatr Cardiol 2000; 21: 80–98.

22. Fogelman R, Nykanen D, Smallhorn JF et al. Clinical impact on management and medium-term follow-up. Circulation 1995; 92(4): 881–5.

23. Duke C, Rosenthal E, Qureshi SA. The efficacy and safety of stent redilatation in congenital heart disease. Heart 2003; 89(8): 905–12.

24. Chau AK, Leung MP. Management of branch pulmonary artery stenosis: balloon angioplasty or endovascular stenting. Clin Exp Pharmacol Physiol 1997; 24(12): 960–2.

25. Hosking MC, Thomaidis C, Hamilton R et al. Clinical impact of balloon angioplasty for branch pulmonary arterial stenosis. Am J Cardiol 1992; 69(17): 1467–70.

26. Soongswang J, McCrindle BW, Jones TK et al. Outcomes of transcatheter balloon angioplasty of obstruction in the neo-aortic arch after the Norwood operation. Cardiol Young 2001; 11(1): 54–61.

27. Tworetzky W, McElhinney DB, Burch GH et al. Balloon arterioplasty of recurrent coarctation after the modified Norwood procedure in infants. Cathet Cardiovasc Interven 2000; 50(1): 54–8.

28. Zeltser I, Menteer J, Gaynor JW et al. Impact of re-coarctation following the Norwood operation on survival in the balloon angioplasty era. J Am Coll Cardiol 2005; 45(11): 1844–8.

Section XIV

Left atrial appendage closure

63

PLAATO device

Yves Laurent Bayard, Reinhardt M Becht, Stephan H Ostermayer, and Horst Sievert

Anatomy and pathology

The left atrial appendage (LAA) is a small, muscular saccu-lation of the left atrium (LA) located between the left upper pulmonary vein and the left ventricle, overlapping the prox-imal left circumflex artery. It is a derivative of the primitive atrium and has a wide anatomic variability. Its size ranges from 20 to 45 mm in length and 15 to 35 mm in orifice diameter.[1] In more than two-thirds of the population the LAA consists of two or more lobes originating from one common orifice. Among other cardiac structures the left atrial appendage releases atrionatriuretic peptide (ANP), a polypeptide promoting diuresis.

Whereas the LAA plays a rather minor role under physio-logic circumstances, it gains in importance in patients with atrial fibrillation. Several surgical, echocardiographic, and autopsy studies have shown that more than 90% of all thrombi in patients with non-rheumatic atrial fibrillation forming in the LA are isolated to, or originate in the LAA.[2] Therefore, occluding this anatomic structure is a logical approach to preventing thrombus formation and subse-quent cardioembolic events in these patients.

Indication for treatment and alternative options

Despite other therapeutic options such as cardioversion, catheter ablation, or long term antiplatelet therapy, antico-agulation still remains the treatment of choice in the major-ity of atrial fibrillation patients who are at high risk for ischemic stroke.[3] Warfarin or coumadin reduces the inci-dence of stroke significantly. However, many patients have contraindications for this treatment or do not receive war-farin due to various other reasons.[4,5] Thus, transcatheter closure of the LAA should be considered in high risk atrial fibrillation patients who cannot receive or refuse to take long term anticoagulation treatment.

History

The first surgical attempt to remove the LAA as a possible source for a thromboembolic event was made by Madden in 1948.[6] Nowadays, surgical obliteration or resection of the LAA is usually not performed as a stand-alone procedure because of its invasive character. However, it is part of the Maze procedure, a surgical approach to interrupt the con-duction of abnormal impulses of atrial fibrillation to the atrioventricular node, and also recommended by the American College of Cardiology and the American Heart Association guidelines during mitral valve surgery.[7,8] Percutaneous LAA closure was introduced into clinical practice in 2001 using the PLAATO™ system (Percutaneous Left Atrial Appendage Transcatheter Occlusion) (ev3, Inc., Plymouth, MN, USA).[9] The results of the PLAATO™ feasibility study published in July 2005 showed that this new procedure is feasible and that it can be performed at acceptable risk.[10]

Patient screening and preparations

Prior to the procedure it is mandatory to perform trans-esophageal echocardiography (TEE) in order to exclude thrombi in the LAA. Furthermore, information regarding the size and morphology of the LAA should be obtained. The orifice diameter of the appendage must be in the range between 13.6 mm and 26.5 mm for a safe positioning of the occluder. As for pre-procedure medication, we recommend aspirin 300 mg twice a day 48 hours prior to the procedure and a loading dose of clopidogrel 300 mg (or, if not suitable,

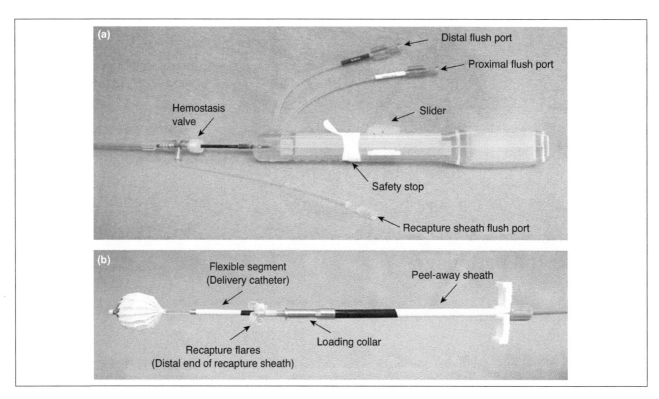

Figure 63.1
(a) Proximal part of the delivery system. (b) Distal part of the delivery system.

ticlopidine 250 mg). Endocarditis prophylaxis should be administered one hour prior to the intervention.[11]

Procedure

The PLAATO™ system consists of three different components: the implant, its delivery catheter, and an especially designed 12 Fr transseptal sheath (Figure 63.1a,b). The implant comprises a self-expanding nitinol cage laminated with impermeable expanded polytetrafluoroethylene (ePTFE) in order to exclude the appendage from circulation. It is available in diameters ranging from 20 to 32 mm. Three rows of small hooks along the struts provide a stable position of the device post-implantation (Figure 63.2). The delivery catheter offers proximal and distal dye injection ports as well as a control mechanism to expand, collapse, and release the implant throughout the procedure. It also includes a recapture sheath which may be used to safely withdraw the device if necessary. The 12 Fr transseptal sheath contains a Mullins-like primary curve to cross the septum and a distal anterior curve to reach the distal part of the LAA.

Percutaneous appendage occlusion can be performed under either general or local anesthesia. After venous groin access transseptal puncture is performed using standard techniques. Septal puncture should be performed as inferior

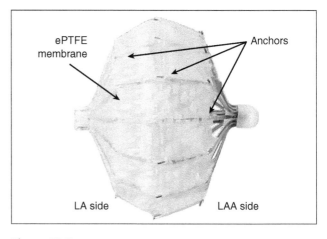

Figure 63.2
The PLAATO™ implant: nitinol framework, ePTFE covering, small anchors along the struts stabilize the occluder in the orifice of the appendage. LA, left atrium; LAA, left atrial appendage.

as safely possible (Figure 63.3). After successful puncture verified by pressure monitoring, 10 000 units of heparin are administered in order to keep the activated clotting time above 250 seconds. For the first dye injection into the appendage ('appendogram') we suggest a 4 Fr angulated pigtail catheter. It allows for deep and safe positioning of the

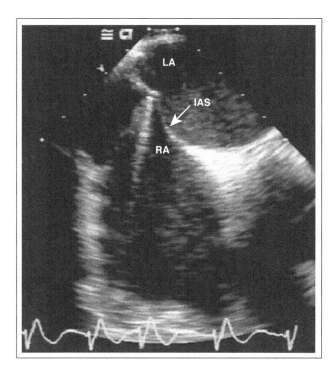

Figure 63.3
Transesophageal echocardiogram: transseptal puncture should be performed as inferior as safely possible using standard techniques. IAS, interatrial septum; LA, left atrium; RA, right atrium.

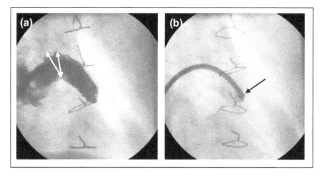

Figure 63.4
Angiogram of the LAA. (a) After venous and transseptal puncture a specially designed transseptal sheath is advanced into the LAA; dye injection provides information on the diameter of the ostium (arrows) and the morphology of the LAA. (b) The radio-opaque marker at the distal end of the sheath (diameter 4.4 mm) is used for calibration (arrow). LAA, left atrial appendage.

Table 63.1 *Implant selection*	
LAA orifice diameter (mm)	PLAATO™ implant (mm)
13.6–15.5	20
15.6–17.5	23
17.6–19.5	26
19.6–21.5	29
21.6–26.5	32

catheter and reduces the risk of perforation. An extra stiff J-tip 0.035 inch exchange guidewire is inserted into the LAA via the pigtail catheter and remains in the appendage during the positioning of the 12 Fr PLAATO™ transseptal sheath. After carefully advancing the tip of the sheath into the appendage, additional dye injections in several planes allow for assessment of the maximum diameter within the proximal part (5–10 mm) of the LAA. According to our experience the most helpful views are 30° right anterior oblique (RAO)/15° cranial (CRAN), RAO, caudal (CAUD) and anterior posterior (AP) (Figure 63.4a). The sheath's diameter (4.4 mm) serves as a reference for calibration (Figure 63.4b). According to the appendogram a suitable device is chosen (Table 63.1). The occluder should be oversized by 20–50%. A too large device results in incomplete seal of the LAA since the ePTFE membrane is not completely stretched between the struts of the device.

Preparation of the device requires loading the implant and flushing the entire delivery system. To load the implant the device has to be collapsed by entirely retracting the slider of the control handle. In order to move the slider it has to be mildly pressed down. Small detents in the control handle with increments of approximately 1 to 2 mm inhibit the slider from spontaneous movement. After retracting the slider, the implant is pulled through the loading collar into the introducer so the distal hub of the occluder matches the

black portion of the introducer. Now the loading collar can be removed and discarded. Before flushing the system with heparinized saline, three-way stopcocks are attached to all flush ports. The ports are flushed in the order of recapture sheath, distal port, and proximal port with 20 ml of saline, respectively. While flushing the proximal port the black portion of the introducer should be squeezed to mobilize air pockets from the collapsed occluder. Before the delivery system is introduced into the transseptal sheath, it is helpful to fill the sheath with dye to confirm a proper sheath position in the distal portion of the appendage. Thereby small amounts of contrast are emitted from the sheath while the occluder is advanced, confirming a stable sheath position. Saline injection into the proximal flush port during insertion of the delivery system prevents air bubbles from entering the sheath. After advancing the entire delivery system 20 cm into the sheath, fluoroscopy is used to assess for remaining bubbles. If necessary, they can be aspirated via the distal and/or proximal injection port with regard to the position of the bubbles. In this case, it is important to flush the system again to avoid blood clotting in the sheath. Insert the delivery catheter completely into the recapture sheath until the delivery handle is in contact with the hemostasis valve. The hemostasis valve has to be opened a quarter turn whenever the delivery system is manipulated and closed thereafter to avoid air insertion.

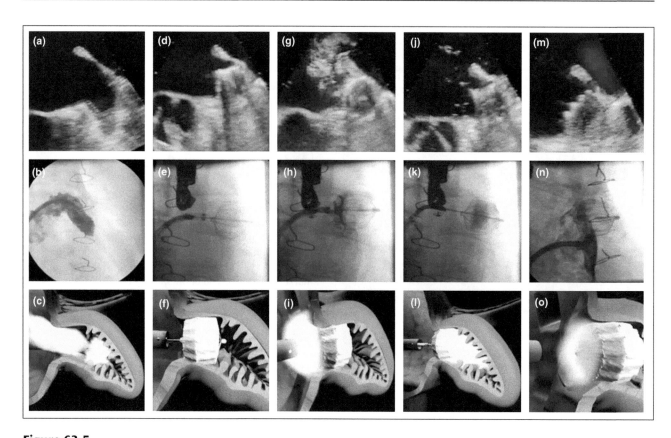

Figure 63.5

Device implantation step by step. (a)–(c) Assessment of LAA morphology. Measure the LAA orifice diameter by TEE (a) and angiography (b) to choose appropriate device size (see Table 63.1). Exclude possible thrombi in the LAA. (d)–(f) Positioning and expansion of the device. Make sure that at least two rows of anchors are engaged in the LAA tissue. Perform proximal (g–i) and distal (j–l) dye injections to assess the seal quality of the occluder (see Table 63.3). After a successful device stability test, the PLAATO™ occluder is released from its delivery catheter. To assess the final leak status, color Doppler (m) is used and a final dye injection (n, o) is performed. LAA, left atrial appendage; TEE, transesophageal echocardiogram. (See also color plate section.)

The occluder is advanced towards the tip of the sheath within the LAA so that the tip of the device reaches the marker band of the PLAATO™ sheath. Distal contrast injections are useful to reconfirm the optimal position of the device before the sheath is retrieved, exposing the occluder. The device is expanded under fluoroscopy by slowly advancing the slider of the control handle until no further expansion is noticed. Five criteria must be met before releasing the device: (1) position of the occluder, (2) anchor engagement in LAA tissue on TEE, (3) residual compression of the device, (4) seal quality, and (5) stability of the occluder.

TEE immediately shows the initial position of the implant in relation to the LAA (criterion 1) (Figure 63.5d). To ensure a stable position of the device, at least two rows of anchors must be engaged in the tissue (criterion 2). For an objective measurement of the residual compression, it is important to relieve tension of the delivery system. Therefore, the slider is retracted until an increase in resistance is felt. Now the slider is re-advanced by three detents. The hemostasis valve of the recapture sheath is opened.

Applying gentle tension on the delivery handle will mobilize a dot marker at the distal end of the delivery catheter within the implant. This indicates that the compression of the device is no longer applied by the catheter, but its surrounding structures (tissue of the appendage). Measurement of the maximum expanded diameter of the implant at the central row of anchors must show a minimum residual compression of 10% (Table 63.2) (criterion 3). Before performing the proximal dye injection to evaluate the seal quality (Figure 63.5h), the transseptal sheath is slightly advanced towards the occluder to provide for optimal visualization. To prepare the distal contrast injection (Figure 63.5k), the transseptal sheath is withdrawn beyond the radio-opaque flexible catheter section. The distal injection has to be performed very gently to avoid LAA perforation. Successful occlusion of the LAA is defined as 'mild' to 'absent leak' (Table 63.3) (criterion 4).

If sealing quality is adequate, a stability test is performed under angiography and TEE control. To avoid any interference with the occluder, the distance between its proximal

Table 63.2 *Residual compression guidelines*

Implant size (mm)	Maximum expanded implant diameter (mm)
20	18
23	20.7
26	23.4
29	26.1
32	28.8

Table 63.3 *Graduation of LAA seal quality after proximal dye injection over five or fewer ventricular beats*

Trace to absent leak	Barely or no detectable blush of dye flowing into the LAA
Mild leak	Well defined dye flow filling one-third of the LAA
Moderate leak	Well defined dye flow filling two-thirds of the LAA
Severe leak	Single or multiple sources of dye flow completely filling the LAA

LAA, left atrial appendage.

hub and the tip of the transseptal sheath must be at least 10 mm. While maintaining the position of the sheath, the deployment handle is now alternately retracted and advanced 5–10 mm. There should be no movement of the device within the LAA, whereas there might be some movement of the device and its surrounding structures as a whole (criterion 5).

To release the implant from the delivery system, the transseptal sheath is re-advanced to the proximal hub of the device. The safety stop (white plastic clip) is removed from the control handle and the slider completely advanced. Thereafter the delivery system is retracted so that the recapture shaft is completely withdrawn from the LA into the transseptal sheath. This may result in a minor change of device alignment within the LAA. Now the delivery system can be completely removed through the transseptal sheath. A final proximal dye injection (Figure 63.5n) as well as transesophageal Doppler color flow (Figure 63.5m) assess the degree of LAA occlusion.

If the implant position or occlusion of the LAA is suboptimal, the device can be collapsed and repositioned in the LAA. Under fluoroscopy, advance the deployment handle to place the recapture shaft radio-opaque marker at the distal hub of the implant. Align the distal end of the transseptal sheath with the distal end of the flexible segment and retract the slider until the implant has been collapsed to approximately one-third or less of its expanded diameter. The implant can now be repositioned and re-expanded. Do not attempt to reposition the device without first collapsing it!

If the result after repositioning is not satisfying, the device can be recaptured and an occluder of different size can be chosen. For recapture, the introducer is split up to its black portion and advanced completely towards the valve of the transseptal sheath. After the hemostasis valve is opened, the recapture sheath is advanced into the transseptal sheath while the delivery catheter remains in its stable position. When the half marker band of the recapture sheath is on a level with the marker band of the transseptal sheath, the flares of the recapture sheath are exposed out of the transseptal sheath. Thereafter, the device is collapsed completely and removed into the recapture sheath until increased resistance is noticed. The occluder is then approximately half way inside the recapture sheath (Figure 63.6). After the hemostasis valve is locked again, the entire delivery system can be withdrawn from the transseptal sheath. While this is done the flares will fold over the anchors of the device and allow secure recovery of the occluder. It is important to maintain access of the transseptal sheath within the LA for additional attempts. The 4 Fr pigtail catheter in combination with the extra stiff guidewire may be used once again to access the distal portion of the LAA before another occluder is inserted.

Follow-up and medication

Patients should be followed with chest X-ray, transthoracic echocardiogram, and clinical examination before hospital discharge, at 1 and 6 months' follow-up. Furthermore, we recommend TEE after 1 and 6 months to assess for implant position, LAA occlusion, and exclusion of thrombus formation on the device.

Post-procedure, we suggest clopidogrel (75 mg) and an endocarditis prophylaxis for the first 6 months. Aspirin (300–325 mg) should be prescribed on a continuing basis.

Complications and management

Pericardial effusion (2.5%) and *tamponade* (2.5%) are the most common complications. They are mainly observed in centers that are beginning their learning curve with the PLAATO™ procedure and are seen less frequently as experience increases. Transesophageal echocardiographic guidance can be very helpful to assure a safe transseptal puncture site. After needle crossing, pressure monitoring is useful to confirm LA position before the transseptal sheath is advanced. We avoid the use of end-hole catheters to approach the LAA and routinely use a pigtail catheter for safe and deep insertion into the LAA. In addition, only J-tip guidewires are used for catheter exchange.

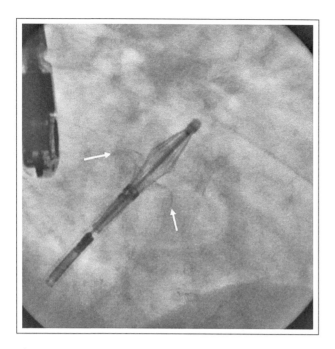

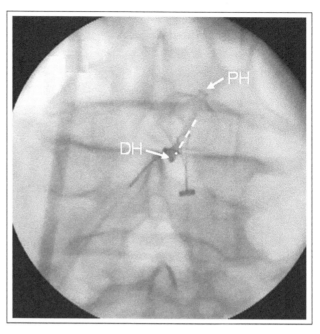

Figure 63.6

Device recapture: the recapture sheath is advanced into the transseptal sheath while the delivery catheter remains in a stable position. The flares of the recapture sheath (arrows) are exposed and the device is completely collapsed and removed half way into the recapture sheath. The flares cover the anchors at the surface of the occluder and allow a secure retraction of the implant.

Figure 63.7

In case of embolization, the device's inner guide tube (dashed line) and distal hub (no ePTFE covering) may be snared. It is important not to capture the proximal hub since the device anchors point in its direction. DH, distal hub; PH, proximal hub. In this picture, the second snare is not attached to the occluder.

Standard management consists of the administration of protamin and/or pericardiocentesis. However, if the device is already positioned in the LAA, the procedure may still be completed after adequate protamin administration.

Thrombi of a filiform, floating character were occasionally noted during the procedure for two reasons. In the cases observed so far, heparin was not given immediately after successful transseptal puncture while the procedure was continued with the 12 Fr transseptal sheath. The thrombi seen were located between the tip of the sheath and the surface of the occluder. It is obvious that adequate heparin administration and timing play an important role. The other cause was that the sheath was not flushed with saline after successful aspiration of an air bubble and blood through the delivery system. While the device was advanced within the sheath afterwards, a fresh thrombus was pushed out of the sheath.

If the thrombus is detected while the device is still within the transseptal sheath, we recommend retrieving the device from the sheath and attempting aspiration of the thrombus by applying a gentle vacuum in order not to destroy it. It can be helpful to slightly advance the sheath towards the thrombus to allow for aspiration. If the thrombus is located between the sheath and the surface of the occluder we do not recommend collapsing the device before the thrombus

has been removed. If these attempts fail, thrombolysis should be initiated.

Embolization of the PLAATO™ occluder represents a possible, but rare complication. In the total experience of more than 350 procedures performed worldwide this occurred only in two patients in whom the release criteria were not fully met. It seems that the residual compression (Table 63.2) in particular plays a major role since in both cases the compression of the occluder was less than 10% during measurement. The devices ended up in the aorta and were retrieved in the cath lab. We recommend using a large introducer sheath with a minimum of 13 Fr placed into the femoral artery. The distal end of the introducer should be dilated using a 5 mm balloon catheter to create a mouth-like entry for the device. The device should be retrieved with a snare. It is important to snare the distal hub of the device in order to allow retrieval into the sheath (Figure 63.7). A second snare introduced either from the same or contralateral femoral artery side may be useful to center the device during its retrieval into the arterial introducer sheath. The device can be withdrawn into the introducer and removed from the patient.

Thrombus formation on the occluder during the healing process is a rare complication that may be detected by TEE during early follow-up. In our experience, these thrombi were firmly attached to the device surface and not of a mobile or floating character (Figure 63.8). Continuous administration of aspirin and clopidogrel or low-molecular-weight heparin alone was effective in resolving these thrombi.

Tips and tricks

In bent appendages, or when the angle of the transseptal sheath is not coaxial to the LAA, the transition catheter (part of the transseptal sheath kit) can be used to induce a round and less traumatic shape of the tip of the sheath when advancing it.

Besides the orifice diameter, the length and shape of the appendage can influence device selection as well. In the case of a wide, but short appendage, a smaller device could potentially be introduced further than the device which is recommended by the sizing table (Table 63.1). However, the implant release criteria, in particular the residual compression of the occluder, must be met before the device can be released!

Advancing the sheath too far into the LA usually directs the device downwards and may result in a malalignment of the implant within the LAA. If the device is tilted downwards after expansion, too much catheter load in the left atrium could be the cause. We recommend recollapsing the device partially and retracting the entire delivery system including the sheath. During re-expansion of the device, traction should be maintained on the sheath until the first anchors become engaged within the tissue of the LAA.

In our experience, it is also possible to use a patent foramen ovale (PFO) or an atrial septal defect (ASD) to access the left atrium. However, in this case, the curve of the transseptal sheath might be more acute than crossing through a mid to low puncture of the fossa ovalis. Kinks in the sheath due to this curve can be eliminated while advancing the delivery system into the LAA very cautiously.

References

1. Veinot JP, Harrity PJ, Gentile F et al. Anatomy of the normal left atrial appendage. Circulation 1997; 96: 3112–15.
2. Blackshear JL, Odell JA. Appendage obliteration to reduce stroke in cardiac surgical patients with atrial fibrillation. Ann Thorac Surg 1996; 61: 755–9.

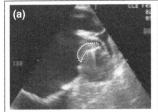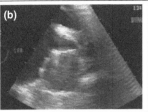

Figure 63.8
(a) Thrombus formation (dashed line) on the occluder noted at the 6-month follow-up TEE. It was firmly attached to the device surface and not of a mobile or floating character. (b) It was resolved without sequelae for the patient under continuous clopidogrel and aspirin administration at the 12-month follow-up. TEE, transesophageal echocardiogram.

3. Fuster V, Rydén LE, Asinger RW et al. ACC/AHA/ESC guidelines for the management of patients with atrial fibrillation: executive summary. A report of the American College of Cardiology/American Heart Association Task Force on practice guidelines and the European Society of Cardiology Committee for practice guidelines and policy conferences (Committee to develop guidelines for the management of patients with atrial fibrillation). Circulation 2001; 104: 2118–50.
4. Stafford RS, Singer DE. National patterns of warfarin use in atrial fibrillation. Arch Intern Med 1996; 156: 2537–41.
5. Bungard TJ, Ghali WA, Teo KK et al. Why do patients with atrial fibrillation not receive warfarin? Arch Intern Med 2000; 160: 41–6.
6. Madden J. Resection of the left auricular appendix. JAMA 1948; 140: 769–72.
7. Cox JL. The surgical treatment of atrial fibrillation. IV. Surgical technique. J Thorac Cardiovasc Surg 1991; 101: 584–92.
8. Bonow RO, Carabello B, de Leon AC et al. ACC/AHA guideline for the management of patients with valvular heart disease: A report of the American College of Cardiology/American Heart Association Task Force on practice guidelines (Committee on management of patients with valvular heart disease). J Am Coll Cardiol 1998; 32: 1486–1582.
9. Sievert H, Lesh MD, Trepels T et al. Percutaneous left atrial appendage transcatheter occlusion to prevent stroke in high-risk patients with atrial fibrillation – early clinical experience. Circulation 2002; 105: 1887–9.
10. Ostermayer SH, Reisman M, Kramer PH et al. Percutaneous left atrial appendage transcatheter occlusion (PLAATO system) to prevent stroke in high-risk patients with non-rheumatic atrial fibrillation: results from the international multi-center feasibility trials. J Am Coll Cardiol 2005; 46: 9–14.
11. Dajani AS, Taubert KA, Wilson W et al. Prevention of bacterial endocarditis: recommendations by the American Heart Association. Circulation 1997; 96: 358–66.

64

Amplatzer devices

Bernhard Meier

Introduction

The quest is obvious to combine the excellent idea of percutaneous exclusion of the left atrial appendage to obviate the need for chronic oral anticoagulation[1] with the general ease of Amplatzer (AGA Medical Corporation, Golden Valley, Minnesota, USA) shunt closure device implantations. After initial experiments with cadaver hearts (Figure 64.1) a first clinical case was performed on 15 June, 2002.[2] This constituted the first left atrial appendage closure worldwide in an awake patient without transesophageal echocardiographic guidance (Figure 64.2).

Technique for left atrial appendage occlusion using Amplatzer devices

A transesophageal echocardiogram excluding mobile thrombi in the left atrial appendage is a prerequisite before embarking on a percutaneous left atrial appendage occlusion. Absence of thrombus is once more ascertained by an angiogram before entering the left atrial appendage (Figure 64.3). The intervention is carried out from a right femoral vein puncture under local anesthesia without echocardiographic guidance; 5000 units of heparin are given at the beginning of the procedure. Intravenous antibiotics are recommended during and once or twice after the procedure (unless it is done as an outpatient intervention).

Save in the presence of a patent foramen ovale, which should be closed on the way out (Figure 64.4), a transseptal puncture is carried out.

The transseptal technique recommended is explained in Figure 64.5. Injection of contrast medium through the puncture needle is used to identify the proper site for puncture and also stain the interatrial septum for a landmark during the procedure. This avoids the need to look

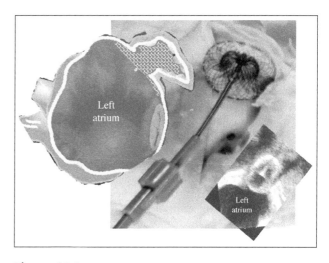

Figure 64.1
Principle of occluding a left atrial appendage with Amplatzer atrial septal defect occluders, patent foramen ovale occluders, or ventricular septal defect occluders using the pacifier approach. The proximal disk is used like the pacifier plate in front of the mouth of a baby to make sure the entire left atrial appendage is excluded from the circulation. The distal disk is supposed to conform to the variable left atrial appendage anatomy acting at the same time as an anchor or retainer (left insert). The photograph shows an aspect of an implanted device from the left atrium in a cadaver heart. The insert at the bottom right displays the transesophageal echocardiographic appearance 6 months after implantation in a patient, with the circumference of the proximal disk dotted.

for specific markers on an X-ray still frame, hook the needle up to an ECG, or observe pressures during the procedure.

In many cases the slightly curved Amplatzer introducer advanced over a wire placed in the left atrium will directly cannulate the left atrial appendage. In case of failure to do

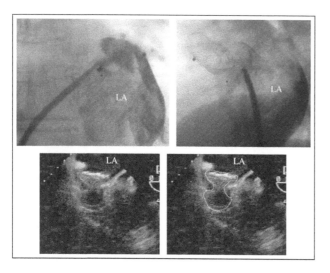

Figure 64.2

First Amplatzer left atrial appendage occlusion in a 63-year-old butcher with chronic atrial fibrillation who declined oral anticoagulation for professional reasons. The top panel shows the 30 mm Amplatzer atrial septal defect occluder implanted in the left atrial appendage in a frontal (left) and lateral (right) projection with faint dye opacification of the left atrium delineating the snug position of the proximal disk (pacifier principle). The bottom panels show a transesophageal echocardiographic follow-up examination at 1 year revealing a perfect fit with complete occlusion of the left atrial appendage (LA). The device is outlined in the right panel for clarification.

so or inability to avoid a pulmonary vein originating opposite the transseptal puncture site, a right Judkins or multi-purpose diagnostic coronary catheter can be inserted through the introducer to selectively look for the left atrial appendage (Figure 64.6).

For small left atrial appendages the devices can be introduced through steerable, large bore, coronary guiding catheters (Figure 64.7).

Before releasing the device from the pusher cable it is fairly vigorously wiggled (Kurt Amplatz refers to this as the 'Minnesota wiggle'). If the proximal but not the distal part of the device wiggles or if the entire left atrial appendage participates in the motion with the device, the position is considered stable.

An alternative approach to the pacifier position is a perpendicular double disk position in the neck of the left atrial appendage (Figures 64.7–64.9). The double disk position has the advantage of no material in the left atrium itself, but the disadvantage of leaving part of the neck of the left atrial appendage open. It will probably also have a higher risk of residual shunt, as shown in Figure 64.9.

The position of the device can be checked at all times with hand injections of contrast medium through the introducer. Care has to be taken to keep the introducer bubble-free and clot-free.

After the intervention the patient is ambulated within a few hours. Before discharge, which may be the same day, a chest X-ray is obtained to exclude device embolization following the procedure. Acetylsalicylic acid is prescribed for 5 months and clopidogrel for 1 month; prophylaxis against endocarditis is instructed for a few months. A transesophageal echocardiogram is recommended at 6 months. If the left atrial appendage is completely occluded (Figure 64.10), no further anticoagulation or platelet inhibition is required.

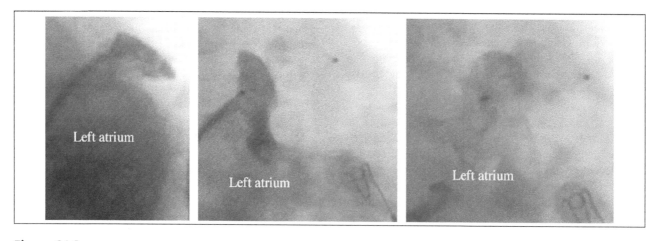

Figure 64.3

Left: angiogram by hand injection through the introducer of the left atrial appendage of a 72-year-old male, currently in sinus rhythm. Center: repeat contrast injection before release of an 18 mm Amplatzer atrial septal defect occluder. Note that the peripheral disk assumes the shape of the left atrial appendage ('Snoopy' shape). Right: final injection through the introducer before removing it after release of the device.

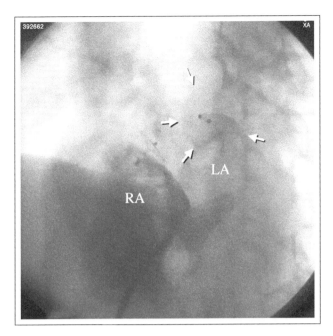

Figure 64.4
Left atrial appendage occlusion with a 20 mm Amplatzer atrial septal defect occluder (arrows) and incidental patent foramen ovale occlusion with an 18 mm Amplatzer patent foramen ovale occluder through the same 8 Fr introducer. LA, left atrium; RA, Right atrium.

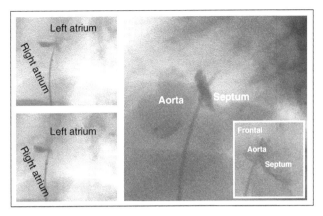

Figure 64.5
Transseptal technique using a 6 Fr curved Mullins sheath without side-arm and a transseptal needle. The Mullins sheath is placed below the aortic valve and advanced against the septum in a lateral projection. The needle is advanced to the end of the sheath and a small amount of contrast medium is injected through it. When tenting of the interatrial septum is observed with a direction of the needle towards 1 o'clock in a lateral view (top left), the needle is passed through the septum and an additional dye injection used to confirm the position in the left atrium (bottom left). Further confirmation can be obtained by the pressure tracing or by aspirating arterial blood. The Mullins sheath is then placed in the left atrium to allow for a regular guidewire to be advanced into the left atrium. The advantage of a lateral projection is shown in the right panel, which shows a lateral view of the anatomy of the interatrial septum stained with contrast medium and its relation to the aortic root also stained during initial attempts to puncture the interatrial septum. In contrast to the frontal view (insert at the bottom right), there is no overlap in the lateral projection.

Device selection for Amplatzer left atrial appendage occlusion

Figure 64.11 depicts standard shapes of Amplatzer shunt occluders. Devices created for closure of an atrial septal defect, a patent foramen ovale, a ventricular septal defect, a patent ductus arteriosus, or other arteriovenous fistulae can be employed for occlusion of the left atrial appendage (Figure 64.12). However, none of these devices appears ideal for that indication.

A recently developed tissue-free left atrial appendage plug is currently under clinical investigation (Figure 64.13). A clinical application of the dedicated Amplatzer left atrial appendage occluder is depicted in Figure 64.9.

The idea of featuring hooks that will disengage in case the device has to be removed for replacement (Figure 64.14) has been discarded because of the risk of perforation and pericardial bleeding. This complication, germane to other devices for left atrial appendage closure is less of a threat with Amplatzer devices.

Complications with Amplatzer left atrial appendage occlusion

In the first 40 cases, complications encountered were restricted to device embolizations. Three embolizations occurred due to technical errors. In two, the device unfolded awkwardly. This was recognized in one case but thought to be of no importance (Figure 64.15) and not recognized in the other (Figure 64.16).

The only embolization that did not occur during implantation due to poor technique or malfunction, was found in an asymptomatic patient at 7 months after an initially successful implantation. The routine follow-up transesophageal echocardiogram showed no device in an otherwise clean left atrial appendage (the patient had only been taking acetylsalicylic acid). At fluoroscopy the device was detected in the descending aorta below the renal arteries (Figure 64.17),

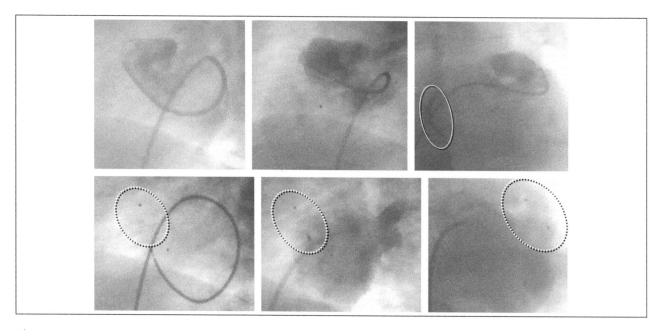

Figure 64.6
Awkward orientation of a left atrial appendage in a 64-year-old man with chronic atrial fibrillation and a contraindication to oral anticoagulation. Left top: the appendage could only be catheterized with the help of a diagnostic right Judkins coronary catheter (advanced to the very tip of the left atrial appendage). Over this catheter, the 7 Fr Amplatzer introducer was successfully advanced (top center). Top right: the frontal projection shows even more conspicuously the retroverted position of the left atrial appendage. At the left border of this panel the staining of the interatrial septum is visible overlying the spine (circle). Bottom left: the implantation of the device (dotted circle) was carried out forming a large loop in the left atrium with the introducer. Bottom center and bottom right: final position of the device (dotted circles) in the projections corresponding to the panels above.

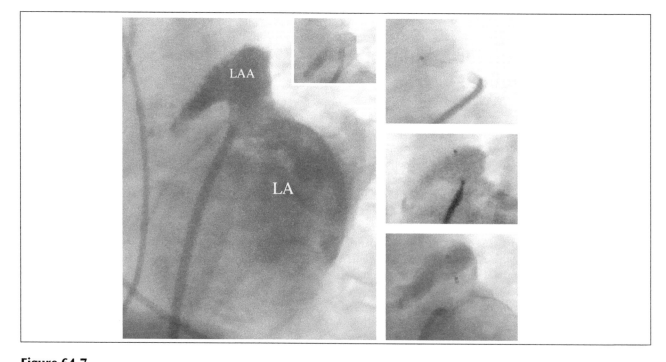

Figure 64.7
Small retroverted left atrial appendage (LAA) in a 62-year-old man with chronic atrial fibrillation and a history of coumadin necrosis. Left panel, the regular Amplatzer introducer could only reach the base of the left atrial appendage. A 9 Fr right Judkins coronary guiding catheter afforded deployment of a device in a more correct trajectory (insert and right hand panels). A 10 mm Amplatzer atrial septal defect occluder was used and parked as a double disk completely inside the left atrial appendage.

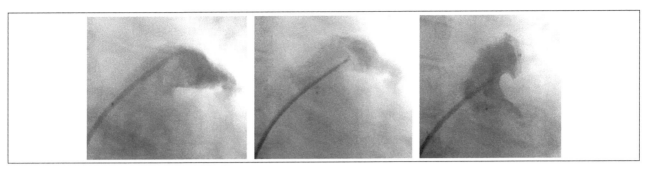

Figure 64.8
Double disk position of a 19 mm Amplatzer atrial septal defect occluder in a left atrial appendage of a 67-year-old male with Osler's disease and paroxysmal atrial fibrillation. The left panel shows the anatomy, the central panel an initial attempt with a 15 mm Amplatzer atrial septal defect occluder which proved too small, and the right panel the final occlusion with the 19 mm device. The fact that the long neck of the left atrial appendage is still open to the left atrium is acceptable as this portion contains but few pectinate muscles. There is good hope that this somewhat peripheral exclusion of the left atrial appendage serves the purpose fully.

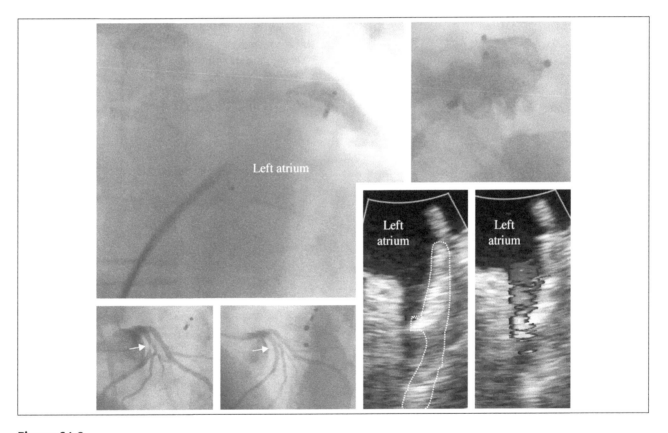

Figure 64.9
Incomplete closure of a left atrial appendage due to a non-perpendicular double disk position. Left top panel: The non-optimal position of the 15 mm Amplatzer atrial septal defect occluder was recognized at the end of implantation. Not to risk embolization of this device, a second device (top panel, dedicated Amplatzer left atrial appendage occluder 32/18 mm) was inserted only after a follow-up transesophageal echocardiogram had confirmed the incomplete occlusion of the left atrial appendage (bottom right inserts: the left depicts the non-perpendicular position of the Amplatzer device in the left atrial appendage and the right shows the continuous flow into the left atrial appendage by color Doppler). The inserts at the bottom left show that during the second intervention an incidental coronary angiography revealed a tight stenosis of the left anterior descending coronary artery (arrow) at the takeoff of the first diagonal branch which was successfully stented with additional balloon angioplasty of the diagonal branch. The left picture shows only 1 left atrial appendage closure device while the right picture shows both. Coronary angiography was carried out before, coronary angioplasty after implantation of the second device.

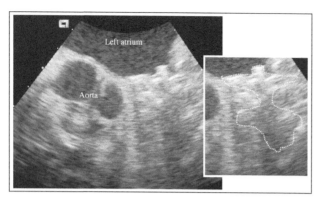

Figure 64.10
Transesophageal echocardiography 6 months after implantation of a 15 mm Amplatzer atrial septal defect occluder in the left atrial appendage of a 64-year-old man. The device is nicely embedded and completely filling in the left atrial appendage. The right insert outlines the device for clarification.

from where it could be pulled down to the femoral artery and removed with a local cut-down. It had not been obstructive in the aorta. The device was nicely endothelialized. It was assumed that the device had embolized early after implantation, possibly before discharge from the hospital. A chest X-ray at discharge had not been done.

Outlook

The Amplatzer device provides the easiest method to occlude the left atrial appendage. However, a high rate of device embolization with the commercially available shapes is a major problem about to be solved by dedicated shape adaptations and a safety tether within the pusher cable. Although embolizations have caused no subjective clinical problems so far, they are a potential threat to the patient and may impose cardiac or vascular surgery that would otherwise not be necessary.

Left atrial appendage closure, in general, has not yet proved its efficacy. In the advent of novel oral anticoagulants such as the recently withdrawn direct thrombin inhibitor ximelagatran, the incentive or need to protect patients with atrial fibrillation from stroke by non-medical means may decrease. Nevertheless, some patients will persist who are unwilling or unable to take any type of oral anticoagulation. Moreover, catheter interventions needed for other indications, such as closure of atrial septal defects or patent foramen ovale, or electrophysiologic ablations in

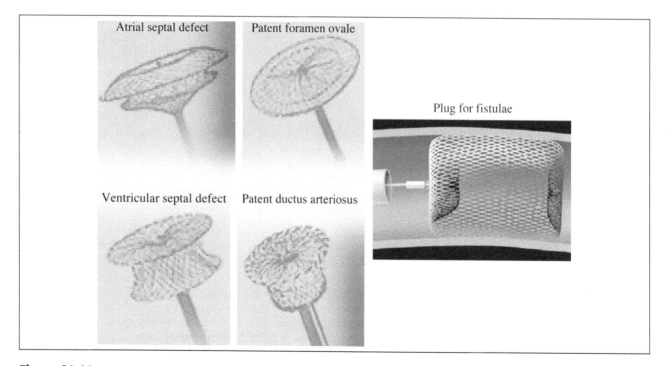

Figure 64.11
Commercially available Amplatzer devices for shunt closure. All except for the plug for fistulae have been used for left atrial appendage closure. (Courtesy of Kurt Amplatz.)

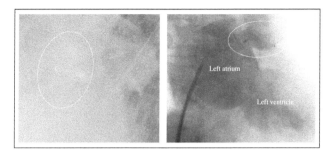

Figure 64.12
Left: 25 mm Amplatzer patent foramen ovale occluder (circle) in the double disk position in a left atrial appendage (lateral chest X-ray 2 weeks after implantation). Right: 18 mm Amplatzer membranous ventricular septal defect occluder (circle) in a left atrial appendage.

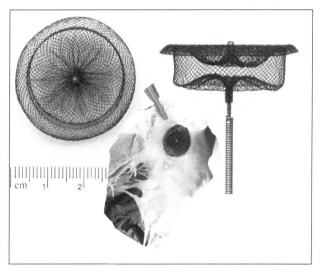

Figure 64.13
Amplatzer left atrial appendage occluder with 144 0.004 inch nitinol wires and no tissue fitting in two perpendicular views, and implanted in a cadaver left atrial appendage (center insert). (Courtesy of Kurt Amplatz.)

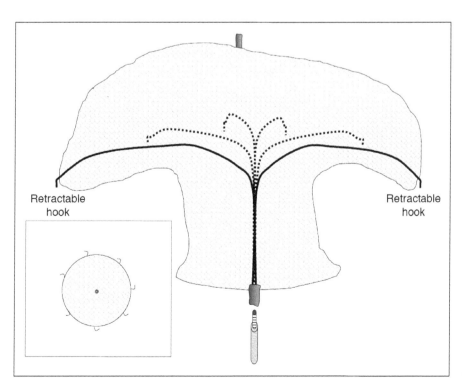

Retractable hook

Retractable hook

Figure 64.14
Prototype of an Amplatzer left atrial appendage occluder with hooks. The insert shows the view from the fundus of the left atrial appendage.

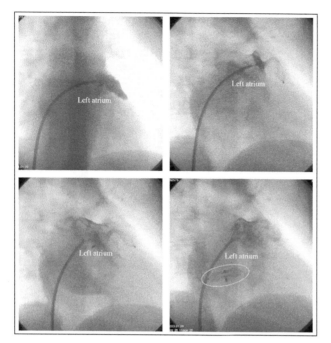

Figure 64.15

Embolized 20 mm Amplatzer atrial septal defect occluder implanted into the left atrial appendage of a 58-year-old woman with chronic atrial fibrillation who was catheterized for closure of a large atrial septal defect. Top left: initial angiogram of the left atrial appendage which is free of thrombus. Top right: the device is deployed but exhibits the cobra sign (unilateral unfolding) of the distal disk. Bottom left: mistakenly it was assumed that this shape would retain the device in the left atrial appendage like a coat hanger hook. After releasing it from the cable, it immediately became unstable and embolized a few seconds later into the left atrium, where it assumed its original double disk shape (bottom right, circle). The patient had no clinical symptoms but was referred for semi-elective cardiac surgery the next day to occlude both atrial appendages, remove the device from the left atrium, and close the atrial septal defect.

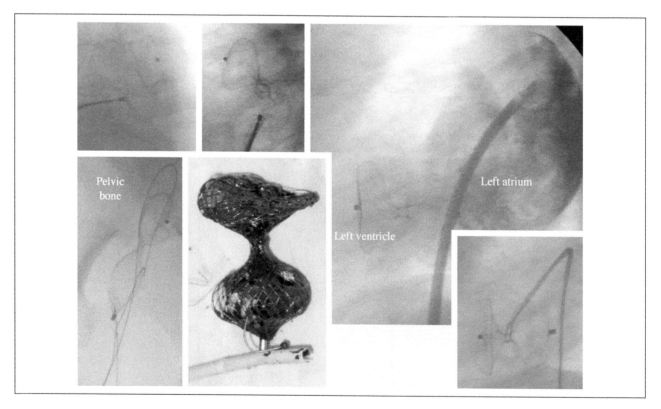

Figure 64.16

Attempt to occlude the left atrial appendage and a large atrial septal defect in a 78-year-old man. The 30 mm Amplatzer atrial septal defect occluder deployed in the left atrial appendage showed a tight constriction of the middle part (top left: frontal view, top center: lateral view). It was assumed that the constriction was due to a narrow part of the left atrial appendage and that deployment would hence be secure. Immediately after deployment the device embolized and got stuck in the mitral valve without obstructing it (top right). It maintained its distorted configuration. It was snared in that position (bottom right) and percutaneously removed through the atrial septal defect and the femoral vein. Even outside the body it retained its incompletely unfolded shape (bottom center).

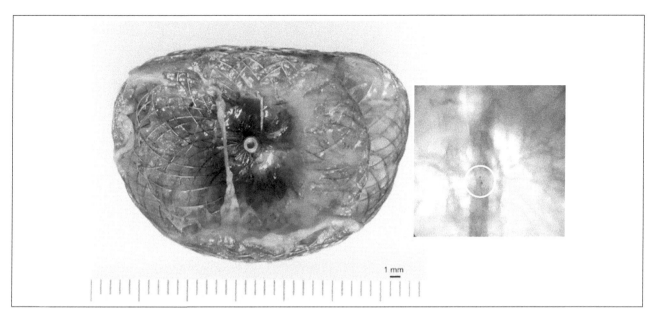

Figure 64.17
Amplatzer atrial septal defect occluder implanted 7 months earlier into the left atrial appendage in a patient in chronic atrial fibrillation. The device was found embolized in the descending aorta (circle on the right insert) during routine follow-up echocardiography. The device was pulled down to the femoral artery and removed with a surgical cut-down. The device was fully endothelialized and no thrombi were attached. The patient had been on acetylsalicylic acid only.

the left atrium, are an invitation to incidentally plug the left atrial appendage in patients with established atrial fibrillation or a high propensity for it.

It is likely that the technical improvements with Amplatzer and other devices will render percutaneous left atrial appendage closure sufficiently safe and easy to make it a competitive method for patients with atrial fibrillation, even considering the fact that not all risk for embolization emanates from the left atrial appendage.

References

1. Sievert H, Lesh MD, Trepels T et al. Percutaneous left atrial appendage transcatheter occlusion to prevent stroke in high-risk patients with atrial fibrillation: early clinical experience. Circulation 2002; 105: 1887–9.
2. Meier B, Palacios I, Windecker S et al. Transcatheter left atrial appendage occlusion with Amplatzer devices to obviate anticoagulation in patients with atrial fibrillation. Cathet Cardiovasc Interven 2003; 60: 417–22.

65

Left atrial appendage closure with the Watchman® device

Peter Sick

Introduction

An alternative procedure for closure of the left atrial appendage (LAA) to prevent arterial embolism in chronic or paroxysmal atrial fibrillation without anticoagulation is the implantation of a Watchman® device (Atritech Company, Plymouth, Minnesota; Figure 65.1). The first procedure was performed in August 2002, and currently a total of 63 patients have been implanted. Indications for implantation of the device are patients with chronic or paroxysmal atrial fibrillation with a principal indication for anticoagulation and without definitive contraindications for coumadine therapy, as coumadine therapy is recommended for the first 45 days to allow endothelialization of the device.

Anatomically the LAA is positioned in the anterior-superior part of the left atrium, just superior to the mitral valve. It can be best visualized angiographically in a right anterior oblique (RAO) 30° and lateral view.

Technique for left atrial appendage occlusion using the Watchman® device

Performing a transesophageal echocardiogram within 48 hours before the procedure is mandatory to exclude thrombi in the LAA, to measure the LAA ostium, proximal part and length of the body, as well as to see the shape of the LAA, which may have multiple lobes, leading to difficulties in placing the device. It is recommended for several reasons to have transesophageal echo as well during the implantation procedure to assure the correct placement of the device in the LAA. The procedure is therefore performed in general short term anesthesia with midazolam and propofol.

The Watchman® device is implanted using a three-part system consisting of a transseptal access sheath (Figure 65.2),

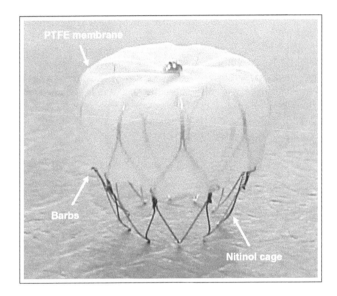

Figure 65.1
Watchman® device with the nitinol cage and the polyethylene membrane spanned over the surface in contact with the left atrium. The barbs prevent the device from embolization by fixing in the left atrial appendage wall.

a delivery catheter, and an implantable nitinol device as already shown in Figure 65.1. The principal method and location of the device are shown in Figure 65.3. The (14 Fr) access system and (12 Fr) delivery catheter are designed to facilitate device placement via femoral venous access and to cross into the left atrium via the interatrial septum for final device implantation. The delivery catheter is designed to allow for retrieval of a deployed Watchman® device, prior to implant release, if the placement is not optimal.

For pressure control and introduction of a pigtail catheter in the ascending aorta, an arterial 5 Fr sheath is introduced through the right or left femoral groin. To get into the left atrium, a transseptal puncture has to be performed with a transseptal needle and the Brockenbrough

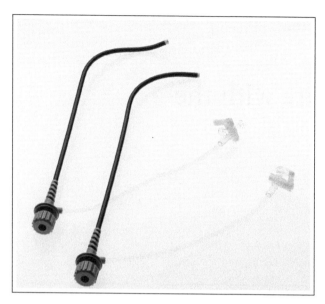

Figure 65.2
Transseptal introduction sheath, which is directed after transseptal puncture over a stiff wire to the LAA. There are two different shapes available, one with a single curve and one with a double curve, which is used in over 90% of the cases. The side branch is used for continuous saline infusion to avoid air suction during pullback of the device.

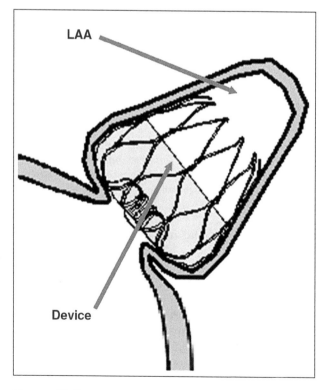

Figure 65.3
The device is implanted into the left atrial appendage upside down, with the polyethylene membrane covering the orifice of the LAA.

catheter. It is best performed under pressure control in a pa and lateral view to assure the correct puncture site. The site of the puncture should be in the upper part of the foramen ovale of the interatrial septum. The reason for this is that the LAA is located in the superior part of the left atrium. If the puncture site is chosen too low (comparable with transseptal puncture to reach the left ventricle via the mitral valve, i.e, in mitral valvuloplasty or a diagnostic procedure for aortic stenosis) it is very difficult to get to the top of the left atrium into the LAA. After successful transseptal puncture the Brockenbrough catheter has to be exchanged over a wire. The best wire to use is the Inoue wire, which is hard to get on the free market. Alternatively a stiff wire like the Amplatzer has to be placed into a pulmonary vein, the Brockenborough catheter has to be removed, and the introduction sheath (Figure 65.2) of the Watchman® device has to be introduced. There are two shapes available, one with a single curve and one with a double curve, which is very often the sheath of choice, as in most cases it fits quite well to the LAA ostium. It is very important to have a continuous saline infusion through the side-arm of the sheath and to remove the dilator of the sheath very slowly to avoid negative pressure in the sheath, which might lead to air embolism in case of air suction through the valve of the sheath at the moment of removal of the dilator. In the near future, side holes in the tip of the catheter will provide a backward flow of blood to avoid this problem, at least in part, if the tip of the catheter is in direct contact with the atrial wall.

The principal procedure is shown in Figure 65.4(a–c) with measurement of the LAA, implantation of the device, and late results with complete endothelialization of the surface of the device.

The first step is to measure the size of the LAA body, orifice, and length in two planes by contrast injection through the introduction sheath (see Figure 65.5a,b). This is mostly best performed in an RAO 30° and lateral view. The measured size of the LAA has to be about 80% of the nominal size of the device to be implanted. The 20% compression of the device after implantation is necessary due to the fixation barbs of the device, that have to be in good contact with the wall of the LAA to avoid embolization of the device. The Watchman® device itself (see Figure 65.1) consists primarily of a nitinol frame structure with fixation barbs along the frame surface and a thin permeable polyester material that covers the atrial facing surface of the device. The device is implanted at or slightly distal to the ostium of the left atrial appendage. The device is constrained within a delivery sheath until deployment into the left atrial appendage. It is available in various diameter sizes of 21, 24, 27, 30, and 33 mm to accommodate the unique anatomy of each patient's LAA.

After positioning of the introduction sheath deep in the LAA confirmed by contrast injections, the delivery system is introduced with rinsing of saline solution through the system with a syringe to avoid air bubbles. After another

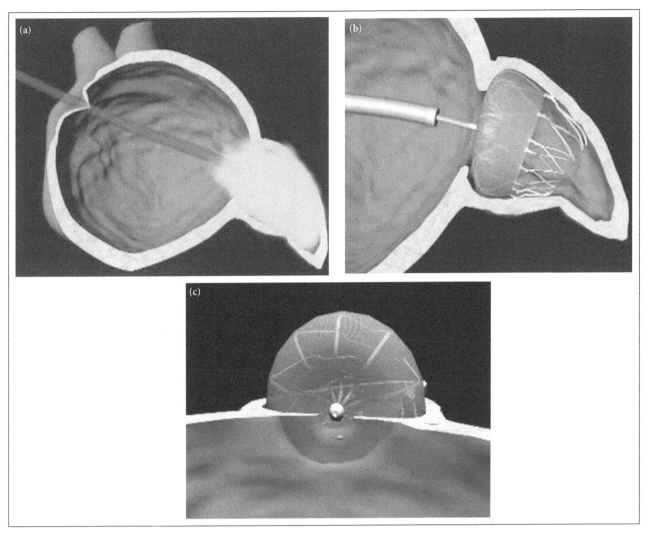

Figure 65.4
Schematic implantation of the Watchman® device in the LAA. (a) Injection of contrast dye in the left atrial appendage to measure the size of the body to select the correct size of the device. (b) The implanted device still connected to the delivery system. (c) Schematic endothelialization of the device with complete coverage of the surface to the LA, thus leading to complete occlusion of the LAA usually within 6 months.

contrast injection through the delivery device to confirm correct placement, the sheath is pulled back while the delivery system is held stable in position. The self-expanding device is folded up, still fixed at the delivery system (Figure 65.6). Angiographic control with dye injection (Figure 65.7a) and transesophageal echocardiography (Figure 65.7b) confirm correct positioning of the device. Another proof of stability is to wiggle the catheter to test device stability in the LAA. As the atrial wall is very thin and mobile, it is recommended to inject some dye into the LAA for the wiggle procedure, then the whole LAA can be seen moving, otherwise it may not be possible to demonstrate device stability in the LAA except with TEE. The device can now be released from the delivery system by turning it counterclockwise 5 times

(Figure 65.8). A last contrast injection has to be performed, then the introduction sheath can be removed from the LAA (Figure 65.9).

Post-interventional medical treatment

As we know from animal trials with this device, patients should be set on coumadine at least for 45 days with an INR between 2 and 3 in parallel to aspirin 100 mg, until the endothelialization process is terminated. If there is no flow behind the device in the LAA, or a flow jet below 3 mm around the margins of the device (Figure 65.10),

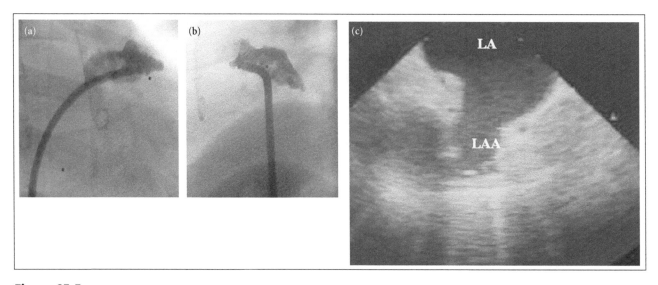

Figure 65.5
(a) and (b) Angiographic measurement of the LAA in two planes for correct selection of the size of the device. (c) In parallel to angiographic measurements of the LAA, size is also measured by transesophageal echocardiography. The LAA is also screened in different projections to visualize its variable anatomy, which can be lobed in two or more segments, sometimes leading to difficulties in placing the device to cover all lobes completely.

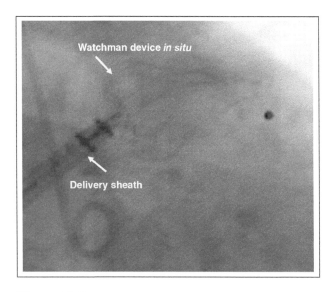

Figure 65.6
Implanted device still connected to the delivery system.

coumadine therapy can be ceased after 45 days, continued by clopidogrel therapy 75 mg daily until 6-month follow-up. This is due to the fact that 4 patients in the feasibility study had thrombus formation on the device at 6-month follow up; one example is demonstrated in Figure 65.10. On the other hand, there is evidence for complete endothelialization in a patient who died after 6 months due to aortic aneurysm. Figure 65.11 shows the pathologic state of the Watchman® device at the time of autopsy. If

there are good results on top of the device with no thrombus or flow in or into the LAA at 6-month TEE control, clopidogrel therapy is stopped and aspirin therapy 100 mg per day is continued lifelong. In case of thrombus formation, clopidogrel is stopped and coumadine therapy has to be restarted.

Device-specific possible complications

The possible complications of heart catheterization and transseptal puncture will not be discussed here, only device-specific complications will be metioned.

One device-specific complication may be relevant air embolism, especially in case of retrieval of the device. If the catheter tip is in tight contact with the atrial wall, underpressure can develop in the introduction sheath during pullback of the device. When removing the delivery system from the introduction sheath, air might be sucked into the sheath, which could be injected into the left atrium with the next contrast medium injection. A continuous infusion of saline solution through the side branch of the introduction sheath helps to avoid this problem, if the delivery system is pulled back slowly. In the near future, the introduction sheath will have some side holes at the tip of the catheter to allow retrograde blood flow into the introduction sheath.

Another complication could be a perforation of the LA wall with the catheter as well as with the device itself, leading to pericardial tamponade. The wiggling procedure in particular may be dangerous if performed without

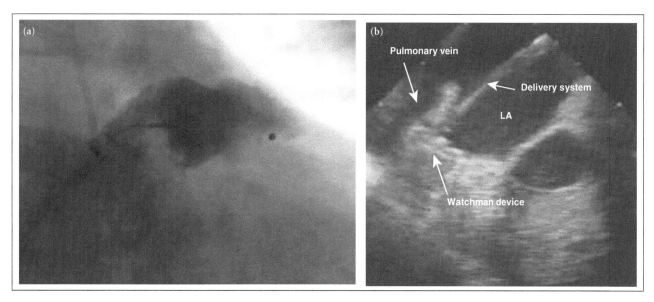

Figure 65.7
(a) Angiographic control of the device implanted in the LAA. Contrast dye is injected through the delivery system and shows the barrier between the left atrium and the LAA due to the membrane of the device. The 'wiggling' test is performed during dye injection to visualize the movement of the complete LAA. (b) Echocardiographic control shows complete coverage of the LAA by the device. The wiggling test can also be controlled by echocardiography.

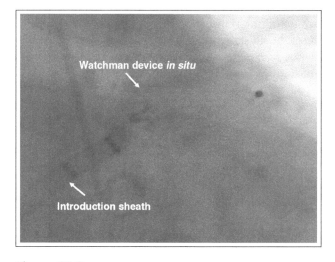

Figure 65.8
After control of device stability has been achieved, the delivery system is removed by counterclockwise rotation. The released device is in a stable position in the LAA.

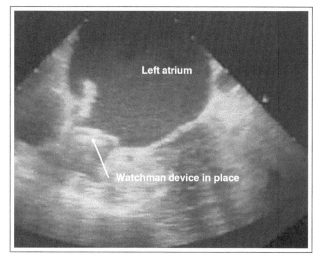

Figure 65.9
Echocardiographic control also shows a well positioned device with complete coverage of the entrance of the LAA.

angiographic or echocardiographic control, as the movement of the LAA tissue cannot be felt by the operator; it has to be visualized by contrast injection or by TEE to see the movement of the whole LAA.

Embolizations of the device were seen with the first generation devices, which had very small fixation barbs around the body. All of the embolized devices could be retrieved percutaneously by snaring in the descending aorta and pulling out through a femoral sheath. With the second generation devices after modification of the barbs, no further embolizations were recognized.

Bleeding complications in the femoral groin are quite comparable to other interventional procedures with large introduction sheaths, but for the arterial sheath the size is only 5 Fr and in the low pressure venous system the problem with 14 Fr is not very important.

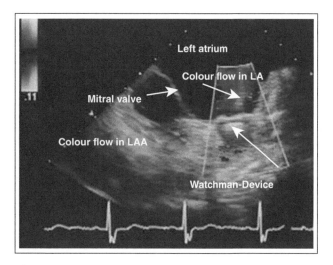

Figure 65.10
Echocardiographic control 45 days after implantation of the device. The color Doppler demonstrates very little flow behind the device in the LAA, thus coumadine therapy can be stopped. (See also color plate section.)

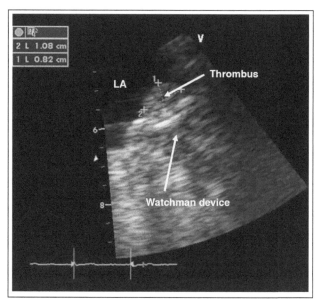

Figure 65.12
Smooth thrombus formation on the surface of a Watchman® device in a patient with non-compliance to coumadine therapy. LA, left atrium.

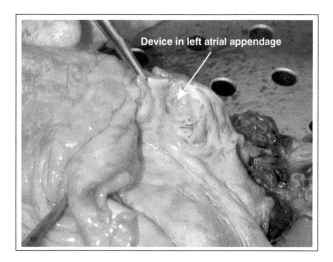

Figure 65.11
Pathologic anatomy in a patient who died 9 months after implantation of a Watchman® device due to aortic aneurysm. There is complete coverage of the device with new endothelium.

Overall results of the device in a pivotal trial

Preliminary data of the feasibility data are published as an abstract in TCT 2004 and the German Congress of Cardiology.[1,2] To date, 63 patients (50 Europeans and 13 in the United States) have had the device implanted successfully with a mean follow-up of 211 days. The mean age was 68.2 years (range 47–82 years) and 63% were male. Two patients with a first generation device experienced device embolization; both were successfully retrieved percutaneously. No embolizations have occurred since the fixation barbs were enhanced. Five procedural events occurred, including two pericardial effusions; both could be treated interventionally. One hematoma and one pseudoaneurysm were also treated conservatively. A major air embolism led to acute malignant rhythm disorders; the patient had to be resuscitated. After 3 hours, however, the patient could be weaned from the respirator and was discharged from hospital without remnant symptoms of hypoxia. Two delivery system issues were reported, one requiring surgical intervention due to a broken delivery system wire. The delivery system was therefore modified and no further events have been reported. At 6-month follow-up 41/46 (89.1%) patients had ceased device-related coumadine therapy. No ischemic stroke or systemic embolism has occurred. One patient died after 9 months due to an ascending aortic dissection. Autopsy documented a stable, well endothelialized device with complete LAA occlusion (Figure 65.11). One patient with a history of transient ischemic attacks (TIAs) experienced a TIA at 4 months without LAA thrombus visible; another patient had a TIA at 6-month follow-up, showing a smooth layer of thrombus formation on the surface of the device (Figure 65.12). Three additional patients showed thrombus formation on the atrial surface of the device without neurologic symptoms. One of these 4 patients was incompliant with medical treatment already in the early state after implantation with regard to anticoagulation. Compared with spontaneous thrombus formation even under anticoagulation therapy, one can also find quite a number of patients representing with thrombus in the LAA under therapeutic use of coumadine.

Outlook

As left atrial appendage closure has not yet proved its efficacy in comparison with coumadine therapy in a long term run, a randomized trial was started in February 2005 to show non-inferiority of the device compared with anticoagulation therapy. This is the first trial really comparing both modes of therapy, without all the other closure devices. If non-inferiority can be proved with an acceptable rate of procedural complications, this device-related therapy might be a good alternative for long term anticoagulation in patients with relative contraindications for coumadine therapy, and might have some advantage with

regard to quality of life, as patients are more independent from anticoagulation checks and are at less risk for potential bleeding complications.

References

1. Sick P, Ulrich M, Muth G. University of Leipzig, Heart Center; Hauptmann KE, Klinikum der Barmherzigen Brueder Trier; Schuler G, University of Leipzig, Heart Center; Grube E, Klinikum Rhein-Sieg, Siegburg. Left atrial appendage filter device for prevention of embolization in patients with nonvalvular atrial fibrillation: initial results of a multicenter feasibility trial. Am J Cardiol 2004; 94(6): 95E, TCT-208.
2. Sick P, Ulrich M, Muth G et al. Universität Leipzig, Herzzentrum GmbH, Leipzig; Herzzentrum Siegburg; Krankenhaus der Barmherzigen Brüderk, Trier. Erste klinische Erfahrungen mit dem WATCHMAN® Verschlußsystem für das linke Vorfohr zur Verhinderung thrombo-embolischer Komplikationen bei Patienten mit nicht valvulärem Vorhofflimmern. Z Kardiol 2005; 94(Suppl 1), abstract V241.

Index

Note: Page references in *italics* refer to Figures; those in **bold** refer to Tables. Plates are indicated by Pl.